BASIC AND CLINICAL ASPECTS OF NEUROENDOCRINE IMMUNOLOGY IN RHEUMATIC DISEASES

ANNALS OF THE NEW YORK ACADEMY OF SCIENCES
Volume 1069

BASIC AND CLINICAL ASPECTS OF NEUROENDOCRINE IMMUNOLOGY IN RHEUMATIC DISEASES

Edited by
Maurizio Cutolo, Robert G. Lahita, Johannes W.J. Bijlsma, Alfonse T. Masi, and Rainer H. Straub

Published by Blackwell Publishing on behalf of the New York Academy of Sciences
Boston, Massachusetts
2006

Library of Congress Cataloging-in-Publication Data

Basic and clinical aspects of neuroendocrine immunology in rheumatic diseases / edited by Maurizio Cutolo. . . [et al.].
p. ; cm. – (Annals of the New York Academy of Sciences, ISSN 0077-8923 ; v. 1069)
Includes bibliographical references and index.
ISBN-13: 978-1-57331-593-7 (alk. paper)
ISBN-10: 1-57331-593-1 (alk. paper)
1. Rheumatism–Immunological aspects. 2. Rheumatism–Endocrine aspects. 3. Neuroendo-crinology. 4. Rheumatoid arthritis–Pathophysiology. I. Cutolo, M. (Maurizio) II. New York Academy of Sciences. III. Series.
[DNLM: 1. Rheumatic Diseases–drug therapy. 2. Rheumatic Diseases–immunology. 3. Glu- cocorticoids–therapeutic use. 4. Neurosecretory Systems–immunology. 5. Neurosecretory Systems–physiopathology. 6. Tumor Necrosis Factor-alpha–antagonists & inhibitors.
W1 AN626YL v.1069 2006 / WE 544 B311 2006]
Q11.N5 vol. 1069
[RC927]
500 s–dc22
[616.7'23079]

2006013805

The *Annals of the New York Academy of Sciences* (ISSN: 0077-8923 [print]; ISSN: 1749-6632 [online]) is published 28 times a year on behalf of the New York Academy of Sciences by Blackwell Publishing, with offices located at 350 Main Street, Malden, Massachusetts 02148 USA, PO Box 1354, Garsington Road, Oxford OX4 2DQ UK, and PO Box 378 Carlton South, 3053 Victoria Australia.

Information for subscribers: Subscription prices for 2006 are: Premium Institutional: $3850.00 (US) and £2139.00 (Europe and Rest of World).
Customers in the UK should add VAT at 5%. Customers in the EU should also add VAT at 5% or provide a VAT registration number or evidence of entitlement to exemption. Customers in Canada should add 7% GST or provide evidence of entitlement to exemption. The Premium Institutional price also includes online access to full-text articles from 1997 to present, where available. For other pricing options or more information about online access to Blackwell Publishing journals, including access information and terms and conditions, please visit www.blackwellpublishing.com/nyas.

Membership information: Members may order copies of the *Annals* volumes directly from the Academy by visiting www.nyas.org/annals, emailing membership@nyas.org, faxing 212-888-2894, or calling 800-843-6927 (US only), or +1 212 838 0230, ext. 345 (International). For more information on becoming a member of the New York Academy of Sciences, please visit www.nyas.org/membership.

Journal Customer Services: For ordering information, claims, and any inquiry concerning your institutional subscription, please contact your nearest office:
UK: Email: customerservices@blackwellpublishing.com; Tel: +44 (0) 1865 778315; Fax +44 (0) 1865 471775
US: Email: customerservices@blackwellpublishing.com; Tel: +1 781 388 8599 or 1 800 835 6770 (Toll free in the USA); Fax: +1 781 388 8232
Asia: Email: customerservices@blackwellpublishing.com; Tel: +65 6511 8000; Fax: +61 3 8359 1120
Members: Claims and inquiries on member orders should be directed to the Academy at email: membership@nyas.org or Tel: +1 212 838 0230 (International) or 800-843-6927 (US only).

Printed in the USA.
Printed on acid-free paper.

Mailing: The *Annals of the New York Academy of Sciences* are mailed Standard Rate. **Postmaster:** Send all address changes to *Annals of the New York Academy of Sciences*, Blackwell Publishing, Inc., Journals Subscription Department, 350 Main Street, Malden, MA 01248-5020. Mailing to rest of world by DHL Smart and Global Mail.

Annals are available to subscribers online at the New York Academy of Sciences and also at Blackwell Synergy. Visit www.annalsnyas.org or www.blackwell-synergy.com to search the articles and register for table of contents e-mail alerts. Access to full text and PDF downloads of *Annals* articles are available to nonmembers and subscribers on a pay-per-view basis at www.annalsnyas.org.

The paper used in this publication meets the minimum requirements of the National Standard for Information Sciences Permanence of Paper for Printed Library Materials, ANSI Z39.48_1984.

ISSN: 0077-8923 (print); 1749-6632 (online)
ISBN-10: 1-57331-593-1 (paper); ISBN-13: 978-1-57331-593-7 (paper)

A catalogue record for this title is available from the British Library.

ANNALS OF THE NEW YORK ACADEMY OF SCIENCES

Volume 1069
June 2006

BASIC AND CLINICAL ASPECTS OF NEUROENDOCRINE IMMUNOLOGY IN RHEUMATIC DISEASES

Editors

MAURIZIO CUTOLO, ROBERT G. LAHITA, JOHANNES W. J. BIJLSMA, ALFONSE T. MASI, AND RAINER H. STRAUB

This volume is the result of a conference entitled **Third International Conference on Neuroendocrine Immune Basis of the Rheumatic Diseases**, held on September 10–12, 2005, in Genova, Italy.

CONTENTS

Part II. The Central Nervous System: Stimulation Tests of the Stress Axis and Its Involvement in Rheumatic Diseases

Part III. The Peripheral Nervous System: Nerve Fibers, Neuropeptides, and Clinical Links in Arthritis

Part IV. The Role of Gonadal Hormones: Sex Hormones and Rheumatic Diseases

Part V. Glucocorticoids as Endogenous Neuroendocrine Immune Modulators: New Perspectives in the Therapy of Rheumatic Diseases

Part VI. Clinical Aspects: The Neuroendocrine and Immune Systems in Rheumatology

Part VII. Clinical Evidence: Anti-TNF Strategies and Effects on Neuroendocrine Immune Mechanisms in Rheumatic Diseases

Part VIII. Clinical Perspectives: Lipid Metabolism in Rheumatic Diseases

Part IX. Metabolic/Inflammatory Effects

Financial assistance was received from:

Supporters

- Abbott Spa
- Schering-Plough Spa
- Wyeth Lederle Spa

Contributors

- Abbott B.V. Netherlands
- Actelion Pharmaceuticals Italia Srl
- Aventis Pharma Spa-Gruppo Sanofi-Aventis
- Eli Lilly Italia Spa
- Italfarmaco Spa
- Novartis Farma Spa
- Otsuka Pharmaceutical Sa
- Pfizer Italia Srl
- Procter & Gamble Srl
- Rottapharm Spa

Overview Article for Basic and Clinical Aspects of Neuroendocrine Immunology in Rheumatic Diseases

The Third International Conference on the Neuroendocrine Immune Basis of the Rheumatic Diseases brought together scientists from all over the world to discuss matters relating to a variety of topics. These topics ranged from stress and the immune system to sex steroids and their effects on cytokines and certain disease states. There was much cutting-edge material within this meeting, and this overview touches on the many areas covered in this book in far more detail. The purpose of this overview is to give you the breadth and depth of the topics discussed at this international meeting.

At this meeting and in our past meetings, the issue of stress and disease has played a prominent role. Tarricone *et al.* presented a paper that dealt with the stress response in skeletal muscle myofibers and, therefore, with the role of stress in certain musculoskeletal diseases. On a related note, Maestroni *et al.* focused on the effects of the sympathetic nervous system and dendritic cells of the immune system, contending that there was an important relationship regarding stress. Dr. Maestroni speaks of adrenergic receptors in the dendritic cells and toll-like receptors within the cells, that when stimulated respond differently because of cytokines released. The cytokines may be different depending on the stimuli and evoke a Th1 or Th2 response. Harbuz *et al.* followed up on the Maestroni paper by talking about stress in autoimmune disease models. Here in the rat model of rheumatoid arthritis (RA) (adjuvant-induced disease), there is an activation of the hypothalamic-pituitary-adrenal (HPA) axis associated with the development of inflammation. The surprising idea is that stress may not be bad for inflammatory disease, suggesting beneficial effects after exposure to a particular stressor. Using RA as a specific model of HPA axis and stress, Geenen *et al.* show clearly that the HPA and the autonomic nervous system are activated by stress and that these effects might affect the clinical manifestations of RA. These authors reviewed 56 publications of the past 15 years to get insight into the possible roles of stress on the disease of RA. Finally stress, innate and T helper cytokines, and disease susceptibility were the topics for a paper by Calcagni *et al.* They discussed the role of stress on disease outcomes and conclude that stress hormones inhibit or upregulate innate and T helper cytokine production and affect the manifestations and ultimate outcomes for patients with these diseases.

Autoantibodies were mentioned in several abstracts. Harel and Shoenfeld describe the presence of autoantibodies as predictors of diseases like lupus

Ann. N.Y. Acad. Sci. 1069: xiii–xvii (2006).
doi: 10.1196/annals.1351.050

months or years in advance of symptoms. They mention early antibodies like anti-islet cell or anticyclic citrullinic antibodies, which were found in the sera of both diabetics and RA patients 5 and 4.5 years, respectively, before the onset of illness. They propose a method of screening patients with these syndromes through the use of autoantibodies. These autoantibodies were also the substance of a paper by Valesini *et al.* who described a firm association of antiendothelial antibodies in patients with neuropsychiatric systemic lupus erythematosus (SLE). More specifically, these antibodies were against a specific protein in the septin family of intracytoplasmic proteins called Nedd5. Tincani *et al.* described in another study the role of antiphospholipid antibodies, anti-Ro, and antiplatelet antibodies in pregnancy. In this insightful study, the authors describe the various clinical manifestations of such antibodies in pregnancy like heart block, thrombosis, and thrombocytopenia, most of which have catastrophic implications for the mother. Finally, in the autoantibody area, Di Simone *et al.* deal with the topic of β2-glycoprotein antibodies and apoptosis. Their contention is that such antibodies, which are related to the phospholipid syndrome, might enhance apoptosis of the trophoblastic cells during a pregnancy. While a reaction between these cells and antibodies was found, no association with enhanced apoptosis was found.

One whole aspect of this volume involves a discussion of various disease entities like RA and SLE as they relate to the neuroendocrine system. There was much interest at this meeting in tumor necrosis factor (TNF) inhibition and various associated neuroendocrine mediators of inflammation. Del Porto *et al.* reported on TNF inhibitors and levels of nerve growth factor and brain-derived neurotrophic factors that did not change with the advent of TNF therapy. Gabriele studied similar changes in chromogranin A, another neuroendocrine analyte that mirrored the levels of TNF and TNF receptor in patients with RA. Seriolo *et al.* even looked at TNF inhibition and bone metabolism in active RA patients. They offer data that bone growth increased and resorption decreased during TNF therapy. TNF therapy was also implicated in lipid metabolism, which is particularly important in RA patients because of their propensity for accelerated vascular disease, which has been linked to the inflammatory reaction. After treatment with TNF inhibitors, the total cholesterol increased, as did the HDL levels. Both of these lipid increases correlated with decreased disease activity and ameliorated some key vascular risk factors.

A paper by Traverse *et al.* dealt with the antiphospholipid syndrome (APLS) and neuroendocrine interactions. This study was designed to see whether patients with APLS might evolve into other diseases as a result of neuroendocrine reactions. The conclusions were that some patients with APLS might acquire inflammatory diseases triggered by pregnancy. There were also pilot studies of oral pulse dexamethasone (DEX) therapy in RA by Kroot *et al.* who suggested that DEX might be a good bridging therapy in early RA in contradistinction to oral high-dose corticosteroids. Other papers on RA dealt with the sex ratios of patients who acquire it. Kvien *et al.* found that females with RA had lesser responses to disease-modifying drugs like methotrexate. Romanovsky *et al.* discussed the very interesting area of common therapeutic targets in all forms of arthritis, particularly osteoarthritis (OA) and RA. These investigators found that erythropoietin-producing hepatocellular (Eph) receptor kinases and their ligands called ephrins, which are stimulated in inflammation, played a major role in the pathogenesis of the arthritides.

There were two papers on polymyalgia rheumatica (PMR). One paper dealt with the fact that women have more severe PMR than men. In that paper, Cimmino claimed that the female sex was a risk factor and needed a long course of steroid therapy. The second paper by Sulli *et al.* deals with the difficulties surrounding PMR and elderly onset RA. The distinctions made are essential to the appropriate treatment of such patients with glucocorticoids. Moreover, the cytokine and hormone responses in such patients were shown to be different. Rovensky *et al.* studied prolactin and growth hormone responses to lowered blood glucose in patients with psoriatic arthritis and scleroderma and found very little difference. Sarzi-Puttini *et al.* looked at the very perplexing fibromyalgia syndrome and suggested that the HPA axis and the autonomic nervous systems played a major role in this condition. Most important to this paper is the review of the cardiovascular aspects of this important illness, said to be based largely on neuroendocrine phenomena.

A significant part of this meeting is always devoted to sex hormones. Dulos *et al.* discuss dehydroepiandrosterone (DHEA) metabolism and arthritis and the role for the p450 enzymes Cyp7b at the "immune endocrine crossroad." These authors suggest that DHEA does not work via the glucocorticoid receptor but rather the Cyp7b oxidase, an enzyme that has enhanced activity and expression in RA patients. Both TNF and IL-1β stimulate Cyp7b activity, which also has downstream implications for the efficacy of this hormone. Cutolo *et al.* studied sex hormones and anti-TNF effects. His suggestion that TNF stimulates aromatase activity in the joints of patients with RA is a major finding. Anti-TNF antibody had no effect on the levels of serum sex hormones, however, and more research is needed. There were also two papers on inflammation and sex hormone metabolism. One was by Schmidt *et al.* which dealt with inhibition of selective sex pathway enzymes that had consequent actions on inflammatory events in RA, and another paper was by Capellino *et al.* who suggest that estrogens, through their functional receptors, modulate macrophage function. Doria *et al.* in an elegant paper discussed estrogens and pregnancy in SLE. The finding of low IL6 and lower than expected serum estradiol levels in such patients, they contend, might account for the lowered humoral response in such patients during pregnancy.

The sex hormone papers culminate with two brief papers on disease severity and risk. One by Masi *et al.* discussed the risks of RA development and environmental influences by sex hormones. The other paper was by Mirone *et al.* who discuss altered levels of prolactin and androgen in patients with scleroderma, which they relate directly to the chronicity of disease.

A great deal of attention was paid to the corticosteroids in this NeuroImmunoEndocrinology meeting, and that is common to all of these congresses. The first paper (Negrini *et al.*) was directed toward the glucocorticoid-induced TNF receptor (GITR). These receptors present on regulatory T cells upregulate the immune system. A role for these receptors is given on $CD8^+$ T suppressor cells, which if true could have a substantial role in diseases like RA. Cutolo *et al.* describe circadian rhythms in their abstract, which reviews glucocorticoids and arthritis. In this interesting paper, the right timing of glucocorticoid therapy—mainly in the morning—is stressed as appropriate for patients with RA. Cutolo also notes that melatonin has the opposite effects of naturally produced corticosteroids. DaSilva *et al.* discuss the lack of toxicity of low-dose corticosteroids in the treatment of RA. Their paper makes the use of low-dose steroids in the treatment of certain diseases acceptable, since the fears of added toxicity are really unfounded. Bjilsma makes a case for glucocorticoids as true disease modifying antirheumatic drugs (DMARDS), a point that can hardly be argued. Janele *et al.* discuss the stimulatory roles of estrogens and the inhibitory roles of androgens in the presence of glucocorticoids. Surprising is his belief that estrogens increase TNF secretion and are dependent on physiological concentrations of cortisol. Ferone *et al.* reports on the cortistatin/somatostatin system in various immune diseases. He provides an interesting discussion of somastostatin receptors and their binding to corticostatin in certain immune disorders. This might be a whole new way of looking at these pharmacologically important compounds in lymphoid tissues. Imrich looked at insulin-induced shock and its effects on the adrenomedullary hormone system (AMHS) in patients with scleroderma and RA. He suspects that there are defects in the AMHS response in those disease groups. Lewis-Tuffin *et al.* discusses the phenomenon of glucocorticoid resistance in some patients who fail to respond to steroids. The author discusses two kinds of glucocorticoid receptors, their ratios, and their relationship to this form of resistance. There are two additional molecular papers dealing with corticosteroids. Guiducci *et al.* discuss scleroderma and endothelial injury, wherein they discuss polymorphisms of the genes for angiotensin-converting enzymes and their roles in macrovascular disease. This is followed by studies of Wagner *et al.* which investigate polymorphisms of the corticotrophin-releasing hormone, the binding properties of nuclear proteins, and gene expression.

There were also quite a few miscellaneous papers about such things as thiopurine methyltransferase (TMTP) and azathioprine therapy. Schedel *et al.* looked at adverse events in some 139 patients prospectively. He found a normal gaussian distribution of those patients who had some toxicity to azathioprine common to patients with low levels of the TMTP enzyme.

Three papers were directed to lipid metabolism. The first was a paper by Michel-Dayer *et al.* which measured IL-1 receptor antagonists in obese patients and found them to be a significant factor in local inflammatory processes.

Montecucco *et al.* studied the induction of neutrophil chemotaxis by leptin, which is a little known fact about this amazing molecule. Finally, H. Garle *et al.* confirm the previous data by discussing leptin as a link between fat tissue and inflammation, facts that might place leptin in position as a key molecule that influences diabetes and vascular disease.

Particularly relevant to this congress were papers on neuropeptides. There were two papers on this topic. First was one by Konttinen *et al.*, who discuss the role of neuropeptides in the innervation of the joint in RA compared to normals with particular attention to proprioception. The second paper by Levine *et al.* discusses similar issues of neuropeptides and inflammation. However, here the sexual dimorphism of the pain response is discussed, and some very interesting conclusions are drawn.

Endothelin plays a major role in vascular disease and pulmonary hypertension. Paolo Rossi *et al.* explore the genetic variation in the endothelin system and cardiovascular homeostasis. Single nucleotide polymorphisms of this gene are explored and discussed in the context of therapeutic regimens for these conditions.

Lastly, the cytokines and their roles in the neuroendocrine networks are considered. The first paper by Ostensen *et al.* deals with her favorite topic, that of cytokines and pregnancy in rheumatic disease. A new concept of gestationally induced cytokine inhibitors is introduced, and it is a concept that is of interest to all physicians who follow the remission of RA disease during the gestational period. Bruni *et al.* discuss alexithymia (a disorder of emotional regulation mechanisms in disease) and the neuroendocrine immune response in diseases, such as RA and SLE. The authors are looking for a common pathogenetic pathway for integration of alexithymic phenomena and autoimmune inflammatory disease.

These topics formed the basis for a most stimulating meeting and are those discussed in this fascinating book. We hope that you will derive inspiration and new information from your reading of these proceedings.

ROBERT G. LAHITA
New York, N. Y.
e-mail: RLahita@Libertyhcs.org
MAURIZIO CUTOLO
Genova, Italy

Neuroendocrine Immune System Involvement in Rheumatology

JOHANNES W.J. BIJLSMA,[a] ALFONSE MASI,[b] RAINER H. STRAUB,[c] ROBERT LAHITA,[d] AND MAURIZIO CUTOLO[e]

[a]*Department of Rheumatology and Clinical Immunology, University Medical Center Utrecht, 3508 GA Utrecht, The Netherlands*

[b]*Division of Medicine, University of Illinois College of Medicine, Peoria, Illinois 61605, USA*

[c]*Department of Internal Medicine I, University Hospital Regensburg, Regensburg 93042, Germany*

[d]*Department of Medicine, Jersey City Medical Center, Mount Sinai School of Medicine, New York 10029, USA*

[e]*Division of Rheumatology, Department of Internal Medicine, University of Genova, Genova 16126, Italy*

INTRODUCTION

The purpose of the Third International Conference was to bring together people from all over the world that were interested in the complex interactions of the nervous system, the endocrine system, the vascular system, and of course the immune system that lead to inflammatory processes, ultimately resulting in clinical symptoms of rheumatic diseases. Being interested in these complex interactions means formulating a hypothesis and then seeking evidence in basic or clinical research, to refute or to confirm that hypothesis. In other words, finding evidence with the ultimate goal to discover ways to decrease the burden of rheumatic diseases. During the Congress we had exactly done this: we discussed the hypotheses, the models derived from our research, explained the relevance of each hypothesis, and showed the evidence that we have collected. Of course this introduction can only be very incomplete; for a more comprehensive review see references.[1–6]

SOME HISTORICAL NOTES

Since 1930 observations have been made regarding the role of the endocrine system in rheumatoid arthritis: women have a clearly increased risk for this disease compared to men, but pregnancy ameliorates rheumatoid arthritis.

Address for correspondence: J.W.J. Bijlsma, Department of Rheumatology and Clinical Immunology, University Medical Center Utrecht, Box 85 500, 3508 GA Utrecht, The Netherlands. Voice: + 31-30-250-7357; fax: 31-30-252-3741.
e-mail: j.w.j.bijlsma@umcutrecht.nl

Ann. N.Y. Acad. Sci. 1069: xviii–xxiv (2006). © 2006 New York Academy of Sciences.
doi: 10.1196/annals.1351.049

Since the work of Selye and Fortier in the 1940s, the sympathetic nervous system and the hypothalamic-pituitary-adrenal axis were believed to play an important supportive role in the fight-and-flight reaction during stress. Selye's work on the general adaptation syndrome and the diseases of adaptation have made a clear link between the nervous system and inflammation.[7] In the same time frame (1948), the American rheumatologist Philip S. Hench was the first to administer cortisone to a patient with rheumatoid arthritis; consequently, Hench discovered the therapeutic effects of glucocorticoids.[8] This observation confirmed the clear link between the endocrine system and inflammation.

In the following years, additional data on estrogens and different rheumatic diseases were collected. From epidemiological data, it was suggested that oral contraceptives might prevent rheumatoid arthritis, but that the use of estrogens did not ameliorate rheumatoid arthritis.[9] Masi reported in 1984 that women with early rheumatoid arthritis, and even before they developed rheumatoid arthritis, had low adrenal androgenic anabolic steroid levels compared to controls.[10] Studies were performed by Cutolo, and later by Straub, looking at the synovial tissue level into the role of gonadal hormones. On the basis of these data, clinical studies were performed looking at the effect of replacement therapy with oral testosterone undecanoate to male rheumatoid arthritis patients: slight improvement in the number of affected joints and decreased daily intake of nonsteroidal anti-inflammatory drugs were noted.[11] In a double-blind, placebo-controlled study of testosterone administration as an adjuvant treatment in 57 postmenopausal rheumatoid arthritis patients, this androgen was found to improve pain score, erythrocyte sedimentation rate, and disability; 21% of the patients showed clinically relevant improvement.[12] At that time, so many people were working in this field that it was decided to start a formal study group at the American College of Rheumatology and to organize the First International Conference on the Neuroendocrine Immune Basis of the Rheumatic Diseases, which was held in Genova, Italy from September 18–20, 1998.

THE FIRST INTERNATIONAL CONFERENCE

On account of the relentless activities of Maurizio Cutolo, nearly everybody who was working in this field came together in Genova. There were seven topics at the conference:

1. the hypothalamic-pituitary-adrenal and gonadal axis and immune response;
2. sex hormones, prolactin, and immune response;
3. glucocorticoid effects on the immune response;
4. cytokines and neuroimmune response;
5. *in vitro* models of neuroendocrine–immune interaction;

6. clinical aspects of the relationships between gonadal hormones and autoimmune rheumatic diseases; and
7. stress effects on autoimmune rheumatic diseases.

It is impossible to give a real flavor of what transpired during those 3 energetic days. As an example, here is mentioned the emphasis that was put on the modulation by gonadal hormones of the cytokine release by immune cells,[13] in which Ian Chikanza and Bob Lahita led the way. Also, an effort was made to translate the NEI findings to the pathogenesis of rheumatoid arthritis. The interaction between sex hormones and glucocorticoids was another topic.[14]

All the lectures and ensuing discussions were published by the New York Academy of Sciences[2] and a report of the conference was published in the "Trends" section of *Immunology Today*.[3]

Many of the researchers involved in the first conference were also involved in the publication of a nice volume of *Rheumatic Disease Clinics of North America*, in November 2000, *Neuroendocrine Mechanisms in Rheumatic Diseases*.[1]

THE SECOND INTERNATIONAL CONFERENCE

In the following years, the joint efforts of many researchers led to the need to organize a second conference, which was held also in Genova, in September 2001.

One week before our conference started, the disaster of 9/11 happened in New York and unfortunately quite a number of our American friends were unable to attend this conference.

The themes of the second conference were:

1. state-of-the-art;
2. glucocorticoids and rheumatic diseases;
3. androgens and estrogens in rheumatic diseases;
4. prolactin in rheumatic diseases;
5. melatonin and rheumatoid arthritis;
6. effects of stress;
7. the hypothalamic-pituitary-adrenal axis and arthritis;
8. the nervous system and arthritis; and
9. neuroendocrine immune aspects of various rheumatic diseases.

In this Congress, Rainer H. Straub had an important impact on the theme of nervous system/stress and rheumatic diseases.[15–17]

During that conference, interactive poster sessions were held in order to also stimulate the involvement of fellows in research. There were many highlights during this conference, both in basic research, such as further elucidating how cytokines influence gonadal hormones, and also more clinical data on conditions like the antiphospholipid syndrome.

More general overviews were given discussing the balance of the immune system, in which immune stimulation may lead to autoimmunity, and immune suppression to infection and cancer. This balance is influenced by stress and glucocorticoids, leading to immune suppression, while certain cytokines and prolactin may lead to immune stimulation. In chronic arthritis, altered function of the hypothalamus-pituitary-adrenal and hypothalamus-pituitary-gonadal axis is further elucidated. This was illustrated in patients with very early rheumatoid arthritis that were shown to have a dysregulation of the diurnal cortisol rhythm, inappropriate for the ongoing inflammation.[18] The role of adrenal and gonadal hormones in immune modulation was summarized and the clinical use in rheumatic diseases was evaluated. An important observation was the Utrecht experience with glucocorticoids in rheumatoid arthritis, showing not only a clear symptomatic relief, but also showing retardation of erosions.[19]

Apart from the science and discussions, friendship has become an important way to improve science. The surroundings of Genoa and Santa Margherita Ligure made this very easy.

Again, all the lectures and the discussions and also the extended posters were published in the Annals of the New York Academy of Sciences.[4] Also, the activities of many researchers in this field led to the second volume of *Rheumatic Disease Clinics of North America: Clinical aspects of immune neuroendocrine mechanisms in rheumatic diseases.*[6]

THE THIRD INTERNATIONAL CONFERENCE

After 4 years, the Third International Conference was held again in Genova, Santa Margherita Ligure, in September 2005, supported by the active cooperation of the editors of the present issue of the Annals of the New York Academy of Sciences.

The growing interest for an evidence-based medicine in neuroendocrine–immune mechanisms in rheumatic diseases, suggested to the organizers a more "clinical" approach to the conference.

Therefore, the eight topics of the meeting were the following:

1. anti-TNF strategies and effects on neuroendocrine immune mechanisms in rheumatic diseases;
2. glucocorticoids—new perspectives in the therapy of rheumatic diseases;
3. nerve fibers and rheumatoid arthritis;
4. stimulation tests and the stress response;
5. sex hormones and rheumatic diseases;
6. lipid metabolism in rheumatic diseases;
7. gene polymorphisms and the neuroendocrine immune system in rheumatic diseases; and
8. neuroendocrine immune aspects of autoimmune diseases.

The participation of researchers and clinicians from over 25 different countries has been the best confirmation of the interest for the "neuroendocrine immune" approach to the rheumatic diseases.

Interestingly, first controlled studies with anti-TNF antibodies demonstrate positive effects on the endocrine and nervous system and were presented during the conference.[20,21] In addition, this therapy may shed new light on pathophysiological processes in rheumatoid arthritis.

Additional data from the randomized controlled clinical trials showed that the incidence, severity, and impact of adverse effects of low-dose glucocorticoid therapy in rheumatoid arthritis trials are modest, and often not statistically different to those of placebo.[22] Glucocorticoids in rheumatoid arthritis might exert disease modifying effects. Stimulating reports on gene polymorphisms and the neuroendocrine–immune system in rheumatic diseases were related to the angiotensin-converting enzyme and endothelin system changes in scleroderma. A link between lipids and inflammation was discussed, in particular, referring to the adipose tissue as having immunomodulatory properties and leptin as a link between adipose tissue and inflammation. Sex hormones were confirmed as modulators of the immune inflammatory reactions in different presentations.[23,24]

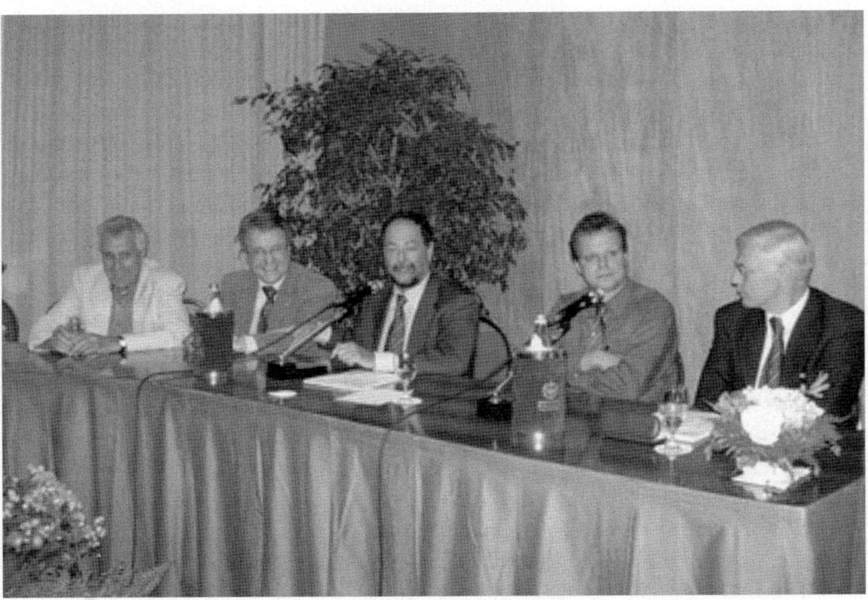

FIGURE 1. The Board of Editors of the Third International NEI Conference (Genova, September 2005). From left to right: Alfonse Masi, Robert Lahita, Maurizio Cutolo, Rainer H. Straub, and Johannes W.J. Bijlsma.

Again, this Congress was very fruitful, and the organizers (FIG. 1) are proud to present the results from this Congress in this volume of the *Annals of the New York Academy of Sciences*.

REFERENCES

1. MASI, A.T., J.W.J. BIJLSMA, I.C. CHIKANZA & M. CUTOLO, Eds.: 2000. Neuroendocrine mechanisms in rheumatic diseases. Rheum. Dis. Clin. North Am. **26:** 693–1042.
2. CUTOLO, M., A.T. MASI, J.W.J. BIJLSMA, *et al.*Eds.: 1999. Neuroendocrine immune basis of the rheumatic diseases. Ann. N. Y. Acad. Sci. **876:** 1–429.
3. BIJLSMA, J.W.J., M. CUTOLO, A.T. MASI & I.C. CHIKANZA. 1999. The neuroendocrine immune basis of rheumatic diseases. Immunol. Today **20:** 298–301.
4. CUTOLO, M., J.W.J. BIJLSMA, R.G. LAHITA, *et al.*, Eds.: 2002. Neuroendocrine immune basis of the rheumatic diseases II. Ann. N. Y. Acad. Sci. **966:** 1–511.
5. BIJLSMA, J.W.J., R.H. STRAUB, A.T. MASI, *et al.* 2002. Neuroendocrine immune mechanisms in rheumatic diseases. Trends Immunol. **23:** 59–61.
6. BIJLSMA, J.W.J., M. CUTOLO, R.H. STRAUB & A.T. MASI, Eds.: 2005. Clinical aspects of immune neuroendocrine mechanisms in rheumatic diseases. Rheum. Dis. Clin. North Am. **31:** 1–210.
7. SELYE, H. 1946. The general adaptation syndrome and the diseases of adaptation. J. Clin. Endocrin. **6:** 117–230.
8. HENCH, P.S., E.C. KENDALL, C.H. SLOCUMB, *et al.* 1949. The effect of a hormone of the adrenal conrtex and of pituitary adrenocorticotropic hormone on rheumatoid arthritis: preliminary report. Proc. Staff Meet Mayo Clin. **24:** 181–197.
9. BIJLSMA, J.W.J. & H.J. VAN DEN BRINK. 1992. Estrogens and rheumatoid arthritis. Am. J. Reprod. Immunol. **28:** 231–236.
10. MASI, A.T., D.B. JOSIPOVIC & W.E. JEFFERSON. 1984. Low adrenal androgenic-anabolic steroids in women with rheumatoid arthritis. Semin. Arthritis Rheum. **14:** 1–23.
11. CUTOLO, M., F. BALLEARI, M. GINSTI, *et al.* 1991. Androgen replacement therapy in male patients with RA. Arthritis Rheum. **34:** 1–6.
12. BOOIJ, A., A.M. BIEWENGA-BOOIJ, O. HUBER-BRUNING & J.W.J. BIJLSMA. 1996. Androgens as adjuvant treatment in postmenopausal patients with RA. Ann. Rheum. Dis. **55:** 811–817.
13. CHIKANZA, I.C. & A.B. GROSSMAN. 2000. Reciprocal interactions between the neuro-endocrine and immune systems during inflammation. Rheum. Dis. Clin. North Am. **26:** 693–711.
14. DA SILVA, J.A.P. 1993. Sex steroids affect glucocorticoid response to chronic inflammation and to interleukin-1. J. Endocrinol. **136:** 389–397.
15. STRAUB, R.H. 1998. Dialogue between CNS and immune system in lymphoid organs. Immunol. Today **19:** 409–413.
16. STRAUB, R.H. & H.O. BESEDOWSKY. 2003. Integrated evolutionary, immunological, and neuroendocrine framework for the pathogenesis of chronic disabling inflammatory diseases. FASEB J. **17:** 2176–2183.
17. STRAUB, R.H., F.S. DHABBAR, J.W.J. BIJLSMA & M. CUTOLO. 2005. How psychological stress via hormones and nerve fibers may exacerbate rheumatoid arthritis. Arthritis Rheum. **52:** 16–26.

18. DEKKERS, J.C., R. GEENEN, G.C.R. GODAERT & J.W.J. BIJLSMA. 2000. Diurnal rhythm of salivary cortisol in patients with RA of recent onset. Arthritis Rheum. **43:** 465–466.
19. BIJLSMA, J.W.J., A.A. VAN EVERDINGEN, M. HUISMAN, *et al.* 2002. Glucocorticoids in RA, effects on erosions and bone. Ann. N. Y. Acad. Sci. **966:** 82–90.
20. STRAUB, R.H., G. PONGRATZ , J. SCHÖLMERICH, *et al.* 2003. Long-term anti-tumor necrosis factor antibody therapy in rheumatoid arthritis patients sensitizes the pituitary gland and favors adrenal androgen secretion. Arthritis Rheum. **48:** 1504–1512.
21. WOLFE, F. & K. MICHAUD. 2004. Fatigue, rheumatoid arthritis, and anti-tumor necrosis factor therapy: an investigation in 24831 patients. J. Rheumatol. **31:** 2115–2120.
22. DA SILVA, J.A., J.W. JACOBS, J.R. KIRWAN, *et al.* 2006. Low-dose glucocorticoid therapy in rheumatoid arthritis. A review on safety: published evidence and prospective trial data. Ann. Rheum. Dis. **65:** 285–293.
23. CUTOLO, M., S. CAPELLINO, P. MONTAGNA, *et al.* 2003. New roles for estrogens in rheumatoid arthritis. Clin. Exp. Rheumatol. **21:** 687–690.
24. CUTOLO, M., S. CAPELLINO, P. MONTAGNA, *et al.* 2004. Sex hormone modulation of cell growth and apoptosis of the human monocytic/macrophage cell line. Arthritis Res. Ther. **7:** R1124–R1133.

The Physiology of Human Glucocorticoid Receptor β (hGRβ) and Glucocorticoid Resistance

LAURA J. LEWIS-TUFFIN[a,b] AND JOHN A. CIDLOWSKI[a]

[a]*Laboratory of Signal Transduction, National Institute of Environmental Health Sciences, National Institutes of Health, Department of Health and Human Services, Research Triangle Park, North Carolina, 27709, USA*

[b]*Department of Cancer Cell Biology, Mayo Clinic, Jacksonville, Florida 32224, USA*

ABSTRACT: The development of glucocorticoid (GC) resistance is a serious problem that complicates the treatment of immune-related diseases, such as asthma, ulcerative colitis, and hematologic cancers. hGRα and hGRβ are two isoforms of the human glucocorticoid receptor, which differ in the structural composition of the carboxy-terminal end of the ligand-binding domain and therefore in their ability to bind glucocorticoid ligand and in their physiological function. hGRα is the classically functional GR, while hGRβ seems to act mainly as a dominant negative to the function of hGRα. Because of the ability of hGRβ to antagonize the action of hGRα, it has been hypothesized that changes in the expression of hGRβ may underlie the development of glucocorticoid resistance. In this article we review what is known about the expression and physiological action of hGRβ in normal cells and tissue as well as in several disease states. Taken together, the evidence suggests that the ratio of hGRα:hGRβ expression is indeed critical to the glucocorticoid responsiveness of various cells. This ratio can be altered by changing the expression level of hGRα, hGRβ, or both receptors simultaneously. Higher ratios correlate with glucocorticoid sensitivity, while lower ratios correlate with glucocorticoid resistance. Thus hGRβ can be an important modulator of glucocorticoid responsiveness.

KEYWORDS: glucocorticoid receptor beta (GRβ); glucocorticoid resistance; insensitivity; asthma; ulcerative colitis; leukemia; nasal polyps

INTRODUCTION

Glucocorticoids (GC) are a class of naturally occurring and synthetic steroid hormones that affect virtually every aspect of human physiology. Their actions

Address for correspondence: John A. Cidlowski, Laboratory of Signal Transduction, National Institute of Environmental Health Sciences, National Institutes of Health, Department of Health and Human Services, 111 TW Alexander Drive, P.O. Box 12233, Research Triangle Park, NC 27709, USA. Voice: 919-541-1564; fax: 919-541-1367.
e-mail: cidlowski@niehs.nih.gov

Ann. N.Y. Acad. Sci. 1069: 1–9 (2006). © 2006 New York Academy of Sciences.
doi: 10.1196/annals.1351.001

include important roles in the development of the lung and nervous system,[1–3] the modulation of skeletal metabolism,[4] the maintenance of homeostasis,[5–7] and the modulation/regulation of behavior.[8–12] Perhaps their most important effects, however, are highly effective anti-inflammatory and immunomodulatory actions that are exploited in the treatment of such diseases as arthritis, asthma, allergic rhinitis, and leukemia/lymphoma.[13–18] The broad involvement of glucocorticoids in both normal and pathologic physiological processes makes them one of the most important and commonly prescribed classes of drugs available,[19] but also underlies the side effects commonly experienced with glucocorticoid treatment.[20,21] In particular, the development of glucocorticoid resistance is a serious complication that can occur during chemotherapy regimens for hematologic cancers and chronic asthma therapy, making treatment of those conditions more difficult.[22,23] The mechanisms that underlie the development of glucocorticoid resistance are poorly understood and likely vary with disease type, treatment regimen, and the genetic background of the patient. However, an increasing number of reports indicate that changes in the relative expression of the glucocorticoid receptor (GR) isoforms hGRα and hGRβ are associated with glucocorticoid resistance, and may contribute to its development. Here, we review what is known about hGRβ and its relationship to glucocorticoid resistance.

GLUCOCORTICOID RECEPTOR α AND β: STRUCTURAL DIFFERENCES

Glucocorticoid actions are mediated by the glucocorticoid receptor, which is a member of the large steroid/thyroid/retinoic acid receptor superfamily that regulates gene transcription in a ligand-dependent manner. The gene for human GR (hGR) was originally cloned in 1985.[24] It is located on chromosome 5 (region 5q31)[25,26] and consists of nine exons.[24,27] Through alternative splicing of exon 9, two isoforms of the hGR gene, hGRα and hGRβ, are produced.[28]

The nuclear receptor superfamily has a common, modular domain structure that includes a variable-length amino terminus, a centrally located, zinc-finger DNA-binding domain (DBD), and a carboxy terminus ligand-binding domain (LBD).[19,29] In addition to these domains, GR has two transcription-activating regions, one in the amino terminal domain of the protein (AF-1 or τ1) that appears to act somewhat independently of ligand binding, and a second in the ligand-binding domain (AF-2 or τ2) whose function is dependent on ligand binding.[30,31] Additionally, the hGR LBD contains nuclear localization signals and sites for interaction with other transcription factors, cofactors, and protein chaperones.[32–34] Analysis of the crystal structure of the hGRα LBD indicates that it is a 12-helix bundle consisting of three layers, with the ligand-binding pocket located in the center.[35] Comparison of the GR LBD structure with the LBD structures of other nuclear receptors suggests that the ligand-dependent conformation of the final, 12th helix is critical to the AF-2 transactivation function of GR.[36,37]

The alternately spliced exon 9 of the hGR coding sequence encodes the extreme carboxy terminal end of the GR ligand-binding domain, as well as the 3′ UTR. Thus the hGRα and β isoforms are identical proteins up through amino acid 727 corresponding to the C-terminal end of helix 10 of the LBD, but the remainder of the ligand-binding domain differs between the two receptors. hGRα has an additional 50 amino acids that encode helices 11 and 12 to complete a functional domain capable of binding ligand and transactivating gene expression. In contrast, hGRβ has only an additional 15 distinct amino acids. Consequently, hGRβ is missing helix 12 of the ligand-binding domain and possesses a unique sequence in helix 11 when compared to hGRα. The shortened, distinct LBD of hGRβ is reported to be unable to bind ligand,[24,28,30] resulting in a receptor that is unable to directly activate glucocorticoid responsive promoters.[24,30] Sequential mutation of the 15 unique amino acids within the hGRβ LBD suggests that amino acids 733 and 734 (unique amino acids 6 and 7) play an important role in determining the biological activity of hGRβ.[38]

GLUCOCORTICOID RECEPTOR α AND β: FUNCTIONAL DIFFERENCES

Because the α isoform of hGR binds ligand and affects gene expression, while the β isoform does not, far more is known about the mechanisms of hGRα than hGRβ action. In the absence of ligand, hGRα is maintained in the cytoplasm in a multiprotein complex that includes heat-shock protein 90 and several immunophilins. Upon ligand binding, this complex dissociates, exposing the nuclear localization signal of hGRα and allowing it to translocate to the nucleus. Once in the nucleus, hGRα affects gene transcription, either by binding to specific DNA elements known as glucocorticoid response elements (GRE), or by protein–protein interactions with other transcription factors, such as AP-1, NF-κB, or STAT family members.

In contrast, hGRβ is found constitutively in the nucleus and is not thought to bind ligand. [28,39] In addition, hGRβ cannot affect gene expression by itself. Instead, evidence suggests that hGRβ may act as a dominant negative to repress the transcriptional activity of hGRα. Reporter gene experiments carried out using exogenously expressed hGRα and hGRβ in cells that do not express endogenous GR have shown that (1) hGRβ is not able to activate reporter gene expression by itself[28,40] and (2) when hGRβ is overexpressed relative to hGRα, hGRβ represses the transcriptional activity of hGRα.[40,41] In addition, exogenous expression of hGRβ can repress the activity of transiently transfected reporter genes driven by endogenous hGRα expression.[28] It is believed that hGRβ's dominant negative activity is the combined result of (1) differences in the identity of amino acid residues 733 and 734 between the hGRα and hGRβ LBDs, which cause hGRβ's Helix 11 to be disordered, and (2) the constitutively nuclear localization of the hGRβ receptor.[38]

The dominant negative activity of hGRβ in cell culture has led to the hypothesis that changes in hGRβ expression relative to hGRα could underlie the development of glucocorticoid (GC) resistance in several human diseases. This hypothesis has been partially tested in cell culture using HeLa S_3 cells that express endogenous hGR. It has been demonstrated in these cells that hGRβ protein levels increase in response to treatment with the proinflammatory cytokine tumor necrosis factor α (TNF-α).[42] This increase was correlated with the development of GC resistance in these cells, as measured by reporter gene assay. A more direct test of the idea that hGRβ expression underlies GC resistance comes from a study in which mouse hybridoma cells, which are naturally devoid of the GRβ isoform, were virally transduced with cDNA for hGRβ.[43] The proliferation of these cells was then compared to nontransduced cells in the presence of hydrocortisone. In contrast to the nontransduced cells, the cells that expressed hGRβ were resistant to the antiproliferative effects of hydrocortisone. Although these studies do not prove that increased expression of hGRβ directly underlies glucocorticoid resistance in humans, they do provide evidence that such expression could contribute to this desensitized state of hormone responsiveness. Consequently, there have been a number of investigations into the expression of hGRβ in disease states that have become GC resistant.

EXPRESSION OF HGRβ IN NORMAL AND DISEASED CELLS AND TISSUE

The distribution of hGRβ has been examined in both normal and diseased human cells and tissues, as well as in a number of human cell lines. However, direct comparisons of the levels of the hGRα and hGRβ isoforms, especially for protein expression in normal tissues, have not been done as often or as rigorously as one would like. In addition, few attempts have been made to analyze the expression of hGRβ in different cell types within the same organ (e.g., neurons vs. glia in brain tissue). Therefore, the actual extent of hGRα versus β expression in both normal and diseased cells and tissues is in many cases still unclear. Having said that, the mRNA for hGRβ has been found in almost every normal human tissue and cell type examined, including adult brain, lung, liver, heart, placenta, skeletal muscle, kidney, pituitary, pancreas, thymus, spleen, bone marrow, nasal mucosa, abdominal fat, leukocytes, eosinophils, peripheral blood mononuclear cells (PBMCs), macrophages, and neutrophils, as well as fetal brain, lung, and liver.[28,40,44] In contrast, hGRβ protein has been shown to have a more restricted distribution. Most frequently, hGRβ protein has been found in normal T lymphocytes, macrophages, neutrophils, eosinophils, and PBMCs.[45–47] In addition, hGRβ protein has been reported in brain, lung, and heart tissue,[39] although there is a contradictory report.[44] Finally, human lung carcinoma, breast carcinoma, endometrial carcinoma, and bladder carcinoma cell lines, as well as HeLa S_3 cervical carcinoma cells, CEM-C7 leukemia cells, JAR choriocarcinoma cells, HEK-293 embryonic kidney cells, and normal lung epithelial cells have all been shown to express hGRβ protein.[39]

The expression of hGRβ in diseased tissue has been studied primarily in the context of GC-resistant forms of asthma, ulcerative colitis, nasal polyposis, and leukemia, including chronic lymphocytic and acute lymphoblastic leukemias. Of these, GC-resistant chronic asthma has been the most extensively studied. Increased numbers of hGRβ immunoreactive PBMCs and CD3+ T cells from the airways of patients with GC-resistant versus GC-sensitive asthma have been reported.[45,48] Extending these findings, greater numbers of hGRβ immunoreactive cells, primarily CD3+ T cells, have also been found in the lungs of fatal asthma cases as compared to cases of emphysema, mild asthma, or normal subjects.[49] Furthermore, using a cutaneous tuberculin inflammation model, the expression of hGRβ was greater in T cells and macrophages from GC-resistant versus GC-sensitive asthma patients.[50] Taken together, these reports suggest that increased expression of hGRβ in inflammatory cells, especially T cells, may be related to the development of GC-insensitive asthma.

Three studies have examined the expression of hGRβ in GC-resistant forms of ulcerative colitis. Two of these studies, examining hGRα and β mRNA expression in PBMCs from patients with ulcerative colitis versus normal subjects, found that PBMCs from patients with active ulcerative colitis were more likely to express hGRβ mRNA.[51,52] In addition, quantitative comparison of hGRβ mRNA levels in PBMCs from patients with GC-resistant versus GC-sensitive ulcerative colitis revealed higher expression of hGRβ mRNA in the GC-resistant cases. Furthermore, examination of hGRβ mRNA levels longitudinally in patients whose ulcerative colitis relapsed revealed increased hGRβ levels during the relapse.[52] There was no difference in the expression of hGRα mRNA between normal subjects and any of the ulcerative colitis patients in these studies. Finally, examination of hGRβ protein levels in PBMCs by Western blot and in colonic mucosal cells by immunocytochemistry confirmed increased expression of hGRβ in GC-resistant versus GC-sensitive ulcerative colitis.[51,53] Taken together, these studies suggest that increased expression of hGRβ in inflammatory cells is predictive of GC resistance, which is reduced patient response to GC treatment, in ulcerative colitis.

The expression of hGRβ protein in inflammatory cells found in nasal polyps as opposed to normal middle olfactory turbinate tissue has also been examined.[47] This study found increased hGRβ expression in nasal polyp inflammatory cells, particularly in T cells, eosinophils, and macrophages. Furthermore, although the number of subjects was small, an inverse correlation was noted between the baseline level of hGRβ expression and the response to the glucocorticoid fluticasone propionate. High levels of hGRβ expression correlated with a poor response to treatment with fluticasone propionate.

Finally, hGRβ expression associated with GC resistance has been examined in several cases of leukemia. The first such report concerned the relative expression of hGRα and β isoforms in a single case of GC-resistant chronic lymphocytic leukemia.[54] In cultured lymphocytes from this patient, the level of hGRα protein was found to be severely reduced and the level of hGRβ protein was elevated, resulting in a 20-fold excess of hGRβ compared to hGRα. A second report examined the relative levels of hGRα and β in 13 cases of acute lymphoblastic leukemia (ALL), including 8 ALL cases with pre-B cell lineage and 5 ALL cases with T cell lineage versus EBV-transformed lymphocytes from normal controls.[55] This study found no changes in the expression of hGRβ protein in ALL versus normal controls, but did find significant decreases in the expression of hGRα protein, especially in the T cell lineage ALL cells. As a result, the ratio of hGRα:hGRβ expression was reduced, from 1.4 in controls to 0.86 in ALL with pre-B lineage, and to 0.09 in ALL with T cell lineage. Interestingly, lymphoblasts of the T cell lineage are known to have reduced GC sensitivity.[56] A similar study also correlated the ratio of hGRβ:hGRα to ALL-phenotype and GC sensitivity.[57] In that study, hGRβ:hGRα ratios were lower in cases of pre-B ALL, which responds well to GC treatment, compared to other types of ALL, which have with a poorer prognostic phenotype and response to GC treatment. Taken together, the results of these studies indicate that the relative expression of hGRα to hGRβ in leukemia cells correlates with their sensitivity to GCs. Lymphoblasts/lymphocytes with lower hGRα:hGRβ ratios are less sensitive to the apoptosis-inducing effects of GC treatment and are associated with a poorer prognosis.

When the results of all these studies on hGRβ expression in different disease states are taken together, a picture begins to emerge in which a reduction in the relative expression of hGRα:hGRβ protein is associated with a poor response to GC treatment. Thus decreased expression of hGRα and/or increased expression of hGRβ in inflammatory cells appears to be a common mechanism for the development of glucocorticoid resistance in multiple organs.

CONCLUSIONS

There is general agreement that the expression of hGRα is much greater than the expression of hGRβ in most cells and tissues, in both normal and diseased states. Consequently, there is some disagreement as to whether hGRβ makes an important contribution to either normal or disease physiology. Some authors have argued that, with such low starting levels, small increases in hGRβ expression are unlikely to be physiologically relevant because they cannot substantially affect the hGRα:hGRβ ratio. However, it has been demonstrated for a growing number of immune-related disease states that decreases in the expression of hGRα and/or increases in the expression of hGRβ do result in substantial changes to the hGRα:hGRβ ratio and are correlated with the development of GC resistance. When taken together, these results suggest that hGRβ does have an important role to play in the development of GC resistance. Thus, even if we do not currently understand the mechanistic details, hGRβ is potentially a key modulator of the progression of certain immune-related diseases. It is up to future investigators to determine the mechanisms of hGRβ function in both normal and disease states.

REFERENCES

1. JOBE, A.H. 2001. Glucocorticoids, inflammation and the perinatal lung. Sem. Neonatol. **6:** 331–342.
2. KOENIG, J.I., B. KIRKPATRICK & P. LEE. 2002. Glucocorticoid hormones and early brain development in schizophrenia. Neuropsychopharmacology. **27:** 309–318.
3. MATTHEWS, S.G. *et al.* 2002. Glucocorticoids, hypothalamo-pituitary-adrenal (HPA) development, and life after birth. Endocr. Res. **28:** 709–718.
4. CANALIS, E., R.C. PEREIRA & A.M. DELANY. 2002. Effects of glucocorticoids on the skeleton. J. Pediat Endocrinol. Metab. **15:** 1341–1345.
5. DALLMAN, M.F. *et al.* 2000. Bottomed out: metabolic significance of the circadian trough in glucocorticoid concentrations. Int. J. Obes. Rel. Metab. Disord: J. Int. Assoc. Study Obes. **24:** S40–S46.
6. JEANRENAUD, B. & F. ROHNER-JEANRENAUD. 2000. CNS-periphery relationships and body weight homeostasis: influence of the glucocorticoid status. Int. J. Obes. Rel. Metab. Disord: J. Int. Assoc. Study Obes. **24:** S74–S76.
7. RABER, J. 1998. Detrimental effects of chronic hypothalamic-pituitary-adrenal axis activation: from obesity to memory deficits. Mol. Neurobiol. **18:** 1–22.
8. FUCHS, E. *et al.* 2001. Psychosocial stress, glucocorticoids, and structural alterations in the tree shrew hippocampus. Physiol. Behav. **73:** 285–291.
9. MACCARI, S. *et al.* 2003. Prenatal stress and long-term consequences: implications of glucocorticoid hormones. Neurosci. Biobehav. Rev. **27:** 119–127.
10. MARINELLI, M. & P.V. PIAZZA. 2002. Interaction between glucocorticoid hormones, stress and psychostimulant drugs. Eur. J.Neurosci. **16:** 387–394.
11. REUS, V.I. & O.M. WOLKOWITZ. 2001. Antiglucocorticoid drugs in the treatment of depression. Exp. Opin. Invest. Drugs **10:** 1789–1796.
12. STECKLER, T., F. HOLSBOER & J.M. REUL. 1999. Glucocorticoids and depression. Best Prac. Res. Clin. Endocrinol. Metab. **13:** 597–614.
13. ALMAWI, W.Y., M.M. ABOU JAOUDE & X.C. LI. 2002. Transcriptional and post-transcriptional mechanisms of glucocorticoid antiproliferative effects. Hem. Oncol. **20:** 17–32.
14. BARNES, P.J. 1998. Anti-inflammatory actions of glucocorticoids: molecular mechanisms. Clin. Sci. **94:** 557–572.
15. NACLERIO, R.M. 1988. The pathophysiology of allergic rhinitis: impact of therapeutic intervention. J. Allergy Clin. Immunol. **82:** 927–934.
16. RICCARDI, C., S. BRUSCOLI & G. MIGLIORATI. 2002. Molecular mechanisms of immunomodulatory activity of glucocorticoids. Pharmacol. Res. **45:** 361–368.
17. PERRETTI, M. & A. AHLUWALIA. 2000. The microcirculation and inflammation: site of action for glucocorticoids. Microcirculation **7:** 147–161.
18. SZEFLER, S.J. 2000. Asthma: the new advances. Advan. Pediat. **47:** 273–308.

19. EVANS, R.M. 1988. The steroid and thyroid hormone receptor superfamily. Science **240:** 889–895.
20. SCHACKE, H., W.D. DOCKE & K. ASADULLAH. 2002. Mechanisms involved in the side effects of glucocorticoids. Pharm. Therap. **96:** 23–43.
21. WHELAN, C.J. 2003. Will non-steroid approaches to the treatment of inflammation replace our need for glucocorticoids? Curr. Opin. Invest. Drugs **4:** 536–543.
22. SCHAAF, M.J. & J.A. CIDLOWSKI. 2002. Molecular mechanisms of glucocorticoid action and resistance. J. Steroid Biochem. Mol. Biol. **83:** 37–48.
23. KINO, T. *et al.* 2003. Tissue glucocorticoid resistance/hypersensitivity syndromes. J. Steroid Biochem. Mol. Biol. **85:** 457–467.
24. HOLLENBERG, S.M. *et al.* 1985. Primary structure and expression of a functional human glucocorticoid receptor cDNA. Nature **318:** 635–641.
25. FRANCKE, U. & B.E. FOELLMER. 1989. The glucocorticoid receptor gene is in 5q31-q32 [erratum appears in Genomics 1989 5(2):388]. Genomics **4:** 610–612.
26. THERIAULT, A. *et al.* 1989. Regional chromosomal assignment of the human glucocorticoid receptor gene to 5q31. Hum. Gen. **83:** 289–291.
27. ENCIO, I.J. & S.D. DETERA-WADLEIGH. 1991. The genomic structure of the human glucocorticoid receptor. J. Biol. Chem. **256:** 7182–7188.
28. OAKLEY, R.H., M. SAR & J.A. CIDLOWSKI. 1996. The human glucocorticoid receptor beta isoform: expression, biochemical properties, and putative function. J. Biol. Chem. **271:** 9550–9559.
29. KUMAR, R. & E.B. THOMPSON. 1999. The structure of the nuclear hormone receptors. Steroids **64:** 310–319.
30. GIGUERE, V. *et al.* 1986. Functional domains of the human glucocorticoid receptor. Cell **46:** 645–652.
31. HOLLENBERG, S.M. & R.M. EVANS. 1988. Multiple and cooperative *trans*-activation domains of the human glucocorticoid receptor. Cell **55:** 899–906.
32. DEFRANCO, D.B. 1999. Regulation of steroid receptor subcellular trafficking. Cell Biochem. Biophys. **30:** 1–24.
33. JENKINS, B.D., C.B. PULLEN & B.D. DARIMONT. 2001. Novel glucocorticoid receptor coactivator effector mechanisms. Trends Endocrinol. Metab. **12:** 122–126.
34. PRATT, W.B. 1993. The role of heat shock proteins in regulating the function, folding, and trafficking of the glucocorticoid receptor. J. Biol. Chem. **268:** 21455–21458.
35. BLEDSOE, R.K. *et al.* 2002. Crystal structure of the glucocorticoid receptor ligand binding domain reveals a novel mode of receptor dimerization and coactivator recognition. Cell **110:** 93–105.
36. WEATHERMAN, R.V., R.J. FLETTERICK & T.S. SCANLAN. 1999. Nuclear-receptor ligands and ligand-binding domains. Annu. Rev. Biochem. **68:** 559–581.
37. STEINMETZ, A.C.U., J.-P. RENAUD & D. MORAS. 2001. Binding of ligands and activation of transcription by nuclear receptors. Annu. Rev. Biophys. Biomol. Struct. **30:** 329–359.
38. YUDT, M.R. *et al.* 2003. Molecular origins for the dominant negative function of human glucocorticoid receptor beta. Mol. Cell Biol. **23:** 4319–4330.
39. OAKLEY, R.H. *et al.* 1997. Expression and subcellular distribution of the beta-isoform of the human glucocorticoid receptor. Endocrinology **138:** 5028–5038.
40. BAMBERGER, C.M. *et al.* 1995. Glucocorticoid receptor β, a potential endogenous inhibitor of glucocorticoid action in humans. J. Clin. Invest. **95:** 2435–2441.

41. OAKLEY, R.H. *et al.* 1999. The dominant negative activity of the human glucocorticoid receptor beta isoform: specificity and mechanisms of action. J. Biol. Chem. **274:** 27857–27866.
42. WEBSTER, J.C. *et al.* 2001. Proinflammatory cytokines regulate human glucocorticoid receptor gene expression and lead to the accumulation of the dominant negative beta isoform: a mechanism for the generation of glucocorticoid resistance. Proc. Natl. Acad. Sci. USA. **98:** 6865–6870.
43. HAUK, P.J. *et al.* 2002. Increased glucocorticoid receptor β expression converts mouse hybridoma cells to a corticosteroid-insensitive phenotype. Am. J. Resp. Cell Mol. Biol. **27:** 361–367.
44. PUJOLS, L. *et al.* 2002. Expression of glucocorticoid receptor alpha- and beta-isoforms in human cells and tissues. Am. J. Physiol. Cell Physiol. **283:** C1324–C1331.
45. HAMID, Q. *et al.* 1999. Increased glucocorticoid receptor β in airway cells of glucocorticoid-insensitive asthma. Am. J. Resp. Crit. Care Med. **159:** 1600–1604.
46. STRICKLAND, I. *et al.* 2001. High constitutive glucocorticoid receptor β in human neutrophils enables them to reduce their spontaneous rate of cell death in response to corticosteroids. J. Exp. Med. **193:** 585–593.
47. HAMILOS, D.L. *et al.* 2001. GRβ expression in nasal polyp inflammatory cells and its relationship to the anti-inflammatory effects of intranasal fluticasone. J. Allergy Clin. Immunol. **108:** 59–68.
48. LEUNG, D.Y.M. *et al.* 1997. Association of glucocorticoid insensitivity with increased expression of glucocorticoid receptor β. J. Exp. Med. **186:** 1567–1574.
49. CHRISTODOULOPOULOS, P. *et al.* 2000. Increased number of glucocorticoid receptor-β-expressing cells in the airways in fatal asthma. J. Allergy Clin. Immunol. **106:** 479–484.
50. SOUSA, A.R. *et al.* 2000. Glucocorticoid resistance in asthma is associated with elevated in vivo expression of the glucocorticoid receptor β-isoform. J. Allergy Clin. Immunol. **105:** 943–950.
51. HONDA, M. *et al.* 2000. Expression of glucocorticoid receptor β in lymphocytes of patients with glucocorticoid-resistant ulcerative colitis. Gastroenterology **118:** 859–866.
52. ORII, F. *et al.* 2002. Quantitative analysis for human glucocorticoid receptor α/β mRNA in IBD. Biochem. Biophys. Res. Commun. **296:** 1286–1294.
53. ZHANG, H. *et al.* 2005. Significance of glucocorticoid receptor expression in colonic mucosal cells of patients with ulcerative colitis. World J. Gastroenterol. **11:** 1775–1778.
54. SHAHIDI, H. *et al.* 1999. Imbalanced expression of the glucocorticoid receptor isoforms in cultured lymphocytes from a patient with systemic glucocorticoid resistance and chronic lymphocytic leukemia. Biochem. Biophys. Res. Commun. **254:** 559–565.
55. LONGUI, C.A. *et al.* 2000. Low glucocorticoid receptor alpha/beta ratio in T-cell lymphoblastic leukemia. Horm. Metab. Res. **32:** 401–406.
56. PIETERS, R. *et al.* 1998. Relation between age, immunophenotype and in vitro drug resistance in 395 children with acute lymphoblastic leukemia: implications for treatment of infants. Leukemia **12:** 1344–1348.
57. KOGA, Y. *et al.* 2005. Differential mRNA expression of glucocorticoid receptor alpha and beta is associated with glucocorticoid sensitivity of acute lymphoblastic leukemia in children. Pediat. Blood Cancer **45:** 121–127.

Angiotensin-Converting Enzyme in Systemic Sclerosis

From Endothelial Injury to a Genetic Polymorphism

SERENA GUIDUCCI,[a] CINZIA FATINI,[b] VERONICA ROGAI,[a] MARINA CINELLI,[a] ELENA STICCHI,[b] ROSANNA ABBATE,[b] AND MARCO MATUCCI CERINIC[a]

[a]*Division of Medicine I and Rheumatology, Department of Medicine and Surgery, University of Florence, Florence, Italy*

[b]*Department of Clinical and Surgical Critical Care, Section of Clinical Medicine, Thrombosis Centre, University of Florence, Florence, Italy*

ABSTRACT: The main pathologic hallmark of systemic sclerosis (SSc) is endothelial derangement; the pathologic alterations of the vessel wall in SSc are strikingly similar to the modification detected in the atherosclerotic lesions, and it is now evident that SSc is also characterized by accelerated macrovascular disease. Peptides related to angiotensin II, the final product of the renin–angiotensin system (RAS), play a role as regulators of endothelial cell function. Angiotensin-converting enzyme (ACE), the key enzyme in the RAS, is the predominant pathway of angiotensin II formation in blood and tissues. In intron 16 of the gene encoding for ACE an insertion/deletion (I/D) polymorphism, consisting of the presence or absence of a 287–base pair Alu sequence, has been identified. This polymorphism has been related to ACE enzyme levels, and data from experimental studies reported a functional role for this polymorphism in modulating the angiotensin II levels. We previously documented a high ACE D allele frequency in SSc patients and its role in increasing the risk of SSc, thus suggesting that the I/D polymorphism might be a useful genetic marker to identify SSc patients at risk to develop a severe vascular disease, frequently leading to gangrene. Moreover, our preliminary data, besides supporting the role of ACE I/D polymorphism as a predisposing factor to SSc, demonstrated its involvement in accelerated macrovascular disease by increasing the intima media thickness. Therefore, in SSc, not only endothelial dysfunction, but also vascular damage, linked to ACE I/D polymorphism, may significantly contribute to accelerated macrovascular disease, as the ACE D allele, by regulating both the production of angiotensin II and the degradation of bradykinin,

Address for correspondence: Serena Guiducci, Division of Medicine I and Rheumatology, Villa Monna Tessa, Viale Pieraccini 18, 50139, Florence, Italy. Voice/fax: 00390557949271.
e-mail: serena16@libero.it

Ann. N.Y. Acad. Sci. 1069: 10–19 (2006). © 2006 New York Academy of Sciences.
doi: 10.1196/annals.1351.002

contributes to mechanisms involved in the induction and maintenance of vessel wall modification.

Keywords: systemic sclerosis; atherosclerosis; macrovascular disease; renin–angiotensin system; angiotensin; angiotensin-converting enzyme; ACE; polymorphism

INTRODUCTION

The main pathologic hallmark of systemic sclerosis (SSc) is endothelial derangement, which is the main cause of such vascular disorders as Raynaud's phenomenon and pulmonary hypertension. The endothelial injury is the main sign of the microvascular involvement in SSc associated with smooth muscle cell migration in the intima.[1] This event induces the progressive reduction of the vessel lumen, thereby determining tissue ischemia, tissue anoxia, and gangrene. Endothelium-dependent vasodilatation is also deeply impaired in SSc. Endothelial cells (ECs) play a critical role in the control of vascular tone by releasing vasorelaxing and vasoconstricting substances that interact with microvascular smooth muscle cells.[2] EC functions are also controlled by molecules derived from the bloodstream and microenvironment. Moreover, regulation of vascular smooth cell growth is critical to the maintenance of normal blood flow and vessel patency. In SSc, some reports focused on the relevance of some molecules of the renin–angiotensin system (RAS), especially angiotensin-converting enzyme (ACE), for either pathogenetic implications or therapeutic options, given the outstanding importance of ACE inhibitors in preventing and treating the SSc renal crisis.[3–5] All components of the RAS are present in the vessel wall, and the endothelium, which is the target of SSc, is relevant in modulating smooth muscle cell function and growth.

THE RENIN–ANGIOTENSIN SYSTEM

To date, the RAS plays a pivotal role in controlling cardiovascular homeostasis and blood pressure, and in the pathogenesis of vascular disease, by modulating key components at both molecular and cellular levels. Two distinct, functionally similar and perhaps interrelated RASs have been identified. They are the circulating and the local RAS.

In the circulating RAS, renin, which is released into circulation by the juxtaglomerular apparatus of the kidney in response to decreased glomerular perfusion, catalyzes the first cleavage-producing angiotensin I (Ang I).

The tissue RAS produces local angiotensin II (Ang II), which is involved in autocrine and paracrine signaling within organs and tissues, and is present in all of the major body organs, including heart, blood vessels, and kidneys. The tissue RAS may operate similarly to the circulating RAS, except that all the components necessary to generate Ang II are present within the tissue, such as an isolated blood vessel. Thus, tissue renin generates tissue Ang I, which is subsequently catalyzed by tissue ACE into tissue Ang II.

The ACE catalyzes Ang I into Ang II, a potent vasoconstrictor, and degrades bradykinin (BK) at the endothelial surface,[6] thereby regulating its biological functions, which include an influence on fibrinolysis, platelet aggregation, and blood-clotting activation.[7] Recently, an experimental study demonstrated that ACE is the predominant pathway of Ang II formation in blood and tissue of mice, and plays a major role in BK metabolism.[8] Moreover, in addition to its enzymatic activities, ACE exerts numerous actions on the endothelium by regulating the release of the protective substance nitric oxide (NO).[9] ACE is expressed at the EC membrane, and created Ang II may activate endothelial receptors, which are linked to the production of endothelin and many other molecules, including free radicals, thereby contributing to endothelial dysfunction, which is considered to play an important role in the pathogenesis of vascular disease.

Ang II (452–amino acid protein), produced by the liver, is an oligopeptide produced by two enzymatic cleavages of angiotensinogen, and plays a relevant role in controlling the growth of vascular smooth muscle cells and in promoting the growth of transgenic cardiomyocytes;[10] Ang II also interacts with vasoactive substances, thereby playing a significant role in the regulation of vascular tone.[11]

Recently, a homologue of ACE, termed ACE-related carboxypeptidase (ACE2), has been identified.[12] ACE2 is a membrane-associated, zinc metalloprotease expressed predominantly in the endothelium in heart, kidney, and testis. ACE2 has been shown to convert Ang I and Ang II into Ang (1–9) and Ang (1–7), respectively.[12] Ang (1–7) is an active peptide that has been demonstrated to be a potent vasodilator. It potentiates BK actions through the release of prostaglandins, NO, or endothelium-derived hyperpolarizing factor.[13] It also possesses antitrophic and anti-inflammatory effects. Although Ang II is a potent stimulus for the plasminogen activator inhibitor-1 (PAI-1), Ang (1–7) decreases PAI-1 expression in EC.[14] Deletion of ACE2 results in a severe cardiac contractility defect that may be associated with changes in the cardiac RAS. These results suggest that ACE2 interacts with Ang II and BK pathways and may modulate the RAS by multiple mechanisms.

ACE is a major link between the RAS and the kinin systems, because it not only converts Ang I to Ang II, but also degrades kinins. ECs are an important site for the effects of BK and have been shown to express both its receptors B1R and B2R.[15] ACE inhibitors potentiate the actions of BK by reducing its degradation, which causes an increase in BK binding to EC receptors.[9] In addition, ACE inhibitors alter B2R binding site affinities and targeting to caveolin-rich areas of the membrane, illustrating another regulatory link between the RAS and the kinin system.[16]

Ang II exerts its functions through two receptors, type 1 (AT1R) and type 2 (AT2R). The AT1R is ubiquitously and abundantly distributed in adult tissues, including blood vessels, heart, kidney, adrenal gland, liver, brain, and lungs.[17]

The effects mediated by the AT1R are currently well understood and include promoting cell growth and regulating the expression of bioactive substances such as vasoconstrictive hormones, growth factors, cytokines, aldosterone, and extracellular matrix components. The AT1R also initiates several autoregulatory feedback loops of the RAS. Through one positive loop, Ang II stimulates expression of its precursor, angiotensinogen. This feedback occurs via a multihormone-responsive enhancer, called the acute-phase response element, in the promoter of angiotensinogen.[18,19] The AT1R pathways may similarly result in enhanced ACE activity. However, via the AT1R, Ang II also engages in a negative feedback loop by inhibiting the secretion of renin.[20] The AT2R in the adult is limited mainly to the myocardium, vascular epithelium, uterus, ovary, brain, pancreas, and adrenal medulla. It is upregulated with atherosclerosis, vascular injury, MI, and heart failure.[21] In the human heart, the AT2R is predominantly located in interstitial fibroblasts, suggesting that it may be involved in the progression of inflammation and fibrosis. Although the AT2R often counterbalances the effects of the AT1R by favoring apoptosis and inhibiting the growth of vascular smooth muscle and cardiac myocytes, it may also have a role in cell growth. Ultimately, the ratio of AT1R:AT2R expression may mediate the effects of Ang II.[22] Although Ang II seems to be the ligand responsible for most signal transduction through the AT1R and the AT2R, newly described components of the RAS indicate that it is not the only ligand, and the AT1R and the AT2R are not its only receptors. Ang II may be cleaved into Ang III, which stimulates aldosterone synthesis and inflammation, and Ang IV, which binds to the AT1R, resulting in vasoconstriction, and to the receptor type 4 (AT4R), promoting PAI production.

ANGIOTENSIN II, ACE INHIBITORS, AND SYSTEMIC SCLEROSIS

Initially, Ang II was identified as a hormone which controls blood pressure by regulating renal salt and water metabolism, central nervous system mechanisms (thirst and sympathetic outflow), and vascular smooth muscle cell (VSMC) tone.[17] Later, Ang II was found to exert long-term effects on tissue structure, including cardiac hypertrophy, vascular remodeling, and renal fibrosis. Interestingly, recent human studies with ACE inhibitors and Ang receptor blockers (ARBs) have yielded exciting clinical benefits such as decreased incidence of stroke, diabetes mellitus, and end-stage renal disease.[23,24] The endothelium-specific effects of these drugs and Ang II are based on the concept of diverse signals and effects mediated by multiple Ang receptors (AT1R, AT2R, and AT4R), multiple Ang I- and Ang II-derived peptides (Ang III, Ang IV and Ang [1–7]), and vascular bed–specific events. The enzymes that control generation of these peptides, including ACE, ACE2, endopeptidases, and aminopeptidases, interact with each other. In addition, drugs such as ACE inhibitors inhibit formation of Ang II, and binding to its receptor also modify the expression of receptors for Ang II and for other vasoactive hormones, including BK. This complex interplay of pathways helps to explain the findings that Ang II can have both beneficial and detrimental effects on vascular function.

There is strong evidence that the inhibition of ACE activity has clinical benefits to limit cardiovascular events including myocardial infarction, congestive heart failure, and stroke.[25,26]

ACE inhibitors work in part by improving endothelial dysfunction,[27] and by increasing arterial dilation via B2R-NO-pathways;[28] ACE inhibitors also improve EC survival after hypoxic injury via B2R-NO–dependent pathways.[29]

In addition, these drugs induce B1R in the renal vasculature and increase NO production from ECs expressing these receptors.[30] Recently, a novel mechanism for ACE inhibitors has been discovered involving signal transduction by ACE itself. Specifically, the protein kinase CK2 was found to phosphorylate the cytoplasmic tail of ACE, thereby activating intracellular signaling via jun N-terminal kinase (JNK). ACE inhibitors potentiate this signaling, which may be another mechanism by which these drugs produce their beneficial effects.[31]

Inhibition of ACE has revolutionized the management of scleroderma renal crisis, which previously had an almost invariably fatal outcome.[32] ACE inhibition has also been reported to be effective in treating complications due to myocardial and pulmonary artery involvement. Since the first report of the successful use of captopril to reverse scleroderma renal crisis, the early treatment with ACE inhibitors has dramatically improved the outcome of patients with this complication.[33] In some reports of successful treatment of the renal complication with ACE inhibition,[34] amelioration of skin conditions and Raynaud's phenomenon occurred, thus suggesting that this treatment might have long-term beneficial effects on other manifestations of the disease. Several studies have suggested that ACE inhibition is capable of producing an acute and sustained decrease in pulmonary vascular resistance in patients with pulmonary hypertension in association with SSc.[35] ACE inhibition may also have a role in controlling the primary myocardial involvement, which represents another serious complication of SSc, [36,37] and data from the literature reported a sustained improvement in ventricular function and thallium myocardial perfusion with ACE inhibition.[37] We could hypothesize that long-term ACE inhibition will ameliorate manifestations of microvascular disease in SSc, such as Raynaud's phenomenon and ischemic digital lesions, and will reduce the progression of visceral organ involvement and the occurrence of macrovascular complications including pulmonary hypertension.

ACE AND ENDOTHELIAL INJURY

In SSc, the derangement of EC function induces a decrease of endothelial ACE production, thus suggesting that the ACE activity reduction may represent a reliable and sensible marker of EC injury in SSc.[38,39] Our data published in 1990 showed increased levels of circulating vWF:Ag and decreased ACE plasma activity in SSc patients.[40] Results were in agreement with the reports that indicated ACE and vWF:Ag levels were useful marker for the clinician in evaluating the degree of endothelial injury in SSc.

We have demonstrated that in SSc patients a significant reduction of plasma angiotensin peptide levels, concomitant with the decrease of neutral endopeptidase (NEP) and ACE levels, is present.[41] Thus, both the levels of the single components of tissue RAS, and the whole activity of the system seems to be downregulated in SSc.[42] The downregulation of the RAS system in SSc may be explained by the severe and widespread endothelial damage typical of the disease. In fact, ACE is produced in large quantity by ECs that are severely damaged in SSc. Therefore, in SSc a whole downregulation of RAS components is present, with the prevalence of the vasoconstricting Ang II over the vasodilating Ang (1–7). The dysregulation of RAS components, by favoring vasoconstriction, may have a role in the impaired endothelium-dependent vasodilatation.

ACE I/D POLYMORPHISM AND SSC

ACE is encoded by a 21-kilobase, 26-exon gene localized on chromosome 17 (17q23). The insertion/deletion (I/D) polymorphism in intron 16 of the gene consists of three genotypes: DD and II homozygotes, and ID heterozygote. The ACE I/D polymorphism has been related to vascular disorders (coronary artery disease, hypertension, cerebrovascular disease, hypertrophic cardiomyopathy, and diabetic or nondiabetic nephropathy). In particular, the ACE D allele has been associated with an increased risk of malignant vascular injury[43,44] and SSc.[45] Therefore, the discrepancy between the high prevalence of D allele and reduced ACE plasma levels in SSc calls into question the current knowledge on the regulation and function of the RAS in SSc.

Actually, the ACE I/D polymorphism has been related to ACE enzyme levels, with a dose-dependent effect, and data from experimental studies reported a functional role for this polymorphism in modulating the Ang II levels. An experimental study provides evidence of its functional role by demonstrating the direct effect of this polymorphism on human cells *in vitro*.[46] It has been demonstrated that ACE DD cells had higher levels of Ang II and were more prone to cell death than ACE II cells, which suggested their survival advantage during stress. To date, the ID polymorphism modulates serum ACE activity,[47] and expression of ACE mRNA from the D allele is suspected to be greater than that from the I allele, or the polymorphism may affect the stability of the ACE mRNA. Recently, it has been demonstrated that the amount of ACE mRNA from the D allele is greater than that from the I allele in white blood cells,[48] even if the ID polymorphism itself does not affect or is not linked to the polymorphisms in the promoter region. ACE has been demonstrated to be expressed not only in ECs, but also in macrophages and intimal smooth muscle cells in the atheromatous arterial plaques,[49] and the above-mentioned observations substantiate the role of ACE D allele in pathogenesis of vascular disease.

Our data documented a high ACE D allele frequency in Italian SSc patients and suggested that the ACE D allele of the I/D polymorphism was associated with an increased risk of SSc.[45]

Recently, we observed a significant difference in ACE D allele frequency between Italian and Greek healthy subjects, and an association between ACE D allele and the predisposition to SSc in Italians, but not in Greeks.[50] The perplexities about the role of ACE I/D polymorphism were increased by the recent evidence that ACE I/D polymorphism is not significantly different in SSc patients and controls in a U.S. population.[51] These different results concerning the role of this polymorphism as a predisposing factor to SSc could suggest a potential influence of different ethnic origins in these populations from different geographic areas to the predisposition to a complex disease such as SSc, Further studies addressing ACE genotypes and phenotypes would be needed in order to understand the "real" role of this polymorphism in SSc, in which the study of the phenotype may be clinically more relevant.

THE ACE PARADOX: AN UNSOLVED PROBLEM

In SSc the ACE I/D polymorphism should induce the increase of the circulating levels of the enzyme, and therefore SSc patients should be characterized by elevated circulating ACE levels. However, this does not seem the case in SSc patients in whom low ACE circulating activity and low ACE circulating levels have been demonstrated.[40] In SSc patients a high prevalence of the ACE D allele has been observed,[45] thus allowing the hypothesis of high ACE circulating levels. The discrepancy between the high prevalence of D allele and reduced ACE plasma levels in SSc may be explained by chronic endothelial injury, which enables ECs to produce sufficient circulating ACE levels. But in SSc, ACE inhibition has always provided a clinical benefit to SSc patients in renal crisis or pulmonary hypertension. Thus, it remains unexplained why ACE inhibition is effective in SSc despite low levels of the quantity and activity of ACE. ACE inhibition may improve vascular NO activity by a reduction in Ang II-dependent vascular superoxide anion generation or by an interaction with BK. To date, it has been suggested that genetically determined differences in the levels of ACE activity modulated the responsiveness of the RAS via the differential generation of Ang II. In SSc, the impact of the ACE I/D polymorphism on disease development, endothelial injury, and response to ACE inhibitors warrants studies on a larger number of patients and clinical trials to demonstrate the link between ACE I/D polymorphism and disease features, and to determine whether the treatment of endothelial dysfunction can exert a beneficial effect on vascular events in patients with SSc.

REFERENCES

1. LeRoy, E.C. 1996. Systemic sclerosis: a vascular prespective. Rheum. Dis. Clin. N. Amer. **22:** 675–695.
2. Matucci Cerinic, M., S. Generini & A. Pignone. 1997. New approaches to Raynaud's phenomenon. Curr. Opin. Rheumatol. **9:** 544–554.
3. Matucci Cerinic, M., A. Jaffa & B. Kahaleh. 1992. Angiotensin converting enzyme: an in vivo marker of endothelial injury. J. Lab. Clin. Med. **120:** 428–433.
4. Matucci-Cerinic, M., F. Iannone, A. Carossino, *et al.* 1999. Discrepant expression of neprilysin on fibroblasts in diffuse systemic sclerosis. J. Rheumatol. **26:** 347–351.
5. Steen, V.D., J.P. Costantino, A.P. Shapiro, *et al.* 1990. Outcome of renal crisis in systemic sclerosis: relation to availability of angiotensin converting enzyme (ACE) inhibitors. Ann. Intern. Med. **113:** 352–357.
6. Soubrier, F., C. Hubert, P. Testut, *et al.* 1993. Molecular biology of the angiotensin I converting enzyme: biochemistry and structure of the gene. J. Hypertens. **11:** 471–476.
7. Nishimura, H., H., Tsuji, H. Masuda, *et al.* 1999. The effects of angiotensin metabolites on the regulation of coagulation and fibrinolysis in cultured rat aortic endothelial cells. Thromb. Haemost. **82:** 1516–1521.
8. Campbell, D.J., T. Alexiou, H.D. Xiao, *et al.* 2004. Effect of reduced angiotensin-converting enzyme gene expression and angiotensin-converting enzyme inhibition on angiotensin and bradykinin peptide levels in mice. Hypertension **43:** 854–859.
9. Linz, W., G. Wiemer & B.A. Scholkens. 1992. ACE-inhibition induces NO-formation in cultured bovine endothelial cells and protects isolated ischemic rat hearts. J. Mol. Cell Cardiol. **24:** 909–919.
10. Cook, J.L., S. Bhandaru, J.F. Giardina, *et al.* 1995. Identification and antisense inhibition of a renin-angiotensin system in transgenic cardiomyocytes. Am. J. Physiol. **268:** H1471–H1482.
11. Patel, J.M., F.R. Yarid, E.R. Block, *et al.* 1989. Angiotensin receptors in pulmonary arterial and aortic endothelial cells. Am. J. Physiol. **256:** C987–C993.
12. Donoghue, M., F. Hsieh, E. Baronas, *et al.* 2000. A novel angiotensin-converting enzyme-related carboxypeptidase (ACE2) converts angiotensin I to angiotensin 1–9. Circ. Res. **87:** E1–E9.
13. Ferrario, C.M. 2003. Contribution of angiotensin-(1–7) to cardiovascular physiology and pathology. Curr. Hypertens. Rep. **5:** 129–134.
14. Yoshida, M., Y. Naito, T. Urano, *et al.* 2002. L-158,809 and (D-Ala(7))-angiotensin I/II (1–7) decrease PAI-1 release from human umbilical vein endothelial cells. Thromb. Res. **105:** 531–536.
15. Seegers, H.C., P.S. Avery, D.F. McWilliams, *et al.* 2004. Combined effect of bradykinin B2 and neurokinin-1 receptor activation on endothelial cell proliferation in acute synovitis. FASEB J. **18:** 762–764.
16. Benzing, T., I. Fleming, A. Blaukat, *et al.* 1999. Angiotensin-converting enzyme inhibitor ramiprilat interferes with the sequestration of the B2 kinin receptor within the plasma membrane of native endothelial cells. Circulation **99:** 2034–2040.
17. Kim, S. & H. Iwao. 2000. Molecular and cellular mechanisms of angiotensin II-mediated cardiovascular and renal diseases. Pharmacol. Rev. **52:** 11–34.

18. JAMALUDDIN, M., T. MENG, J. SUN, *et al.* 2000. Angiotensin II induces nuclear factor (NF)-kB1 isoforms to bind the angiotensinogen gene acute phase response element: a stimulus-specific pathway for NF-kB activation. Mol. Endocrinol. **14:** 99–113.
19. LI, J. & A.R. BRASIER. 1996. Angiotensinogen gene activation by angiotensin II is mediated by the rel A (nuclear factor-kb p65) transcription factor: one mechanism for the renin angiotensin system positive feedback loop in hepatocytes. Mol. Endocrinol. **10:** 252–264.
20. KURTZ, A. & C. WAGNER. 1999. Regulation of renin secretion by angiotensin II-AT1 receptors. J. Am. Soc. Nephrol. **10:** S162–S168.
21. UNGER, T. 2000. Neurohormonal modulation in cardiovascular disease. Am. Heart J. **139:** S2–S8.
22. SADOSHIMA, J. 2000. Cytokine actions of angiotensin II. Circ. Res. **86:** 1187–1189.
23. YUSUF, S., P. SLEIGHT & J. POGUE. 2000. Effects of an angiotensin-converting-enzyme inhibitor, ramipril, on cardiovascular events in high-risk patients. The Heart Outcomes Prevention Evaluation Study Investigators (comment). [erratum appears in 2000 May 4;342(18):1376]. N. Engl. J. Med. **342:** 145–153.
24. DAHLOF, B., R.B. DEVEREUX, S.E. KJELDSEN, *et al.* 2002. Cardiovascular morbidity and mortality in the Losartan Intervention for Endpoint reduction in hypertension study (LIFE): a randomised trial against atenolol. Lancet **359:** 995–1003.
25. THE CONSENSUS TRIAL STUDY GROUP. 1987. Effects of enalapril on mortality in severe congestive heart failure. Results of the Cooperative North Scandinavian Enalapril Survival Study (CONSENSUS). N. Engl. J. Med. **316:** 1429–1435.
26. THE SOLVD INVESTIGATORS. 1991. Effect of enalapril on survival in patients with reduced left ventricular ejection fractions and congestive heart failure. N. Engl. J. Med. **325:** 293–302.
27. SCHLAIFER, J.D., T.J. WARGOVICH, B. O'NEILL, *et al.* 1997. Effects of quinapril on coronary blood flow in coronary artery disease patients with endothelial dysfunction. TREND Investigators—Trial on Reversing Endothelial Dysfunction. Am. J. Cardiol. **80:** 1594–1597.
28. HORNIG, B., C. KOHLER & H. DREXLER. 1997. Role of bradykinin in mediating vascular effects of angiotensin-converting enzyme inhibitors in humans. Circulation **95:** 1115–1118.
29. FUJITA, N., H. MANABE, N. YOSHIDA, *et al.* 2000. Inhibition of angiotensin-converting enzyme protects endothelial cell against hypoxia/reoxygenation injury. Biofactors **11:** 257–266.
30. IGNJATOVIC, T., F. TAN, V. BROVKOVYCH, *et al.* 2002. Novel mode of action of angiotensin I converting enzyme inhibitors: direct activation of bradykinin B1 receptor. J. Biol. Chem. **277:** 16847–16852.
31. KOHLSTEDT, K., R.P. BRANDES, W. MULLER-ESTERL, *et al.* 2004. Angiotensin-converting enzyme is involved in outside-in signaling in endothelial cells. Circ. Res. **94:** 60–67.
32. WASNER, C., R.C. COOKE & J.F. FRIES. 1978. Successful medical treatment of scleroderma renal crisis. N. Engl. J. Med. **299:** 873–875.
33. LOPEZ-OVEJERO, J.A., S.D. SAAL, W.A. D'ANGELO, *et al.* 1979. Reversal of vascular and renal crises of scleroderma by oral angiotensin-converting-enzyme blockade. Am. J. Med. **300:** 1417–1421.
34. WHITMAN, H.H. III, D.B. CASE, J.H. LARAGH, *et al.* 1982. Variable response to oral angiotensin-converting-enzyme blockade in hypertensive scleroderma patients. Arthritis Rheum. **25:** 241–248.

35. ALPERT, M.A., T.A. PRESSLY, V. MUKERJI, *et al.* 1992. Short- and long-term hemodynamic effects of captopril in patients with pulmonary hypertension and selected connective tissue disease. Chest **102:** 1407–1412.
36. KAZZAM, E., K. CAIDAHL, R. HALLGREN, *et al.* 1991. Non-invasive evaluation of long-term cardiac effects of captopril in systemic sclerosis. J. Intern. Med. **230:** 203–212.
37. KAHAN, A., J.Y. DEVAUX, B. AMOR, *et al.* 1990. The effect of captopril on thallium 201 myocardial perfusion in systemic sclerosis. Clin. Pharmacol. Ther. **47:** 483–489.
38. PIGNONE, A., S. GENERINI & M. MATUCCI-CERINIC. 2001. Prostaglandin E1 restores the levels of vWF and ACE in chronic critical limb ischemia in systemic sclerosis. Clin. Exp. Rheumatol. **19:** 358–359.
39. MATUCCI CERINIC, M., A. JAFFA & B. KAHALEH. 1992. Angiotensin converting enzyme: an in vivo marker of endothelial injury. J. Lab. Clin. Med. **120:** 428–433.
40. MATUCCI-CERINIC, M., A. PIGNONE, T. LOTTI, *et al.* 1990. Reduced angiotensin converting enzyme plasma activity in scleroderma: a marker of endothelial injury? J. Reumatol. **17:** 328–330.
41. PIGNONE, A., A. DEL ROSSO, N. FERRARIO, *et al.* 2006.Angiotensin 1-7 in systemic sclerosis: a potential key molecule in the pathogenesis of endothelial dysfunction? Clin. Exp. Rheumatol. Submitted for publication.
42. CHAPPELL, M.C., A.J. ALLRED & C.M. FERRARIO. 2001. Pathways of angiotensin-(1-7) metabolism in the kidney. Nephrol. Dial. Transplant. **16** (Suppl 1): 2–6.
43. FATINI, C., G. PRATESI, F. SOFI, *et al.* 2005. ACE DD genotype: a predisposing factor for abdominal aortic aneurysm. Eur. J. Vasc. Endovasc. Surg. **29:** 227–232.
44. MAYER, N.J., A. FORSYTH, S. KANTACHUVESIRI, *et al.* 2002. Association of the D allele of the angiotensin I converting enzyme polymorphism with malignant vascular injury. Mol. Pathol. **55:** 29–33.
45. FATINI, C., F. GENSINI, E. STICCHI, *et al.* 2002. High prevalence of polymorphisms of angiotensin-converting enzyme (I/D) and endothelial nitric oxide synthase (Glu298Asp) in patients with systemic sclerosis. Am. J. Med. **112:** 540–544.
46. HAMDI, H.K. & R. CASTELLON. 2004. A genetic variant of ACE increases cell survival: a new paradigm for biology and disease. Biochem. Biophys. Res. Commun. **318:** 187–191.
47. RIGAT, B., C. HUBERT, F. ALHENC-GELAS, *et al.* 1990. An insertion/deletion polymorphism in the angiotensin I-converting enzyme gene accounting for half the variance of serum enzyme levels. J. Clin. Invest. **86:** 1343–1346.
48. SUEHIRO, T., T. MORITA, M. INOUE, *et al.* 2004. Increased amount of the angiotensin-converting enzyme (ACE) mRNA originating from the ACE allele with deletion. Hum. Genet. **115:** 91–96.
49. OHISHI, M., M. UEDA, H. RAKUGI, *et al.* 1999. Relative localization of angiotensin-converting enzyme, chymase and angiotensin II in human coronary atherosclerotic lesions. J. Hypertens. **17:** 547–553.
50. GUIDUCCI, S., A. GEORGOUNTZOS, C. FATINI, *et al.* Etrurians vs. Greeks: shadows on the role of ACE I/D polymorphism in systemic sclerosis. Submitted for publication.
51. ASSASSI, S., M. MAYES, T. MCNEARNEY, *et al.* 2005. Polymorphism of endothelial nitric synthase and angiotensin converting enzyme in systemic sclerosis. Am. J. Med. **117:** 908–911.

Sequence Variants of the CRH 5′-Flanking Region

Effects on DNA–Protein Interactions Studied by EMSA in PC12 Cells

UTA WAGNER, MATTHIAS WAHLE, OLGA MALYSHEVA, ULF WAGNER, HOLM HÄNTZSCHEL, AND CHRISTOPH BAERWALD

Department of Internal Medicine IV, Division of Rheumatology, Neuroendocrine-Immunology Laboratory, University Hospital Leipzig, 04103 Leipzig, Germany

ABSTRACT: **Recently, studies in adult rheumatoid arthritis patients have shown an association with four single-nucleotide polymorphisms (SNPs) in the 3.7-kb regulatory region of human corticotropin-releasing hormone (hCRH) gene located at positions −3531, −3371, −2353, and −684 bp. Three of these novel polymorphisms are in absolute linkage disequilibrium, resulting in three combined alleles, named A1B1, A2B1, and A2B2. To study whether the described polymorphic nucleotide sequences in the 5′ region of the hCRH gene interfere with binding of nuclear proteins, an electric mobility shift assay (EMSA) was performed. At position −2353 bp, a specific DNA protein complex was detected for the wild-type sequence only, possibly interfering with a binding site for the activating transcription factor 6 (ATF6). In contrast, no difference could be detected for the other SNPs. However, at position −684, a quantitative difference in protein binding due to cAMP incubation could be observed. To further investigate whether these SNPs in the CRH promoter are associated with an altered regulation of the CRH gene, we performed a luciferase reporter gene assay with transiently transfected rat pheochromocytoma cells PC12. Incubation with 8-Br-cAMP alone or in combination with cytokines enhanced significantly the promoter activity in PC12 cells. The promoter haplotypes studied exhibited a differential capacity to modulate CRH gene expression. In all our experiments, haplotype A1B1 showed the most pronounced influence on promoter activity. Taken together, our results demonstrate a differential binding capacity of nuclear proteins of the promoter polymorphisms resulting in a different gene regulation. Most probably the SNP at position −2,353 plays a major role in mediating these differences.**

Address for correspondence: Uta Wagner, Medizinische Klinik und Poliklinik IV, Universitaetsklinikum Leipzig, Liebigstr. 22, 04103 Leipzig. Germany. Voice: +49-0-341-972-4710; fax: +49-0-341-972-4709.

e-mail: Uta.Wagner@medizin.uni-leipzig.de

Ann. N.Y. Acad. Sci. 1069: 20–33 (2006).
doi: 10.1196/annals.1351.003

KEYWORDS: EMSA; corticotropin-releasing hormone (CRH); reporter gene assay; PC12 cells; SNP; rheumatoid arthritis; gene regulation; CRH 5′ gene polymorphisms

INTRODUCTION

Corticotropin-releasing hormone (CRH) is a 41-amino-acid primary hypothalamic neuropeptide synthesized in the parvocellular subdivision of the paraventricular nucleus (PVN).[1] The human CRH (hCRH) gene and its regulatory region have been sequenced and finally localized to chromosome 8q13, identifying two exons and one intron.[2–4] The peptide and proximal promoter sequences are highly conserved in the human, rat, and mouse.[5,6] However, four polymorphisms in the human 3.7-kb regulatory region of CRH have been characterized as a T → C base substitution located at position −2353 and at position −684 bp, a C → G base substitution at position −3531, and a T → G base substitution located at position −3371 bp.[7,8] Three of these polymorphisms co-segregate absolutely, resulting in two alleles *A1* and *A2*. Compound alleles named A1B1, A2B1, and A2B2, respectively, could be assigned by taking into account the biallelic polymorphism at position −3371 bp in the CRH promoter. In the Caucasian population, the common haplotype represents A1B1, with the other two being rare combined alleles. So far no functional differences could be attributed to the described polymorphisms. Potent modulators of CRH gene expression are proinflammatory cytokines[9,10] and cAMP-dependent transcriptional activation of the CRH promoter.[11,12]

To determine whether the described polymorphic nucleotide sequences in the 5′ region of the hCRH gene interfere with binding of nuclear proteins, electric mobility shift assay (EMSA) was performed using nuclear extracts of untreated/treated PC12 cells to detect nuclear protein DNA complexes. To further investigate whether the detected polymorphisms in the regulatory region of the CRH gene might result in different promoter reactivity upon various stimuli, we transiently transfected pheochromocytoma rat PC12 cells with a 3625 bp human CRH 5′-promoter-luciferase fusion gene and studied the effects of IL-1β, IL-6, TNF-α, and IFN-γ, either alone or combined with 8-Br-cAMP (cAMP), on CRH gene 5′-promoter activity.

MATERIALS AND METHODS

Preparation of Nuclear Extracts

PC12 cells grown on 6-well polystyrene plates were treated with media containing reagents. Cytokines and 8-Br-cAMP were added to cell culture alone or in combination as described above. Nuclear extracts were prepared by the procedure as described by Andrews and Faller.[13] Their protein concentration was determined with the BCA protein assay kit (Pierce, Rockford, IL, USA) using bovine serum albumin as standard. The nuclear extracts were stored at −80°C in aliquots until further use.

Synthesis and Labeling of Oligonucleotides

Oligonucleotide pairs were designed to have a complementary sequence with 5′ extension. Single-stranded human oligomers: *position −3531* (5′ ggactgttgtgttgg***c***tctgttttaatttacc 3′) and mutated (5′ ggactgttgtgttgg***g***tctgttttaattta 3′), *position −3371* (5′ ggctcctttccagaagtta***t***tcttacatgtaagat 3′) and mutated (5′ ggctcctttccagaagtta***g***tcttacatgtaagat 3′), *position −2353* (5′ ggccaccatgtaagacgtg***t***ctttgcttctccatt 3′) and mutated (5′ ggccaccatgtaagacgtg***c***ctttgcttctccatt 3′), *position −684* (5′ ggctgcattttgagaga***t***ttattggccttgcttc 3′) and mutated (5′ ggctgcattttgagaga***c***ttattggccttgcttc 3′) oligomers, and their complementary strands were synthesized and purified at a concentration of 50 pmol/μL (BioTeZ, Berlin, Germany). Oligomers and their complementary strands (10 μL each) were mixed with 70 μL water and 10 μL of 500 mM Tris/HCl pH 7.5, 100 mM $MgCl_2$, 10 mM DTT and 1,000 mM NaCl and annealed by heating at 95°C for 5 min, followed by cooling down to room temperature (RT) such that the final concentration of the oligomers was 5 pmol/μL. Double-stranded oligomers (10 μl each) were end-labeled with 20 μCi of [^{32}P] dCTP (3000 Ci/mmol, MP Biomedicals Europe, Eschwege, Germany) using a Klenow fragment of *Escherichia coli*, DNA polymerase I (Roche Applied Science, Mannheim, Germany) in a 25-μL reaction mixture for 1 h at 37°C. Radiolabeled probes (specific activity 1–5 × 10^5 cpm/μg) were purified by Qiagen Nucleotide Removal Kit (Qiagen, Hilden, Germany).

Electrophoretic Mobility Shift Assay

For EMSA, equal amounts (5 μg) of nuclear extracts were incubated in 10 μL of binding buffer containing 12.5 mM HEPES (pH 7.9), 10% glycerol, 100 mM KCL, 1 mM EDTA, 1 mM DTT, and 1 μg Poly-dAdT for 10 min at RT. For competition experiments, nuclear extracts were incubated with 20-fold molar excess of the cold (unlabeled) oligomers having wild-type (wt) or mutant (mt) sequences for 10 min at RT in the binding buffer prior to the addition of the labeled oligo. The mixtures were then incubated with 1 μL of ^{32}P-labeled probe for 20 min at RT before being applied to 5% nondenaturing polyacrylamide gels that were run at 150 V in 0.5 Tris-borate/EDTA buffer at 4°C for 2.5 h. The gels were dried, autoradiographed, and visualized using a Phosphor Imaging System.

Cell Culture

The rat adrenal pheochromocytoma PC12 cells were obtained from the German Collection of Microorganisms and Cell Cultures (ACC 159; Braunschweig, Germany). PC12 cells were cultured on either flat-bottom wells in 6-well plates of 10 cm^2 surface area/well (TPP Schubert, Germany) or on flasks of 75 cm^2 surface area, at an initial concentration of 2×10^5 cells/mL. PC12 cells were maintained in RPMI 1640 medium containing Glutamax supplemented with 10% heat-inactivated fetal calf serum, 5% horse serum (Gibco, Invitrogen Corporation, Paisley, Scotland, UK), 100 U/mL penicillin and 0.1 mg/mL streptomycin (Sigma, St Louis, MO) in a humidified atmosphere at 5% CO_2 and 37°C.

Preparation of CRH Promoter-Driven Luciferase Reporter Construct $phCRH_{3625}LUC$ by a Two-Step Cloning Method

To examine the potentially altered regulation of the human CRH gene, we cloned the three polymorphic nucleotide fragments, previously sequenced and described as two biallelic polymorphic sequences resulting in compound alleles A1B1, A2B1, and A2B2, respectively,[14] of the proximal 3625 nucleotides 5′-flanking the major mRNA start site of the hCRH gene[15] in a sense orientation upstream of luc+ into the promoterless luciferase reporter plasmid pGL3-Basic. The luciferase construct (8.5 kb) was used to transform *E. coli* JM109 competent cells (Promega Corporation, Madison, WI). Transformants were grown overnight in a small volume of LB medium (Becton Dickinson, San Jose, CA) with ampicillin (Sigma), and miniprep DNA (Qiagen, Hilden, Germany) was fractionated in agarose gel to screen for $phCRH_{3625}LUC$ incorporation. The identity of the candidate clone was further verified by digestion and the integrity of all reporter constructs was confirmed by DNA sequencing using DNA Sequencing Kit, BigDye™ Terminator Cycle Sequencing (Applied Biosystems, Warrington, UK). We transfected cells with these constructs and examined the response of luciferase activity to potential stimulants and inhibitors.

Transfection and Reporter Gene Assay

Each treatment was performed in duplicate, and each experiment was repeated six times.

One day before transfection, the PC12 cells were plated in normal growth medium without antibiotics at an initial density of 4×10^5 cells/well in 6-well poly-L-lysine (Sigma), coated plates resulting in 50–70% confluent cells at the time of transfection. The medium was replaced with a fresh medium without antibiotics for following transfection experiments. Transient transfection was performed with Lipofectamin 2000 (Invitrogen^{TM}, Life Technologies, Carlsbad, CA) according to the manufacturer's instruction using Opti-MEM I reduced serum medium to dilute Lipofectamin 2000. To set up transfection efficiency, pilot experiments were performed by transfecting plated PC12 with 3 μg EGFP-C1 vector (Clontech, Palo Alto, CA). After 24 h, expression of enhanced green fluorescent protein (EGFP) was determined either by inversion fluorescence microscopy (DMIRB, Leica, Wetzlar) or by FACScan^{TM} analysis utilizing the software CellQuest^{TM} (Becton Dickinson). Transfection efficiency reached 50% at least.

For luciferase activity assay, a total of 3 μg of DNA (ratio $phCRH_{3625}LUC$ firefly : pRL-null Renilla as co-transfected vector 30:1) and 10 μL of Lipofectamin 2000 per transfection/well were used. In each experiment, the pGL3-Basic plasmid was also transfected in separate wells in order to determine the basic activity of the promoterless plasmid. Cells were incubated with the transfection mixture for 6 h. Transfectants were then switched to the initial serum-containing medium with antibiotics and left overnight in culture before cells were washed and exposed for 36 h to the indicated compounds and their combinations. The experiments were performed using the following concentrations: 5 mM 8-Br-cAMP; recombinant IL-1β 40 ng/mL, IL-6 20 ng/mL, IFN-γ 10 U/mL (R&D Systems, Minneapolis, MN, USA*)*, and TNF-α 10 ng/mL (Sigma). Cells were washed twice with PBS and lysed in 500 μL passive lysis buffer (Promega Corporation) for 20 min at RT. Activities of the firefly luciferase and the Renilla luciferase in cell lysates were measured sequentially by using the dual-luciferase reporter (DRL) assay system (Promega Corporation) according to the manufacturer's instructions. The light output from the firefly luciferase or the *Renilla* luciferase was recorded for 15 sec following a 3-sec premeasurement delay using a TD-20/20 luminometer (Turner Designs, Sunnyvale, CA, USA). The luciferase activity closely reflects real-time changes in promoter activity; thus the reporter protein activity indicates changes in the transcription rate. Initial experiments revealed that *Renilla* luciferase activity in cell lysate was not affected by cAMP or cytokines. The variation in transfection efficiency was normalized by dividing the firefly luciferase activity with the Renilla luciferase activity. The transcriptional activity of the promoter–reporter construct was determined as relative fluorescence units to that of the untreated transfectants.

STATISTICAL ANALYSES

Values in figures are presented as the mean ± SEM if not otherwise indicated from at least six independent experiments. Data were compared by the repeated measures analysis of variance (ANOVA) followed by Bonferroni's *t*-test, using the software package SigmaStat (SPSS, Inc., Chicago, IL, USA). When normality test failed, Kruskal–Wallis repeated measures ANOVA on ranks and the Dunnett's method for calculation of multiple comparisons versus the control group were used. Differences between groups were calculated by one-way ANOVA, followed by pair-wise multiple comparison Tukey's test and multiple comparison versus the control group (Dunn's method). The difference between experimental conditions was considered to be significant at $P < 0.05$.

RESULTS

Nuclear Protein Complex Analyses by EMSA

To determine whether transcription factors interact with the described polymorphic nucleotide sequences in the 5′ region of the hCRH gene, EMSA was performed using nuclear extracts of untreated/treated PC12 cells.

At position *−2353 bp* (T→C base substitution, A allele) a specific DNA protein complex is detected using ^{32}P-labeled wt but not the mt oligonucleotide probe (FIG. 1, lanes 7 and 11). Differences in complex formation were observed with nuclei isolated from PC12 cells exposed to cytokines (10 U/mL INF-γ; 10 ng/mL TNF-α, 20 ng/mL IL6, 40 ng/mL IL1), cytokines in combination with 5 mM 8-Br-cAMP for 36 h, or no treatment. The binding intensity of DNA protein complexes increased in cells exposed to cAMP and cytokines (FIG. 1; compare lanes 2, 3, 7, and 11).

For the polymorphisms at positions –3531 bp (C→G base substitution, A allele), –3371 bp (T→G base substitution, B allele), and –684 bp (T→C base substitution, A allele), EMSA did not reveal any significant differences in the binding of nuclear protein complexes between the respective wt and mt oligonucleotides.

However, at position –684 bp, the visual impression again suggests a differential modulation of the binding intensity due to incubation conditions (FIG. 2). Cyclic AMP (lanes 10 and 12) increased the intensity of binding for the complex compared to binding induced by cytokines (lanes 6 and 8). This DNA protein complex was prevented from binding by competition with an excess (20-fold) of wt and mt nonradiolabeled oligonucleotides, respectively.

At position –3531 bp, EMSA revealed that cAMP increases the binding intensity of a specific complex using PC12 nuclear proteins (FIG. 3, lanes 10 and 12).

DLR Gene Assay

Incubation with 5 mM 8-Br-cAMP for 36 h caused a strong increase in luciferase activity in CRH 5′- pLUC transfected PC12 cells. Haplotype A1B1 exhibited a 13.1 ± 3.1-fold induction compared to unstimulated controls ($P < 0.05$, $n = 6$), thus representing maximal stimulatory effect. In contrast,

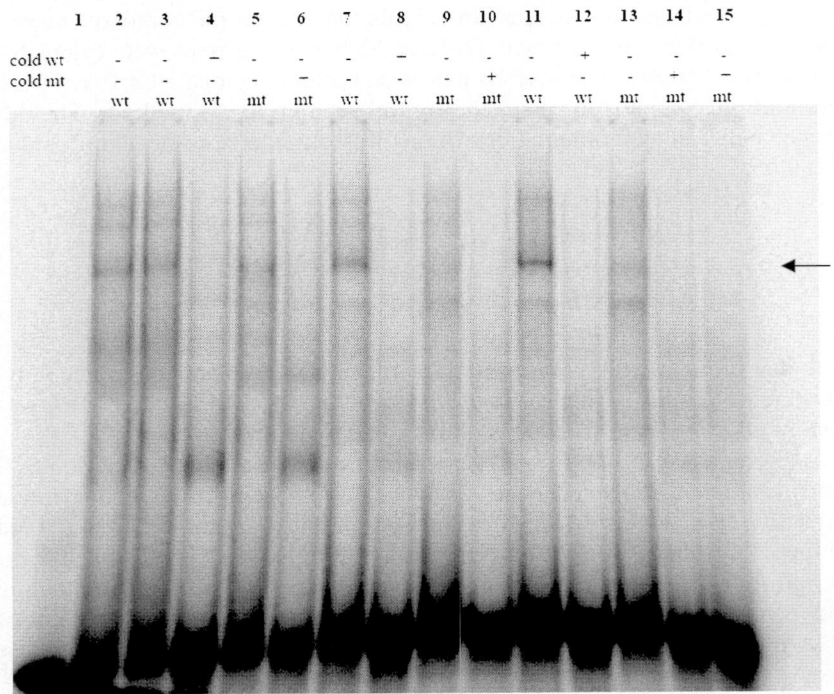

FIGURE 1. Electric mobility shift assay (EMSA) was performed from nuclear proteins of PC12 cells bound to ^{32}P-labeled oligonucleotides containing the T→C polymorphism at position –2353 bp in the 5′-flanking region of the hCRH gene. The *top rows* indicate the radioactive-labeled oligonucleotides (wild-type [wt] and mutant [mt]) and the addition of cold wt and mt oligonucleotides, respectively. Nuclear protein was extracted from untreated PC12 cells (*lanes* 2–6), PC12 cells exposed for 36 h to cytokines alone (10 U/mL INF-γ; 10 ng/mL TNF-α, 20 ng/mL IL6, 40 ng/mL IL1, *lanes* 7–10) or in combination with 5 mM 8-Br-cAMP (*lanes* 11–14). Indicated with an *arrow* is the position of the specific protein: DNA complex that can be detected as ^{32}P-labeled wt oligonucleotide only (*lanes* 2, 3, 7, and 11). Binding of this complex can be specifically inhibited by cold wt oligonucleotide (20-fold; *lanes* 4, 8, and 12). Differences in complex formation were observed in nuclei isolated from untreated PC12 cells (*lanes* 2 and 3), PC 12 cells exposed to cytokines (*lane* 7) and cytokines in combination with 5 mM 8-Br-cAMP (*lane* 11). The visual impression suggests a difference in the intensity of the bands due to the incubation conditions with the strongest band observed for co-incubation with cytokines and 8-Br-cAMP (*lane* 11). *Lane* 1 contains no nuclear protein extract. The same incubation conditions apply for *lanes* 2 and 3, respectively. + = addition of cold wt and mt oligonucleotides, respectively, in excess (20-fold) for competitive binding.

for A2B1 and A2B2, the studies revealed a 6.0 ± 1.3- and 8.1 ± 2.0-fold increase, respectively, in promoter activity compared to controls (n = 6, P < 0.05; FIG. 4). There was a statistically significant difference in 8-Br-cAMP-induced stimulatory effect between A1B1 and A2B1 (P < 0.05).

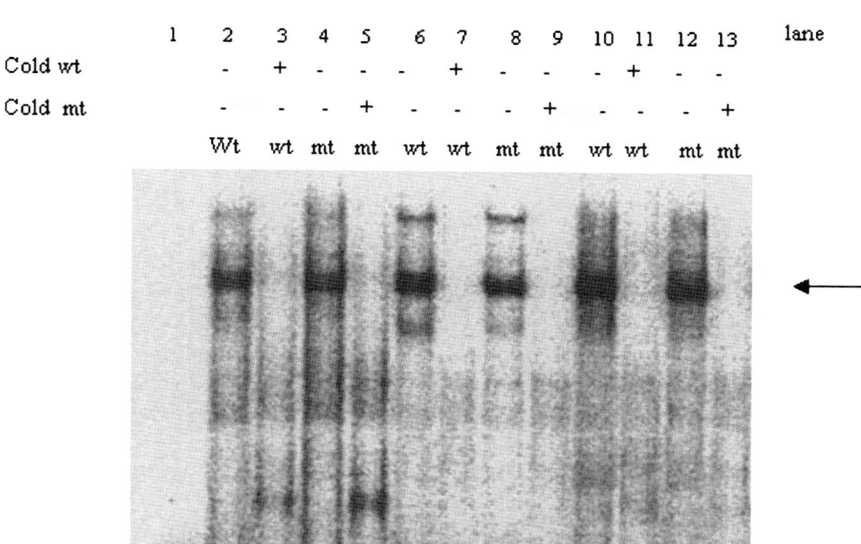

FIGURE 2. Electric mobility shift assay (EMSA) was performed from nuclear proteins of PC12 cells bound to ^{32}P-labeled oligonucleotides containing the T→C polymorphism at position –684 bp (5′ ggctgcatttgagaga***t***ttattggccttgcttc 3′) in the 5′-flanking region of hCRH gene. The top rows indicate the radioactive-labeled oligonucleotides (wild-type [wt] and mutant [mt]) and the addition of cold wt and mt oligonucleotides, respectively. Nuclear protein was extracted from untreated PC12 cells (*lanes* 2–5), PC12 cells exposed for 36 h to cytokines alone (10 U/mL INF-γ; 10 ng/mL TNF-α, 20 ng/mL IL6, 40 ng/mL IL1; (*lanes* 6–9) or in combination with 5 mM 8-Br-cAMP (*lanes* 10–13) bound to ^{32}P-labeled wt oligonucleotides (*lanes* 2, 3, 6, 7, 10, and 11) or to ^{32}P-labeled mt oligonucleotides (*lanes* 4, 5, 8, 9, 12, and 13). The position of the specific protein:DNA complex is indicated with an *arrow*. Protein:DNA complex formation was competed with cold (20-fold) wt oligonucleotide or cold mt oligonucleotide. Differences in complex formation were observed in nuclei isolated from treated PC12 cells. The visual impression suggests a difference in the intensity of the bands due to the incubation conditions with the strongest band observed for co-incubation with cytokines and 8-Br-cAMP (*lanes* 10 and 12). *Lane* 1 contains no nuclear protein extract. + = addition of cold wt and mt oligonucleotides, respectively, in excess (20-fold) for competitive binding.

Compared to respective unstimulated controls, treatment of transfected PC12 cells with a combination of cytokines IL-1β, IL-6, TNF-α, and IFN-γ for 36 h exhibited a slight increase (3-fold) in luciferase activity in all three haplotypes studied ($P < 0.05$). There was no statistically significant difference in induced promoter activity between the haplotypes A1B1, A2B1, and A2B2 (FIG. 4).

However, co-incubation of PC12 cells with 8-Br-cAMP and cytokines yielded an additional enhancement in luciferase reporter activity as depicted in FIGURE 4. Compared to untreated controls, the maximal stimulatory effect on

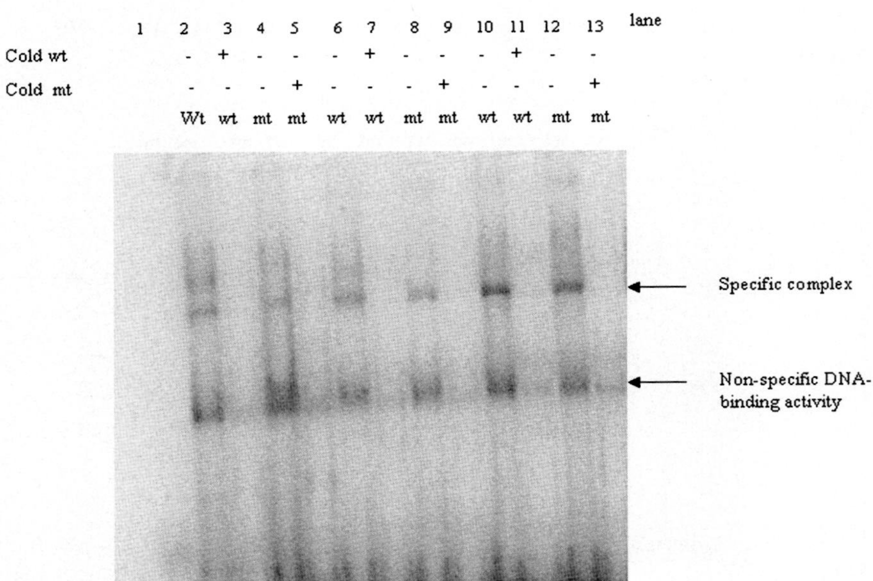

FIGURE 3. EMSA showing PC12 cell nuclear protein interaction with hCRH DNA sequence. EMSA was performed for nuclear protein from PC12 cells bound to ^{32}P-labeled oligonucleotides containing the C→G polymorphism at position −3531bp (5′ ggactgttgtgttggctctgttttaatttacc 3′) and mutated (5′ ggactgttgtgttgggtctgttttaattta 3′) in the 5′-flanking region of hCRH gene. Nuclear protein was extracted from untreated (*lanes* 2–5) or PC12 cells exposed for 36 h to cytokines (10 U/mL INF-γ; 10 ng/mL TNF-α, 20 ng/mL IL6, 40 ng/mL IL1; (*lanes* 6–9) alone or in combination with 5 mM 8-Br-cAMP (*lanes* 10–13) and bound to ^{32}P-labeled wild-type (wt) oligonucleotides (*lanes* 2, 3, 6, 7, 10, and 11) or to ^{32}P-labeled mutant (mt) oligonucleotides (*lanes* 4, 5, 8, 9, 12, and 13). *Lane* 1 contains no nuclear protein extract. + = addition of cold wt and mt oligonucleotides, respectively, in excess (20-fold) for competitive binding.

CRH 5′-promoter activity (22.5 ± 7.5-fold increase) was detected in A1B1. For A2B2, a 14.0 ± 5.5-fold increase was determined followed by a 9.4 ± 2.3-fold increase for A2B1 ($n = 6$; $P < 0.05$ vs. baseline controls). Analysis showed that for all three haplotypes studied the promoter activity was significantly enhanced by cAMP compared to cytokines alone ($P < 0.05$).

DISCUSSION

In this report, we investigated whether genetic variation at the CRH locus has any functional consequence on the CRH promoter activity in response to various stimuli. EMSA was performed to investigate the influence of the promoter polymorphisms on nuclear protein-binding intensity. Furthermore,

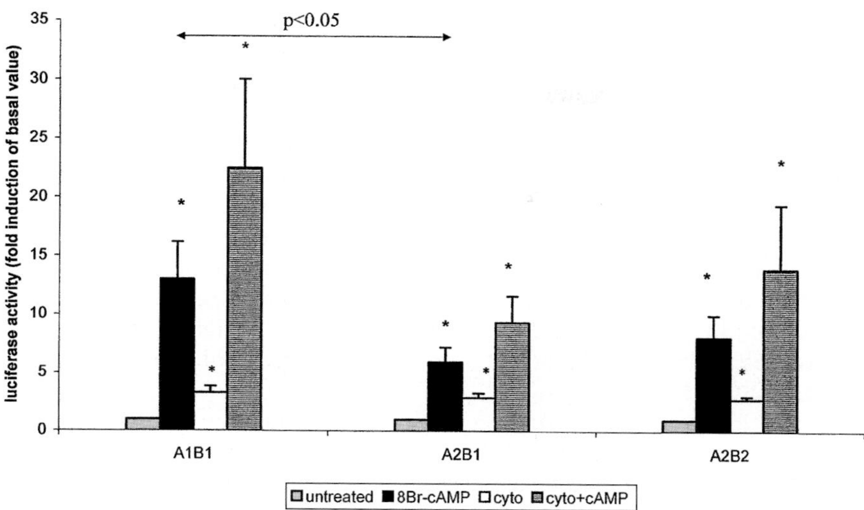

FIGURE 4. The human CRH promoter variants A1B1, A2B1, and A2B2, respectively, were fused to the luciferase gene and transiently transfected into rat pheochromocytoma PC12 cells. Incubation with cytokines alone had a subtle stimulatory effect only (3-fold, *white bars*). The construct drove high transcriptional activity after 36 h of treatment with 5 mM 8-Br-cAMP (*black bars*), resulting in a 6- to 13-fold increase compared to controls (*gray bars*). Luciferase activity was further enhanced upon co-incubation of cAMP and cytokines (9- to 22.5-fold induction, *striped* bars). The results represent the mean ± SEM of six separate experiments done in duplicate. * Denotes a significant difference compared to unstimulated transfected cells (controls, $P < 0.05$).

we studied the effects of cytokines and cAMP on CRH gene expression using PC12 rat pheochromocytoma cells transiently transfected with the CRH 5′-promoter luciferase reporter gene construct.

EMSA studies revealed specific binding of nuclear proteins at position −2353 for the wt sequence only. Furthermore, the incubation conditions modulated the binding intensity of nuclear proteins with cAMP, increasing the binding intensity at various CRH gene 5′positions. PC12 cells posses the capacity to mediate signals to the CRH promoter, resulting in a differential modulation of CRH gene expression by the combined haplotypes of the CRH promoter, A1B1, A2B1, and A2B2.

The transcription factors and signaling molecules that are critical for the induction of hCRH gene expression are poorly understood. Analysis of the 3625-bp 5′ flanking region of the hCRH gene DNA sequence using the TRANSFAC database revealed that the region contains some consensus sites for transcription factors overlapping identified described polymorphisms. It is of importance that the polymorphism at position –2353 results in a base exchange for the binding site of the transcription factor activating transcription factor 6 (ATF6). ATF6 is a member of the human basic leucine zipper (bZIP) protein family and participates in two independent signaling pathways, both of which lead to transcriptional activation in the nucleus and interact with cAMP responsiveness.[16,17] Interestingly, EMSA of PC12 cell nuclear extracts demonstrated different protein–DNA interactions between the wt (allele A1) and mt (allele A2) sequence at position −2353. Treating PC12 with cytokines or cAMP led to a specific binding of nuclear protein for wt sequence only. The binding site for another transcription factor also overlaps this −2353 bp position, the X-box-binding protein 1 (XBP-1), a basic-region leucine zipper protein in the (CREB/ATF) family of transcription factors, could be shown to be involved in different cell-differentiation processes.[18] Hence, the observed differences in the response of CRH promoter activity might be mediated by this motif.

Several lines of evidence suggest that a major stimulation of CRH gene expression is mediated via the cAMP-dependent protein kinase signal pathway. cAMP analogues stimulate gene transcription through PKA, a serine/threonine kinase that activates CREB-, fos-, and Jun-related factors.[19] We, as other investigators,[20–22] demonstrated that cAMP strongly increases gene expression in reporter constructs with the 5′ regulatory region of CRH fused to luciferase (LUC) in transient transfection assays using PC12 cell line. The studied haplotype A1B1 exhibited higher LUC activity which was significant compared to that of A2B1, following cAMP treatment of PC12 cells. It was demonstrated that cAMP-dependent transcriptional activation is mediated largely through a classical, highly conserved consensus sequence, that is, a cAMP-responsive element (CRE) within the proximal CRH promoter.[6,23] It locates at –224 bp and its binding protein, CREB, a member of bZIP or leucine zipper family of transcription factors, plays an important role in the regulation of the activity of the CRH promoter.[24,25] Members of the AP-1 family of transcription factors bind to the hCRH CRE site and AP-2α induces hCRH promoter activity by its interaction with CREB.[12,23,26,27] Recently, additional elements were described for cell-type-specific cAMP-dependent enhancement of gene transcription, in particular nuclear factor Y (NF-Y).[28] NF-Y together with other nuclear proteins exhibits enormous potential to affect transcription. Interestingly, the polymorphism at position –684 is located at a consensus sequence for a NF-Y-box-binding factor (−687 to −673) that might be responsible for the differences we could observe for the cAMP-induced LUC activity. Interestingly, we found a variation of the binding intensity due to incubation conditions in the EMSA, with cAMP being the most potent inducer of nuclear protein binding, indicating the importance of this region for CRH gene regulation. However, we could not detect a difference in the EMSA between the wt and mt sequence at position –684.

In addition to cAMP, inflammatory cytokines can cause stimulation of the HPA axis via direct and indirect mechanisms[29] acting through regulation of nuclear factor-kB (NF-kB) and the mitogen-activated protein kinase pathways.[30]

Interestingly, it could be shown that cytokines stimulate the CRH promoter via interactions with the CREB/CRE system,[31] revealing an avenue for cross-talk between both signaling systems. In this respect, our results underline the modulating capacity of cytokines on cAMP-induced LUC activity in PC12 cells. Results demonstrate that cAMP mediates stimulation of the CRH promoter activity, and that cAMP analogues enhance cytokine action on this promoter in PC12. Our findings are in agreement with other studies that suggest that the site of action of cytokines is at least in part distant to cAMP.[10,32] There may be some compounding effects on intracellular signaling pathways below receptor level pointing to a modulation of neuropeptide-regulated CRH gene expression by cytokines. Therefore, a dynamic communication between immune and endocrine systems at the molecular level within the hormone glands can be postulated.

In conclusion, the promoter haplotypes studied exhibited a differential capacity to modulate CRH gene expression, probably because of differential binding of nuclear factors resulting in altered cAMP signaling. In all our experiments and cell lines studied, haplotype A1B1 showed the most pronounced influence on promoter activity, probably mediated via differential binding of the transcription factor ATF6 at position −2353. Studies are under way to evaluate the clinical significance of these findings in various disease states.

ACKNOWLEDGMENTS

This work was supported by Grant BA 1770/2-1 from the Deutsche Forschungsgemeinschaft (DFG).

REFERENCES

1. VALE, W., J. SPIESS, C. RIVIER, *et al.* 1981. Characterization of a 41-residue ovine hypothalamic peptide that stimulates secretion of corticotropin and beta-endorphin. Science **213:** 1394–1397.
2. SHIBAHARA, S., Y. MORIMOTO, Y. FURUTANI, *et al.* 1983. Isolation and sequence analysis of the human corticotropin-releasing factor precursor. EMBO J. **2:** 775–779.
3. ARBISER, J.L., C.C. MORTON, G.A. BRUNS, *et al.* 1988. Human corticotropin-releasing hormone gene is located on the long arm of chromosome 8. Cytogenet. Cell. Genet. **47:** 113–116.
4. VAMVAKOPOULOS, N.C. & G.P. CHROUSOS. 1993. Structural organization of the 5′ flanking region of the human corticotropin-releasing hormone gene. DNA Seq. **4:** 197–206.
5. THOMPSON, R.C., A.F. SEASHOLTZ & E. HERBERT. 1987. Rat corticotropin-releasing hormone gene: sequence and tissue specific expression. Mol. Endocrinol. **1:** 363–370.

6. Vamvakopoulos, N.C. & G.P. Chrousos. 1993. Regulated activity of the distal promoter-like element of the human corticotropin-releasing hormone gene and secondary structural features of its corresponding transcripts. Mol. Cell. Endocrinol. **94:** 73–78.
7. Baerwald, C.G.O., G.S. Panayi & J.S. Lanchbury. 1996. A new *Xmn*I polymorphism in the regulatory region of the corticotropin-releasing hormone gene. Hum. Genet. **97:** 697–698.
8. Baerwald, C.G., C.C. Mok, M.S. Fife, *et al.* 1999. Distribution of corticotropin-releasing hormone promoter polymorphism in different ethnic groups: evidence for natural selection in human populations. Immunogenetics **49:** 894–899.
9. Makrigiannakis, A., A.N. Margioris, E. Zoumakis, *et al.* 1999. The transcription of corticotropin-releasing hormone in human endometrial cells is regulated by cytokines. Neuroendocrinology **70:** 451–459.
10. Katahira, M., Y. Iwasaki, Y. Aoki, *et al.* 1998. Cytokine regulation of the rat proopiomelanocortin gene expression in AtT-20 cells. Endocrinology **139:** 2414–2422.
11. Cheng, Y.H., R.C. Nicholson, B. King, *et al.* 2000. Glucocorticoid stimulation of corticotropin-releasing hormone gene expression requires a cyclic adenosine 3′,5′-monophosphate regulatory element in human primary placental cytotrophoblast cells. J. Clin. Endocrinol. Metab. **85:** 1937–1945.
12. King, B.R., R. Smith & R.C. Nicholson. 2002. Novel glucocorticoid and cAMP interactions on the CRH gene promoter. Mol. Cell Endocrinol. **194:** 19–28.
13. Andrews, N.C. & D.V. Faller. 1991. A rapid micropreparation technique for extraction of DNA-binding proteins from limiting numbers of mammalian cells. Nucleic Acids Res. **19:** 2499.
14. Baerwald, C.G., C.C. Mok, M. Tickly, *et al.* 2000. Corticotropin releasing hormone (CRH) promoter polymorphisms in various ethnic groups of patients with rheumatoid arthritis. Z. Rheumatol. **59:** 29–34.
15. Vamvakopoulos, N.C. & G.P. Chrousos. 1993. Evidence of direct estrogenic regulation of human corticotropin-releasing hormone gene expression: potential implications for the sexual dimorphism of the stress response and immune/inflammatory reaction. J. Clin. Invest. **92:** 1896–1902.
16. Yoshida, H., K. Haze, H. Yanagi, *et al.* 1998. Identification of the *cis*-acting endoplasmic reticulum stress response element responsible for transcriptional induction of mammalian glucose-regulated proteins: involvement of basic leucine zipper transcription factors. J. Biol. Chem. **273:** 33741–33749.
17. Fawcett, T.W., J.L. Martindale, K.Z. Guyton, *et al.* 1999. Complexes containing activating transcription factor (ATF)/cAMP-responsive-element-binding protein (CREB) interact with the CCAAT/enhancer-binding protein (C/EBP)-ATF composite site to regulate Gadd153 expression during the stress response. Biochem. J. **339:** 135–141.
18. Zambelli, A., E. Mongiardini, S.N. Villegas, *et al.* 2005. Transcription factor XBP-1 is expressed during osteoblast differentiation and is transcriptionally regulated by parathyroid hormone (PTH). Cell Biol. Int. **29:** 647–653.
19. Bousquet, C., V. Chesnokova, A. Kariagina, *et al.* 2001. cAMP neuropeptide agonists induce pituitary suppressor of cytokine signaling-3: novel negative feedback mechanism for corticotroph cytokine action. Mol. Endocrinol. **15:** 1880–1890.

20. ADLER, G., C.M. SMAS & J.A. MAJZOUB. 1988. Expression and dexamethasone regulation of the human corticotropin releasing hormone gene in a mouse anterior pituitary cell line. J. Biol. Chem. **263:** 5846–5852.
21. SEASHOLTZ, A.F., R.C. THOMPSON & J.O. DOUGLAS. 1988. Identification of a cyclic adenosine monophosphate-responsive element in rat corticotropin-releasing hormone gene. Mol. Endocrinol. **2:** 1311–1319.
22. GUARDIOLA-DIAZ, H.M., C. BOSWELL & A.F. SEASHOLTZ. 1994. The cAMP-responsive element in the corticotropin-releasing hormone gene mediates transcriptional regulation by depolarization. J. Biol. Chem. **269:** 14784–14791.
23. NICHOLSON, R.C., B.R. KING & R. SMITH. 2004. Complex regulatory interactions control CRH gene expression. Front. Biosci. **9:** 32–39.
24. WOLFL, S., C. MARTINEZ & J.A. MAJZOUB. 1999. Inducible binding of cyclic adenosine 3′,5′-monophosphate (cAMP)-responsive element binding protein (CREB) to a cAMP-responsive promoter in vivo. Mol. Endocrinol. **13:** 659–669.
25. KING, B.R., R. SMITH & R.C. NICHOLSON. 2001. The regulation of human corticotropin-releasing hormone gene expression in the placenta. Peptides **22:** 1941–1947.
26. CHENG, Y.H. & S. HANDWERGER. 2002. AP-2alpha modulates human corticotropin-releasing hormone gene expression in the placenta by direct protein–protein interaction. Mol. Cell Endocrinol. **191:** 127–136.
27. SCATENA, C.D. & S. ADLER. 1998. Characterization of a human-specific regulator of placental corticotropin-releasing hormone. Mol. Endocrinol. **12:** 1228–1240.
28. KAPATOS, G., S.L. STEGENGA & K. HIRAYAMA. 2000. Identification and characterization of basal and cyclic AMP response elements in the promoter of the rat GTP cyclohydrolase I gene. J. Biol. Chem. **275:** 5947–5957.
29. TSIGOS, C. & G.P. CHROUSOS. 2002. Hypothalamic-pituitary-adrenal axis, neuroendocrine factors and stress. J. Psychosom. Res. **53:** 865–871.
30. KISHIMOTO, T., T. TAGA & S. AKIRA. 1994. Cytokine signal transduction. Cell **76:** 253–262.
31. DIBBS, K.I., E. ANTEBY, M.A. MALLON, *et al.* 1997. Transcriptional regulation of human placental corticotropin-releasing factor by prostaglandins and estradiol. Biol. Reprod. **57:** 1285–1292.
32. CHESNOKOVA, V. & S. MELMED. 2002. Neuro-immuno-endocrine modulation of the hypothalamic-pituitary-adrenal (HPA) axis by gp130 signaling molecules. Endocrinology **143:** 1571–1574.

Genetic Variation in the Endothelin System

Do Polymorphisms Affect the Therapeutic Strategies?

GIAN PAOLO ROSSI AND GISELLA PITTER

Department of Clinical and Experimental Medicine, Clinica Medica 4, University of Padova, 235126 Padova, Italy

ABSTRACT: Endothelin-1 (ET-1) exerts multiple biological effects, including vasoconstriction and the stimulation of cell proliferation in tissues both within and outside of the cardiovascular system. ET-1 is synthesized by ET-converting enzymes (ECE), chymases (CMAs), and non-ECE metalloproteases through a process regulated in an autocrine fashion in vascular and nonvascular cells. ET-1 acts through the activation of $G_i$protein–coupled receptors. ET_A receptors mediate vasoconstriction and cell proliferation, whereas ET_B receptors are important for aldosterone secretion, endothelial cell (EC) migration, the release of nitric oxide (NO) and prostacyclin, the clearance of ET-1, and the inhibition of *ECE-1*. ET is activated in scleroderma, hypertension, atherosclerosis, restenosis, heart failure, idiopathic cardiomyopathy, and renal failure. Tissue concentrations more reliably reflect the activation of the ET system because of the predominantly abluminal secretion of the peptide. Experimental studies and clinical trials have demonstrated that ET-1 plays a major role in normal cardiovascular homeostasis and in the functional and structural changes observed in arterial and pulmonary hypertension, glomerulosclerosis, atherosclerosis, and heart failure. Accordingly, ET antagonists are promising new agents in the treatment of cardiovascular diseases. Single nucleotide polymorphisms (SNPs) of the genes of *preproET-1*, *ECE-1*, CMA, ET_A and ET_B receptors have been identified and can be important for their functional regulation. However, for most of them the association with disease conditions and the evidence for a functional role remain controversial. Thus, even though ET antagonists are being used for the treatment of pulmonary hypertension, there is no convincing evidence for a role of SNPs in affecting the therapeutic strategies.

Address for correspondence: Prof. Gian Paolo Rossi, M.D., F.A.C.C., D.M.C.S., Internal Medicine 4, University Hospital, via Giustiniani, 235126 Padova, Italy. Voice: +39-49-821-3304; fax: +39-49-880-2252.

e-mail: gianpaolo.rossi@unipd.it

Ann. N.Y. Acad. Sci. 1069: 34–50 (2006). © 2006 New York Academy of Sciences.
doi: 10.1196/annals.1351.004

KEYWORDS: endothelin-1; G protein–coupled receptors; cardiovascular system; cardiovascular disease; genetic polymorphisms

INTRODUCTION

In March 1988, a paper in *Nature* by Prof. Masaki's laboratory reported the isolation and chemical identification of a peptide, named endothelin (ET).[1] This was followed by a *deluge* of studies that have enormously improved our mechanistic understanding of most cardiovascular and some noncardiovascular diseases and have led to the development of a novel effective strategy for the treatment of pulmonary hypertension.

ISOFORMS, FUNCTION, BIOSYNTHESIS, AND REGULATION

Endothelin-1 (ET-1) is the prototype of a larger family of structurally similar isopeptides that comprise ET-1, ET-2, and ET-3. They are encoded by genes that have been mapped on chromosomes 6, 1, and 20, for ET-1, ET-2, and ET-3, respectively. The most widely studied isopeptide is ET-1 that entails a 21-amino acid residue peptide predominantly made by endothelin cells (ECs) from which it is released abluminally toward the vascular smooth muscle cells (SMCs), where it acts in a paracrine fashion.[2] Other cells involved in cardiovascular disease, such as SMCs,[3] leukocytes, macrophages, cardiomyocytes, and mesangial cells, can also produce ET-1 under disease conditions.[4]

Transcription of the *preproET-1* gene is regulated through binding sites for nuclear factor-1, GATA-2, AP-1, the phorbol-ester–sensitive *c-fos* and *c-jun* complexes, and acute phase reactant regulatory elements.[2] The translation of preproET mRNA results in the formation of a 212-amino acid preproET peptide, which undergoes a further intracellular processing as described below. The *preproET-1* is cleaved by a furin convertase, to the 38-amino acid inactive precursor big (pro)ET-1_{1-38}. This is followed by a cleavage of the Trp_{21}–Val_{22} bond by a specific ET-converting enzyme-1 (*ECE-1*) that is partially inhibited by phosphoramidon and is ubiquitously expressed in human tissues.[5] The *ECE-1* gene has been finely mapped on chromosome 1p36,[6] and its expression is regulated through protein kinase C-dependent mechanisms, ET_B-receptors, the transcription factor ets-1, and cytokines.[2]

ECE-independent pathways also contribute to ET-1 production, because in *ECE-1* knockout mice the tissue levels of ET-1 are reduced by only about 30%.[7] Indeed, chymase A (CMA), a major angiotensin II-forming enzyme in the human cardiovascular system,[8] can generate ET-1_{1-21}.[2] It also cleaves big ET-1 at the Tyr_{31}–Gly_{32} bond, resulting in the formation of ET-1_{1-31}, which acts as a selective ET_A receptor agonist.

ET synthesis is regulated by physicochemical factors, such as pulsatile stretch, shear stress, hypoxia, and pH (see Ref. 2) (FIGURE 1). Exercise

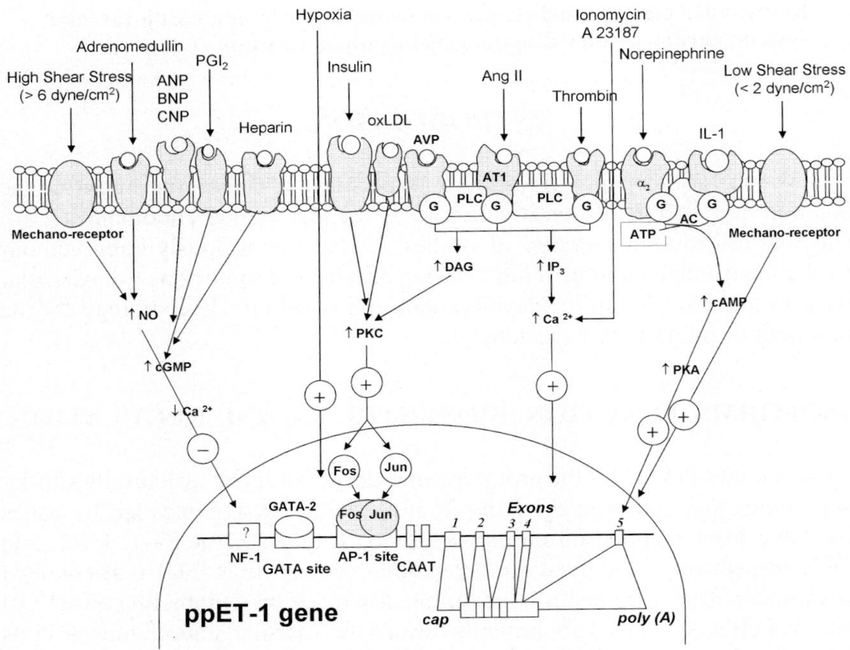

FIGURE 1. The cartoon summarizes the factors affecting ET-1 synthesis and related intracellular signaling pathways. Shear stress affects ppET-1 expression in a bidirectional way depending on its values. The factors acting via activation of the phospholypase C (PLC)–protein kinase C (PKC) pathway, as insulin, LDL, AVP, angiotensin II, and thrombin, enhance ET-1 production by binding of the heterodimer *fos-jun* forming the AP-1 complex to the specific motif in the *ppET-1* promotor. Natriuretic peptides, prostacyclin (PGI_2), oxLDL, and heparin, blunt *ppET-1* gene transcription by increasing cGMP, whereas adrenomedullin acts by increasing NO production, and norepinephrine- and IL-1 by acting via cAMP and PKA. Exons and consensus sequences in the promotor are schematically depicted in the nucleus.

upregulates myocardial ET-1 expression, thus suggesting that ET-1 intervenes in the functional cardiac adaptation to exercise.[9] ET-1 biosynthesis is stimulated by most cardiovascular risk factors (see Ref. 2). Vasoconstrictors, growth factors, cytokines, and adhesion molecules also stimulate ET production. Inhibitors of ET-1 synthesis include nitric oxide (NO), prostacyclin, atrial natriuretic peptides, homocysteine, and estrogens,[2] and alcohol-free extracts of red wine.[10]

ET RECEPTOR

The biological effects of ET are mediated by two different G_i protein–coupled, 7-transmembrane domain receptors, termed ET_A, and ET_B, which are encoded by different genes and characterized by distinct tissue distribution and pharmacological properties. In the vasculature, ET_A receptors are in SMCs, whereas ET_B receptors are on ECs and, to some extent, in SMCs, and macrophages.[2] The binding of ET-1 to ET_A receptors activates phospholypase C, which leads to an accumulation of inositol triphosphate (IP_3) and intracellular Ca^{2+} and thereby to long-lasting vasoconstriction.[1,11] The activation of ET_A receptors by ET-1 or ET-1_{1-31} also induces cell proliferation in different tissues, including the adrenal cortex, which express CMA and therefore can synthesize ET-1_{1-31}.[2] By contrast, the activation of endothelial ET_B subtype mediates the release of endothelial-derived relaxing factors (EDRFs), like NO, adrenomedullin and prostacyclin, prevents apoptosis, and inhibits *ECE-1* expression in ECs.[2] ET_B receptors also mediate the pulmonary clearance of circulating ET-1, the reuptake of ET-1 by ECs and the release of aldosterone.[12] However, under disease conditions ET_B receptors can also be expressed in vascular SMCs and mediate vasoconstriction.[13]

ET-1-MEDIATED MECHANISMS OF DISEASES

ET-1 is much more than an extremely potent vasoconstrictor: it has mitogenic effects, stimulates cytokines and growth factors production, and promotes the formation of reactive oxygen species (ROS) including superoxide anion ($O_2^{\circ -}$), in cells of the vascular wall (see Ref. 2), and monocyte-macrophage infiltrating the atherosclerotic plaques. $O_2^{\circ -}$ scavenges NO, activates the family of nuclear transcription factor (NF)–κB, which triggers the expression of genes coding for proatherogenic and pro-inflammatory molecules as adhesins (VCAM-1, ICAM-1, E-selectin) and inflammatory cytokines (interleukin [IL-6 and IL-8]), and activates matrix metalloproteases (MMPs). Therefore, ET-1-induced NF-κB activation is instrumental for the induction and progression of atherosclerosis, as well as for atherosclerotic plaque destabilization. ET-1 also enhances extracellular matrix proteins deposition and collagen I gene activity, promotes expression of fibronectin and potentiates the effects of transforming growth factor-ß and platelet-derived growth factor, a number of actions that are important for remodeling of small resistance arteries and left ventricular hypertrophy in arterial hypertension, renal damage, tissue fibrosis, and in scleroderma. ET-1 also interacts with the blood cells stimulating neutrophil adhesion, and platelet aggregation, and is a chemiotactic factor for macrophages. ET-1 promotes cell-cycle progression in an autocrine fashion (see Ref. 2). Finally, the mature ET-1 peptide stimulates synthesis and secretion of hormones and autacoids, such as aldosterone, arginin-vasopressin, NO, adrenomedullin, and prostacyclin (see Ref. 2 and 14). Accordingly, the ET-1 system plays a role in inducing cardiovascular damage and accelerated atherogenesis in hypertension, in triggering cardiovascular events, and in promoting tissue fibrosis in scleroderma, and possibly other disease conditions (see later).

BLOCKADE OF THE ET SYSTEM AND THERAPEUTIC TARGETS

Peptides and nonpeptide ET receptor blockers are available as research tools and for clinical development (see Ref. 15). Among them, bosentan has been approved for clinical use (see later). A detailed discussion of the general properties of ET receptor blockers and of the strategy underlying their development and use in different diseases is available.[15]

ET-1 AND DISEASES

Since ET-1 synthesis can be triggered by several factors that can be involved in arterial hypertension and atherosclerosis and since picomolar concentrations of ET-1 induce a sustained and dose-dependent vasoconstriction, the peptide has been implicated in the pathogenesis of conditions that feature excess vasoconstriction and cell proliferation, including arterial hypertension, atherosclerosis, acute myocardial ischemia, pulmonary hypertension, systemic arterial hypertension, congestive heart failure, renal diseases, hemangioendothelioma, and Conn's syndrome. Furthermore, based on the consideration that ET-1 plays an important role in regulating collagen and extracellular matrix deposition, the peptide has been associated also with scleroderma and its complications, including tissue and pulmonary fibrosis.

ARTERIAL HYPERTENSION, RENAL DAMAGE, AND ATHEROSCLEROSIS

The role of ET-1 differs markedly across the experimental models of hypertension (see Ref. 16 and 17) and this heterogeneity is mirrored in human hypertension. ET-1 undoubtedly plays a crucial pathophysiologic role in the rare patients with ET-1-producing hemangioendothelioma, but its role is more controversial in primary (essential) hypertension (see Ref. 2). Nonetheless, ET receptor blockade with bosentan lowered blood pressure in patients with mild-to-moderate hypertension as effectively as the ACE inhibitor enalapril.[18] Furthermore, combined ET_A/ET_B receptor blockade with TAK 044 induced a greater vasodilatory response in hypertensive patients than in normal subjects.[19] Infusion of low doses of the ET_A receptor antagonist BQ-123, alone or combined with the ET_B receptor antagonist BQ-788, induced a fall of blood pressure in hypertensive patients regardless of the degree of activation of the renin–angiotensin system.[20] Thus, overall available data suggest that ET-1 contribute to maintaining raised blood pressure values in a wide range of hypertensive patients.

ET-1 promotes vasoconstriction and cell growth in the vasculature and in the kidney, mainly via ET_A receptors. Accordingly, in experimental models, chronic ET receptor blockade inhibits vascular injury, reduces renal and vascular injury associated with hypertension and other forms of renal diseases, and prolongs renal survival.[21]

Hypercholesterolemia and the atherogenic-oxidized low-density lipoproteins (LDL) upregulate *ET-1* gene expression in ECs and enhance vascular SMCs proliferation via ET_A receptors.[22] As mentioned, ET-1 stimulates the synthesis of growth factors and adhesins that are implicated in atherogenesis. ET-1 also increases neutrophil and platelet adhesion, thereby promoting plaque growth and coronary thrombosis.[23] In experimental hypercholesterolemia, ET_A receptor blockade reduced macrophage infiltration in fatty streaks,[24] and combined ET_A/ET_B receptor blockade improved the impaired endothelium-dependent vasodilatation.[25] ET-1 also contributes to myocardial infarction in atherosclerotic mice and in apolipoprotein E-deficient mice, long-term ET_A blockade reduces the extent of atherosclerosis, corrects endothelial dysfunction and prevents increased vascular ET-1, even without affecting blood pressure or plasma cholesterol.[26]

In patients with coronary artery disease and myocardial infarction, ET-1 plasma levels are increased and the expression of ET-1 and ECE is enhanced in human atherosclerotic lesions.[3,27] Tissue ET-1 likely plays a substantial functional role in coronary artery disease, because the extent of immunoreactive staining for ET-1 in atheromatous lesions is related to angina class and the plasma levels of ET-1 correlate with number of coronary artery diseased vessels.[28] Moreover, combined ET receptor blockade causes vasodilation in patients with coronary atherosclerosis. ET-1 also plays a role in determining the severity of stroke and its sequelae, because ET receptor blockade reduces ischemic brain injury and vasospasm.[29]

ET-1 AND TRANSPLANT-ASSOCIATED VASCULOPATHY

Organ transplantation is associated with raised circulating ET-1 levels, because of the upregulation of the ET system in the transplanted organ vasculature. Accelerated arteriosclerosis of coronary vessels of transplanted heart contributes to worsening the outcome of heart transplant recipients. Immunologic mechanisms leading to chronic nonspecific inflammatory changes and EC activation (induced by cytokines released by infiltrating mononuclear cells and lymphocytes) can be major underlying mechanisms. Enhanced local synthesis of ET-1, with ensuing ROS production, NF-κB activation, and stimulation of adhesins and proinflammatory cytokines expression, contributes to SMCs proliferation. The effectiveness of treatment with bosentan in preventing the development of arteriolar narrowing of transplanted rat hearts indicates a causal role of ET-1 upregulation in this context.[30]

CONGESTIVE HEART FAILURE

ET-1 is an important player in congestive heart failure (CHF), where the increased ET-1 plasma levels predict survival and the upregulation of the *ECE-1*, *preproET-1* and ET_A receptor genes is instrumental for impairing ventricular function. However, ET-1 likely plays a dual role: it maintains cardiac function in early stages of CHF,[31] but can be detrimental in chronic CHF, because ET blockade improves hemodynamics, reduces ventricular dilatation, and prolongs survival (see Ref. 2). Although ET receptor blockade induces beneficial hemodynamic and clinical effects in CHF patients, clinical trials have failed to improve outcome.[32–36] Thus, to date there is no evidence for clinical efficacy for ET-1 receptor antagonists in patients with CHF. For a discussion of the possible explanations of these negative studies, the readers are referred elsewhere.[2]

PULMONARY HYPERTENSION

The vasculature of the lung is a site of intense NO and ET-1 production and clearance, which can be altered in lung disease and pulmonary hypertension. In fact, in both primary and secondary pulmonary hypertension ET-1 synthesis overcomes NO production.[37,38] Furthermore, the ET_A receptor is highly expressed in both conduit and resistance arteries of the lung, which can explain why they are so exquisitely sensitive to the vasoconstrictor effect of ET-1. ET-1 also exerts a clear-cut proliferative effect on pulmonary artery SMC via ET_A receptors.[39] Hypoxia can turn on the transcription of the *ppET-1* gene; furthermore, an activation of the ET-1 system and a beneficial effect of ET receptor blockade on the course of pulmonary hypertension have both been documented.[2] Thus, compelling evidence indicates a role for ET-1 in raising pulmonary artery pressure and causing adverse structural changes in the vasculature. A pilot study[40] in patients with primary and scleroderma-induced pulmonary hypertension showed impressive hemodynamic improvement. A larger multicenter study thereafter conclusively demonstrated an impressive amelioration of the clinical course of this serious disease.[41] Based on these findings, bosentan has been approved in both North America and Europe for the treatment of pulmonary hypertension in patients in NYHA class III/IV. An open label 2-year follow-up study of patients on bosentan indicated a doubling of the survival as compared to the survival rate expected on the basis of the NHI equation (M. Clozel personal communication).

POLYMORPHISMS OF GENES OF THE ET SYSTEM

Several single nucleotide polymorphisms (SNPs) of the genes of prepro ET-1, *ECE-1*, CMA, ET_A and ET_B receptors were identified.[42–72] Some of these SNPs have been investigated in terms of functional relevance and association with cardiovascular (TABLE 1) and noncardiovascular (TABLE 2) phenotypes and/or diseases. Overall, studies relating these SNPs to functional effects

TABLE 1. Identified SNPs of the ET system, location and functional relevance for cardiovascular phenotypes

Gene	SNP	Functional relevance (gain/loss of function)	Associated phenotype/ disease	Significant association	Reference
preproET-1	–1370 T>G	ND	UAE, GFR	Yes	62
		ND	LVMI	Yes	47
		ND	BP	No	
	T –37/in2C	ND	BP (men)	Yes	47
		ND	LVMI	No	
	+138/ex1 del/ins	ND	IDCM	No	45
		ND	CHF	Yes	67
		Yes/gain	Plasma ET-1 levels	Yes	64
		ND	BP, LVMI	No	47
	+862 G>T/Ala288Ser (exon 5)	ND	HT	No	57
	+5665 G>T/ Lys198Asn (exon 5)	ND	IDCM	No	45
		ND	BP	Yes	75
		ND	UAE, GFR	Yes	62
		ND	BP, LVMI	No	47
		ND	BP (women)	Yes	48
		No	ET-1 level *in vitro*, plasma ET-1 level	No	64
		ND	SVD	No	51
	IVS4 + 8002 G>A	ND	CHF	Yes	67
ECE-1	–839 T>G (isoform b)	ND	BP (women)	Yes	49
	–338 C>A	Yes/gain	BP (women)	Yes	49
	(Isoform b)	ND	BP (women)	Yes	48
Chymase A (CMA)	–3255 G>A (CMA/B)	ND	HCM	Yes	61
		ND	ACEI cough	No	71
		ND	CRF	No	52

Continued.

TABLE 1. Continued

Gene	SNP	Functional relevance (gain/loss of function)	Associated phenotype/ disease	Significant association	Reference
		ND	Pregnancy-induced HT	No	58
		ND	Nephropathy in DM2	No	72
		ND	LVMI in DM2	Yes	53
		ND	LVMI	No	54
	−1905 A>G	ND	Atherosclerosis in venous CABG	Yes	60
ET_A receptor	−231 A>G	ND	IDCM	No	45
		ND	BP, MI	No	59
		ND	BP	Yes	43
		ND	SVD	No	51
	+69 C>T/ His323His (exon 6)	ND	HT	No	63
		ND	BP, MI	No	59
	+105 A>G/Glu335Glu (exon 6)	ND	BP, MI	No	59
	+211 C>G (exon 8)	ND	BP	Yes	59
		ND	MI	No	59
	+1222 C>T (exon 8)	ND	SVD	No	51
	+1363 C>T (exon 8)	ND	IDCM	Yes	45
		ND	BP	Yes	59
		ND	MI	No	59
		ND	HT	Yes	43
	3′ *52 T>C	ND	BP, MI	No	59
ET_B receptor	5′ −544 G>A	ND	BP, MI	No	59
	+307 G>A/Gly57Ser (exon 1)	ND	BP, MI	No	59
		ND	SVD	No	51
	+30 G>A/Leu277Leu (exon 4)	ND	IDCM	No	45
		ND	BP, MI	No	59
		ND	SVD	No	51

UAE = urinary albumin excretion; GFR = glomerular filtration rate; LVMI = left ventricular mass index; BP = blood pressure; IDCM = idiopathic dilated cardiomyopathy; CHF = congestive heart failure; HT = arterial hypertension; HCM = hypertrophic cardiomyopathy; CRF = chronic renal failure; SVD = cerebral small vessel disease; DM2 = diabetes mellitus type 2; CABG = coronary artery bypass graft; MI = myocardial infarction.

NOTE: The SNPs were defined according to the suggested recommendations,[76] whenever possible, or according to the quoted references when unfeasible.

are limited and have not been independently replicated. Likewise, most studies associating the SNPs with phenotypes and/or diseases were cross-sectional and/or limited to small series of patients and therefore were prone to the possibility of selection biases. The use in many studies of restriction fragment length polymorphism (RFLP) analysis, which is a suboptimal and sometimes inaccurate technique for genotyping, has further limited the weight of their conclusions. Biological plausibility has also been neglected in a few studies that attempted to relate SNPs with phenotypes. Thus, caution is strongly advised before drawing either positive or negative conclusions, and both an independent replication and a mechanistic explanation of results are much necessary.

As regards cardiovascular phenotypes/diseases, most studies have investigated the association of SNPs with blood pressure and hypertension-related cardiovascular damage. Of interest, the *ET-1* gene exon 5 Lys198Asn SNP was reported to be significantly associated with a steeper increase of systolic blood pressure with increasing body mass index (BMI),[65] but this finding still remains an isolated observation. SNPs in the *ECE-1*, ET_A and ET_B receptor genes have also been associated with blood pressure-related phenotypes.[43,59] However, studies are isolated and findings have not been independently confirmed. Moreover, no data indicate any functional relevance of these SNPs and therefore the interpretation of these findings remains unclear. A C-338A SNP found in the *ECE-1B* gene was associated with BP levels in women but not in men.[48] Specifically, females homozygous for the A allele had significantly higher systolic, diastolic, and mean BP levels, after adjustment for age and BMI. Genotyping of the ET-1 Lys198Asn polymorphism showed that this variant was not associated with BP values in either men or women, but interacted with the *ECE-1* variant to influence systolic and mean BP levels in women.[48]

As relates to noncardiovascular disease/phenotypes, studies have investigated the association of ET_A receptor gene SNPs with migraine and glaucoma,[56,66] and of ET_B receptor gene SNPs with Hirschprung disease. The latter studies were triggered by the observations that ET_B receptor gene mutations produce megacolon in mice[73] and that a G–>T missense mutation in exon 4 that substitutes the highly conserved Trp-276 residue in the fifth transmembrane helix of the G protein–coupled receptor with a Cys residue (W276C) implies a blunting of ligand-induced Ca^{2+} transient levels in transfected cells and an increased risk of Hirschprung disease.[74] Overall, these studies have not given consistent results (Table 2).

Thus, even though ET antagonists proved to be extremely useful for the treatment of pulmonary hypertension and are being exploited for other indications, there is no convincing evidence for a role of SNPs in the genes of the ET system in affecting the therapeutic strategies. Therefore, further research efforts should be devoted to this field.

TABLE 2. Identified SNPs of the ET system, location and functional relevance for noncardiovascular phenotypes

Gene	SNP	Functional relevance (gain/loss of function)	Associated phenotype/ disease	Significant association	Reference
preproET-1	–1398 T>A	ND	ND		42
	–1396 G>A	ND	ND		42
	–1370 T>G	ND	Glaucoma	No	56
	G –46/in1A	ND	ND		42
	+138/ex1 del/ins	ND	Glaucoma	No	56
	IVS1 + 1932 G>A	ND	ND		42
	IVS2 + 3539 T>C	ND	ND		42
	+5665 G>T/ Lys198Asn (exon 5)	ND	Glaucoma	No	56
	IVS4 + 8002 G>A	ND	Psoriasis	No	68
		ND	Glaucoma	No	56
ET_A receptor	–231 A>G	ND	Migraine	Yes	66
		ND	Glaucoma	No	56
	+69 C>T/His323His (exon 6)	ND	Glaucoma	No	56
	+70 C>G (exon 8)	ND	Glaucoma	Yes	56
	+1222 C>T (exon 8)	ND	Glaucoma	No	56
ET_B receptor	5′ –148 A>G (exon 1)	ND	IND, HSCR	No	50

Continued.

TABLE 2. Continued

Gene	SNP	Functional relevance (gain/loss of function)	Associated phenotype/ disease	Significant association	Reference
	+178 G>A/Ala60Thr (exon 1)	ND	HSCR, HSCR/Down's syndrome	No	70
	+ 307 G>A/Gly57Ser (exon 1)	ND	IND, HSCR	No	50
	+552 C>T/(exon 2)	ND	HSCR/Down's syndrome	Yes	70
		ND	HSCR	No	
	+561 C>T/(exon 2)	ND	HSCR/Down's syndrome	Yes	70
		ND	HSCR	No	
	+702 C>T/(exon 3)	ND	HSCR, HSCR/Down's syndrome	No	70
	+ 30 G>A/Leu277Leu (exon 4)	ND	HSCR/Down's syndrome	?Yes	70
		ND	HSCR	No	56
		ND	Glaucoma	No	
	+818 A>G/Lys273Arg (exon 4)	ND	IND, HSCR	No	50
	875 T>G/Phe292Cys (exon 4)	ND	IND, HSCR	No	50
	IVS3 -6 C>T	ND	HSCR, HSCR/Down's syndrome	No	70
	IVS4 +3 A>G	ND	HSCR, HSCR/Down's syndrome	No	70

IND = intestinal neuronal dysplasia; HSCR = Hirschsprung disease; the others as inTable 1.

CONCLUSIONS

The ET system is upregulated in most conditions associated with generation of ROS, and blunted NO bioactivity, such as hypertension, atherosclerosis, and heart failure, where it plays a crucial role in the progression of the disease. It is conceivable that the complex interplay of the underlying mechanisms with variation of genes of the ET system may account for the different individual susceptibility to cardiovascular disease. At a time when ET receptor blockade has been shown to have therapeutic potential in hypertension, atherosclerosis, heart failure, pulmonary disease, and renal damage, further studies are necessary to determine whether variation of these genes can affect the responses to these novel agents, which appear to be powerful tools in cardiovascular and noncardiovascular medicine.

REFERENCES

1. Yanagisawa, M., H. Kurihara, *et al.* 1988. A novel potent vasoconstrictor peptide produced by vascular endothelial cells. Nature **332:** 411–415.
2. Rossi, G.P. & A.C. Pessina. 2005. Endothelins: molecular mechanisms in hypertension and cardiovascular diseases. *In* Molecular Mechanisms of Hypertension. D. Di Pette, E.L. Schiffrin & J.H. Sowers, Eds.: XX.Taylor & Francis Medical Books. London.
3. Rossi, G.P., S. Colonna, *et al.* 1999. Endothelin-1 and its mRNA in the wall layers of human arteries Ex vivo. Circulation **99:** 1147–1155.
4. Rubanyi, G.M. & M.A. Polokoff. 1994. Endothelins: molecular biology, biochemistry, pharmacology, physiology, and pathophysiology. Pharmacol. Rev. **46:** 325–415.
5. Rossi, G.P., G. Albertin, *et al.* 1995. Expression of the endothelin-converting enzyme gene in human tissues. Biochem. Biophys. Res. Commun. **211:** 249–253.
6. Albertin, G., G.P. Rossi, *et al.* 1996. Fine mapping of the human ECE gene by fluorescent in situ hybridization and radiation hybrids. Biochem. Biophys. Res. Commun. **221:** 682–687.
7. Yanagisawa, H., M. Yanagisawa, *et al.* 1998. Dual genetic pathways of endothelin-mediated intercellular signaling revealed by targeted disruption of endothelin converting enzyme-1 gene. Development **125:** 825–836.
8. Urata, H., A. Kinoshita, *et al.* 1990. Identification of a highly specific chymase as the major angiotensin II-forming enzyme in the human heart. J. Biol. Chem. **265:** 22348–22357.
9. Maeda, S., T. Miyauchi, *et al.* 1998. Prolonged exercise causes an increase in endothelin-1 production in the heart in rats. Am. J. Physiol. **275:** H2105–H2112.
10. Corder, R., J.A. Douthwaite, *et al.* 2001. Endothelin-1 synthesis reduced by red wine. Nature **414:** 863–864.
11. Pollock, D.M., T.L. Keith, *et al.* 1995. Endothelin receptors and calcium signaling. FASEB J. **9:** 1196–1204.

12. Rossi, G., G. Albertin, *et al.* 1994. Gene expression, localization, and characterization of endothelin A and B receptors in the human adrenal cortex. J. Clin. Invest. **94:** 1226–1234.
13. Teerlink, J.R., V. Breu, *et al.* 1994. Potent vasoconstriction mediated by endothelin ETB receptors in canine coronary arteries. Circ. Res. **74:** 105–114.
14. Nussdorfer, G.G., G.P. Rossi, *et al.* 1999. Autocrine-paracrine endothelin system in the physiology and pathology of steroid-secreting tissues. Pharmacol. Rev. **51:** 1–35.
15. Luscher, T.F. & M. Barton. 2000. Endothelins and endothelin receptor antagonists: therapeutic considerations for a novel class of cardiovascular drugs. Circulation **102:** 2434–2440.
16. Rossi, G.P., A. Sacchetto, *et al.* 1999. Interactions between endothelin-1 and the renin-angiotensin-aldosterone system. Cardiovasc. Res. **43:** 300–307.
17. Schiffrin, E.L. 2001. Role of endothelin-1 in hypertension and vascular disease. Am. J. Hypertens. **14:** 83S–89S.
18. Krum, H., R.J. Viskoper, *et al.* 1998. The effect of an endothelin-receptor antagonist, bosentan, on blood pressure in patients with essential hypertension. Bosentan Hypertension Investigators. N. Engl. J. Med. **338:** 784–790.
19. Taddei, S., A. Virdis, *et al.* 1999. Vasoconstriction to endogenous endothelin-1 is increased in the peripheral circulation of patients with essential hypertension. Circulation **100:** 1680–1683.
20. Rossi, G.P., C. Ganzaroli, *et al.* 2003. Endothelin receptor blockade lowers plasma aldosterone levels via different mechanisms in primary aldosteronism and high-to-normal renin hypertension. Cardiovasc. Res. **57:** 277–283.
21. Orth, S.R., J.P. Esslinger, *et al.* 1998. Nephroprotection of an ETA-receptor blocker (LU 135252) in salt-loaded uninephrectomized stroke-prone spontaneously hypertensive rats. Hypertension **31:** 995–1001.
22. Lerman, A., D.R. Holmes, Jr., *et al.* 1995. Endothelin in coronary endothelial dysfunction and early atherosclerosis in humans. Circulation **92:** 2426–2431.
23. Lopez Farre, A., A. Riesco, *et al.* 1993. Effect of endothelin-1 on neutrophil adhesion to endothelial cells and perfused heart. Circulation **88:** 1166–1171.
24. Kowala, M.C., P.M. Rose, *et al.* 1995. Selective blockade of the endothelin subtype A receptor decreases early atherosclerosis in hamsters fed cholesterol. Am. J. Pathol. **146:** 819–826.
25. Best, P.J.M., C.J. McKenna, *et al.* 1999. Chronic endothelin receptor antagonism preserves coronary endothelial function in experimental hypercholesterolemia. Circulation **99:** 1747–1752.
26. Barton, M., C.C. Haudenschild, *et al.* 1998. Endothelin ETA receptor blockade restores NO-mediated endothelial function and inhibits atherosclerosis in apolipoprotein E-deficient mice. Proc. Natl. Acad. Sci. USA **95:** 14367–14372.
27. Zeiher, A.M., H. Goebel, *et al.* 1995. Tissue endothelin-1 immunoreactivity in the active coronary atherosclerotic plaque. A clue to the mechanism of increased vasoreactivity of the culprit lesion in unstable angina. Circulation **91:** 941–947.
28. Salomone, O.A., P.M. Elliott, *et al.* 1996. Plasma immunoreactive endothelin concentration correlates with severity of coronary artery disease in patients with stable angina pectoris and normal ventricular function. J. Am. Coll. Cardiol. **28:** 14–19.

29. BLEZER, E.L.A., K. NICOLAY, *et al.* 1999. Early-onset but not late-onset endothelin-A-receptor blockade can modulate hypertension, cerebral edema, and proteinuria in stroke-prone hypertensive rats. Hypertension **33:** 137–144.
30. OKADA, K., Y. NISHIDA, *et al.* 1998. Role of endogenous endothelin in the development of graft arteriosclerosis in rat cardiac allografts: antiproliferative effects of bosentan, a nonselective endothelin receptor antagonist. Circulation **97:** 2346–2351.
31. SAKAI, S., T. MIYAUCHI, *et al.* 1996. Endogenous endothelin-1 participates in the maintenance of cardiac function in rats with congestive heart failure: marked increase in endothelin-1 production in the failing heart. Circulation **93:** 1214–1222.
32. KALUSKI, E., I. KOBRIN, *et al.* 2003. RITZ-5: randomized intravenous TeZosentan (an endothelin-A/B antagonist) for the treatment of pulmonary edema: a prospective, multicenter, double-blind, placebo-controlled study. J. Am. Coll. Cardiol. **41:** 204–210.
33. O'CONNOR, C.M., W.A. Gattis, *et al.* 2003. Tezosentan in patients with acute heart failure and acute coronary syndromes: design of the fourth Randomized Intravenous Tezosentan Study (RITZ-4). Am. Heart J. **145:** S58–S59.
34. RICH, S. & V.V. MCLAUGHLIN. 2003. Endothelin receptor blockers in cardiovascular disease. Circulation **108:** 2184–2190.
35. LOUIS, A.A., I.R. MANOUSOS, *et al.* 2002. Clinical trials update: the heart protection study, IONA, CARISA, ENRICHD, ACUTE, ALIVE, MADIT II and REMATCH. Impact of nicorandil on angina. Combination assessment of ranolazine in stable angina. Enhancing recovery in coronary heart disease patients. Assessment of cardioversion using transoesophageal echocardiography. azimilide post-infarct survival evaluation. Randomised evaluation of mechanical assistance for treatment of chronic heart failure. Eur. J. Heart Fail. **4:** 111–116.
36. LUSCHER, T.F., F. ENSELEIT, *et al.* 2002. Hemodynamic and neurohumoral effects of selective endothelin A (ET(A)) receptor blockade in chronic heart failure: the Heart Failure ET(A) Receptor Blockade Trial (HEAT). Circulation **106:** 2666–2672.
37. DUPUIS, J., P. CERNACEK, *et al.* 1998. Reduced pulmonary clearance of endothelin-1 in pulmonary hypertension. Am. Heart J. **135:** 614–620.
38. GIAID, A., R.P. MICHEL, *et al.* 1993. Expression of endothelin-1 in lungs of patients with cryptogenic fibrosing alveolitis. Lancet **341:** 1550–1554.
39. ZAMORA, M.A., E.C. DEMPSEY, *et al.* 1993. BQ123, an ETA receptor antagonist, inhibits endothelin-1-mediated proliferation of human pulmonary artery smooth muscle cells. Am. J. Respir. Cell. Mol. Biol. **9:** 429–433.
40. WILLIAMSON, D.J., L.L. WALLMAN, *et al.* 2000. Hemodynamic effects of Bosentan, an endothelin receptor antagonist, in patients with pulmonary hypertension. Circulation **102:** 411–418.
41. RUBIN, L.J., D.B. BADESCH, *et al.* 2002. Bosentan therapy for pulmonary arterial hypertension. N. Engl. J. Med. **346:** 896–903.
42. Available at: http://genecanvas.idf.inserm.fr/
43. BENJAFIELD, A.V., K. KATYK, *et al.* 2003. Association of EDNRA, but not WNK4 or FKBP1B, polymorphisms with essential hypertension. Clin. Genet. **64:** 433–438.
44. BROWN, M.J., P. SHARMA, *et al.* 2000. Association between diastolic blood pressure and variants of the endothelin-1 and endothelin-2 genes. J. Cardiovasc. Pharmacol. **35:** S41–S43.

45. CHARRON, P., F. TESSON, *et al.* 1999. Identification of a genetic risk factor for idiopathic dilated cardiomyopathy. Involvement of a polymorphism in the endothelin receptor type A gene. CARDIGENE group. Eur. Heart J. **20:** 1587–1591.
46. DIEFENBACH, K., F.A. NAHAD, *et al.* 2004. Identification of twelve polymorphisms in the endothelin-1 gene by use of fluorescently labeled oligonucleotides and PCR with restriction fragment polymorphism analysis. Clin. Chem. **50:** 448–451.
47. DONG, Y., X. WANG, *et al.* 2004. Endothelin-1 gene and progression of blood pressure and left ventricular mass: longitudinal findings in youth. Hypertension **44:** 884–890.
48. FUNALOT, B., D. COURBON, *et al.* 2004. Genes encoding endothelin-converting enzyme-1 and endothelin-1 interact to influence blood pressure in women: the EVA study. J. Hypertens. **22:** 739–743.
49. FUNKE-KAISER, H., F. REICHENBERGER, *et al.* 2003. Differential binding of transcription factor E2F-2 to the endothelin-converting enzyme-1b promoter affects blood pressure regulation. Hum. Mol. Genet. **12:** 423–433.
50. GATH, R., A. GOESSLING, *et al.* 2001. Analysis of the RET, GDNF, EDN3, and EDNRB genes in patients with intestinal neuronal dysplasia and Hirschsprung disease. Gut **48:** 671–675.
51. GORMLEY, K., S. BEVAN, *et al.* 2005. Polymorphisms in genes of the endothelin system and cerebral small-vessel disease. Stroke **36:** 1656–1660.
52. GUMPRECHT, J., M.J. ZYCHMA, *et al.* 2000. Angiotensin I-converting enzyme gene insertion/deletion and angiotensinogen M235T polymorphisms: risk of chronic renal failure. End-Stage Renal Disease Study Group. Kidney Int. **58:** 513–519.
53. GUMPRECHT, J., M. ZYCHMA, *et al.* 2002. Angiotensin I-converting enzyme and chymase gene polymorphisms—relationship to left ventricular mass in type 2 diabetes patients. Med. Sci. Monit. **8:** CR603–CR606.
54. HE, H., L.M. LI, *et al.* 2005. A study of the relationships between angiotensin- converting enzyme gene, chymase gene polymorphisms, pharmacological treatment with ACE inhibitor and regression of left ventricular hypertrophy in essential hypertension patients treated with benazepril. Ann. Hum. Biol. **32:** 30–43.
55. HERRMANN, S., K. SCHMIDT-PETERSEN, *et al.* 2001. A polymorphism in the endothelin-A receptor gene predicts survival in patients with idiopathic dilated cardiomyopathy. Eur. Heart J. **22:** 1948–1953.
56. ISHIKAWA, K., T. FUNAYAMA, *et al.* 2005. Association between glaucoma and gene polymorphism of endothelin type A receptor. Mol. Vis. **11:** 431–437.
57. KAETSU, A., T. KISHIMOTO, *et al.* 2004. The lack of relationship between an endothelin-1 gene polymorphism (Ala288ser) and incidence of hypertension: a retrospective cohort study among Japanese workers. J. Epidemiol. **14:** 129–136.
58. NALOGOWSKA-GLOSNICKA, K., B.I. LACKA, *et al.* 2000. Angiotensin II type 1 receptor gene A1166C polymorphism is associated with the increased risk of pregnancy-induced hypertension. Med. Sci. Monit. **6:** 523–529.
59. NICAUD, V., O. POIRIER, *et al.* 1999. Polymorphisms of the endothelin-A and -B receptor genes in relation to blood pressure and myocardial infarction: the Etude Cas-Temoins sur l'Infarctus du Myocarde (ECTIM) Study Am. J. Hypertens. **12:** 304–310.
60. ORTLEPP, J.R., U. JANSSENS, *et al.* 2001. A chymase gene variant is associated with atherosclerosis in venous coronary artery bypass grafts. Coron. Artery Dis. **12:** 493–497.

61. PFEUFER, A., K.J. OSTERZIEL, *et al.* 1996. Angiotensin-converting enzyme and heart chymase gene polymorphisms in hypertrophic cardiomyopathy. Am. J. Cardiol. **78:** 362–364.
62. PINTO-SIETSMA, S.J., S.M. HERRMANN, *et al.* 2003. Role of the endothelin-1 gene locus for renal impairment in the general nondiabetic population. J. Am. Soc. Nephrol. **14:** 2596–2602.
63. STEVENS, P.A. & M.J. BROWN. 1995. Genetic variability of the ET-1 and the ETA receptor genes in essential hypertension. J. Cardiovasc. Pharmacol. (26 Suppl.) **3:** S9–S12.
64. TANAKA, C., K. KAMIDE, *et al.* 2004. Evaluation of the Lys198Asn and -134delA genetic polymorphisms of the endothelin-1 gene. Hypertens. Res. **27:** 367–371.
65. TIRET, L., O. POIRIER, *et al.* 1999. The Lys198Asn polymorphism in the endothelin-1 gene is associated with blood pressure in overweight people. Hypertension **33:** 1169–1174.
66. TZOURIO, C., M. EL AMRANI, *et al.* 2001. Association between migraine and endothelin type A receptor (ETA -231 A/G) gene polymorphism. Neurology **56:** 1273–1277.
67. VASKU, A., L. SPINAROVA, *et al.* 2002. The double heterozygote of two endothelin-1 gene polymorphisms (G8002A and -3A/-4A) is related to big endothelin levels in chronic heart failure. Exp. Mol. Pathol. **73:** 230–233.
68. VASKU, V., A. VASKU, *et al.* 2002. Genotype association of C(-735)T polymorphism in matrix metalloproteinase 2 gene with G(8002)A endothelin 1 gene with plaque psoriasis. Dermatology **204:** 262–265.
69. WARPEHA, K.M., F. AH-FAT, *et al.* 1999. Dinucleotide repeat polymorphisms in EDN1 and NOS3 are not associated with severe diabetic retinopathy in type 1 or type 2 diabetes. Eye **13:** 174–178.
70. ZAAHL, M.G., P.L. DU, *et al.* 2003. Significance of novel endothelin-B receptor gene polymorphisms in Hirschsprung's disease: predominance of a novel variant (561C/T) in patients with co-existing Down's syndrome. Mol. Cell. Probes. **17:** 49–54.
71. ZEE, R.Y., V.S. RAO, *et al.* 1998. Three candidate genes and angiotensin-converting enzyme inhibitor-related cough: a pharmacogenetic analysis. Hypertension **31:** 925–928.
72. ZYCHMA, M.J., E. ZUKOWSKA-SZCZECHOWSKA, *et al.* 2000. Angiotensinogen M235T and chymase gene CMA/B polymorphisms are not associated with nephropathy in type II diabetes Nephrol. Dial. Transplant. **15:** 1965–1970.
73. HOSODA, K., R.E. HAMMER, *et al.* 1994. Targeted and natural (Piebald-lethal) mutations of endothelin-B receptor gene produce megacolon associated with spotted coat color in mice. Cell **79:** 1267–1276.
74. PUFFENBERGER, E.G., K. HOSODA, *et al.* 1994. A missense mutation of the endothelin-B receptor gene in multigenic Hirschsprung's disease. Cell **79:** 1257–1266.
75. TIRET, L. 2002. Gene-environment interaction: a central concept in multifactorial diseases. Proc. Nutr. Soc. **61:** 457–463.
76. DEN DUNNEN, J.T. & S.E. ANTONARAKIS. 2001. Nomenclature for the description of human sequence variations. Hum. Genet. **109:** 121–124.

Stress in Autoimmune Disease Models

M.S. HARBUZ,[a] L.J. RICHARDS,[a] A.J. CHOVER-GONZALEZ,[b]
O. MARTI-SISTAC,[c] AND D.S. JESSOP[a]

[a]*HW LINE, Dorothy Hodgkin Building, Whitson Street, Bristol, United Kingdom*

[b]*Facultad de Medicina, Universidad de Cadiz, Spain*

[c]*Dept. de Biologia Cellular de Fisiologia i d'Immunologia, Sphere Universitat Autonoma de Barcelona, Barcelona, Spain*

ABSTRACT: The release of endogenous glucocorticoids is critical in regulating the severity of disease activity in patients with inflammatory conditions such as rheumatoid arthritis (RA). Blocking cortisol production results in a flare-up in disease activity in RA patients, and surgical removal of the adrenals in patients with Cushing's disease has been reported to exacerbate autoimmune disease. In adjuvant-induced arthritis (AA; a rat model of RA), there is an activation of the hypothalamo-pituitary-adrenal (HPA) axis associated with the development of inflammation. In addition, there are profound changes in peptides within the paraventricular nucleus, which are responsible for regulating the HPA axis. These changes have profound implications on the ability of AA rats to respond to acute stress. Understanding the regulation of the HPA axis in health and disease holds out the promise of targeted therapy to alleviate inflammatory conditions. This article will consider the impact of stress on an individual and his or her susceptibility to inflammation. We wish to question the idea that stress is "all bad." As we shall see, exposure to a single acute stressor can alter the phenotype of the rat to change it from being susceptible to resistant in autoimmune disease models. This alteration in susceptibility takes days to manifest itself, but can last for weeks, suggesting beneficial effects of exposure to an acute stressor.

KEYWORDS: stress; HPA axis; CRF; AVP; inflammation

INTRODUCTION

Despite a considerable amount of research, a definition of stress remains as elusive today as when Hans Selye first coined the term in the 1930s. Recently, Bruce McEwen wrote, "Stress may be defined as a real or interpreted threat to the physiological or psychological integrity of an individual that results in physiological and/or behavioral responses."[1] Other authors have defined stress

Address for correspondence: Dr. D. S. Jessop, HW LINE, Dorothy Hodgkin Building, Whitson Street, Bristol BS1 3NY, UK. Voice: +44-117-3313050; fax: +44-117-3313049.
e-mail: David.Jessop@bristol.ac.uk

**Ann. N.Y. Acad. Sci. 1069: 51–61 (2006). © 2006 New York Academy of Sciences.
doi: 10.1196/annals.1351.005**

as a "state of disharmony or threatened homeostasis."[2] More recently, the concept of allostasis has broadened this idea to include variations that reflect the situation of the individual, for example, time of day, whether the individual is rested, etc. Implicit in many of the definitions in the literature is the idea of stress as being a disturbance or threat, essentially a negative event that homeostatic and allostatic mechanisms are designed to counter. These homeostatic and allostatic mechanisms are considered to return the systems back to their starting point.

For the purposes of this review, we will consider the definition provided by McEwen.[1] "In biomedicine, stress often refers to situations in which adrenal glucocorticoids . . . are elevated because of an experience." The elevation in glucocorticoids from the adrenal cortex is under the control of ACTH released from the anterior pituitary. ACTH is in turn regulated by the release of corticotropin-releasing factor (CRF) and arginine vasopressin (AVP) from the median eminence into the hypophysial portal blood. CRF and AVP are synthesized in the parvocellular cells of the paraventricular nucleus (PVN). Following acute stress, the hypothalamo-pituitary-adrenal (HPA) axis is activated, resulting in the release of corticosterone into the blood. Glucocorticoids (corticosterone in the rat, cortisol in man) have a negative feedback action at the pituitary, hypothalamus, and other brain areas to restore homeostasis.[3,4] The termination of the stress response is important for long-term health and survival. In addition to glucocorticoids, a number of other factors have been identified, which are also able to inhibit HPA axis activity (for review, see Ref. 5). Failure of these systems to effectively terminate the stress response at an appropriate time following activation may result in the development of disease.

The activation and termination of the HPA axis response to acute stress is relatively well understood. The situation with chronic stress is much more complex. In practice, many chronic stress studies in rodents have utilized repeated acute stress paradigms to mimic chronic stress. When stressors are repeated over a period of time, then habituation or adaptation of the ACTH and corticosterone response to the repeated stress occurs. Studies have shown that immobilization or restraint stress, ethanol administration, i.p. administration of hypertonic saline solution or footshock stress all elevate corticosterone acutely. However, with repeated administration, the elevated levels begin to lower toward base line despite repeated exposure to the stressor. This is not to say that the animals become refractory to stress. Indeed, the response to a novel heterotypic stressor will be normal or even exaggerated. This is reflected by increases in pro-opiomelanocortin (POMC) mRNA in the anterior pituitary and in adrenal weight in repeated/chronically stressed rats, suggesting an increase in the capacity of these rats to respond to heterotypic stress, but not to a homotypic stressor. This alteration in the HPA axis responsiveness to homotypic stressors is mediated at a central level through coordination, at the level of the PVN, of signals from different afferent pathways. A number of studies have highlighted the importance of AVP in maintaining HPA axis responsiveness in chronic stress situations when CRF is often refractory (for review, see Ref. 6). We have recently reported that chronic treatment with the selective serotonin reuptake inhibitor citalopram preferentially upregulates AVP mRNA in the parvocellular cells of the PVN.[7] The data suggest that vasopressin is crucial in maintaining HPA axis responsiveness in chronic stress situations when CRF may be downregulated.

An area that has received comparatively little attention concerns the long-term effects of a single acute stressor. Following an acute stress, ACTH and corticosterone concentrations are elevated for a matter of minutes to hours before returning to base line. There is a subsequent elevation in mRNA encoding for AVP and/or CRF in the PVN and POMC in the anterior pituitary. These return to base line after a few hours. The underlying assumption is that within hours of the termination of an acute stressor, the HPA axis will be returned to its original state. However, an area of increasing interest concerns the ability of a single acute stress to alter responsiveness to a variety of stressors several days or even weeks after the initial exposure. A number of stressors have been used, including physical stressors such as footshock and immobilization, predominantly psychological stressors such as social defeat, immune challenges such as interleukin-1 and lipopolysaccharide (LPS; endotoxin), and drugs like amphetamine and alcohol.[8–14] This long-term alteration in stress responsiveness appears to be partially, but not fully, mediated by glucocorticoids.[15,16] However, at a central level, there is evidence for plasticity in the noradrenergic innervation of the PVN following single administration of IL-1α or amphetamine,[17] and that these long-term adaptations to IL-1 involve CRF signaling in the PVN.[18] A number of other brain areas in addition to the PVN have also been implicated in the long-term effects of LPS administration including the central amygdala, lateral division of the bed nucleus of the stria terminalis, and the locus coeruleus.[19] Together, these reports highlight the importance of the stress history of individuals for stress studies and for the critical need for contemporary controls in all such investigations.

The adjuvant-induced arthritis (AA) model has been used as a model of pain, inflammation, and rheumatoid arthritis (RA).[20,21] In the rat, the model involves a single intradermal injection of a suspension of ground, heat-killed *Mycobacterium butyricum* in paraffin oil. Typically, the animals show a reddening of the paws at around day 12 or 13 after adjuvant injection, and hind paw inflammation is usually apparent at day 14. Maximum severity occurs at around day 21, after which the inflammation begins to subside. Associated with the development of inflammation there is an increase in adrenal weight, circulating corticosterone and ACTH, and increased POMC mRNA in the anterior pituitary. Paradoxically, there is a decrease in CRF mRNA in the PVN although AVP mRNA levels are increased in the parvocellular subdivision of the PVN.[22,23] The data suggest that in this chronic inflammatory stress model, there is an alteration in hypothalamic regulation of the HPA axis with an increased role for AVP similar to the situation with other chronic/repeated stressors. Indeed, the paradoxical decrease in CRF mRNA and/or an increase in AVP has been noted in a variety of immune-mediated disease models, including experimental allergic encephalomyelitis (EAE; model of choice for multiple sclerosis research) and eosinophilia myalgia syndrome in the rat, leishmaniasis and systemic lupus erythematosus in mice, and multiple sclerosis in humans (for review, see Ref. 4). The alteration in hypothalamic control appears to be a feature of a wide range of autoimmune disease models in rats and mice and may also be a feature of autoimmune disease in humans. It would appear that the major drive to the pituitary–adrenal axis is provided by AVP, while CRF acts in a secondary, permissive role. The role of the HPA axis in patients with RA has recently been reviewed.[24] The role of AVP in RA, MS, and other autoimmune diseases in humans has also been reviewed.[25,26]

The integrity of the HPA axis is critical for survival following immune activation. Adrenalectomized rodents do not survive injection of cytokines or LPS at doses tolerated in the adrenal-intact animal. Similarly, chronic immune activation associated with the development of AA and EAE is fatal in adrenalectomized rats, where animals develop the disease more rapidly than adrenal-intact individuals. Symptoms can be prevented by steroid replacement.[27,28] Supporting evidence has been provided by observations in patients. Metyrapone treatment, which blocks cortisol synthesis, results in an exacerbation of disease activity in patients with RA.[29] Furthermore, removal of the adrenal gland in patients with Cushing's syndrome has exacerbated RA and autoimmune thyroid disease.[30,31]

These changes in hypothalamic regulation have a profound influence on the ability of AA rats to respond to acute stress. Indeed, we have noted an inability of AA rats to respond either to predominantly psychological stressors, such as restraint and noise stress, or to a physical stressor such as i.p. hypertonic saline.[28,32,33] A similar inability to mount a cortisol response to joint replacement surgery has been reported in patients with RA,[34] although a further study reported a normal response,[35] suggesting that more work will be required to tease out these discrepancies in humans. In contrast to the hyporesponsiveness to predominantly psychological and physical stressors, AA rats are able to mount a response to LPS injection at all levels of the HPA axis.[36] Clearly, there are different pathways mediating these different stressors. An inability to damp down the immune response provoked by LPS injection, by stimulating corticosterone release, has been shown to be fatal. It would appear that there are secondary mechanisms to override the inhibition of the CRF neuron at the level of the PVN, preventing the response to nonfatal stimuli that ensure an HPA axis response to potentially fatal immune stimuli.

A fundamental question is, "what determines whether an individual is likely to develop an autoimmune disease?" Genetic susceptibility has been invoked. A defect in HPA axis responsivity to acute stress has been suggested as underlying susceptibility to disease.[37,27] The hypothesis suggested that an inability to mount an appropriate HPA axis response to the onset of disease allowed the disease to develop unchecked. It was assumed that the systems involved were hard-wired and susceptibility predetermined. These observations acted as a spur to further research and as the decade progressed, numerous studies explored this hypothesis. The original studies had noted that the Lewis strain of rat with poor HPA axis responsiveness was susceptible to disease, whereas the Fischer and PVG strains with a good response were resistant. However, comparison of different strains showed that HPA axis responsiveness and severity of disease were not always related.[4] A number of studies showed that differences in housing/environmental conditions could alter development of experimental arthritis. Germ-free rats are highly susceptible to experimental arthritis, whereas conventionally housed rats of the same strain are resistant.[38–40] We have noted that rats kept in clean (but not germ-free) conditions are resistant to AA and remain so for 48 h after transfer to a stock room. However, after a week in the stock room, they become susceptible.[4] These data suggest an inherent plasticity in the system in that bacterial microflora present in the environment may alter resistance and reactivation of experimental arthritis.[40,41]

It is well established that HPA axis and immune plasticity exist during the neonatal period, whereby intervention during this early developmental period can alter adult responses.[42] We decided to investigate whether neonatal treatments, known to alter HPA axis responsivity, could alter susceptibility to AA. We compared the effects of neonatal handling (pups removed from their home cage for 15–20 min each day for the first 21 days after birth until the pups were weaned) and exposure to LPS.[43] Handling has previously been shown to decrease HPA axis responsiveness in later life.[44] Pups exposed to handling and challenged with adjuvant as adults did not show an alteration in susceptibility or severity of inflammation. In contrast, the rats treated with LPS as pups were completely protected and showed no evidence of inflammation. Of interest was the observation that the HPA axis activation seen in rats with inflammation was also present in those rats that were protected, suggesting that other factors besides the HPA axis were involved in the protective effects.

The plasticity in the neonatal rat is well established. However, beyond the neonatal period, it is generally thought that systems become hard-wired and no longer have that same adaptability. In order to investigate this, we determined whether the effects of acute stress could modify the susceptibility or severity of AA in adults. Rats were exposed to either footshock or LPS, and returned to their home cages for a period of 3 wk prior to the induction of AA. The development of inflammation in the rats exposed to footshock was normal.[45] In contrast, however, rats injected with LPS 3 wk prior to adjuvant injection were completely protected and showed no signs of inflammation even at 3 wk after adjuvant injection, the time of maximum severity in this model (FIG. 1). In addition to the generalized immune response evoked by LPS, a single administration of interleukin (IL)-1β 1 wk prior to induction of EAE was shown to markedly suppress the neurological symptoms of EAE.[46] A shift to enhanced AVP stores in the median eminence was observed in this study,

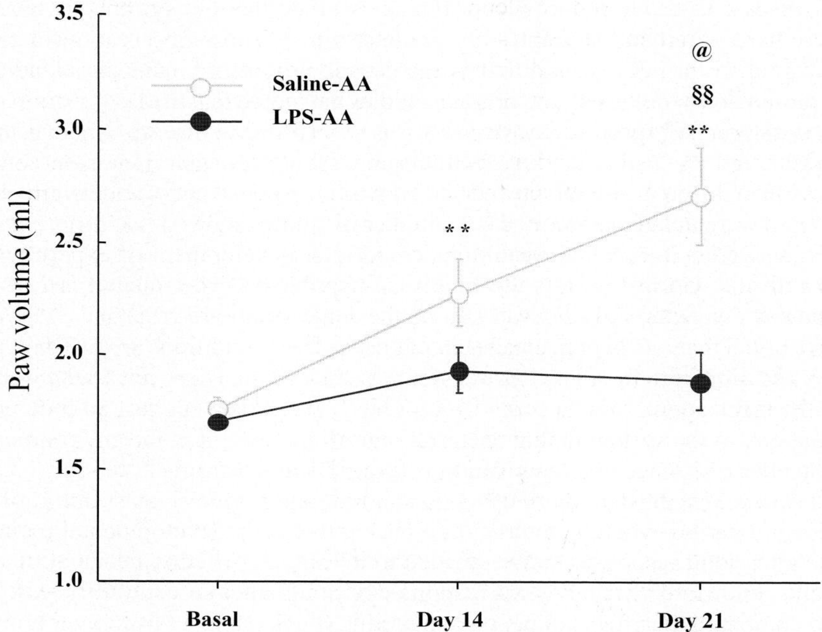

FIGURE 1. Paw volume (mL) of rats on day 0 (basal), day 14 and day 21 following injection of adjuvant (AA). The rats had previously been exposed to either saline (Saline-AA) or LPS (LPS-AA), three weeks prior to injection of adjuvant. Data represent means ± SEM (n = 8 rats/group). $^{**}P < 0.01$, compared to basal levels. §§$P < 0.01$ Saline-AA compared to LPS-AA at day 21. @$P < 0.05$ Saline-AA at day 21 compared to Saline-AA at day 14. Reprinted from reference 45. Copyright (2002), with permission from Elsevier Press.

suggesting alterations at a central level mediating these effects. However, morning corticosterone levels were unaffected following immunization or during the clinical phase, suggesting that the mechanisms underlying IL-1-induced suppression of EAE were not related to enhanced HPA axis responses.

A number of studies have investigated the mechanisms underlying the observed protective effects of stress and have looked at HPA axis and immune responsiveness at various times following the initial exposure to the acute immune challenge. Huitinga *et al.*[46] noted that 11 days after initial exposure to IL-1β, a repeated exposure to IL-1β resulted in an attenuated ACTH response. An attenuated ACTH and corticosterone response to LPS were noted 1 wk and 4 wk after initial exposure to LPS, providing further evidence for an inherent plasticity in the adult system [47]. Also observed in this study was an attenuation in the tumor necrosis factor (TNF)-α response to the second LPS challenge when compared with the first exposure. A concern in these studies is the possibility of habituation to the initial challenge, as the same stimulus was used for the second challenge. In order to address this issue, we have recently determined the HPA axis and immune system responsiveness to a second LPS challenge of a different serotype to that used for the initial challenge. We have observed that injection of adjuvant 1 wk after first exposure to LPS only partially protects the rats and that although there is a slight reduction in the severity of inflammation, the rat's paws do become inflamed. This suggests that the protective effects take between 1 and 3 wk to develop. We therefore gave a second challenge of a different serotype of LPS at 1 wk and 3 wk after the first challenge. Using this experimental paradigm, we have confirmed the above observations of an attenuated ACTH and corticosterone response to the second exposure to LPS when given 1 wk after the initial LPS challenge. This is consistent with the idea that decreased HPA axis responsiveness at this time contributes to the inflammatory process. In addition, a reduced activation of pro-inflammatory cytokines (IL-1β, TNF-α, and IFN-γ), both *in vivo* and *in vitro*, was observed while anti-inflammatory cytokine release (IL-10) was maintained. However, at 3 wk after the first LPS exposure, in addition to the decrease in pro-inflammatory cytokines and maintained levels of IL-10, there was a robust and rapid response of ACTH and corticosterone to the second LPS injection. This combination of decreased pro-inflammatory cytokines and increased anti-inflammatory cytokines and hormones may together contribute to the overall anti-inflammatory milieu seen 3 wk after initial exposure to LPS.

Recently, we have observed two subpopulations of patients with RA that differ in their ability to escape from dexamethasone suppression in response to challenge with CRF.[48] It remains to be determined whether an early escape from dexamethasone suppression is associated with altered pathology. However, use of the dexamethasone-CRF test holds out great prospect for the targeted treatment of RA patients who may, or may not, be receptive to glucocorticoid treatment.

In summary, the development of inflammation in the rat model of AA is associated with a profound alteration in hypothalamic regulation of the HPA axis, with a switch to AVP over CRF in the PVN. This decrease in CRF activity is also observed in a number of immune-mediated disease models. This paradoxical decrease in CRF activity occurs despite an increase in the release of ACTH and corticosterone. This alteration in hypothalamic regulation has a major effect on the ability of the HPA axis to respond to acute stress. Animals with AA have a reduced or absent response to predominantly psychological and physical stressors that are nonfatal, while response to the potentially fatal challenge of bacterial infection remains intact. While acute exposure to LPS is pro-inflammatory, the long-term effects of LPS exposure have a protective beneficial role in AA that is not fully present at 1 wk after LPS injection, but is present at 3 wk. This protective effect is associated with alterations in both HPA axis and immune parameters, with an overall shift to an anti-inflammatory milieu that prevents inflammation in this model. These changes reveal the inherent plasticity in the systems, which alters the phenotype of rats from AA-susceptible to AA-resistant. These data add to the accumulating evidence to suggest that susceptibility to disease is modulated by environment and is not entirely dependent on genetic factors.

ACKNOWLEDGMENT

We would like to acknowledge the support of The Wellcome Trust.

REFERENCES

1. McEwen, B. 2000. Stress, definition and concepts of. *In* Encylcopedia of Stress, Vol 3. G. Fink, Ed.: 508–509. Academic Press. San Diego.
2. Chrousos, G.P. & P.W. Gold. 1992. The concepts of stress and stress systems disorders. JAMA **267:** 1244–1252.
3. Buckingham, J.C., A.-M. Cowell, G. Gillies, *et al.* 1998. The neuroendocrine system: anatomy, physiology and responses to stress. *In* Stress, Stress Hormones and the Immune System. J.C. Buckingham, G. Gillies & A.-M. Cowell, Eds.: 9–47. John Wiley. New York.
4. Harbuz, M. 2002. Neuroendocrinology of autoimmunity. Int. Rev. Neurobiol. **52:** 133–161.
5. Jessop, D.S. 1999. Central non-glucocorticoid inhibitors of the hypothalamo-pituitary-adrenal axis. J. Endocrinol. **160:** 169–180.
6. Aguilera, G. & C. Rabadan-Diehl. 2000. Vasopressinergic regulation of the hypothalamic-pituitary-adrenal axis: implications for stress adaptation. Regul. Pept. **96:** 23–29.
7. Hesketh, S., D.S. Jessop, S. Hogg & M.S. Harbuz. 2005. Differential actions of acute and chronic citalopram on the rodent hypothalamic-pituitary-adrenal axis response to acute restraint stress. J. Endocrinol. **185:** 373–382.
8. Schmidt, E.D., A.W. Janszen, F.G. Wouterlood, *et al.* 1995. Interleukin-1-induced long-lasting changes in hypothalamic corticotropin-releasing hormone (CRH)-neurons and hyperresponsiveness of the hypothalamus-pituitary-adrenal axis. J. Neurosci. **15:** 7417–7426.
9. Schmidt, E.D., A.N. Schoffelmeer, T.J. De Vries, *et al.* 2001. A single administration of interleukin-1 or amphetamine induces long-lasting increases in evoked noradrenaline release in the hypothalamus and sensitization of ACTH and corticosterone responses in rats. Eur. J. Neurosci. **13:** 1923–1930.
10. Tilders, F.J., E.D. Schmidt, W.J. Hoogendijk & D.F. Swaab. 1999. Delayed effects of stress and immune activation. Baillieres Best Pract. Res. Clin. Endocrinol. Metab. **13:** 523–540.
11. Vanderschuren, L.J., E.D. Schmidt, T.J. De Vries, *et al.* 1999. A single exposure to amphetamine is sufficient to induce long-term behavioral, neuroendocrine, and neurochemical sensitization in rats. J. Neurosci. **19:** 9579–9586.
12. Lee, S., E.D. Schmidt, F.J. Tilders & C. Rivier. 2001. Effect of repeated exposure to alcohol on the response of the hypothalamic-pituitary-adrenal axis of the rat: I. Role of changes in hypothalamic neuronal activity. Alcohol Clin. Exp. Res. **25:** 98–105.

13. MARTI, O., A. GARCIA, A. VALLES, *et al.* 2001. Evidence that a single exposure to aversive stimuli triggers long-lasting effects in the hypothalamus-pituitary-adrenal axis that consolidate with time. Eur. J. Neurosci. **13:** 129–136.
14. VALLES, A., O. MARTI & A. ARMARIO. 2003. Long-term effects of a single exposure to immobilization stress on the hypothalamic-pituitary-adrenal axis: transcriptional evidence for a progressive desensitization process. Eur. J. Neurosci. **18:** 1353–1361.
15. DAL-ZOTTO, S., O. MARTI & A. ARMARIO. 2003. Glucocorticoids are involved in the long-term effects of a single immobilization stress on the hypothalamic-pituitary-adrenal axis. Psychoneuroendocrinology **28:** 992–1009.
16. DAL-ZOTTO, S., O. MARTI, R. DELGADO & A. ARMARIO. 2004. Potentiation of glucocorticoid release does not modify the long-term effects of a single exposure to immobilization stress. Psychopharmacology **177:** 230–237.
17. JANSEN, A.S., E.D. SCHMIDT, P. VOORN & F.J. TILDERS. 2003. Substance induced plasticity in noradrenergic innervation of the paraventricular hypothalamic nucleus. Eur. J. Neurosci. **17:** 298–306.
18. SCHMIDT, E.D., G. AGUILERA, R. BINNEKADE & F.J. TILDERS. 2003. Single administration of interleukin-1 increased corticotropin releasing hormone and corticotropin releasing hormone-receptor mRNA in the hypothalamic paraventricular nucleus which paralleled long-lasting (weeks) sensitization to emotional stressors. Neuroscience **116:** 275–283.
19. VALLES, A., O. MARTI & A. ARMARIO. 2005. Mapping the areas sensitive to long-term endotoxin tolerance in the rat brain: a c-fos mRNA study. J. Neurochem. **93:** 1177–1188.
20. BOMHOLT, S.F., M.S. HARBUZ, G. BLACKBURN-MUNRO & R.E. BLACKBURN-MUNRO. 2004. Involvement and role of the hypothalamo-pituitary-adrenal (HPA) stress axis in animal models of chronic pain and inflammation. Stress **7:** 1–14.
21. ROSENTHALE, M.E. & R.J. CAPETOLA. 1982. Adjuvant arthritis: immunopathological and hyperalgesic features. Fed. Proc. **41:** 2577–2582.
22. HARBUZ, M.S., R.G. REES, D. ECKLAND, *et al.* 1992. Paradoxical responses of hypothalamic CRF mRNA and CRF-41 peptide and adenohypophyseal POMC mRNA during chronic inflammatory stress. Endocrinology **130:** 1394–1400.
23. CHOWDREY, H.S., P.J. LARSEN, M.S. HARBUZ, *et al.* 1995. Evidence for arginine vasopressin as the primary activator of the HPA axis during adjuvant-induced arthritis. Br. J. Pharmacol. **116:** 2417–2424.
24. JESSOP, D.S. & M.S. HARBUZ. 2005. A defect in cortisol production in rheumatoid arthritis: why are we still looking? Rheumatology **44:** 1097–1100.
25. CHIKANZA, I.C. & A.S. GROSSMAN. 1998. Hypothalamic-pituitary-mediated immunomodulation: arginine vasopressin is a neuroendocrine immune mediator. Br. J. Rheumatol. **37:** 131–136.
26. CHIKANZA, I.C., P. PETROU & G. CHROUSOS. 2000. Perturbations of arginine vasopressin secretion during inflammatory stress: pathophysiologic implications. Ann. N. Y. Acad. Sci. **917:** 825–834.
27. MASON, D., I. MACPHEE & F. ANTONI. 1990. The role of the neuroendocrine system in determining genetic susceptibility to experimental encephalomyelitis in the rat. Immunology **70:** 1–5.
28. HARBUZ, M.S., R.G. REES & S.L. LIGHTMAN. 1993. Hypothalamo-pituitary responses to acute stress and changes in circulating glucocorticoids during chronic adjuvant-induced arthritis in the rat. Am. J. Physiol. **264:** R179–R185.

29. PANAYI, G.S. 1992. Neuroendocrine modulation of disease expression in rheumatoid arthritis. Eular Congress Rep. **2:** 2–12.
30. TAKASU, N., I. KOMIYA, Y. NAGASAWA, *et al.* 1990. Exacerbation of autoimmune thyroid dysfunction after unilateral adrenalectomy in patients with Cushing's syndrome due to an adrenocortical adenoma. N. Engl. J. Med. **322:** 1708–1712.
31. YAKUSHIJI, F., M. KITA, N. HIROI, *et al.* 1995. Exacerbation of rheumatoid arthritis after removal of adrenal adenoma in Cushing's syndrome. Endocr. J. **42:** 219–223.
32. AGUILERA, G., D.S. JESSOP, M.S. HARBUZ, *et al.* 1997. Biphasic regulation of hypothalamic-pituitary corticotropin releasing hormone receptors during development of adjuvant-induced arthritis in the rat. J. Endocrinol. **153:** 185–191.
33. WINDLE, R.J., S.A. WOOD, Y.M. KERSHAW, *et al.* 2001. Increased corticosterone pulse frequency during adjuvant-induced arthritis and its relationship to alterations in stress responsiveness. J. Neuroendocrinol. **13:** 905–911.
34. CHIKANZA, I.C., P. PETROU, G. KINGSLEY, *et al.* 1992. Defective hypothalamic response to immune and inflammatory stimuli in patients with rheumatoid arthritis. Arthritis Rheum. **35:** 1281–1288.
35. EIJSBOUTS, A., F. VAN DEN HOOGEN, R. LAAN, *et al.* 1998. Similar response of adrenocorticotrophic hormone, cortisol and prolactin to surgery in rheumatoid arthritis and osteoarthritis. Br. J. Rheumatol. **37:** 1138–1139.
36. HARBUZ, M.S., C. ROONEY, M. JONES & C.D. INGRAM. 1999. Hypothalamo-pituitary-adrenal axis responses to lipopolysaccharide in male and female rats with adjuvant-induced arthritis. Brain Behav. Immun. **13:** 335–347.
37. STERNBERG, E.M., W.S. YOUNG, R. BERNARDINI, *et al.* 1989. A central nervous system defect in biosynthesis of corticotropin-releasing hormone is associated with the susceptibility to streptococcal cell wall-induced arthritis in Lewis rats. Proc. Natl. Acad. Sci. USA **86:** 4771–4775.
38. VAN DEN BROEK, M.F., M.C. VAN BRUGGEN, J.P. KOOPMAN, *et al.* 1992. Gut flora induces and maintains resistance against streptococcal cell wall-induced arthritis in F344 rats. Clin. Exp. Immunol. **88:** 313–317.
39. GRIPENBERG-LERCHE, C. & P. TOIVANEN. 1993. Yersinia associated arthritis in SHR rats: effect of the microbial status of the host. Ann. Rheum. Dis. **52:** 223–228.
40. VAN DE LANGERIJT, A.G., P.L. VAN LENT, A.R. HERMUS, *et al.* 1993. Susceptibility to adjuvant arthritis: relative importance of adrenal activity and bacterial flora. Clin. Exp. Immunol. **94:** 150–155.
41. LICHTMAN, S.N., J. WANG, R.B. SARTOR, *et al.* 1995. Reactivation of arthritis induced by small bowel bacterial overgrowth in rats: role of cytokines, bacteria, and bacterial polymers. Infect. Immun. **63:** 2295–2301.
42. FRANCIS, D.D., F.A. CHAMPAGNE, D. LIU & M.J. MEANEY. 1999. Maternal care, gene expression, and the development of individual differences in stress reactivity. Ann. N. Y. Acad. Sci. **896:** 66–84.
43. SHANKS, N., R.J. WINDLE, P.A. PERKS, *et al.* 2000. Early-life exposure to endotoxin alters hypothalamic-pituitary-adrenal function and predisposition to inflammation. Proc. Natl. Acad. Sci. USA **97:** 5645–5650.
44. LEVINE, S. 1967. Maternal and environmental influences on the adrenocortical response to stress in weanling rats. Science **156:** 258–260.
45. HARBUZ, M.S., A.J. CHOVER-GONZALEZ, J. GIBERT-RAHOLA & D.S. JESSOP. 2002. Protective effect of prior acute immune challenge, but not stress, on inflammation in the rat. Brain Behav. Immun. **16:** 439–449.

46. HUITINGA, I., E.D. SCHMIDT, M.J. VAN DER CAMMEN, *et al.* 2000. Priming with interleukin-1beta suppresses experimental allergic encephalomyelitis in the Lewis rat. J. Neuroendocrinol. **12:** 1186–1193.
47. VALLES, A., O. MARTI, M.S. HARBUZ & A. ARMARIO. 2002. A single lipopolysaccharide administration is sufficient to induce a long-term desensitization of the hypothalamic-pituitary-adrenal axis. Neuroscience **112:** 383–389.
48. HARBUZ, M.S., D.S. KORENDOWYCH, D.S. JESSOP, *et al.* 2003. HPA axis dysregulation in patients with rheumatoid arthritis following the dexamethasone-CRF test. J. Endocrinol. **178:** 55–60.

Stress System Activity, Innate and T Helper Cytokines, and Susceptibility to Immune-Related Diseases

EMANUELE CALCAGNI AND ILIA ELENKOV

Laboratory of Neuro-Endocrine-Immunology, San Raffaele Research Center, Rome 00163, Italy

ABSTRACT: Associations between stress and health outcomes have now been carefully documented, but the mechanisms by which stress specifically influences disease susceptibility and outcome remain poorly understood. Recent evidence indicates that glucocorticoids (GCs) and catecholamines (CAs), the major stress hormones, inhibit systemically IL-12, TNF-α, and INF-γ, but upregulate IL-10, IL-4, and TGF-β production. Thus, during an immune and inflammatory response, the activation of the stress system, through induction of a Th2 shift may protect the organism from systemic "overshooting" with T helper lymphocyte 1 (Th1)/proinflammatory cytokines. In certain local responses and under certain conditions, however, stress hormones may actually facilitate inflammation, through induction of IL-1, IL-6, IL-8, IL-18, TNF-α, and CRP production, and through activation of the corticotropin-releasing hormone (CRH)/substance P(SP)-histamine axis. Autoimmunity, chronic infections, major depression, and atherosclerosis are characterized by a dysregulation of the pro/anti-inflammatory and Th1/Th2 cytokine balance. Thus, hyperactive or hypoactive stress system, and a dysfunctional neuroendocrine–immune interface associated with abnormalities of the "systemic anti-inflammatory feedback" and/or "hyperactivity" of the local proinflammatory factors may contribute to the pathogenesis of these diseases. Conditions that are associated with significant changes in stress system activity, such as acute or chronic stress, cessation of chronic stress, pregnancy and the postpartum period, or rheumatoid arthritis (RA) through modulation of the systemic or local pro/anti-inflammatory and Th1/Th2 cytokine balance, may suppress or potentiate disease activity and/or progression. Thus, stress hormones-induced inhibition or upregulation of innate and Th cytokine production may represent an important mechanism by which stress affects disease susceptibility, activity, and outcome of various immune-related diseases.

KEYWORDS: stress; cytokines; innate immunity; T helper 1 and T helper 2 cells; autoimmunity

Address for correspondence: Dr. Ilia Elenkov, Laboratory of Neuro-Endocrine-Immunology, San Raffaele Research Center, via della Pisana 235, 00163 Rome, Italy. Voice: 39-06-661-30422; fax: 39-06-661-30407.
e-mail: elenkovi@mail.nih.gov

Ann. N.Y. Acad. Sci. 1069: 62–76 (2006). © 2006 New York Academy of Sciences.
doi: 10.1196/annals.1351.006

INTRODUCTION

Cytokines, the "immune hormones" mediate and control immune and inflammatory responses. Complex interactions exist between cytokines, inflammation, and the adaptive responses in maintaining homeostasis. During an immune and inflammatory reaction, the release of cytokines, such as tumor necrosis factor-α (TNF-α), interleukin-1 (IL-1), IL-6, and IL-12 results in the activation of the stress system. Two major pathway systems are involved in this regulation: the hypothalamic-pituitary-adrenal (HPA) axis and the systemic/adrenomedullary sympathetic nervous system (SNS). Several studies during the 1970s and 1980s revealed that stress hormones inhibit lymphocyte proliferation, cytotoxicity, and the secretion of certain cytokines, such as IL-2 and interferon-γ (INF-γ). These observations lead to the conclusion that stress was, in general, immunosuppressive. Recent evidence, however, indicates that stress hormones influence the immune response in a less monochromatic way—they selectively inhibit the T helper lymphocyte 1 (Th1)/proinflammatory but potentiate Th2/anti-inflammatory cytokine production, systemically, while locally, in certain conditions they may exert proinflammatory effects. Through this mechanism, stress, that is, hyperactive or hypoactive stress system, may influence the onset and/or course of various common human immune-related diseases. This new concept that has emerged and developed in the last decade is briefly outlined below.

SYSTEMIC EFFECTS OF STRESS HORMONES ON INNATE AND TH CYTOKINE PRODUCTION

Glucocorticoids (GCs) and catecholamines (CAs) systemically mediate a Th2 shift by suppressing antigen-presenting cells (APCs) and Th1 and upregulating Th2-cytokine production.[1] Thus, GCs and the two major CAs, norepinephrine (NE) and epinephrine (EPI), through stimulation of classic cytoplasmic/nuclear GR and β2-ARs, respectively, suppress the production by APCs of IL-12, the main inducer of Th1 responses.[2–5] Since IL-12 is extremely potent in enhancing IFN-γ and inhibiting IL-4 synthesis by T cells, this is also associated with decreased IFN-γ but increased production of IL-4 by T cells.[5–7] GCs also have a direct effect on Th2 cells by upregulating their IL-4, IL-10, and IL-13 production.[5,8] GCs do not affect the production of IL-10 by monocytes,[2,9] yet, lymphocyte-derived IL-10 production is upregulated by GCs.[8] This could be the result of a direct stimulatory effect of GCs on T cell IL-10 production and/or a block on the restraining inputs of IL-12 and IFN-γ on lymphocyte IL-10 production. Both GCs and CAs inhibit the production of IL-1, TNF-α, and IFN-γ, while CAs inhibit the production of TNF-α by monocytes, microglial cells, and astrocytes, and suppress the production of IL-1, an effect that is mostly indirect via inhibition of TNF-α and potentiation of IL-10 production.[10–14] Since β2-ARs are expressed on Th1 cells, but not on Th2 cells,[15] CAs do not affect directly the cytokine production by Th2 cells—in murine and human systems β2-AR agonists inhibit IFN-γ production by Th1 cells, but do not affect IL-4 production by Th2 cells.[15,16] However, CAs through stimulation of β2-AR upregulate the production of the anti-inflammatory cytokine IL-10 and IL-6 by APCs.[2,17–19]

LOCAL EFFECTS OF STRESS HORMONES

The above systemic effects of stress hormones may not pertain to certain conditions or local responses in specific compartments of the body. Thus, steroid treatment results in a significant increase in the number of IL-12$^+$ cells with concurrent reduction in the number of IL-13$^+$-expressing cells in bronchial biopsy specimens of asthmatics. Interestingly, this occurs only in steroid-sensitive but not steroid-resistant asthmatic subjects.[20] The number of IL-4$^+$ cells in the bronchial and nasal mucosa is also reduced by GC treatment.[21,22] Furthermore, the synthesis of transforming growth factor-β (TGF-β), another cytokine with potent anti-inflammatory activities, is enhanced by GCs in human T cells but suppressed in glial cells,[23] and low doses of GCs can indeed activate alveolar macrophages, leading to increased lipopolysaccharide (LPS)-induced IL-1β production.[24] In addition, NE, via stimulation of α_2-ARs can augment LPS-stimulated production of TNF-α from mouse peritoneal macrophages,[25] while hemorrhage, a condition associated with elevations of systemic CA concentrations, increases the expression of TNF-α and IL-1 by lung mononuclear cells via stimulation of α-ARs.[26] Because the response to β-AR agonist stimulation wanes during maturation of human monocytes into macrophages,[27] it is possible that in certain compartments of the body, the α-AR-mediated effect of CAs becomes transiently dominant. CAs also potentiate the production of IL-8 (a chemokine that promotes the recruitment of polymorphonuclear cells to an inflammatory site) by monocytes, epithelial cells of the lung, and endothelial cells, indirectly, via an effect on platelets.[28–31] Furthermore, CAs through β2/β3-ARs upregulate IL-6 production by human adipocytes.[32,33] IL-6 is the major inducer of C-reactive protein (CRP) production by the liver and both GCs and CAs enhance this induction to a greater or lesser extent.[34] Interestingly, chronic β-AR stimulation induces myocardial, but not systemic, elaboration of TNF-α, IL-1β, and IL-6.[35]

CRH/SP-Mast Cell-Histamine Axis

Peripherally produced corticotropin-releasing hormone (CRH) acts as a local auto/paracrine proinflammatory agent (*peripheral* or *immune* CRH).

Immunoreactive CRH is identified locally in experimental carrageenin-induced subcutaneous aseptic inflammation, streptococcal cell wall- and adjuvant-induced arthritis, and in human tissues from patients with rheumatoid arthritis (RA), autoimmune thyroid disease (ATD), and ulcerative colitis. CRH may be produced locally by immune cells but also delivered to inflamed tissues by peripheral nerves.[36,37] Urocortin, a recently identified 40 amino acid peptide that shares 45% sequence homology with CRH is also overexpressed in synovial tissues of RA patients, and both CRH and urocortin stimulate the production of the proinflammatory cytokines IL-1β and IL-6 by human peripheral mononuclear cells.[38] Most of the proinflammatory actions of CRH and urocortin are mediated by CRH-R1 rather than CRH-R2.

Peripheral CRH has vascular permeability enhancing and vasodilatory actions. CRH administration causes major peripheral vasodilatation manifested as flushing and increased blood flow and hypotension.[39] An intradermal CRH injection induces a marked increase of vascular permeability and mast cell degranulation, mediated through CRH-R1.[40] It appears that the mast cell is a major target of immune CRH. Substance P (SP) and peripheral CRH, which are released from sensory peptidergic neurons, are two of the most potent mast cell secretagogues.[40–43] Thus, peripheral CRH and SP activates mast cells via a CRH type 1 and NK1 receptor-dependent mechanism leading to release of histamine and other contents of the mast cell granules that subsequently may cause vasodilatation, increased vascular permeability, and other manifestations of inflammation.

INTRACELLULAR INFECTIONS

A major factor governing the outcome of infectious diseases is the selection of Th1 versus Th2 predominant adaptive responses during and after the initial invasion of the host by the pathogen. Stress-induced Th2 shift may, therefore, have a profound effect on the susceptibility of the host to infections and/or may influence the course of infections, and particularly the intracellular ones, the defense against which is primarily through cellular immunity mechanisms. In the 1950s, Thomas Holmes reported that individuals who had experienced stressful life events were more likely to develop tuberculosis and less likely to recover from it.[cf.44] Although it is still a matter of some speculation, stress hormone-induced inhibition of IL-12 and IFN-γ production and the consequent suppression of cellular immunity, might explain the pathophysiologic mechanisms of these observations.[2]

The *Helicobacter pylori* intracellular infection is the most common cause of chronic gastritis, which in some cases progresses to peptic ulcer disease. The role of stress in promoting peptic ulcers has been recognized for many years.[45] Thus, increased systemic stress hormone levels, in concert with an increased local concentration of histamine, induced by inflammatory or stress-related mediators, may skew the local responses toward Th2 and thus might allow the onset or progression of a *H. pylori* infection.

The innervation (primarily sympathetic/noradrenergic) of lymphoid tissue may be particularly relevant to HIV infection, since lymphoid organs represent the primary site of HIV pathogenesis. In fact, as recently shown, NE, the major sympathetic neurotransmitter released locally in lymphoid organs,[46,47] is able to directly accelerate HIV-1 replication by up to 11-fold in acutely infected human peripheral blood mononuclear cells (PBMCs).[48] The effect of NE on viral replication is transduced via the β-AR-adenylyl cyclase-cAMP-PKA signaling cascade.[48] Progression of HIV infection is also characterized by increased cortisol secretion in both the early and late stages of the disease. Increased GC production, triggered by the chronic infection, was recently proposed to contribute to HIV progression.[49] Kino *et al*. found that one of the HIV-1 accessory proteins, Vpr, acts as a potent co-activator of the host GC receptor rendering lymphoid cells hyperresponsive to GCs.[50]

TH1-RELATED AUTOIMMUNITY

Several autoimmune diseases are characterized by common alterations of the Th1 versus Th2 and IL-12/TNF-α versus IL-10, balance. In RA, multiple sclerosis (MS), type 1 diabetes mellitus, ATD, and Crohn's disease (CD), the balance is skewed toward Th1 and an excess of IL-12 and TNF-α production, whereas Th2 activity and the production of IL-10 are deficient. This appears to be a critical factor that determines the proliferation and differentiation of Th1-related autoreactive cellular immune responses in these disorders.[51] Taking into consideration the Th2-driving effects of stress hormones systemically, one could postulate that a hypoactive stress system may facilitate or sustain the Th1 shift in MS or RA (FIG. 1). Animal studies and certain clinical observations support this hypothesis.

Recent studies suggest that suboptimal production of cortisol is involved in the onset and/or progression of RA.[52–54] Most patients with RA have relatively "inappropriately normal" plasma cortisol levels in the setting of severe, chronic inflammation, characterized by increased production of TNF-α, IL-1, and IL-6. Since these cytokines are powerful stimulants to the HPA axis and cortisol production, we would have expected significantly elevated plasma cortisol levels in RA patients. The available data suggest that the HPA axis response is blunted in these patients. Whether this abnormality is primary or secondary has not been established.[53]

Several lines of evidence indicate that the sympathetic–immune interface is defective in MS and its experimental model, the experimental allergic encephalomyelitis (EAE). Thus, sympathetic skin responses are decreased and lymphocyte β-ARs are increased in progressive MS.[55] The density of β-ARs on $CD8^+$ T cells are increased from two- to threefold, compared with age-matched controls.[56,57] Furthermore, isoproterenol and terbutaline, β-AR- and β_2-AR-agonists, respectively, were reported to suppress chronic/relapsing EAE in Lewis (LEW) rats.[58,59]

Several recent data suggest a "protective" role of the SNS in experimental models of RA in animals. Thus, in the arthritis-prone LEW rats sympathectomy with 6-OHDA enhanced the severity of adjuvant induced-arthritis.[60,61] The "protective" role of SNS is further substantiated by the recent study of Malfait *et al.*[62] demonstrating that the β_2-AR agonist, salbutamol, is a potent suppressor of established collagen-induced arthritis in mice. Recent studies in humans also suggest a defective SNS in RA. In patients with RA, diminished autonomic responses were observed after cognitive discrimination and the Stroop color–word interference tests.[63] Miller *et al.*,[64] demonstrated that patients with long-term RA had a highly significant reduction of sympathetic nerve fibers in synovial tissues, which was dependent on the degree of inflammation. Thus, the reduction of sympathetic nerve fibers in the chronic disease may lead to uncoupling of the local inflammation from the anti-inflammatory input of SNS. Interestingly, in RA synovial tissues it appears there is preponderance of about 10:1 for primary sensory, SP-positive fibers as compared with sympathetic fibers.[64] Since SP is powerful proinflammatory agent, via release of histamine and TNF-α and IL-12, such preponderance may lead to an unfavorable proinflammatory state, supporting the disease process of RA (FIG. 1).

The Lewis/Fischer Paradigm

LEW rats are highly susceptible to type II collagen-induced arthritis, adjuvant-induced arthritis, EAE, and experimental autoimmune uveitis (EAU), whereas Fischer (*F*344) rats are highly resistant to these diseases.[52,65] These experimentally induced diseases are mediated by Th1-dominant immune responses. In ocular tissues of EAU, LEW express type 1/proinflammatory cytokines (IL-12p40, IFN-α and TNF-α), coincident with the peak of the response, whereas *F*344 express high basal IL-10 levels mRNA in the eyes.[66] Recently, Sakamoto *et al.*,[67] have also demonstrated that lymph node cells from LEW rats express high levels of IL-12 p40 and there is upregulation of the expression of IL-12 receptor β1 and β2. These data suggest that LEW mounts a more polarized Th1 response that makes them more susceptible to Th1-mediated diseases, whereas *F*344 overproduces IL-10 that may contribute to a higher resistance to induction of these diseases. LEW have globally blunted stress system responses and fail, in response to a wide variety of stressors, to activate the hypothalamic CRH neuron appropriately.[52] Since *F*344 are known to have hyperresponsiveness stress responses and high corticosteroid production, but LEW rats have blunted stress responses with subnormal corticosteroid production, it is postulated that corticosteroids contribute to the differences in the development of pathogenic T cells in these two strains.[52]

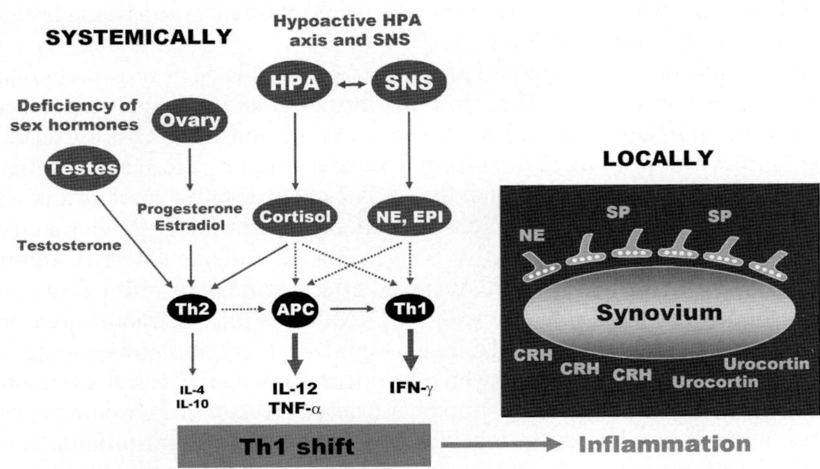

FIGURE 1. Role of systemic and local neuroendocrine factors in the pathogenesis of RA. The hypoactive stress system results in less inhibition of the Th1 responses by GCs and CAs, systemically. In aging men and postmenopausal women, the gonadal deficiency (i.e., less stimulation of the Th2 responses) will further intensify the Th1 shift. These neuroendocrine abnormalities may sustain and facilitate the Th1 shift observed in RA and further promote the local inflammation. Locally, the preponderance of primary sensory, SP-positive fibers as compared with sympathetic fibers and the overexpression of CRH and urocortin results in a dominance of the autocrine and paracrine proinflammatory factors in the synovium of RA patients. Solid lines represent stimulation, while dashed lines inhibition. APC, antigen-presenting cell; CRH, corticotropin-releasing hormone (peripheral); EPI, epinephrine; HPA, hypothalamic-pituitary-adrenal axis; IL, interleukin; NE, norepinephrine; SNS, sympathetic nervous system; SP, substance P; Th, T helper lymphocyte; TNF, tumor necrosis factor.

Pregnancy/Postpartum and Autoimmune Diseases Activity

Some autoimmune diseases like RA and MS often remit during pregnancy, particularly the third trimester but have an exacerbation or their initial onset during the postpartum period.[52,68–71] The risk of developing new onset RA during pregnancy, compared to nonpregnancy, is decreased by about 70%. In contrast, the risk of developing RA is markedly increased in the postpartum period, particularly the first 3 months (odds ratio of 5.6 overall and 10.8 after first pregnancy). In women with MS, the rate of relapses declines during pregnancy, especially in the third trimester, increases during the first 3 months of the post partum, and then returns to the prepregnancy rate.[70]

A decrease in the production of IL-2 and IFN-γ by antigen- and mitogen-stimulated PBMCs, accompanied by an increase in the production of IL-4 and IL-10, is observed in normal pregnancy. The lowest quantities of IL-2 and IFN-γ and the highest quantities of IL-4 and IL-10 are present in the third trimester of pregnancy.[72] Placental tissues from mothers at term express high levels of IL-10,[73] while IL-10 is present in the amniotic fluid of the majority of pregnancies, with higher concentrations found at term compared with the second trimester.[74] We have recently found that during the third trimester of pregnancy, *ex vivo* monocytic IL-12 production was about threefold and TNF-α production approximately 40% lower than postpartum values.[75] These studies suggest that type 1/proinflammatory cytokine production and cellular immunity are suppressed, and there is a Th2 shift during normal pregnancy, particularly, the third trimester. The third trimester of pregnancy and the early postpartum is also known to be associated with abrupt changes in several hormones. Thus, during the third trimester of pregnancy urinary cortisol and NE excretion, and serum levels of 1,25-dihydroxyvitamin D3 are about two- to threefold higher than postpartum values.[75] This is accompanied by the well-known marked elevations of estradiol and progesterone serum concentrations. The data reviewed here are consistent with the view that the increased levels of cortisol, NE, 1,25-dihydroxyvitamin D3, estrogens, and progesterone in the third trimester of pregnancy might orchestrate the improvement in autoimmune diseases, such as RA and MS via suppression of type 1/proinflammatory (IL-12, IFN-γ, and TNF-α) and potentiation of type2/anti-inflammatory (IL-4 and IL-10) cytokine production. Conversely, this particular type of hormonal control of pro/anti-inflammatory cytokine balance might contribute to the flare up of systemic lupus erythematosus (SLE) observed during pregnancy. Post partum, the hormonal state abruptly shifts. The deficit in hormones that inhibit Th1-type cytokines and cell-mediated immunity might permit autoimmune diseases, such as RA and MS to first develop or established disease to flare up.[52,75,76]

MAJOR DEPRESSSION AND ATHEROSCLEROSIS

Recent evidence indicates that proinflammatory cytokines contribute to the biology of depression. First, treatment of patients with chronic hepatitis C and malignant melanoma with high doses of INF-α is often accompanied by symptoms of depression. A full-blown depressive disorder is reported in up to 36% of cases. Second, behavioral changes, resembling the vegetative symptoms of depression are observed in rodents after acute administration of proinflammatory cytokines. Third, recent evidence indicates increased serum levels of proinflammatory cytokines, such as IL-6, in subjects with depressive symptoms and syndromes. Fourth, the involvement of proinflammatory cytokines and specifically IL-6 is further substantiated by reports showing increased plasma levels of acute-phase proteins, such as haptoglobulin and CRP in major depression.[77–79]

Patients with melancholic depression have significantly higher cerebrospinal fluid (CSF) NE and plasma cortisol levels with inappropriately high plasma

TABLE 1. Stress hormones-induced cytokine dysfunction in common human immune-related diseases

Disease group	Disease or condition	Cytokines and Th profiles	Comments	Role of stress hormones
Intracellular infections*	*Mycobacterium tuberculosis* *H. pylori* HIV	Suppressed cellular immunity, deficit of IL-12 and INF-γ, Th2 shift with progression of infection	HIV infection at some stages can express mixed Th1 and Th2 responses	Stress-induced Th2 shift might contribute to increase susceptibility to, or progression of these infections.
Th1-related autoimmunity	RA, MS, ATD, diabetes type 1, CD	Overproduction of IL-12, TNF-α, IFN-γ, deficit of IL-10, Th1 shift	Stress may exacerbate RA through the activation of the CRH-mast-cell-histamine axis (see text for details)	A hypoactive stress system may facilitate or sustain the Th1 shift (see text for details)
Major depression	Melancholic depression	Increased serum levels of IL-1, IL-6, and CRP	Depression is associated with an increased risk of cardiovascular diseases	IL-1 and IL-6 induce hypercortisolemic and hypernoradrenergic state; alternatively CAs upregulate IL-6 production, and thus increase its systemic levels
Atherosclerosis	Myocardial infarction, unstable angina, and stroke	Local overproduction of IFN-γ, TNF-α, IL-1β, IL-8, IL-12, and IL-18; Systemic elevation of IL-6, IL-8, IL-1β, and CRP	The effect of stress hormones on adipose tissue and lipid metabolism may facilitate their local proinflammatory effects	Stress hormones and histamine may induce the production of proinflammatory cytokines by myocardium, endothelium, and adipose tissues

*Modified from Elenkov and Chrousos, 1999 (See Ref. 1).

adrenocorticotropic hormone (ACTH) and CSF CRH levels, considering the degree of their hypercortisolism. These data suggest mutually reinforcing bidirectional links between a central hypernoradrenergic state and the hyperfunctioning of specific central CRH pathways that each are driven and sustained by hypercortisolism.[80] On the other hand, atypical depression might be associated with concomitant hypofunctioning of the CRH and locus ceruleus (LC)–NE systems.[81,82] There is a strong association between depression (melancholic) and osteoporosis. Endocrine factors, such as depression-induced hypersecretion of CRH and hypercortisolism, hypogonadism, growth hormone deficiency, and increased concentration of circulating IL-6, might play a crucial role in the bone loss observed in subjects suffering from major depression (melancholic). Abnormalities of the neuroendocrine system in major depression (melancholic), particularly the hypercortisolism and the central hypernoradrenergic state might be accentuated by the "low-grade" systemic inflammation, and specifically the increase of plasma IL-1 and IL-6.[78] Alternatively, since CAs upregulate IL-6 production, the chronic hypernoradrenergic state may drive the increase in systemic IL-6 levels (TABLE 1).

One of the paradigm shifts in our understanding about atherosclerosis in the last decade is the development of the concept that it is potentially caused by a chronic inflammation. When considering the role of cytokines in inflammation related to atherosclerosis it is important to distinguish between local inflammation within the plaque microenvironment and systemic inflammation, as evident by acute-phase protein production and circulating proinflammatory mediators. Locally produced proinflammatory mediators with atherogenic activity include IFN-γ, TNF-α, IL-1β, IL-8, IL-12, IL-18, and monocyte chemotactic protein-1 (MCP-1). Systemic mediators and markers of inflammation include IL-6, IL-8, and CRP. Increased IL-6 is associated with elevated fibrinogen levels, which leads to an increased tendency to thrombosis, independent of the effects of IL-6.[83] Although a complete discussion is beyond the scope of this article, through a mechanism similar to that in depression, chronic stress-related abnormalities and hyperactivity of the local proinflammatory factors, and particularly the CRH/SP-histamine axis, and the induction of IL-6, IL-8, and CRP, secretion may play a role in the pathogenesis of atherosclerosis (TABLE 1).

REFERENCES

1. ELENKOV, I.J. & G.P. CHROUSOS. 1999. Stress hormones, Th1/Th2 patterns, pro/anti-inflammatory cytokines and susceptibility to disease. Trends Endocrinol. Metab. **10:** 359–368.
2. ELENKOV, I.J., D.A. PAPANICOLAOU, R.L. WILDER & G.P. CHROUSOS. 1996. Modulatory effects of glucocorticoids and catecholamines on human interleukin-12 and interleukin-10 production: clinical implications. Proc. Assoc. Am. Physicians **108:** 374–381.

3. Panina-Bordignon, P., D. Mazzeo, P.D. Lucia, *et al.* 1997. Beta2-agonists prevent Th1 development by selective inhibition of interleukin 12. J. Clin. Invest. **100:** 1513–1519.
4. Hasko, G., C. Szabo, Z.H. Nemeth, *et al.* 1998. Stimulation of beta-adrenoceptors inhibits endotoxin-induced IL-12 production in normal and IL-10 deficient mice. J. Neuroimmunol. **88:** 57–61.
5. Blotta, M.H., R.H. Dekruyff & D.T. Umetsu. 1997. Corticosteroids inhibit IL-12 production in human monocytes and enhance their capacity to induce IL-4 synthesis in CD4+ lymphocytes. J. Immunol. **158:** 5589–5595.
6. Dekruyff, R.H., Y. Fang & D.T. Umetsu. 1998. Corticosteroids enhance the capacity of macrophages to induce Th2 cytokine synthesis in CD4+ lymphocytes by inhibiting IL-12 production. J. Immunol. **160:** 2231–2237.
7. Wu, C.Y., K. Wang, J.F. Mcdyer & R.A. Seder. 1998. Prostaglandin E2 and dexamethasone inhibit IL-12 receptor expression and IL-12 responsiveness. J. Immunol. **161:** 2723–2730.
8. Ramierz, F., D.J. Fowell, M. Puklavec, *et al.* 1996. Glucocorticoids promote a TH2 cytokine response by CD4+ T cells in vitro. J. Immunol. **156:** 2406–2412.
9. Van Der Poll, T., A.E. Barber, S.M. Coyle & S.F. Lowry. 1996. Hypercortisolemia increases plasma interleukin-10 concentrations during human endotoxemia—a clinical research center study. J. Clin. Endocrinol. Metab. **81:** 3604–3606.
10. Hetier, E., J. Ayala, A. Bousseau & A. Prochiantz. 1991. Modulation of interleukin-1 and tumor necrosis factor expression by beta-adrenergic agonists in mouse ameboid microglial cells. Exp. Brain Res. **86:** 407–413.
11. Severn, A., N.T. Rapson, C.A. Hunter & F.Y. Liew. 1992. Regulation of tumor necrosis factor production by adrenaline and β-adrenergic agonists. J. Immunol. **148:** 3441–3445.
12. Nakamura, A., E.J. Johns, A. Imaizumi, *et al.* 1998. Regulation of tumour necrosis factor and interleukin-6 gene transcription by beta2-adrenoceptor in the rat astrocytes. J. Neuroimmunol. **88:** 144–153.
13. Koff, W.C., A.V. Fann, M.A. Dunegan & L.B. Lachman. 1986. Catecholamine-induced suppression of interleukin-1 production. Lymphokine Res. **5:** 239–247.
14. Van Der Poll, T. & S.F. Lowry. 1997. Epinephrine inhibits endotoxin-induced IL-1 beta production: roles of tumor necrosis factor-alpha and IL-10 Am. J. Physiol. **273:** R1885–R1890.
15. Sanders, V.M., R.A. Baker, D.S. Ramer-Quinn, *et al.* 1997. Differential expression of the beta2-adrenergic receptor by Th1 and Th2 clones: implications for cytokine production and B cell help. J. Immunol. **158:** 4200–4210.
16. Borger, P., Y. Hoekstra, M.T. Esselink, *et al.* 1998. Beta-adrenoceptor-mediated inhibition of IFN-gamma, IL-3, and GM-CSF mRNA accumulation in activated human T lymphocytes is solely mediated by the beta2-adrenoceptor subtype. Am. J. Respir. Cell Mol. Biol. **19:** 400–407.
17. Van Der Poll, T., S.M. Coyle, K. Barbosa, *et al.* 1996. Epinephrine inhibits tumor necrosis factor-alpha and potentiates interleukin 10 production during human endotoxemia. J. Clin. Invest. **97:** 713–719.
18. Norris, J.G. & E.N. Benveniste. 1993. Interleukin-6 production by astrocytes: induction by the neurotransmitter norepinephrine. J. Neuroimmunol. **45:** 137–145.

19. MAIMONE, D., C. CIONI, S. ROSA, *et al.* 1993. Norepinephrine and vasoactive intestinal peptide induce IL-6 secretion by astrocytes: synergism with IL-1 beta and TNF alpha. J. Neuroimmunol. **47:** 73–81.
20. NASEER, T., E.M. MINSHALL, D.Y. LEUNG, *et al.* 1997. Expression of IL-12 and IL-13 mRNA in asthma and their modulation in response to steroid therapy. Am. J. Respir. Crit. Care Med. **155:** 845–851.
21. BENTLEY, A.M., Q. HAMID, D.S. ROBINSON, *et al.* 1996. Prednisolone treatment in asthma. Reduction in the numbers of eosinophils, T cells, tryptase-only positive mast cells, and modulation of IL-4, IL-5, and interferon-gamma cytokine gene expression within the bronchial mucosa. Am. J. Respir. Crit. Care Med. **153:** 551–556.
22. BRADDING, P., I.H. FEATHER, S. WILSON, *et al.* 1995. Cytokine immunoreactivity in seasonal rhinitis: regulation by a topical corticosteroid. Am. J. Respir. Crit. Care Med. **151:** 1900–1906.
23. BATUMAN, O.A., A. FERRERO, C. CUPP, *et al.* 1995. Differential regulation of transforming growth factor beta-1 gene expression by glucocorticoids in human T and glial cells. J. Immunol. **155:** 4397–4405.
24. BROUG-HOLUB, E. & G. KRAAL. 1996. Dose- and time-dependent activation of rat alveolar macrophages by glucocorticoids. Clin. Exp. Immunol. **104:** 332–336.
25. SPENGLER, R.N., R.M. ALLEN, D.G. REMICK, *et al.* 1990. Stimulation of α-adrenergic receptor augments the production of macrophage-derived tumor necrosis factor. J. Immunol. **145:** 1430–1434.
26. LETULZO, Y., R. SHENKAR, D. KANEKO, *et al.* 1997. Hemorrhage increases cytokine expression in lung mononuclear cells in mice: involvement of catecholamines in nuclear factor-kappaB regulation and cytokine expression. J. Clin. Invest. **99:** 1516–1524.
27. BAKER, A.J. & R.W. FULLER. 1995. Loss of response to beta-adrenoceptor agonists during the maturation of human monocytes to macrophages in vitro. J. Leukoc. Biol. **57:** 395–400.
28. KAVELAARS, A., D.P. VAN, J. ZIJLSTRA & C.J. HEIJNEN. 1997. Beta 2-adrenergic activation enhances interleukin-8 production by human monocytes. J. Neuroimmunol. **77:** 211–216.
29. LINDEN, A. 1996. Increased interleukin-8 release by beta-adrenoceptor activation in human transformed bronchial epithelial cells. Br. J. Pharmacol. **119:** 402–406.
30. ENGSTAD, C.S., T. LUND & B. OSTERUD. 1999. Epinephrine promotes IL-8 production in human leukocytes via an effect on platelets. Thromb. Haemost. **81:** 139–145.
31. KAPLANSKI, G., R. PORAT, K. AIURA, *et al.* 1993. Activated platelets induce endothelial secretion of interleukin-8 in vitro via an interleukin-1-mediated event. Blood **81:** 2492–2495.
32. MOHAMED-ALI, V., L. FLOWER, J. SETHI, *et al.* 2001. beta-Adrenergic regulation of IL-6 release from adipose tissue: in vivo and in vitro studies. J. Clin. Endocrinol. Metab. **86:** 5864–5869.
33. VICENNATI, V., A. VOTTERO, C. FRIEDMAN & D.A. PAPANICOLAOU. 2002. Hormonal regulation of interleukin-6 production in human adipocytes. Int. J. Obes. Relat. Metab. Disord. **26:** 905–911.
34. BAUMANN, H. & J. GAULDIE. 1994. The acute phase response. Immunol. Today **15:** 74–80.

35. MURRAY, D.R., S.D. PRABHU & B. CHANDRASEKAR. 2000. Chronic beta-adrenergic stimulation induces myocardial proinflammatory cytokine expression. Circulation **101:** 2338–2341.
36. KARALIS, K., H. SANO, J. REDWINE, *et al.* 1991. Autocrine or paracrine inflammatory actions of corticotropin-releasing hormone in vivo. Science **254:** 421–423.
37. ELENKOV, I.J., E.L. WEBSTER, D.J. TORPY & G.P. CHROUSOS. 1999. Stress, corticotropin-releasing hormone, glucocorticoids, and the immune/inflammatory response: acute and chronic effects. Ann. N. Y. Acad. Sci. **876:** 1–11.
38. KOHNO, M., Y. KAWAHITO, Y. TSUBOUCHI, *et al.* 2001. Urocortin expression in synovium of patients with rheumatoid arthritis and osteoarthritis: relation to inflammatory activity. J. Clin. Endocrinol. Metab **86:** 4344–4352.
39. UDELSMAN, R., W.T. GALLUCCI, J. BACHER, *et al.* 1986. Hemodynamic effects of corticotropin releasing hormone in the anesthetized cynomolgus monkey. Peptides **7:** 465–471.
40. THEOHARIDES, T.C., L.K. SINGH, W. BOUCHER, *et al.* 1998. Corticotropin-releasing hormone induces skin mast cell degranulation and increased vascular permeability, a possible explanation for its proinflammatory effects. Endocrinology **139:** 403–413.
41. FOREMAN, J.C. 1987. Substance P and calcitonin gene-related peptide: effects on mast cells and in human skin. Int. Arch. Allergy Appl. Immunol. **82:** 366–371.
42. CHURCH, M.K., M.A. LOWMAN, C. ROBINSON, *et al.* 1989. Interaction of neuropeptides with human mast cells. Int. Arch. Allergy Appl. Immunol. **88:** 70–78.
43. THEOHARIDES, T.C., C. SPANOS, X. PANG, *et al.* 1995. Stress-induced intracranial mast cell degranulation: a corticotropin-releasing hormone-mediated effect. Endocrinology **136:** 5745–5750.
44. LERNER, B.H. 1996. Can stress cause disease? Revisiting the tuberculosis research of Thomas Holmes, 1949–1961. Ann. Intern. Med. **124:** 673–680.
45. LEVENSTEIN, S., S. ACKERMAN, J.K. KIECOLT-GLASER & A. DUBOIS. 1999. Stress and peptic ulcer disease. JAMA **281:** 10–11.
46. ELENKOV, I.J. & E.S. VIZI. 1991. Presynaptic modulation of release of noradrenaline from the sympathetic nerve terminals in the rat spleen. Neuropharmacology **30:** 1319–1324.
47. VIZI, E.S., E. ORSO, O.N. OSIPENKO, *et al.* 1995. Neurochemical, electrophysiological and immunocytochemical evidence for a noradrenergic link between the sympathetic nervous system and thymocytes. Neuroscience **68:** 1263–1276.
48. COLE, S.W., Y.D. KORIN, J.L. FAHEY & J.A. ZACK. 1998. Norepinephrine accelerates HIV replication via protein kinase A-dependent effects on cytokine production. J. Immunol. **161:** 610–616.
49. CLERICI, M., M. BEVILACQUA, T. VAGO, *et al.* 1994. An immunoendocrinological hypothesis of HIV infection [see comments]. Lancet **343:** 1552–1553.
50. KINO, T., A. GRAGEROV, J.B. KOPP, *et al.* 1999. The HIV-1 virion-associated protein vpr is a coactivator of the human glucocorticoid receptor (in process citation). J. Exp. Med. **189:** 51–62.
51. SEGAL, B.M., B.K. DWYER & E.M. SHEVACH. 1998. An interleukin (IL)-10/IL-12 immunoregulatory circuit controls susceptibility to autoimmune disease. J. Exp. Med. **187:** 537–546.
52. WILDER, R.L. 1995. Neuroendocrine-immune system interactions and autoimmunity. Annu. Rev. Immunol. **13:** 307–338.

53. WILDER, R.L. & I.J. ELENKOV. 1999. Hormonal regulation of tumor necrosis factor-alpha, interleukin-12 and interleukin-10 production by activated macrophages. A disease-modifying mechanism in rheumatoid arthritis and systemic lupus erythematosus? Ann. N. Y. Acad. Sci. **876:** 14–31.
54. STRAUB, R.H. & M. CUTOLO. 2001. Involvement of the hypothalamic-pituitary-adrenal/gonadal axis and the peripheral nervous system in rheumatoid arthritis: viewpoint based on a systemic pathogenetic role. Arthritis Rheum. **44:** 493–507.
55. KARASZEWSKI, J.W., A.T. REDER, R. MASELLI, *et al.* 1990. Sympathetic skin responses are decreased and lymphocyte beta-adrenergic receptors are increased in progressive multiple sclerosis. Ann. Neurol. **27:** 366–372.
56. ARNASON, B.G., M. BROWN, R. MASELLI, *et al.* 1988. Blood lymphocyte beta-adrenergic receptors in multiple sclerosis. Ann. N. Y. Acad. Sci. **540:** 585–588.
57. KARASZEWSKI, J.W., A.T. REDER, B. ANLAR & G.W. ARNASON. 1993. Increased high affinity beta-adrenergic receptor densities and cyclic AMP responses of CD8 cells in multiple sclerosis. J. Neuroimmunol. **43:** 1–7.
58. CHELMICKA-SCHORR, E., M.N. KWASNIEWSKI, B.E. THOMAS & B.G. ARNASON. 1989. The beta-adrenergic agonist isoproterenol suppresses experimental allergic encephalomyelitis in Lewis rats. J. Neuroimmunol. **25:** 203–207.
59. WIEGMANN, K., S. MUTHYALA, D.H. KIM, *et al.* 1995. Beta-adrenergic agonists suppress chronic/relapsing experimental allergic encephalomyelitis (CREAE) in Lewis rats. J. Neuroimmunol. **56:** 201–206.
60. LORTON, D., D. BELLINGER, M. DUCLOS, *et al.* 1996. Application of 6-hydroxydopamine into the fatpads surrounding the draining lymph nodes exacerbates adjuvant-induced arthritis. J. Neuroimmunol. **64:** 103–113.
61. FELTEN, D.L., S.Y. FELTEN, D.L. BELLINGER & D. LORTON. 1992. Noradrenergic and peptidergic innervation of secondary lymphoid organs: role in experimental rheumatoid arthritis. Eur. J. Clin. Invest. **22**(Suppl 1)**:** 37–41.
62. MALFAIT, A.M., A.S. MALIK, L. MARINOVA-MUTAFCHIEVA, *et al.* 1999. The beta2-adrenergic agonist salbutamol is a potent suppressor of established collagen-induced arthritis: mechanisms of action. J. Immunol. **162:** 6278–6283.
63. GEENEN, R., G.L. GODAERT, J.W. JACOBS, *et al.* 1996. Diminished autonomic nervous system responsiveness in rheumatoid arthritis of recent onset. J. Rheumatol. **23:** 258–264.
64. MILLER, L.E., H.P. JUSTEN, J. SCHOLMERICH & R.H. STRAUB. 2000. The loss of sympathetic nerve fibers in the synovial tissue of patients with rheumatoid arthritis is accompanied by increased norepinephrine release from synovial macrophages. FASEB J. **14:** 2097–2107.
65. JOE, B., M.M. GRIFFITHS, E.F. REMMERS & R.L. WILDER. 1999. Animal models of rheumatoid arthritis and related inflammation. Curr. Rheumatol. Rep. **1:** 139–148.
66. SUN, B., S.H. SUN, C.C. CHAN & R.R. CASPI. 2000. Evaluation of in vivo cytokine expression in EAU-susceptible and resistant rats: a role for IL-10 in resistance? Exp. Eye Res. **70:** 493–502.
67. SAKAMOTO, S., A. FUKUSHIMA, A. OZAKI, *et al.* 2001. Mechanism for maintenance of dominant T helper 1 immune responses in Lewis rats. Microbiol. Immunol. **45:** 373–381.
68. BUYON, J.P. 1998. The effects of pregnancy on autoimmune diseases. J. Leukoc. Biol. **63:** 281–287.
69. BUYON, J.P., J.L. NELSON & M.D. LOCKSHIN. 1996. The effects of pregnancy on autoimmune diseases. Clin. Immunol. Immunopathol. **78:** 99–104.

70. CONFAVREUX, C., M. HUTCHINSON, M.M. HOURS, *et al.* 1998. Rate of pregnancy-related relapse in multiple sclerosis. Pregnancy in multiple sclerosis group. N. Engl. J. Med. **339:** 285–291.
71. GRIFFITHS, M.M., J. WANG, B. JOE, *et al.* 2000. Identification of four new quantitative trait loci regulating arthritis severity and one new quantitative trait locus regulating autoantibody production in rats with collagen-induced arthritis. Arthritis Rheum. **43:** 1278–1289.
72. MARZI, M., A. VIGANO, D. TRABATTONI, *et al.* 1996. Characterization of type 1 and type 2 cytokine production profile in physiologic and pathologic human pregnancy. Clin. Exp. Immunol. **106:** 127–133.
73. CADET, P., P.L. RADY, S.K. TYRING, *et al.* 1995. Interleukin-10 messenger ribonucleic acid in human placenta: implications of a role for interleukin-10 in fetal allograft protection. Am. J. Obstet. Gynecol. **173:** 25–29.
74. GREIG, P.C., W.N. HERBERT, B.L. ROBINETTE & L.A. TEOT. 1995. Amniotic fluid interleukin-10 concentrations increase through pregnancy and are elevated in patients with preterm labor associated with intrauterine infection. Am. J. Obstet. Gynecol. **173:** 1223–1227.
75. ELENKOV, I.J., R.L. WILDER, V.K. BAKALOV, *et al.* 2001. IL-12, TNF-alpha, and hormonal changes during late pregnancy and early postpartum: implications for autoimmune disease activity during these times. J. Clin. Endocrinol. Metab. **86:** 4933–4938.
76. ELENKOV, I.J., J. HOFFMAN & R.L. WILDER. 1997. Does differential neuroendocrine control of cytokine production govern the expression of autoimmune diseases in pregnancy and the postpartum period? Mol. Med. Today **3:** 379–383.
77. KRONFOL, Z. & D.G. REMICK. 2000. Cytokines and the brain: implications for clinical psychiatry. Am. J. Psychiatry **157:** 683–694.
78. CORCOS, M., O. GUILBAUD, L. HJALMARSSON, *et al.* 2002. Cytokines and depression: an analogic approach. Biomed. Pharmacother. **56:** 105–110.
79. WICHERS, M. & M. MAES. 2002. The psychoneuroimmuno-pathophysiology of cytokine-induced depression in humans. Int. J. Neuropsychopharmacol. **5:** 375–388.
80. WONG, M.L., M.A. KLING, P.J. MUNSON, *et al.* 2000. Pronounced and sustained central hypernoradrenergic function in major depression with melancholic features: relation to hypercortisolism and corticotropin-releasing hormone. Proc. Natl. Acad. Sci. USA **97:** 325–330.
81. GOLD, P.W. & G.P. CHROUSOS. 1999. The endocrinology of melancholic and atypical depression: relation to neurocircuitry and somatic consequences. Proc. Assoc. Am. Physicians **111:** 22–34.
82. GOLD, P.W. & G.P. CHROUSOS. 2002. Organization of the stress system and its dysregulation in melancholic and atypical depression: high vs low CRH/NE states. Mol. Psychiatry **7:** 254–275.
83. GREAVES, D.R. & K.M. CHANNON. 2002. Inflammation and immune responses in atherosclerosis. Trends Immunol. **23:** 535–541.

The Impact of Stressors on Health Status and Hypothalamic-Pituitary-Adrenal Axis and Autonomic Nervous System Responsiveness in Rheumatoid Arthritis

RINIE GEENEN,[a] HENRIËT VAN MIDDENDORP,[a] AND JOHANNES W.J. BIJLSMA[b]

[a]*Department of Clinical and Health Psychology, Utrecht University, Utrecht, the Netherlands*

[b]*Department of Rheumatology and Clinical Immunology, University Medical Center Utrecht, Utrecht, the Netherlands*

ABSTRACT: **The hypothalamic-pituitary-adrenal (HPA) axis and the autonomic nervous system (ANS) are critically involved in inflammation and are activated by stress. This suggests that stressful circumstances may affect the chronic inflammation of rheumatoid arthritis (RA). Fifty-six scientific publications of the past 15 years were reviewed to get insight into the possible impact of stressors (grouped in five categories) on the health status and HPA axis and ANS functioning of adult patients with RA. Our findings in this review were: (1) In response to mental and physical effort and applied physiological stressors, patients demonstrate ANS hyporesponsiveness and "too normal" HPA axis responsiveness considering the elevated immune activity. A premorbid defect, past and current inflammatory activity, past and current stress, and physical deconditioning may explain disturbed physiological responses. (2) After brief naturalistic stressors, self-perceived and clinician's ratings of disease activity are increased; inflammation parameters have been insufficiently examined. (3) Major life events do not univocally affect disease status, but appear able to modify disease activity in a positive or negative way, depending on the nature, duration, and dose of the accompanying physiological stress response. (4) Enduring (e.g., work-related or interpersonal) stressors are associated with perceived health. Because this stressor category mingles with personality variables, the mere observation of a correlation does not prove that chronic stressors provoke health changes, although this might be the case. (5) Not one study rigorously examined the prospective hypothesis that past stressors (e.g., childhood victimization or pre-onset stressful incidents) may trigger RA or aggravate existing RA, which is a realistic belief for some patients.**

Address for correspondence: Dr. Rinie Geenen, Department of Clinical and Health Psychology, Utrecht University, P.O.Box 80140, 3508TC Utrecht, the Netherlands. Voice: +31 30 253 4916; fax: +31 30 253 4718.
e-mail: R.Geenen@home.nl

Ann. N.Y. Acad. Sci. 1069: 77–97 (2006). © **2006 New York Academy of Sciences.**
doi: 10.1196/annals.1351.007

Keywords: rheumatoid arthritis; stress; psychoneuroimmunology; psychophysiology; psychological adaptation; cortisol; norepinephrine; interleukin-6; autonomic nervous system; hypothalamic-pituitary-adrenal axis

INTRODUCTION

The hypothalamic-pituitary-adrenal (HPA) axis and the autonomic nervous system (ANS) are critically involved in inflammation [1,2] and both are activated by physical and psychosocial stressors. This suggests that stressful circumstances may affect the disease process of a chronic inflammatory disease, such as rheumatoid arthritis (RA). In addition, the physiological response to stressful circumstances may change when the HPA axis and ANS stress systems become downregulated or upregulated during or after inflammation.

The HPA axis and ANS respond in a coordinated fashion.[2,3] The release of neurotransmitters, hormones, and immune cells in response to a stressor serves to deal with the taxing situation and to restore adaptation. Cortisol and norepinephrine are main hormones and neurotransmitters of the HPA axis and sympathetic nervous system (SNS), respectively. Immunostimulating or immunosuppressive effects of these stress hormones are dependent on dose and timing: under normal conditions, acute minor stressful stimuli tend to lead to a short-lived rise of cortisol and norepinephrine concentrations as well as to immunostimulation, while major stressful circumstances tend to lead to a huge rise of cortisol and norepinephrine concentrations over days and weeks and to immunosuppression.[2] Inadequate HPA axis and ANS responsiveness to stress may play a role in the etiology, maintenance, and aggravation of rheumatoid arthritis.

To fully understand a possible role of stress in rheumatoid arthritis, one ought to consider that stress is a multi-faceted phenomenon. Most often the stress label refers to a relationship between the person and the environment. The person appraises the environmental demands as endangering to well-being and as taxing or exceeding his or her resources.[4] The current article focuses on the impact of *stressors*, the stimuli that are able to bring about a stress reaction in the person. We are aware that what may affect the health of patients with RA is not the stressor as such (which acts as a trigger), but the appraisal of the stressful situation and the stress response. However, a definition of stress including the perception of and response to the stressor will partly coincide with the perception of and response to health outcome variables, such as pain, joint tenderness, and functional ability. A stimulus definition of stressors fits the assumption that health status and physiological response will partly depend on the type of stressor. We adopt a slightly adapted taxonomy that distinguishes five types of stressors that differ with respect to point in time, duration, and type of the stressor (Table 1)[5,6]: (1) acute time-limited stressors, (2) brief naturalistic stressors, (3) stressful event sequences, (4) chronic and chronic intermittent stressors, and (5) distant stressors.

The aim of the present study was to review the recent literature in order to get insight into the possible impact of divergent stressors on disease activity (pain, joint scores, physical functioning, indicators of inflammation) and on HPA axis and ANS functioning in adult patients with RA.

METHODS

The literature of the past 15 years was reviewed. We used four steps in the selection procedure. First, we selected articles in the Web of Science® (ISI Web of Knowledge℠), with "arthritis" in the title and the words "stress∗" or "life events" anywhere in the fields. Only articles between 1990 and August 2005 were selected. This search resulted in 457 articles.

In a second step, two researchers (R.G. and H.v.M.) independently evaluated all abstracts to judge whether the study fitted one of the five stressor categories (TABLE 1). Other inclusion criteria were that they should be empirical studies with human, adult patients with RA, which were written in English or German. Having read the abstracts, the two judges discussed the not-agreed-upon studies. Forty-six studies were selected.

In a third step, we added eight articles from our archives that were not included in the search at Web of Science. This predominantly concerned studies of reactivity of the ANS and HPA axis to acute time-limited stressors that did not include the words "stress," "stressor," "stressful,'" or "life event" in the title or abstract.

In a final step, we used the "related articles" button in the Web of Science to search for additional articles of the past 15 years within the selected titles of the past 5 years. This resulted in another two articles. Having finished the search and having allocated the studies to the five stressor categories, all articles were collected and reviewed.

RESULTS

The 56 selected studies are shown in TABLE 2. In each section, after a short introduction, we will summarize and discuss the results for each stressor category separately.

Acute Time-Limited Stressors

Acute time-limited stressors involve laboratory challenges, such as mental or physical tasks as well as applied physiological stressors that activate the HPA axis or ANS stress systems.[5] Nineteen studies in the past 15 years

TABLE 1. Typical examples of stressors belonging to the five stressor categories

Stressor category	Examples of stressors
Acute time-limited stressors	Mental and physical tasks (e.g., mental arithmetic, the Stroop test, public speaking, physical exercise, ice-water test, Valsalva maneuver, and orthostatic tests) and physiological stressors (e.g., hypoglycemia, or infusions of acetylcholine, CRH, or epinephrine).
Brief naturalistic stressor [a]	Short-term challenges that are measured on a momentary basis with diaries (e.g., a clinical exam in a hospital, work-related or interpersonal stressors, and other real-life challenges).
Stressful event sequences	A current major incident that gives rise to a series of related challenges (e.g., the death of a close relative, myocardial infarction of a spouse, being fired, and the summation of several life events).
Chronic (intermittent) stressor [b]	Enduring events that pervade a person's life, forcing him or her to restructure his or her identity or social roles (e.g., work-related stressors, interpersonal stressors, and financial problems).
Distant stressors	Traumatic experiences that occurred in the past, yet have a potential to have long-term emotional, cognitive, or physiological consequences (e.g., childhood victimization or an accident, bereavement, or divorce preceding disease onset).

[a]The brief (instantaneous) naturalistic stressors included in the second stressor category refer to an (experimental) *within-person* level of analysis: individual measurements during nonstressor and stressor periods are compared.

[b]This fourth stressor category involves the (correlational) *between-person* level of analysis: the number or extent of enduring stressors is correlated with other variables.

examined in patients with RA the ANS[7–14] and HPA axis[15–25] responsiveness to divergent acute time-limited stressors, such as mental and physical laboratory stressors,[7–11,14,20–22] hypoglycemia,[12,23,24] and infusions of acetylcholine,[13] CRH,[15–19] or epinephrine.[25]

Results

The most common finding with respect to ANS functioning in RA is diminished autonomic responses to mental tasks,[7] deep breathing,[8,9] Valsalva maneuver, and orthostatic tests.[9] This hyporesponsiveness was observed in such varying groups as patients with a recent RA diagnosis,[7] in established RA,[8] and in hospitalized patients with RA.[9] Two studies observed diminished heart rate response to autonomic challenges, which disappeared after elevated pretask levels were defined as a covariate[10,11]; the significance disappeared because patients with RA had both reduced heart rate responses and elevated baseline heart rate levels. Studies using other kinds of stressors also observed ANS hyporeactivity. Reduced epinephrine and norepinephrine responses to insulin-induced hypoglycemia were observed[12] as were reduced vasodilatory

TABLE 2. The 56 studies of our review coded by stressor category

Stressor category	Studies
Acute time-limited stressors (19 studies)	Geenen 1996,[7] Louthrenoo 1999,[8] Toussirot 1993,[9] Perry 1989,[10] Piha 1993,[11] Imrich 2005,[12] Bergholm 2002,[13] Bekkelund 1996,[14] Chikanza 1992,[15] Cutolo 1999,[16] Jorgensen 1995,[17] Gudbjornsson 1996,[18] Harbuz 2003,[19] Dekkers 2001,[20] Pool 2004,[21] Geenen 1998,[22] Rovensky 2002,[23] Gutierrez 1999,[24] Straub 2002.[25]
Brief naturalistic stressors (19 studies)	Chikanza 1992,[15] Stone 1997,[26] Urrows 1994,[27] Cobb 1998,[28] Fifield 2004,[29] Potter 2002,[30] Smith 2002,[31] Zautra 1997,[32] Zautra 1998,[33] Skinner 2004,[34] Crofford 1997,[35] Mastorakos 2000,[36] Hirano 2001,[37] Tanno 2004,[38] Zautra 2004,[39] Catley 2000,[40] Dekkers 2000,[41] Harrington 1993,[42] Affleck 1997.[43]
Stressful event sequences (11 studies)	Cobb 1998,[28] Marcenaro 1999,[44] Potter 1997,[45] Leymarie 1997,[46] Stewart 1994,[47] Dekkers 2001,[48] Haller 1997,[49] Smedstad 1995,[50] Evers 2003,[51] Thomason 1992,[52] Koehler 1993.[53]
Chronic (intermittent) stressors (6 studies)	Marcenaro 1999,[44] Potter 1997,[45] Dekkers 2001,[48] Thomason 1992,[52] Dwyer 1997,[54] Zautra 1994.[55]
Distant stressors (9 studies)	Marcenaro 1999,[44] Stewart 1994,[47] Sakalys 1997,[56] Conway 1994,[57] Carette 2000,[58] Radanov 1996,[59] Radanov 1997,[60] Latman 1996,[61] Kopec 2004.[62]

responses to infusions of acetylcholine and sodium nitroprusside.[13] This vascular dysfunction turned out to be reversible with anti-inflammatory therapy. Only one study found normal ANS responses to stressors, such as deep breathing and orthostatic challenge.[14]

The ongoing scientific attention on HPA axis stress responsiveness is undoubtedly fueled by the observation of improvement of RA after treatment with glucocorticoids. In experimental studies, the type of stressor determines which part of the HPA axis is examined. Studies using CRH infusions as stressor only examine stress responsiveness of the pituitary gland and adrenal cortex, while studies with behavioral challenges or insulin-hypoglycemia stimulation examine the whole HPA axis response including hypothalamic CRH responsiveness. Studies using CRH provocation did not indicate disturbed cortisol and corticotropin responses[15,16] or provided only a weak, marginally significant indication for hyporesponsiveness.[17] Only one study observed a reduced serum cortisol response after CRH stimulation in spite of an intact corticotropin response.[18] Using a CRH challenge after dexamethasone overnight, three of seven patients with RA and none of the control participants escaped from dexamethasone suppression (as in depression) and mounted a cortisol response to CRH challenge, but the implications of this finding are unclear.[19]

Tests examining disturbance at the level of the hypothalamus or higher are inconclusive as well. Two of three studies using mental and physical experimental stressors reported reduced HPA axis responsiveness in patients with RA,[20,21] while the other study observed a normal cortisol response.[22] The cortisol responses to insulin-hypoglycemia of patients with RA as compared to healthy controls was normal in two studies,[12,23] while only a weak indication for HPA axis hyporesponsiveness was found in another study.[24] Analyses tentatively suggested that after epinephrine infusion, patients with RA had a somewhat blunted response of the HPA axis system, which may suggest that real-life stressors that activate the sympathetic nervous system might be relevant for exacerbation of RA.[25]

Conclusion

Studies quite consistently demonstrate ANS hyporesponsiveness to acute time-limited stressors of patients with RA. Results regarding HPA axis responsiveness are inconclusive. Several studies indicate normal corticotropin and cortisol responsiveness, but a few studies provided weak indications for blunted HPA axis responsiveness.

Discussion

Not only for reactivity, but also with respect to baseline levels, the ANS has more often been observed to be deviated than the HPA axis in RA. As summarized elsewhere,[2,63] several studies observed an increased baseline sympathetic tone. Most studies that examined stressor responsiveness of the HPA axis observed normal baseline cortisol levels in patients with RA.[15,17,20,21,23,24] High[22] and low[18,25] cortisol levels have been observed infrequently. One study reported reduced early morning cortisol concentrations and normal cortisol concentrations in the late afternoon.[16]

The hyporeactive ANS response was especially observed in studies using behavioral instead of physiological challenges. A strength of external, behavioral stressors is that the whole person (including cortex and hypothalamus) is stimulated. This is, however, a weakness too. Because individuals may adapt their mental and physical effort to their condition, it is not clear whether the physiological system is hyporeactive or the person is less active. The combination of elevated tonic SNS levels and a hyporeactive ANS response has consistently been found in persons with low physical fitness.[64–66] Also, the recent stress history[67] as well as chronic stress experiences[68] have been shown to be associated with reduced physiological stress responses to acute stressors. Finally, past and current disease activity may explain hyporeactive ANS responses.

We reviewed the selected studies to find possible reasons to explain the discrepancy between studies observing normal and attenuated HPA axis responses to acute stressors, such as gender, age, disease duration, pharmacological treatment, and type of stressor. No clear reasons for the inconsistent findings could be found.

The observation of inconclusive findings with respect to corticotropin and cortisol response to acute stressors is not an isolated finding. Besides, for immunosuppressive hormones such as cortisol, inconsistent results have been observed for immunostimulating hormones, such as prolactin (PRL). The PRL response to acute stressors of patients with RA was observed to be normal,[24] increased,[17] and attenuated.[23,69]

The health consequences of acute time-limited stressors are unclear. A recent study suggested that even acute mental stressors are able to increase C-reactive protein (CRP), and more specifically in those patients with high disease activity.[70] It could be investigated whether increased responsiveness of this inflammation parameter covaries with reduced responsiveness of the HPA axis.

Most likely, the about-normal HPA axis responses give a reflection of the unhealthy status of individual patients only in combination with the diminished ANS responses and increased immune responses.[15,22] Unlike the case in healthy individuals,[71] cortisol levels of patients with RA are inadequately low, considering the high levels of interleukin-6 (IL-6) and tumor necrosis factor-α (TNF-α).[72] Perhaps in a similar fashion, the current observation of reduced or even normal responsiveness to acute stressors indicates that an individual patient is unable to mount an adequate response to real-life psychosocial stressors and inflammation.

Brief Naturalistic Stressors

Brief naturalistic stressors involve short-term challenges that are measured on a momentary basis with diaries.[5,6] Crucial to our definition of brief naturalistic stressors is that, like with the first stressor category, measurements of the research participant during nonstressor periods make up the base line with which to compare the stressor measurements. By emphasizing intra-individual differences, our second stressor category differs from the fourth stressor category (chronic and chronic intermittent stressors), which emphasizes individual differences in enduring daily stress. We will review the results of 19 studies that in the past 15 years described disease activity measures as a function of momentary daily,[26–28] workplace,[29,30] interpersonal,[31–33] and financial stressors,[34] or examined physiological responsiveness to brief naturalistic stressors.[15,32,33,35–43]

Results

Daily life brief naturalistic stressors measured on an hourly,[26] daily,[27] and weekly[28] basis have been shown to be correlated with pain,[26] tender point counts (even when joint tenderness and depression were taken into account),[27] and physical disability.[28] Within-subject analyses observed associations of workplace stressors,[29,30] interpersonal stressors,[31–33] and financial problems[34] with pain (even after controlling for negative mood),[29] health complaints,[34] increases in self-reported arthritis symptoms,[30] self-reported disease activity,[31–33] and clinician's global ratings of disease activity.[32,33] Both instantaneous and prospective correlations were observed.

Some studies examining physiological responsiveness to naturalistic stressors suggest that although immune responsiveness is disturbed, the HPA axis responsiveness is normal.[32,33,35,36]

This finding was partly confirmed in studies that observed normal HPA axis responses to the stress surrounding total knee or hip arthroplasty, while (besides epinephrine levels) the levels of IL-6 were significantly increased just before the operation in one[37] but not the other[38] study. Another study also reported that IL-6 levels of patients with RA increased during a stressful week.[39] A study in a combined sample of patients with RA and patients with fibromyalgia provided neither much evidence of disturbed cortisol reactivity to naturalistic stressors nor of disturbances in the diurnal cycle of cortisol.[40] A significant naturalistic physiological stressor is waking up, which is accompanied by a huge increase of cortisol, the early morning rise. Two studies did observe deviations in the diurnal cycle of cortisol by observing a normal early morning rise of salivary cortisol, but elevated afternoon cortisol levels,[41] and by observing a flattened diurnal cortisol rhythm and a failure to increase cortisol secretion following surgery, despite high levels of interleukin-1β and IL-6.[15]

On the basis of preliminary findings,[42] daily stressors were analyzed in patients with RA in the weeks preceding five clinical examinations across a period of 11 weeks.[43] Pain increased as inflammation increased. Remarkably, within-person analyses demonstrated that daily stressors were associated with increased perceived joint pain as well as decreased joint inflammation. In contrast to the other studies, this study suggested the intriguing possibility that daily stress might alleviate joint inflammation, although this is not echoed in attributions of individuals who blame stress for their increase of pain.

Conclusion

Overall, these studies suggest that brief naturalistic stressors in RA are associated with self-perceived and clinician's global ratings of disease activity (acute-phase reactants have been insufficiently examined) and altered immune reactivity, while HPA-axis functioning is regarded "too normal" considering the elevated immune activity.

Discussion

Our stressor definition referred to within-subject analyses that are relatively free of individual differences in neuroticism or negative affect. Analyses strongly suggested that stressors trigger an increase of self-perceived disease activity. Also, an association between stressors and clinician's rating of disease activity was suggested. Unfortunately, inflammation parameters, such as C-reactive protein (CRP) and erythrocyte sedimentation rate (ESR), were not included. These are necessary to demonstrate that stressors affect health status through changes in inflammation. Although several studies in patients with RA found disturbed immune reactivity to naturalistic stressors, most studies did not find deviations in HPA-cortisol physiology. This suggests that especially the ratio between immune and HPA axis variables is important. The HPA axis appears to react insufficiently to the stressor-induced increase of proinflammatory cytokines. In other words, the HPA axis response in RA is defective precisely because it is normal.[73]

Stressful Event Sequences

Stressful-event sequences involve a current major incident that gives rise to a series of related challenges.[5] An obvious hypothesis is that stressful-event sequences will aggravate the disease. Hypothetically, however, the distress associated with a major life event, such as the death of a relative could, by HPA axis stimulation and an increase of glucocorticoid levels, perhaps inhibit disease activity. Eleven studies in the past 15 years examined health status changes in RA as a function of stressful-event sequences.[28,44–53]

Results

Two single case reports suggested remission of RA after stressful-event sequences: 1 of 15 patients with RA who experienced a major life event while having RA (acute myocardial infarction of the spouse) perceived alleviation of RA[44] and the disease of a 53-year-old female with RA went into a temporary remission the same weeks as the unexpected deaths of her father and daughter.[45] This observation was probed in 25 patients of whom 6 had experienced deaths of meaningful persons during the past 6 months. Lower-joint tenderness for the bereaved patients was observed, while pain intensity did not differ for bereaved and nonbereaved patients.[45] A study in a large sample of 370 patients with RA indicated that major life events do not affect the course of early RA in an obvious manner.[46] Patients were questioned three times at 1-year intervals about life events in the previous year. The occurrence of deaths of relatives or acquaintances did not seem to modify patient status. Positive life events (and at a marginally significant level also negative life events) suggested a protective effect on functional disability, but these life events were not related to disease activity (Ritchie's index) or perceived overall health.[46]

It has also been suggested that major life events may lead to a deterioration of health. Patients (n = 14) who reported to have experienced more severe life events in the past 6 months experienced more current physical disability.[28] In a subgroup of 15 patients with RA with a negative rheumatoid factor, a correlation of $r = 0.34$ was observed between 1-year average levels of negative life events and 1-year average ESR scores; the nonsignificant correlation in a subgroup of 38 patients with RA characterized by a positive rheumatoid factor was in the opposite direction: $r = -0.20$.[47]

Most studies have revealed no association between life events and diverse health aspects. In studies in 54,[48] 48,[49] 238,[50] 78,[51] and 69[52] patients with RA, adverse major life events were not correlated with visual analogue scores of pain and ESR,[48] experiences of acute episodes of the illness,[49] changes in functional limitations,[50] changes in a composite score of ESR and joint-score ratings,[51] and with ESR, global disease status ratings by rheumatologists, and self-reports of pain and disability.[52] Also, a prospective study over 1 year in 30 patients with RA did not support the hypothesis that life events aggravate RA symptoms.[53]

Conclusion

Eleven studies in the past 15 years reported mixed results. Although some studies suggested a possible remission[44–46] or deterioriation,[28,47] most studies suggested no association between major life events and health status.[48–53]

Discussion

In a meta-analysis, it was concluded that to understand opposing immune changes after a major stress event, the nature of the stressor should be considered.[6] Whereas bereavement and depression are generally associated with an increase in cortisol, natural disaster may be associated with a decrease.[74] Although perhaps a major event, such as the loss of a spouse *is able to* establish a temporary remission by an increase in cortisol, our review of studies in large samples did not provide convincing evidence for this hypothesis. Studies generally do not demonstrate that major life events aggravate disease activity, leading to the conclusion that stressful-event sequences as such do not univocally affect the disease status of patients with RA.

However, a prospective study examining the correlation between stressors and disease activity within individual patients reported an equally high number of individuals with positive and negative correlations between major life events and self-reported disease activity, while only a few zero correlations were observed.[53] Perhaps this reflects that major life events *are* able to modify disease activity in a positive or negative way, depending on the nature, duration, and dose of the accompanying physiological stress response.

Chronic and Chronic Intermittent Stressors

Chronic and chronic intermittent stressors involve enduring events that pervade a person's life, forcing him or her to restructure his or her identity or social roles.[5] The number and extent of chronic stressors that are assessed with interviews and questionnaires are usually correlated with divergent health outcome variables. In divergent populations, chronic stressors have been shown to be associated with suppression of both cellular and humoral immune measures,[6] which may be a route to effects on disease activity. Six cross-sectional studies in the past 15 years reported data about a possible correlation between chronic stressors and health status in RA.[44,45,48,52,54,55]

Results

For the patient with decreased symptoms after two unexpected deaths (discussed in the section on stressful-event sequences) and in the between-subjects analyses of 25 patients reported in the article,[45] major events (our third stressor category) were associated with decreased joint tenderness and small events (our fourth stressor category) with increased tenderness. In an explorative interview study, 60% of 15 patients experienced an association between flare-ups of the disease and mild to moderate enduring psychosocial stressors, such as family arguments, job dissatisfaction, and financial problems.[44] In a study in 185 women with RA, "experiences of daily living that were appraised as harmful or threatening to the endorser's well-being" correlated with self-reports of pain severity and reduced physical functioning and global health.[54]

One study (in 69 patients),[52] but not another study (in 54 patients),[48] observed a correlation between minor stressors in the previous weeks and ESR. In both studies, the minor stressors were not correlated with self-reports of pain and in the larger study[52] nor were global disease status ratings by rheumatologists and self-reports of disability. Another study observed that immune-stimulating hormones might explain a relationship between interpersonal-stressors and disease activity. An aggregate measure of the immune-stimulating hormones prolactin and estradiol correlated with interpersonal-conflict events and physician's global illness assessment; a path model suggested that interpersonal-conflict events explained the global illness assessment through depression and these hormones.[55]

Conclusion

It is suggested that enduring interpersonal stressors,[44,45,54] but not daily hassles referring to a short-time frame,[48,52] are associated with perceived health. The finding of a correlation between stressors and ESR needs replication, because it was not confirmed in another study.

Discussion

The above studies used divergent questionnaires and designs to measure chronic stress. Likely more than for the other stressor definitions, the retrospective questionnaire reports of chronic and chronic intermittent stressors mingle with personality variables. Whereas to a certain extent a major event is a rather objective event, the perception of interpersonal stressors and daily hassles in the family and at work will depend on cognitive and affective variables.[48,75] In addition, the study of the association between chronic stressors and health status is so difficult in RA, because the two have a reciprocal influence. Patients mention pain, fatigue, functional limitations, dependency, and difficulties in carrying out activities of daily living as the most severe stressors of RA.[76–78] These disease-related stressors that may be a consequence of past and present inflammatory activity and joint condition will also have consequences for work demands and social roles. The mere cross-sectional observation of a correlation does not prove that the chronic stressors provoke a change in health status, although this might be the case.

Distant Stressors

Distant stressors are traumatic experiences that occurred in the past, yet have a potential to have long-term emotional, cognitive, or physiological consequences.[6] Distant stressors during childhood and preceding the onset of RA have been examined. Nine studies in the past 15 years reported data about the possible role of distant stressors in the etiology[44,47,56–58,62] or aggravation[47,59–61] of RA.

Results

Interviews in 50[56] and 15[44] patients revealed that 74[56] to 86%[44] of the patients observed psychosocial stressors preceding the onset of RA. Specifically asked about the etiology of RA, 27% of 60 patients named emotional stress as a first or second choice.[57] One study suggested that elevated amounts of pre-RA negative life-event stress are more prevalent in patients with a negative than with a positive rheumatoid factor,[47] but another study refuted this suggestion.[57] The above studies perhaps only reflect the beliefs (attributions) of patients, because the designs did not include control groups. A retrospective population-derived study in 55 patients with RA that did include 165 case–controls, did not support the hypothesis that stressful life events and adverse childhood experiences play an etiological role in the development of RA: the retrospectively reported number of historical life stressors was about similar for patients around the onset of RA and for control participants during that time frame.[58] A partly prospective population survey study in 9,159 persons free of arthritis assessed retrospective reports of childhood trauma at baseline.[62] After 4 years, 1,006 new cases of a self-reported rheumatic condition were observed (it was asked "have you been diagnosed by a health professional with arthritis or rheumatism?"). The experience of a childhood trauma predicted an increased risk at a rheumatic condition: persons with two or more traumatic events at baseline were 1.27 times more likely to develop a rheumatic condition than persons who did not experience a childhood trauma. The latter study used a relatively weak self-assessment of a rheumatic condition, but the design is interesting.

Some studies examined the association between retrospective reports of distant stressors and current health variables of patients with RA. Recollections of stress during childhood and adolescence were related to current pain intensity,[59] but not to current functional ability.[60] Distant stressors were not correlated with ESR, self-reported speed of onset of RA, recent pain, or duration of RA,[47] nor with current functional classification score of 128 patients with RA.[61] However, when comparing 26% of 128 patients with RA who reported no stressful life events at the time of disease onset and 50% with more than a few minor life events at the time of onset, the group with more life events exhibited a worse functional classification score.[61]

Conclusion

Some studies observed that several patients retrospectively attribute the onset of their RA to distant stressors in addition to other causes. The few retrospective studies that were done suggest an absent or small correlation between the memory of distant stressors and disease status in RA. None of these studies proves the prospective hypothesis that distant stressors make people more vulnerable to the development of RA or aggravate existing RA. Truly prospective designs of relationships between distant stressors and health status in RA are missing.

Discussion

The load of current circumstances may color the memory of past circumstances. Even more than in RA, stressors in childhood have been suggested to play a role in the etiology of fibromyalgia.[79,80] However, even this hypothesis needs confirmation. Using a prospective cohort design, cases of early childhood abuse or neglect documented between 1967 and 1971 ($n = 676$) and demographically matched controls ($n = 520$) were followed into young adulthood.[81] Assessed prospectively, physically and sexually abused and neglected individuals were not at risk for unexplained pain reported 25 years later (1989–1995). However, in the same group (of 1,196 persons), unexplained pain at the

TABLE 3. Summary of findings: the impact of five types of stressors on health status and hypothalamic-pituitary-adrenal (HPA) axis and autonomic nervous system (ANS) responsiveness in rheumatoid arthritis

Stressor category	Findings
Acute time-limited stressors	All[7–13] studies but one[14] suggest ANS hyporesponsiveness to acute time-limited stressors; normal[12,15,16,22,23] to blunted[18,20,21] HPA axis responsiveness is suggested; the indication for blunted responsiveness in some studies is weak.[17,24,25]
Brief naturalistic stressors	Several studies suggest that brief naturalistic stressors are associated with self-perceived and clinician's global ratings of disease activity[26–34,42,43]; acute-phase reactants have not been examined. HPA axis functioning is appraised "too" normal considering the elevated immune activity.[15,32,33,35–40]
Stressful-event sequences	Although some studies suggest a possible remission[44–46] or deterioriation[28,47] after stressful-event sequences, most studies suggest no association between stressful-event sequences and health status.[48–53]
Chronic (intermittent) stressors	Enduring interpersonal stressors,[44,45,54] but not daily hassles that refer to a short-time frame,[48,52] are associated with perceived health. The finding of a correlation between daily stress and ESR[52] needs replication, because it was not confirmed in another study.[48]
Distant stressors	A number of patients retrospectively attribute the onset of their RA to distant stressors in addition to other causes.[44,47,56,57] An absent[47,60,61] or small[59,61] association between the memory of distant stressors and disease status in RA is suggested. Although some indications were found,[58,62] not one study proves the prospective hypothesis that distant stressors make people more vulnerable to the development of RA or aggravate existing RA.

later assessment was associated with retrospective self-reports of childhood victimization. This study confirmed the relationship between retrospective accounts of distant stressors and chronic pain, but it rejected a prospective relationship.

Similarly, the prospective relationship between distant stressors and the onset or aggravation of RA is unproven. However, the memory of past stressors may be important, because it is a current reality of individuals.

DISCUSSION

Our findings, summarized in TABLE 3, have been discussed in the separate sections. This final section will offer some final considerations with respect to the five stressors.

It is a rather strong finding that ANS responses to *acute time-limited stressors* are reduced, while HPA axis responses are perhaps somewhat blunted or inappropriately normal when considering the abundant cytokine activity in RA.[71–73] The challenge for the future is to find out what the main determinants of this response pattern are. Physical deconditioning may be one explaining factor, because physical exercise training appears to positively affect the ANS,[82] but not the HPA axis.[83] As has been done in diabetes,[67] it would be of interest to examine, by the application of a stressor preceding the experimental stressor, whether the recent stress history partly explains physiological hyporesponsiveness. In addition, effects of current chronic stress experiences[68] and past and current disease activity on ANS and HPA axis responsiveness could be investigated. A final intriguing question is whether ANS hyporesponsiveness or defective HPA axis responses to cytokine activity are present premorbidly. Large samples are needed to examine the possible effects of these multiple determinants.

The longitudinal investigation of instantaneous changes in health status and ANS and HPA axis functioning in response to *brief naturalistic stressors* is a promising line of research. Studies rather consistently show that naturalistic stressors may adversely affect the perceived health of individuals and clinician's global ratings. To be able to examine whether brief naturalistic stressors are able to affect disease activity, future research should include measurements of pro- and anti-inflammatory cytokines and indicators of active disease, such as ESR and CRP.

Seemingly, a possible impact of *stressful-event sequences* on health status of patients with RA is not confirmed (TABLE 3). However, research has been hampered by the choice for between-person designs, while the focus could better be on individuals who will differ in their stress responses. Future research could examine within-person variations in health status as a function of major life sequences as well as the ANS and HPA axis responses that are brought about. Stressful-event sequences might lead to a remission only when, for example, in case of a depressive reaction, the HPA axis is activated and an increase of glucocorticoids inhibits disease activity. Hypothetically, to the extent that stressful-event sequences activate the sympathetic nervous system, for example, in case of an angry or anxious response, active disease may be aggravated.

The association between *chronic (intermittent) stressors* and health status likely depends on personality variables. Events do not just influence persons, but persons also influence events. The perception, selection, and modification of events affect whether a stressor is able to evoke a stress response. Several variables that have been shown to be of relevance to the health status of patients will also be of relevance to the stress response; for example, distress and depression, self-esteem, regulation of emotions, cognition about the illness, coping, self-efficacy, and social support.[84–89] Only studies with repeated measurements in large samples will be able to disentangle the interactions between stressors, disease activity, and these personality variables.

Although patients may link the onset and aggravation of RA to *distant stressors*, prospective research providing evidence for such a causal link is missing. In an experimental animal model of arthritis, it was shown that prior exposure to lipopolysaccharide (LPS), a physiological stressor, protected against inflammation in adjuvant arthritis, while prior exposure to a footshock stressor did not alter susceptibility.[90] Obviously, research in humans does not allow such rigorous testing. However, files of historical stressors like bacterial infections, the death of relatives, or disasters may provide the objective data to examine the prospective relationship between distant stressors and the onset or aggravation of RA.

ACKNOWLEDGMENTS

This research was supported by a grant from the Dutch Arthritis Association.

REFERENCES

1. Elenkov, I.J. & G.P. Chrousos. 2002. Stress hormones, proinflammatory and antiinflammatory cytokines, and autoimmunity. Ann. N.Y. Acad. Sci. **966:** 290–303.
2. Straub, R.H. *et al.* 2005. How psychological stress via hormones and nerve fibers may exacerbate rheumatoid arthritis. Arthritis Rheum. **52:** 16–26.
3. Adler, G.K. & R. Geenen. 2005. Hypothalamic-pituitary-adrenal and autonomic nervous system functioning in fibromyalgia. Rheum. Dis. Clin. North Am. **31:** 187–202.
4. Lazarus, R.S. & S. Folkman. 1984. Stress, Appraisal and Coping. Springer. New York.
5. Elliott, G.R. & C. Eisdorfer. 1982. Stress and Human Health. Analysis and Implications of Research. Springer. New York.
6. Segerstrom, S.C. & G.E. Miller. 2004. Psychological stress and the human immune system: a meta-analytic study of 30 years of inquiry. Psychol. Bull. **130:** 601–630.
7. Geenen, R. *et al.* 1996. Diminished autonomic nervous system responsiveness in rheumatoid arthritis of recent onset. J. Rheumatol. **23:** 258–264.
8. Louthrenoo, W. *et al.* 1999. Cardiovascular autonomic nervous system dysfunction in patients with rheumatoid arthritis and systemic lupus erythematosus. QJM **92:** 97–102.
9. Toussirot, E., G. Serratrice & P. Valentin. 1993. Autonomic nervous system involvement in rheumatoid arthritis. 50 cases. J. Rheumatol. **20:** 1508–1514.
10. Perry, F. *et al.* 1989. Altered autonomic function in patients with arthritis or with chronic myofascial pain. Pain **39:** 77–84.
11. Piha, S.J. & L.M. Voipio-Pulkki. 1993. Elevated resting heart rate in rheumatoid arthritis: possible role of physical deconditioning. Br. J. Rheumatol. **32:** 212–215.
12. Imrich, R. *et al.* 2005. Low levels of dehydroepiandrosterone sulphate in plasma, and reduced sympathoadrenal response to hypoglycaemia in premenopausal women with rheumatoid arthritis. Ann. Rheum. Dis. **64:** 202–206.
13. Bergholm, R. *et al.* 2002. Impaired responsiveness to NO in newly diagnosed patients with rheumatoid arthritis. Arterioscler. Thromb. Vasc. Biol. **22:** 1637–1641.

14. BEKKELUND, S.I. *et al.* 1996. Autonomic nervous system function in rheumatoid arthritis: a controlled study. J. Rheumatol. **23:** 1710–1714.
15. CHIKANZA, I.C. *et al.* 1992. Defective hypothalamic response to immune and inflammatory stimuli in patients with rheumatoid arthritis. Arthritis Rheum. **35:** 1281–1288.
16. CUTOLO, M. *et al.* 1999. Hypothalamic-pituitary-adrenocortical axis function in premenopausal women with rheumatoid arthritis not treated with glucocorticoids. J. Rheumatol. **26:** 282–288.
17. JORGENSEN, C. *et al.* 1995. Dysregulation of the hypothalamopituitary axis in rheumatoid arthritis. J. Rheumatol. **22:** 1829–1833.
18. GUDBJORNSSON, B. *et al.* 1996. Intact adrenocorticotropic hormone secretion but impaired cortisol response in patients with active rheumatoid arthritis: effect of glucocorticoids. J. Rheumatol. **23:** 596–602.
19. HARBUZ, M.S. *et al.* 2003. Hypothalamo-pituitary-adrenal axis dysregulation in patients with rheumatoid arthritis after the dexamethasone/corticotrophin releasing factor test. J. Endocrinol. **178:** 55–60.
20. DEKKERS, J.C. *et al.* 2001. Experimentally challenged reactivity of the hypothalamic pituitary adrenal axis in patients with recently diagnosed rheumatoid arthritis. J. Rheumatol. **28:** 1496–1504.
21. POOL, A.J. *et al.* 2004. Serum cortisol reduction and abnormal prolactin and CD4+/CD8+ T-cell response as a result of controlled exercise in patients with rheumatoid arthritis and systemic lupus erythematosus despite unaltered muscle energetics. Rheumatology **43:** 43–48.
22. GEENEN, R. *et al.* 1998. Experimentally induced stress in rheumatoid arthritis of recent onset: effects on peripheral blood lymphocytes. Clin. Exp. Rheumatol. **16:** 553–560.
23. ROVENSKY, J. *et al.* 2002. Somatotropic, lactotropic and adrenocortical responses to insulin-induced hypoglycemia in patients with rheumatoid arthritis. Ann. N.Y. Acad. Sci. **966:** 263–270.
24. GUTIERREZ, M.A. *et al.* 1999. Hypothalamic-pituitary-adrenal axis function in patients with active rheumatoid arthritis: a controlled study using insulin hypoglycemia stress test and prolactin stimulation. J. Rheumatol. **26:** 277–281.
25. STRAUB, R.H. *et al.* 2002. Infusion of epinephrine decreases serum levels of cortisol and 17-hydroxyprogesterone in patients with rheumatoid arthritis. J. Rheumatol. **29:** 1659–1664.
26. STONE, A.A. *et al.* 1997. The experience of rheumatoid arthritis pain and fatigue: examining momentary reports and correlates over one week. Arthritis Care Res. **10:** 185–193.
27. URROWS, S. *et al.* 1994. Unique clinical and psychological correlates of fibromyalgia tender points and joint tenderness in rheumatoid-arthritis. Arthritis Rheum. **37:** 1513–1520.
28. COBB, S.M.T. *et al.* 1998. Adjustment in patients with rheumatoid arthritis and their children. J. Rheumatol. **25:** 565–571.
29. FIFIELD, J. *et al.* 2004. Chronic strain, daily work stress and pain among workers with rheumatoid arthritis: does job stress make a bad day worse? Work Stress **18:** 275–291.
30. POTTER, P.T. *et al.* 2002. Interpersonal workplace stressors and well-being: a multiwave study of employees with and without arthritis. J. Appl. Psychol. **87:** 789–796.

31. SMITH, B.W. & A.J. ZAUTRA. 2002. The role of personality in exposure and reactivity to interpersonal stress in relation to arthritis disease activity and negative affect in women. Health Psychol. **21:** 81–88.
32. ZAUTRA, A.J. *et al.* 1997. Examination of changes in interpersonal stress as a factor in disease exacerbations among women with rheumatoid arthritis. Ann. Behav. Med. **19:** 279–286.
33. ZAUTRA, A.J. *et al.* 1998. An examination of individual differences in the relationship between interpersonal stress and disease activity among women with rheumatoid arthritis. Arthritis Care Res. **11:** 271–279.
34. SKINNER, M.A., A.J. ZAUTRA & J.W. REICH. 2004. Financial stress predictors and the emotional and physical health of chronic pain patients. Cognit. Ther. Res. **28:** 695–713.
35. CROFFORD, L.J. *et al.* 1997. Circadian relationships between interleukin (IL)-6 and hypothalamic-pituitary-adrenal axis hormones: failure of IL-6 to cause sustained hypercortisolism in patients with early untreated rheumatoid arthritis. J. Clin. Endocrinol. Metab. **82:** 1279–1283.
36. MASTORAKOS, G. & I. ILIAS. 2000. Relationship between interleukin-6 (IL-6) and hypothalamic-pituitary-adrenal axis hormones in rheumatoid arthritis. Z. Rheumatol. **59:** 75–79.
37. HIRANO, D. *et al.* 2001. Serum levels of interleukin 6 and stress related substances indicate mental stress condition in patients with rheumatoid arthritis. J. Rheumatol. **28:** 490–495.
38. TANNO, M. *et al.* 2004. Effect of general anesthesia on the abnormal immune response in patients with rheumatoid arthritis. Clin. Exp. Rheumatol. **22:** 727–732.
39. ZAUTRA, A.J. *et al.* 2004. Immune activation and depression in women with rheumatoid arthritis. J. Rheumatol. **31:** 457–463.
40. CATLEY, D. *et al.* 2000. A naturalistic evaluation of cortisol secretion in persons with fibromyalgia and rheumatoid arthritis. Arthritis Care Res. **13:** 51–61.
41. DEKKERS, J.C. *et al.* 2000. Diurnal rhythm of salivary cortisol levels in patients with recent-onset rheumatoid arthritis. Arthritis Rheum. **43:** 465–467.
42. HARRINGTON, L. *et al.* 1993. Temporal covariation of soluble interleukin-2 receptor levels, daily stress, and disease-activity in rheumatoid-arthritis. Arthritis Rheum. **36:** 199–203.
43. AFFLECK, G. *et al.* 1997. A dual pathway model of daily stressor effects on rheumatoid arthritis. Ann. Behav. Med. **19:** 161–170.
44. MARCENARO, M. *et al.* 1999. Rheumatoid arthritis, personality, stress response style, and coping with illness—a preliminary survey. Ann. N.Y. Acad. Sci. **876:** 419–425.
45. POTTER, P.T. & A.J. ZAUTRA. 1997. Stressful life events' effects on rheumatoid arthritis disease activity. J. Consult. Clin. Psychol. **65:** 319–323.
46. LEYMARIE, F. *et al.* 1997. Life events and disability in rheumatoid arthritis: a European cohort. Br. J. Rheumatol. **36:** 1106–1112.
47. STEWART, M.W. *et al.* 1994. Differential relationships between stress and disease-activity for immunologically distinct subgroups of people with rheumatoid-arthritis. J. Abnorm. Psychol. **103:** 251–258.
48. DEKKERS, J.C. *et al.* 2001. Biopsychosocial mediators and moderators of stress-health relationships in patients with recently diagnosed rheumatoid arthritis. Arthritis Rheum.-Arthritis Care Res. **45:** 307–316.

49. Haller, C. *et al.* 1997. The impact of life events on patients with rheumatoid arthritis: a psychological myth? Clin. Exp. Rheumatol. **15:** 175–179.
50. Smedstad, L.M. *et al.* 1995. Life events, psychosocial factors, and demographic-variables in early rheumatoid arthritis: relations to one-year changes in functional disability. J. Rheumatol. **22:** 2218–2225.
51. Evers, A.W.M. *et al.* 2003. Stress-vulnerability factors as long-term predictors of disease activity in early rheumatoid arthritis. J. Psychosom. Res. **55:** 293–302.
52. Thomason, B.T. *et al.* 1992. The relation between stress and disease-activity in rheumatoid-arthritis. J. Behav. Med. **15:** 215–220.
53. Koehler, T. & U. Verthein. 1993. The influence of life event stress on the course of rheumatoid arthritis: a longitudinal study. Stress Med. **9:** 105–110.
54. Dwyer, K.A. 1997. Psychosocial factors and health status in women with rheumatoid arthritis: predictive models. Am. J. Prevent. Med. **13:** 66–72.
55. Zautra, A.J. *et al.* 1994. Interpersonal stress, depression, and disease activity in rheumatoid arthritis and osteoarthritis patients. Health Psychol. **13:** 139–148.
56. Sakalys, J.A. 1997. Illness behavior in rheumatoid arthritis. Arthritis Care Res. **10:** 229–237.
57. Conway, S.C., F.H. Creed & D.P.M. Symmons. 1994. Life events and the onset of rheumatoid arthritis. J. Psychosom. Res. **38:** 837–847.
58. Carette, S. *et al.* 2000. The role of life events and childhood experiences in the development of rheumatoid arthritis. J. Rheumatol. **27:** 2123–2130.
59. Radanov, B.P. *et al.* 1996. Experience of pain in rheumatoid arthritis—an empirical evaluation of the contribution of developmental psychosocial stress. Acta Psychiatr. Scand. **93:** 482–488.
60. Radanov, B.P. *et al.* 1997. Relationship between self-rated functional status and psychosocial stress in patients suffering from rheumatoid arthritis. Psychother. Psychosom. **66:** 252–257.
61. Latman, N.S. & R. Walls. 1996. Personality and stress: an exploratory comparison of rheumatoid arthritis and osteoarthritis. Arch. Phys. Med. Rehabil. **77:** 796–800.
62. Kopec, J.A. & E.C. Sayre. 2004. Traumatic experiences in childhood and the risk of arthritis: a prospective cohort study. Can. J. Public Health. **95:** 361–365.
63. Dekkers, J.C. *et al.* 2004. Elevated sympathetic nervous system activity in patients with recently diagnosed rheumatoid arthritis with active disease. Clin. Exp. Rheumatol. **22:** 63–70.
64. De Geus, E.J., L.J. Van Doornen & J.F. Orlebeke. 1993. Regular exercise and aerobic fitness in relation to psychological make-up and physiological stress reactivity. Psychosom. Med. **55:** 347–363.
65. Dishman, R.K., E.M. Jackson & Y. Nakamura. 2002. Influence of fitness and gender on blood pressure responses during active or passive stress. Psychophysiology **39:** 568–576.
66. Ueno, L.M. & T. Moritani. 2003. Effects of long-term exercise training on cardiac autonomic nervous activities and baroreflex sensitivity. Eur. J. Appl. Physiol. **89:** 109–114.
67. Davis, S.N. *et al.* 2000. Effects of differing durations of antecedent hypoglycemia on counterregulatory responses to subsequent hypoglycemia in normal humans. Diabetes **49:** 1897–1903.
68. Benschop, R.J. *et al.* 1994. Chronic stress affects immunologic but not cardiovascular responsiveness to acute psychological stress in humans. Am. J. Physiol. **266:** R75–R80.

69. EIJSBOUTS, A.M.M. *et al.* 2005. Decreased prolactin response to hypoglycaemia in patients with rheumatoid arthritis: correlation with disease activity. Ann. Rheum. Dis. **64:** 433–437.
70. VELDHUIJZEN VAN ZANTEN, J.J. *et al.* 2005. Increased C reactive protein in response to acute stress in patients with rheumatoid arthritis. Ann. Rheum. Dis. **64:** 1299–1304.
71. TSIGOS, C. *et al.* 1997. Dose effects of recombinant human interleukin-6 on pituitary hormone secretion and energy expenditure. Neuroendocrinology **66:** 54–62.
72. STRAUB, R.H. *et al.* 2002. Inadequately low serum levels of steroid hormones in relation to interleukin-6 and tumor necrosis factor in untreated patients with early rheumatoid arthritis and reactive arthritis. Arthritis Rheum. **46:** 654–662.
73. JESSOP, D.S. & M.S. HARBUZ. 2005. A defect in cortisol production in rheumatoid arthritis: why are we still looking? Rheumatology **44:** 1097–1100.
74. YEHUDA, R. 2001. Biology of posttraumatic stress disorder. J. Clin. Psychiatry **62**(Suppl): 41–46.
75. BECKHAM, J.C. *et al.* 1991. Pain coping strategies in rheumatoid arthritis.: relationships to pain, disability, depression and daily hassles. Behav. Ther. **22:** 113–124.
76. KATZ, P.P. 1998. The stresses of rheumatoid arthritis: appraisals of perceived impact and coping efficacy. Arthritis Care Res. **11:** 9–22.
77. MAHAT, G. 1997. Perceived stressors and coping strategies among individuals with rheumatoid arthritis. J.Adv. Nurs. **25:** 1144–1150.
78. VAN LANKVELD, W. *et al.* 1993. Stress caused by rheumatoid arthritis: relation among subjective stressors of the disease, disease status, and well-being. J. Behav. Med. **16:** 309–321.
79. AL-ALLAF, A.W. *et al.* 2002. A case-control study examining the role of physical trauma in the onset of fibromyalgia syndrome. Rheumatology **41:** 450–453.
80. VAN HOUDENHOVE, B. *et al.* 2001. Victimization in chronic fatigue syndrome and fibromyalgia in tertiary care: a controlled study on prevalence and characteristics. Psychosomatics **42:** 21–28.
81. RAPHAEL, K.G., C.S. WIDOM & G. LANGE. 2001. Childhood victimization and pain in adulthood: a prospective investigation. Pain **92:** 283–293.
82. BASLUND, B. *et al.* 1993. Effect of 8 wk of bicycle training on the immune system of patients with rheumatoid arthritis. J. Appl. Physiol. **75:** 1691–1695.
83. HAKKINEN, A. *et al.* 2005. Effects of prolonged combined strength and endurance training on physical fitness, body composition and serum hormones in women with rheumatoid arthritis and in healthy controls. Clin. Exp. Rheumatol. **23:** 505–512.
84. EVERS, A.W. *et al.* 2003. Pain coping and social support as predictors of long-term functional disability and pain in early rheumatoid arthritis. Behav. Res. Ther. **41:** 1295–1310.
85. NAGYOVA, I. *et al.* 2005. The impact of pain on psychological well-being in rheumatoid arthritis: the mediating effects of self-esteem and adjustment to disease. Patient Educ. Counsel. **58:** 55–62.
86. SCHARLOO, M. *et al.* 1999. Predicting functional status in patients with rheumatoid arthritis. J. Rheumatol. **26:** 1686–1693.
87. TAAL, E. *et al.* 1993. Health status, adherence with health recommendations, self-efficacy and social support in patients with rheumatoid arthritis. Patient Educ. Couns. **20:** 63–76.

88. VAN MIDDENDORP, H. *et al.* 2005. Styles of emotion regulation and their associations with perceived health in patients with rheumatoid arthritis. Ann. Behav. Med. **30:** 44–53.

89. WALTZ, M., W. KRIEGEL & P. VAN 'T PAD BOSCH. 1998. The social environment and health in rheumatoid arthritis: marital quality predicts individual variability in pain severity. Arthritis Care Res. **11:** 356–374.

90. HARBUZ, M.S. *et al.* 2002. Protective effect of prior acute immune challenge, but not footshock, on inflammation in the rat. Brain Behav. Immun. **16:** 439–449.

Hypoglycemia, an Old Tool for New Findings in the Adrenomedullary Hormonal System in Patients with Rheumatic Diseases

RICHARD IMRICH

Institute of Experimental Endocrinology, Slovak Academy of Sciences, 83306 Bratislava, Slovakia

ABSTRACT: Over the past decades, research in patients with rheumatic disorders showed enormous progress in detecting various perturbations of the neuroendocrine system including those affecting autonomic nervous function. There is, however, a substantial lack of data on adrenomedullary hormonal system (AMHS) function in those patients. Insulin-induced hypoglycemia (IIH) represents a metabolic stressor, which elicits a counterregulatory stress response not only of the hypothalamic-pituitary axis but also of the AMHS. Therefore, in addition to traditional testing of hypothalamic-pituitary function, IIH can be used as a well-controlled functional test of the AMHS. Our recent studies showed, for the first time, attenuated epinephrine and norepinephrine responses to IIH in premenopausal females with rheumatoid arthritis (RA) and systemic sclerosis (SSc). These findings are suggestive of downregulation, or possibly defects, of the AMHS in those patients. This article reviews mechanism of the AMHS activation during IIH and demonstrates applications of the test in neuroendocrine-immune research.

KEYWORDS: insulin-induced hypoglycemia; epinephrine; norepinephrine; adrenomedullary hormonal system

THE ADRENOMEDULLARY HORMONAL SYSTEM AND RHEUMATIC DISEASES

The adaptive response of an organism to changes in the internal and external environment as part of complex homeostatic mechanism involves activation of the several neuroendocrine subsystems including the autonomic nervous system (ANS). Among other important functions, the ANS participates in

Address for correspondence: Richard Imrich, Institute of Experimental Endocrinology, Slovak Academy of Sciences, Vlarska 3, 83306 Bratislava, Slovakia. Voice: +421 2 5477 4942; fax: +421 2 5477 4742.

e-mail: richard.imrich@savba.sk

Ann. N.Y. Acad. Sci. 1069: 98–108 (2006).
doi: 10.1196/annals.1351.008

the development and regulation of the immune system. The ANS consists of at least five distinct subsystems: sympathetic noradrenergic, sympathetic cholinergic, parasympathetic cholinergic, enteric, and the adrenomedullary hormonal system (AMHS). Activation of the latter subsystem leads to secretion of epinephrine and norepinephrine from the adrenal medulla into the bloodstream.[1] Both catecholamines participate in modulation of immune responses by means of binding to adrenergic receptors which are expressed on various subtypes of peripheral blood immune cells.[2]

Several lines of evidence suggest disturbances in the ANS control of the immune system may play a role in the pathogenesis of rheumatic diseases (RD).[3] Regarding the role of the AMHS in the pathogenesis of RD, data indicate altered actions of catecholamines on receptor and post-receptor levels in the immune cells of patients with rheumatoid arthritis (RA), systemic lupus erythematosus (SLE), and Crohn's diseases.[4–7] The current literature, however, does not provide data on AMHS activity in patients with RDs. Such data are not only important for an interpretation of the downstream actions of catecholamines on the immune system, but also for elucidation of ANS alterations in RDs.

The use of tests, which stimulate the AMHS, represents one of the possible approaches to evaluate the system's function. Insulin-induced hypoglycemia (IIH) is a well-controlled metabolic stress stimulus, which elicits complex counterregulatory neuroendocrine responses including AMHS activation.[8] Preliminary studies of the authors group have shown attenuated epinephrine and norepinephrine responses to IIH in premenopausal females with RA,[9] and systemic sclerosis (SSc) (author's personal data), suggesting decreased activity of the AMHS in those patients. The present article summarizes mechanisms and consequences of AMHS activation during IIH and demonstrates application of the IIH as a simple clinical test of AMHS function in neuroendocrine–immune research.

GLUCOSE-SENSING DURING HYPOGLYCEMIA

Glucose is one of the most important metabolic substrates for brain and organ function. Therefore, glucose homeostasis is maintained with high precision by several feedback systems organized in functional hierarchy. These glucose "homeostats" are composed of glucose-sensing comparators (peripheral and central glucose sensors) and multiple effectors, which cooperatively act to maintain glucose steady-state levels. Under physiologic conditions, when glucose stores and plasma levels are sufficient, hepatic and pancreatic glucose-sensing coupled with insulin and glucagon as effectors play a major part in glucose homeostasis. The peripheral regulation of plasma glucose is under central nervous system (CNS) control. Special hypothalamic neurons integrate peripheral metabolic signals, such as glucose, insulin, or leptin, and subsequently regulate a complex adaptive response.[10,11]

Administration of insulin during IIH test is followed by massive transport of glucose from plasma to peripheral tissues. At the same time, insulin blocks endogenous glucose production in the liver, which further participates in a steep decline of plasma and brain glucose concentrations. During this emergency situation, the glucose-sensing ability of the CNS becomes prominent.[12,13] Several types of glucose-sensing neurons located in the hypothalamic ventromedial, arcuate, and paraventricular nuclei, and in the caudal brain stem around the tract of the solitary nucleus change their firing rate in response to decreased brain glucose levels. Their involvement, however, in triggering counterregulatory response to hypoglycemia is not clear.[12,14] It has been suggested that the ventromedial hypothalamus is a key glucose sensor for triggering secretion of the two principal glucose counterregulatory effectors, i.e., glucagon from the pancreas and epinephrine from the adrenal medulla.[15] However, the control of glucagon secretion from pancreatic alpha cells is controlled by multiple systems, including glucose concentration in the periphery, intrapancreatic insulin, and somatostatin levels, in addition to sympathetic regulation.[8]

Some observations suggest that peripheral hepatic glucose-sensing, transmitted to the CNS by sensory fibers of vagus nerve, may participate in an increase in AMHS activity in response to IIH, suggesting the presence of a hepatoadrenal reflex mechanism of glucose control by epinephrine.[16] Recent data from brain/neuron-specific insulin receptor knockout mice also suggest that insulin action in the brain might be important for full activation of AMHS response.[17]

ANS ACTIVATION DURING HYPOGLYCEMIA

In response to IIH, the brain initiates complex neuroendocrine and behavioral response aimed at restoring normal glucose levels, and possibly minimizing hypoglycemia-induced neuronal damage. Neuroendocrine responses to IIH include massive secretion of the hormones involved in acute responses, i.e., glucagon, epinephrine release, or long-term responses which may include glucocorticoids, growth hormone (GH) glucose counterregulation, in addition to the release of other hormones, such as prolactin, β-endorphin or vasopressin. Besides the direct effects of catecholamines on glucose metabolism, ANS activation, especially that of the AMHS, leads to specific hemodynamic changes, which increase efficiency of glucose supply.[10–13]

The signaling from glucose-sensing neurons to centers involved in regulation of hypothalamic–pituitary responses to IIH is very likely mediated by adrenergic neurotransmission.[18] On the other hand, pathways mediating signals from glucose-sensing neurons to autonomic regulatory centers are less clear. It is, however, a widely acknowledged notion that the AMHS is predominantly activated during hypoglycemia. The neural signals are transmitted from ANS centers to the adrenal medulla via the sympathetic cholinergic

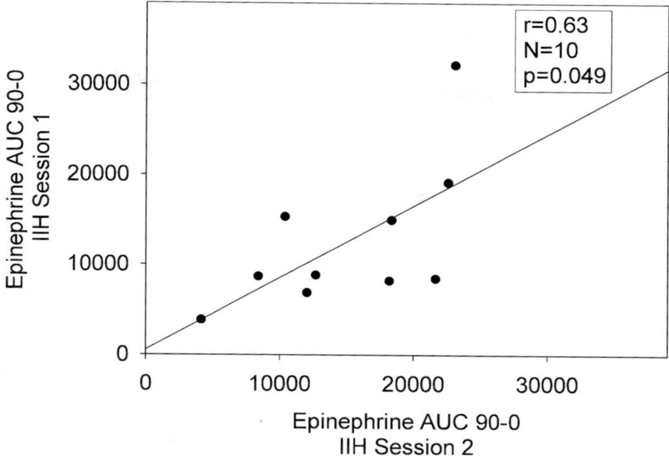

FIGURE 1. A correlation between integrated epinephrine responses to IIH in 10 healthy females tested on two different occasions. Epinephrine responses are expressed as an area under response curve (AUC) from time 0 to 90 min of the test after subtraction of baseline concentration. Pearson's correlation coefficient *r*, number of subjects *N*, and level of statistical significance *P* is displayed in the insert.

preganglionic fibers. In the adrenal medulla, the nervous impulses are transformed into hormonal secretion of epinephrine and norepinephrine.[1] During IIH, plasma epinephrine is increased approximately 5–10 times from the base line reflecting intense activation of the AMHS,[9] and this effect has been consistently reproduced (FIG. 1). While the adrenal medulla does not contribute substantially to the norepinephrine plasma pool under resting conditions, it is however mostly responsible for norepinephrine increase during IIH. Despite this response, the norepinephrine to epinephrine adrenomedullary secretion ratio is relatively low, suggesting that plasma venous norepinephrine increases are only moderate (2–3 times from the base line) in response to IIH, and that they do not usually reach the proportions of the epinephrine response.[1]

In addition to a primary counterregulatory role of glucagon mentioned above, epinephrine is complementary, but not critical, in restoring glucose homeostasis during hypoglycemia.[19,20] In situations when glucagon secretion is disrupted, such as in type 1 diabetes patients, glucose counterregulatory role of epinephrine becomes critical.[21] The mechanisms of the glycemic effects of epinephrine are complex and include stimulation of glucose production and limitation of glucose utilization mediated directly through adrenergic receptors, or via indirect mobilization of nonesterified fatty acids.[11]

Activation of the ANS during IIH has marked hemodynamic effects. Increased muscle sympathetic nervous activity, detected by microneurographic studies during IIH, would normally lead to vasoconstriction.[10] However, epinephrine released in response to IIH causes a β_2-adrenergic receptor-mediated increase in peripheral blood flow, which is believed to offset the increase in muscle sympathetic vasoconstrictor activity. Resulting vasodilatation in skeletal muscles augments glucose delivery and maintains normal glucose uptake despite falls in glucose extraction.[22] Epinephrine-induced vasodilatation during IIH is a likely cause of increased heart rate, systolic pressure, and decreased diastolic blood pressure.[23] Excessive peripheral vasodilatation, which would decrease glucose delivery to the brain, is partially balanced by increased vasoconstrictor alpha-adrenergic activity.[22] Interestingly, patients who underwent surgery affecting the hypothalamic region, had impaired epinephrine and norepinephrine responses to IIH with lack of typical hemodynamic changes, such as increase in heart rate during the test but preserved sympathetic cholinergic and neuroglucopenic symptoms to IIH, and normal cardiovascular and catecholamine responses to orthostatic challenge.[24] The results of the latter study suggest that hemodynamic changes during IIH are predominantly mediated by epinephrine alone, and an increase in cardiac sympathetic noradrenergic activity is secondary, due to epinephrine-mediated vasodilatation. Furthermore, it appears that AMHS responses to IIH are triggered by glucose-sensing centers distinct from those responsible for triggering sympathetic cholinergic responses.

While secreted epinephrine increases heat production during IIH, increased sweating, mediated through sympathetic cholinergic nerve fibers in the skin, increases evaporative heat loss resulting in fall in skin and body core temperature.[25] A shift from sympathetic vasoconstrictor to sudomotor activity is also resulting in increased skin blood flow, which further helps to promote heat loss.[10,25] It has been proposed that changes in skin sympathetic activity during IIH leading to decreased body temperature may be an additional defense mechanism with potentially neuroprotective effects.[25]

A component of the hypoglycemia-induced symptoms occur as a result of the perception of physiologic changes due to sympathetic cholinergic (sweating), adrenomedullary and sympathetic noradrenergic activation (heart pounding, shakiness, anxiousness). Some hypoglycemia symptoms can be also attributed to direct CNS glucose deprivation (tiredness, weakness, dizziness, feeling of warmth).[10] One of the most prominent behavioral symptoms occurring during IIH is hunger, regarded as defense behavior resulting in glucose ingestion.[25]

LIMITATIONS OF INSULIN-INDUCED HYPOGLYCEMIA TESTING

The neuroendocrine system is profoundly involved in metabolic processes, such as regulation of body weight, glucose control, insulin sensitivity, and energy homeostasis. Therefore, a use of IIH for neuroendocrine function assessment has obvious limitations in subjects with metabolic disorders. Indeed, neuroendocrine counterregulatory responses, including that of epinephrine, have shown to be significantly changed in obese patients even after weight loss.[26,27]

Insulin resistance or manifest type 2 diabetes may affect the action of exogenously administered insulin, resulting in an insufficient decrease in plasma glucose, and inadequate neuroendocrine response. Rather than body weight-standardized insulin bolus, use of hyperinsulinemic-hypoglycemic clamp is an alternative approach in order to reach thresholds for neuroendocrine counterregulatory responses. Interestingly, responses of glucagon and epinephrine to IIH were found to be comparable between early type 2 diabetes patients and healthy subjects.[28,29] On the other hand, lower epinephrine responses to IIH have been shown in autoimmune type 1,[21,30] and in type 2 diabetes patients with diminished insulin secretion.[11,30] The changes in counterregulatory responses occurring early in the course of the disease in type 1 diabetes are likely due to changes in CNS activity patterns related to recurrent hypoglycemia but probably not as a result of structural changes, i.e., autonomic neuropathy.[21,30] In experimental models, it was shown that insulin treatment in diabetic rats restored hypothalamic-pituitary-adrenal (HPA) response to IIH but not the deficient epinephrine response.[31]

Treatment with drugs affecting ANS, such as β-adrenergic antagonists can also significantly alter AMHS responses.[18,32,33]

INSULIN-INDUCED HYPOGLYCEMIA IN NEUROENDOCRINE RESEARCH

The fact that IIH elicits a massive release of epinephrine was noted as early as in 1920s and was further studied in 1950s.[34] Hypoglycemia was also known for its stimulatory effects of adrenal corticoids, which was used therapeutically in the dawn of corticoid era in rheumatology.[35] During following decades, clinical use of IIH in rheumatology narrowed to sporadic detection of steroid treatment-induced HPA suppression. In the last two decades of 20th century clinical research, driven by conceptualization of the neuroendocrine–immune relations,[36] observations of altered production of adrenal steroids,[37] and other hormones in RA,[38] have led to the “re-discovery” of IIH as a useful diagnostic tool. Yet, use of IIH has been mostly limited to detection of hypothalamic–pituitary function in RA,[9,39–42] SLE,[43,44] fibromyalgia,[45–48] Behcet’s disease,[49] and ankylosing spondylitis.[49,50]

AMHS PERTURBATIONS IN RA AND SSc

Recently studies conducted by the author’s group have tested counterregulatory responses to IIH (Actrapid, 0.1 IU/kg of body weight i.v. bolus) in 12

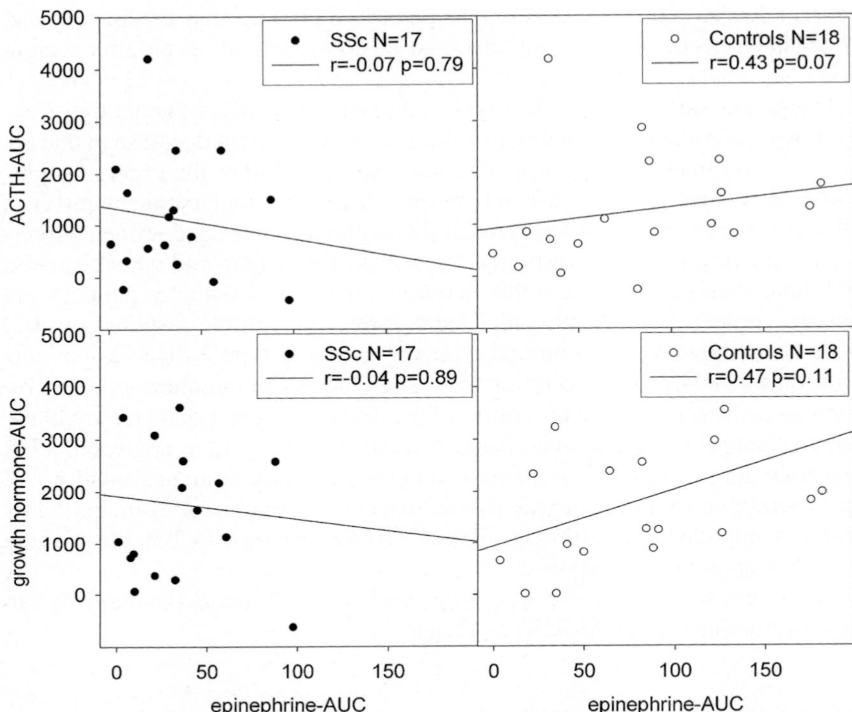

FIGURE 2. Correlations between integrated responses of ACTH and epinephrine (upper panels), and growth hormone and epinephrine (lower panels) to insulin-induced hypoglycemia in 17 SSc females (left-hand panels) and 18 matched healthy controls (right-hand panels). Responses of hormones are expressed as an area under response curve (AUC) from time 0 to 90 min (ACTH and growth hormone) and from time 0 to 60 min (epinephrine) of the test after subtraction of baseline concentration. Pearson's correlation coefficient r, number of subjects N, and level of statistical significance P is displayed in the respective panel inserts.

premenopausal females with RA compared to 11 age-, BMI-matched healthy females[9] and in 17 premenopausal females with SSc compared to 18 age-, BMI-matched healthy females. No differences in baseline catecholamine levels, but lower epinephrine ($P < 0.01$) responses to IIH were found in RA and in SSc patients compared to their respective control groups. The results of lower epinephrine responses to IIH in RA and SSc indicate downregulation or possible defect of the AMHS. Norepinephrine responses in RA and SSc patients were also lower ($P < 0.001$) compared to healthy controls, and unlike healthy controls, there was no significant norepinephrine increase from base line in response to IIH in RA and SSc patients. Considering norepinephrine increase in venous plasma during IIH, a consequence of adrenomedullary secretion, the lack of norepinephrine response to IIH also supports AMHS perturbation in RA and SSc.

Theoretically, the findings of lower catecholamine responses to IIH in RA and SSc patients can be attributed to a perturbation in central, i.e., glucose-sensing centers, downstream ANS regulatory centers, presynaptic sympathetic neurons, and/or peripheral structures, i.e., adrenal medulla. Specific pharmacologic manipulation during IIH testing, e.g., affecting transmission of neural signal to hormonal secretion in the adrenal medulla, may help to discriminate between central and peripheral defects in patients with RDs.

Under normal circumstances, one can anticipate proportional hypothalamic–pituitary and adrenomedullary responses. Indeed, positive relationships between integrated responses of two pituitary hormones and epinephrine, expressed as an area under response curve (AUC) to IIH with subtraction of baseline value, were found in healthy controls. A tendency toward positive correlations between epinephrine-AUC and adrenocorticotropic hormone (ACTH)-AUC ($r = 0.43$, $P = 0.07$), as well as between epinephrine-AUC and GH-AUC ($r = 0.47$, $P = 0.11$) were found in 18 healthy controls. However, there was no similar trend apparent in 17 SSc patients (FIG. 2). The disproportional hypothalamic–pituitary and adrenomedullary responses to IIH in SSc patients may reflect a simple downregulation of the AMHS, or even dissociation between these two neuroendocrine subsystems.

The cohorts in the preliminary studies in RA and SSc females consisted of patients with long-term disease duration. In the future, AMHS testing in early patients with RA and SSc may help to elucidate possible secondary effects of the chronic inflammatory diseases on AMHS activity. Moreover, the results give a rationale for further AMHS testing in other subsets of RA and SSc patients, as well as in patients with different autoimmune disorders.

ACKNOWLEDGMENTS

The study was supported by grant APVT-21-008602. The author wishes to express sincere gratitude to Dr. Milan Vigas and Dr. Susannah Cleary for critical review of the manuscript.

REFERENCES

1. GOLDSTEIN, D.S., G. EISENHOFER & I.J. KOPIN. 2003. Sources and significance of plasma levels of catechols and their metabolites in humans. J. Pharmacol. Exp. Ther. **305:** 800–811.
2. WAHLE, M., A. KRAUSE, M. PIERER, *et al.* 2002. Immunopathogenesis of rheumatic diseases in the context of neuroendocrine interactions. Ann. N. Y. Acad. Sci. **966:** 355–364.

3. STRAUB, R.H., C.G. BAERWALD, M. WAHLE, *et al.* 2005. Autonomic dysfunction in rheumatic diseases. Rheum. Dis. Clin. North Am. **31:** 61–75.
4. BAERWALD, C., C. GRAEFE, C. MUHL, *et al.* 1992. Beta 2-adrenergic receptors on peripheral blood mononuclear cells in patients with rheumatic diseases. Eur. J. Clin. Invest. **22**(Suppl1):42–46.
5. BAERWALD, C.G., M. WAHLE, T. ULRICHS, *et al.* 1999. Reduced catecholamine response of lymphocytes from patients with rheumatoid arthritis. Immunobiology **200:** 77–91.
6. BAERWALD, C.G., M. LAUFENBERG, T. SPECHT, *et al.* 1997. Impaired sympathetic influence on the immune response in patients with rheumatoid arthritis due to lymphocyte subset-specific modulation of beta 2-adrenergic receptors. Br. J. Rheumatol. **36:** 1262–1269.
7. KITTNER, J.M., R. JACOBS, C.R. PAWLAK, *et al.* 2002. Adrenaline-induced immunological changes are altered in patients with rheumatoid arthritis. Rheumatology (Oxford)**41:** 1031–1039.
8. YAMAGUCHI, N. 1992. Sympathoadrenal system in neuroendocrine control of glucose: mechanisms involved in the liver, pancreas, and adrenal gland under hemorrhagic and hypoglycemic stress. Can. J. Physiol. Pharmacol. **70:** 167–206.
9. IMRICH, R., J. ROVENSKY, F. MALIS, *et al.* 2005. Low levels of dehydroepiandrosterone sulphate in plasma, and reduced sympathoadrenal response to hypoglycaemia in premenopausal women with rheumatoid arthritis. Ann. Rheum. Dis. **64:** 202–206.
10. FAGIUS, J. 2003. Sympathetic nerve activity in metabolic control–some basic concepts. Acta Physiol. Scand. **177:** 337–343.
11. CRYER, P.E. 1993. Glucose counterregulation: prevention and correction of hypoglycemia in humans. Am. J. Physiol. **264:** 149–155.
12. LEVIN, B.E. 2002. Metabolic sensors: viewing glucosensing neurons from a broader perspective. Physiol. Behav. **76:** 397–401.
13. MOBBS, C.V., L.M. KOW & X.J. YANG. 2001. Brain glucose-sensing mechanisms: ubiquitous silencing by aglycemia vs. hypothalamic neuroendocrine responses. Am. J. Physiol. Endocrinol. Metab. **281:** 649–654.
14. OOMURA, Y., T. ONO, H. OOYAMA, *et al.* 1969. Glucose and osmosensitive neurones of the rat hypothalamus. Nature **222:** 282–284.
15. BORG, M.A., R.S. SHERWIN, W.P. BORG, *et al.* 1997. Local ventromedial hypothalamus glucose perfusion blocks counterregulation during systemic hypoglycemia in awake rats. J. Clin. Invest. **99:** 361–365.
16. LAMARCHE, L., N. YAMAGUCHI & F. PERONNET. 1996. Selective hypoglycemia in the liver induces adrenomedullary counterregulatory response. Am. J. Physiol. **270:** 1307–1316.
17. FISHER, S.J., J.C. BRUNING, S. LANNON, *et al.* 2005. Insulin signaling in the central nervous system is critical for the normal sympathoadrenal response to hypoglycemia. Diabetes **54:** 1447–1451.
18. TATAR, P. & M. VIGAS. 1984. Role of alpha 1- and alpha 2-adrenergic receptors in the growth hormone and prolactin response to insulin-induced hypoglycemia in man. Neuroendocrinology **39:** 275–280.
19. GARBER, A.J., P.E. CRYER, J.V. SANTIAGO, *et al.* 1976. The role of adrenergic mechanisms in the substrate and hormonal response to insulin-induced hypoglycemia in man. J. Clin. Invest. **58:** 7–15.

20. SCHWARTZ, N.S., S. D. CLUTTER, W.E. SHAH, *et al.* 1987. Glycemic thresholds for activation of glucose counterregulatory systems are higher than the threshold for symptoms. J. Clin. Invest. **79:** 777–781.
21. DAMHOLT, M.B., N.J. CHRISTENSEN & J. HILSTED. 2001. Neuroendocrine responses to hypoglycaemia decrease within the first year after diagnosis of type 1 diabetes. Scand. J. Clin. Lab. Invest. **61:** 531–537.
22. HOFFMAN, R.P., C.A. SINKEY, J.M. DOPP, *et al.* 2002. Systemic and local adrenergic regulation of muscle glucose utilization during hypoglycemia in healthy subjects. Diabetes **51:** 734–742.
23. DEROSA, M.A. & P.E. CRYER. 2004. Hypoglycemia and the sympathoadrenal system: neurogenic symptoms are largely the result of sympathetic neural, rather than adrenomedullary, activation. Am. J. Physiol. Endocrinol. Metab. **287:** 32–41.
24. SCHOFL, C., A. SCHLETH, D. BERGER, *et al.* 2002. Sympathoadrenal counterregulation in patients with hypothalamic craniopharyngioma. J. Clin. Endocrinol. Metab. **87:** 624–629.
25. MAGGS, D.G., A.R. SCOTT & I.A. MACDONALD.1994. Thermoregulatory responses to hyperinsulinemic hypoglycemia and euglycemia in humans. Am. J. Physiol. **267:** 1266–1272.
26. LEIBEL, R.L., E.M. BERRY & J. HIRSCH. 1991. Metabolic and hemodynamic responses to endogenous and exogenous catecholamines in formerly obese subjects. Am. J. Physiol. **260:** 785–791.
27. GULDSTRAND, M., B. AHREN, R. WREDLING, *et al.* 2003. Alteration of the counterregulatory responses to insulin-induced hypoglycemia and of cognitive function after massive weight reduction in severely obese subjects. Metabolism **52:** 900–907.
28. BODEN, G., R.D. SORIANO, M. HOELDTKE, *et al.* 1983. Counterregulatory hormone release and glucose recovery after hypoglycemia in non-insulin-dependent diabetic patients. Diabetes **32:** 1055–1059.
29. HELLER, S.R., I.A. MACDONALD & R.B. TATTERSALL. 1987. Counterregulation in type 2 (non-insulin-dependent) diabetes mellitus. Normal endocrine and glycaemic responses, up to ten years after diagnosis. Diabetologia **30:** 924–929.
30. CRYER, P.E., S.N. DAVIS & H. SHAMOON. 2003. Hypoglycemia in diabetes. Diabetes Care **26:** 1902–1912.
31. CHAN, O., S. CHAN, K. INOUYE, *et al.* 2002. Diabetes impairs hypothalamo-pituitary-adrenal (HPA) responses to hypoglycemia, and insulin treatment normalizes HPA but not epinephrine responses. Diabetes **51:** 1681–1689.
32. SHAMOON, H. & R. SHERWIN. 1984. Beta-adrenergic blockade is more effective in suppressing adrenaline-induced glucose production in Type 1 (insulin-dependent) diabetes. Diabetologia **26:** 183–189.
33. SCHLUTER, K.J. & L. KERP. 1983. Beta-adrenoceptor blocking agents induce different counter-regulatory responses to insulin. J. Pharmacol. **14:** 49–60.
34. GOLDFIEN, A., R. MOORE, S. ZILELI, *et al.* 1961. Plasma epinephrine and norepinephrine levels during insulin-induced hypoglycemia in man. J. Clin. Endocrinol. Metab. **21:** 296–304.
35. WEITZNER, H.A. 1952. The role of insulin induced hypoglycemia in the treatment of rheumatoid arthritis and certain other diseases. Perm. Found. Med. Bull. **10:** 112–118.
36. BESEDOVSKY, H., A. DEL REY & E. SORKIN. 1989. Regulatory links between immune and neuroendocrine systems. Immunol. Ser. **45:** 479–490.

37. MASI, A.T., D.B. JOSIPOVIC & W.E. JEFFERSON. 1984. Low adrenal androgenic-anabolic steroids in women with rheumatoid arthritis (RA): gas-liquid chromatographic studies of RA patients and matched normal control women indicating decreased 11-deoxy-17-ketosteroid excretion. Semin. Arthritis Rheum. **14:** 1–23.
38. CHIKANZA, I.C., P. PETROU, G. CHROUSOS, *et al.* 1993. Excessive and dysregulated secretion of prolactin in rheumatoid arthritis: immunopathogenetic and therapeutic implications. Br. J. Rheumatol. **32:** 445–448.
39. DEMIR, H., F. KELESTIMUR, M. TUNC, *et al.* 1999. Hypothalamo-pituitary-adrenal axis and growth hormone axis in patients with rheumatoid arthritis. Scand. J. Rheumatol. **28:** 41–46.
40. GUTIERREZ, M.A., M.E. GARCIA, J.A. RODRIGUEZ, *et al.* 1999. Hypothalamic-pituitary-adrenal axis function in patients with active rheumatoid arthritis: a controlled study using insulin hypoglycemia stress test and prolactin stimulation. J. Rheumatol. **26:** 277–281.
41. ROVENSKY, J., J. BAKOSOVA, J. KOSKA, *et al.* 2002. Somatotropic, lactotropic and adrenocortical responses to insulin-induced hypoglycemia in patients with rheumatoid arthritis. Ann. N. Y. Acad. Sci. **966:** 263–270.
42. ROVENSKY, J., R. IMRICH, F. MALIS, *et al.* 2004. Prolactin and growth hormone responses to hypoglycemia in patients with rheumatoid arthritis and ankylosing spondylitis. J. Rheumatol. **31:** 2418–2421.
43. GUTIERREZ, M.A., M.E. GARCIA, J.A. RODRIGUEZ, *et al.* 1998. Hypothalamic-pituitary-adrenal axis function and prolactin secretion in systemic lupus erythematosus. Lupus **7:** 404–408.
44. ROVENSKY, J., S. BLAZICKOVA, L. RAUOVA, *et al.* 1988. The hypothalamic-pituitary response in SLE. Regulation of prolactin, growth hormone and cortisol release. Lupus **7:** 409–413.
45. GRIEP, E.N., J.W. BOERSMA & E.R. DE KLOET. 1993. Altered reactivity of the hypothalamic-pituitary-adrenal axis in the primary fibromyalgia syndrome. J. Rheumatol. **20:** 469–474.
46. BERWAERTS, J., G. MOORKENS & R. ABS. 1998. Secretion of growth hormone in patients with chronic fatigue syndrome. Growth Horm. IGF Res. **8:** 127–129.
47. ADLER, G.K., B.T. KINSLEY, S. HURWITZ, *et al.* 1999. Reduced hypothalamic-pituitary and sympathoadrenal responses to hypoglycemia in women with fibromyalgia syndrome. Am. J. Med.**106:** 534–543.
48. DINSER, R., T. HALAMA & A. HOFFMANN. 2000. Stringent endocrinological testing reveals subnormal growth hormone secretion in some patients with fibromyalgia syndrome but rarely severe growth hormone deficiency. J. Rheumatol. **27:** 2482–2488.
49. KORKMAZ, C., O. COLAK, O. ALATAS, *et al.* 2002. Early blunted cortisol response to insulin induced hypoglycaemia in familial Mediterranian fever. Clin. Exp. Rheumatol. **20:** 8–12.
50. IMRICH, R., J. ROVENSKY, M. ZLNAY, *et al.* 2004. Hypothalamic-pituitary-adrenal axis function in ankylosing spondylitis. Ann. Rheum. Dis. **63:** 671–674.

Increased Neural Sympathetic Activation in Fibromyalgia Syndrome

PIERCARLO SARZI-PUTTINI,[a] FABIOLA ATZENI,[a]
ALESSANDRO DIANA,[b] ANDREA DORIA,[c] AND RAFFAELLO FURLAN[b]

[a]*Rheumatology Unit, L. Sacco University Hospital, Milan, Italy*

[b]*Internal Medicine II, L. Sacco University Hospital, Milan, Italy*

[c]*Division of Rheumatology, University of Padua, Italy*

ABSTRACT: Fibromyalgia (FM) is a syndrome characterized by widespread musculoskeletal pain, although the mechanisms underlying the pain have not been fully elucidated. FM patients describe a number of nonspecific symptoms, such as anxiety, depression, fatigue, unrefreshing sleep, and gastrointestinal complaints, which appear after a flu-like illness, or after physical or emotional trauma in half of the patients, and are often exacerbated by exertion, stress, lack of sleep, and weather changes. There may also be symptoms of orthostatic intolerance, which suggests underlying abnormalities in cardiovascular neural regulation. Research suggests that various components of the central nervous system are involved, including the hypothalamic-pituitary-adrenal (HPA) axis, pain-processing pathways, and the autonomic nervous system (ANS). This review discusses the general aspects of the altered HPA and ANS, sympathetic overactivity, and alterations in cardiovascular autonomic responses to gravitational stimuli.

KEYWORDS: hypothalamic-pituitary-adrenal axis; sympathetic overactivity; autonomic nervous system; fibromyalgia syndrome

INTRODUCTION

Fibromyalgia (FM) is a syndrome of unknown etiology that is characterized by chronic widespread pain and discomfort on palpation of specific sites known as tender points, and affects approximately six million people in the United States, with a higher prevalence in women.[1,2] The multicenter study that led to the American College of Rheumatology diagnostic criteria states that, in addition to its defining features, patients with FM have significantly higher rates of diverse clinical manifestations, such as sleep disorders, fatigue, paresthesias,

Address for correspondence: Piercarlo Sarzi-Puttini, M.D., Rheumatology Unit, L Sacco University Hospital, Via GB Grassi 74, 20157 Milano, Italy. Voice: 02-3904-2208; fax: 02-3904-3654.
e-mail: sarzi@tiscali.it

**Ann. N.Y. Acad. Sci. 1069: 109–117 (2006). © 2006 New York Academy of Sciences.
doi: 10.1196/annals.1351.009**

headache, anxiety, sicca symptoms, Raynaud's phenomenon, morning stiffness, and irritable bowel.[3] The symptoms are often exacerbated by exertion, stress, lack of sleep, and weather changes, and appear after a flu-like illness, or after physical or emotional trauma, in half of all patients.[4]

Patients seem to have a generalized abnormality in pain perception, with decreased pain thresholds and tolerance to a variety of stimuli, including pressure, cold, and heat.[5,6] The mechanisms underlying the pain have not been fully elucidated, but research suggests that various components of the central nervous system (CNS) seem to be involved, including the hypothalamic-pituitary-adrenal (HPA) axis, pain-processing pathways, and the autonomic nervous system (ANS).[7–10]

CNS DYSFUNCTION

Disturbances in the neuroendocrine and ANS function can lead to many of the symptoms that are frequently observed in FM patients, including fatigue, weakness, and orthostatic intolerance, and this has prompted many investigators to question whether these systems occur in FM and may be involved in its pathophysiology.[7–10]

The Hypothalamic-Pituitary-Adrenal Axis

One critical component of the neuroendocrine response to stress is the activation of the HPA axis.[11] Individuals with reduced HPA axis activity, such as those undergoing withdrawal from glucocorticoid therapy or who have Addison's disease, often show symptoms of fatigue, depressed mood, myalgias, and disturbed sleep.[12,13] HPA axis activity may also be involved in pain perception, as animal studies suggest that increased central corticotropin-releasing hormone (CRH) levels produce analgesia.[14] Unexplained fatigue has also been reported in subjects whose HPA axis function is genetically altered as a result of glucocorticoid receptor mutations leading to glucocorticoid resistance, or cortisol-binding globulin deficiency leading to low total cortisol but normal active free cortisol levels.[15,16] Activation of the HPA axis stimulates the release of the opioid β-endorphin, corticotrophin, and cortisol, which has anti-inflammatory properties that may reduce pain.[13]

HPA axis alterations have been reported in FM patients.[9,11] Griep *et al.*[17] have shown that, when CRH is released by the hypothalamus, the response is a disproportionately high release of corticotrophin by the pituitary and an unexpectedly small amount of cortisol, possibly released by the adrenal glands into the bloodstream, which suggests that such patients may have a blunted stress response and may not react appropriately to events such as infection or physical or emotional trauma.[18] However, when the same patients are injected with synthetic CRH, the increase in cortisol levels is similar to that observed in healthy control subjects, which shows that adrenal tissue sensitivity to exogenous and endogenous CRH may be different in FM patients.[17]

Studies of the hypothalamic-pituitary-thyroid axis in FM patients suggest that the release of thyrotropin-releasing hormone leads to less thyrotropin, triiodothyronine, and thyroxin secretion than expected, thus implying that the patients have some pituitary dysfunction possibly related to a dampened stress response.[19]

Circulating growth hormone (GH) levels in FM patients tend to normal during waking hours and are only slightly reduced during sleep.[20,21] Stage 4 sleep is often disrupted in patients with FM and, as it stimulates GH secretion, it is unclear whether the decreased GH levels during sleep reflect poor sleep or a sleep-induced reduction in GH stimulation.[22] It has been suggested that this relative GH deficiency may account for poor muscle microtrauma healing, and thus contribute to the nociceptive input.[23] It has been shown that FM patients have increased levels of corticotrophin and that corticotrophin increases hypothalamic somatostatin secretion and, because somatostatin is one of the hormones that inhibit GH via the hypothalamic-pituitary portal system, this may also contribute to their relative GH deficiency.[17,24,25]

A small but systematic study of the hypothalamic-pituitary-gonadal axis found no indication of abnormal gonadotropin secretion or gonadal steroid levels in FM patients.[26]

A number of neurochemical abnormalities are found in FM patients, including low serum serotonin levels, increased levels of substance P in cerebrospinal fluid, norepinephrine deficit, an abnormal dopamine status, and other neurotransmitter abnormalities, and study results suggest that these neurotransmitters play a role in HPA function and control.[27–29]

Finally, although it is not clear how HPA axis dysfunction develops in FM, it has been suggested that HPA axis function is influenced by disturbances in serotonergic neurotransmission and alterations in the activity of arginine vasopressin and CRH.[30]

Autonomic Nervous System

The ANS is an intricate network that works below the level of consciousness to maintain homeostasis, and regulates the functions of various organs and glands by means of antagonistic sympathetic/parasympathetic stimulation. ANS regulation is integrated in the CNS with that of higher brain functions, and so the ANS is the main component of the stress-response system responsible for fight-or-flight reactions.[7]

A large number of studies have evaluated altered pain perception and processing in FM, and it now seems that the neuroendocrine dysfunctions associated with FM can be further considered in terms of central sensitivity.[7–11] Central sensitization of the nociceptive neurons in the dorsal horn due to the activation of *N*-methyl-D-aspartic acid receptors, and the disinhibition of pain due to deficient functioning of the descending inhibitory system, are probably pathogenic factors for hypersensitivity to all kinds of stimuli.[30] However, the potential role of exaggerated neural sympathetic activation in generating and sustaining chronic pain has been postulated on the basis of the similarities between FM and other chronic pain syndromes associated with sympathetic overactivity, such as reflex sympathetic dystrophy and causalgia.[31–34]

Symptoms of orthostatic intolerance may also be present, thus suggesting underlying abnormalities in cardiovascular neural regulation.[32,35,36]

The suggestion that FM is a sympathetically maintained pain syndrome is based on controlled studies showing relentless sympathetic hyperactivity in FM patients, and that their pain is submissive to sympathetic blockade and rekindled by norepinephrine injections.[37]

Dysautonomia may also explain the multisystemic features of FM, although attempts to quantify possible abnormalities of cardiovascular autonomic regulation have so far led to only partial and sometimes contradictory results. For example, a microneurography study by Elam *et al.*[38] found no differences in muscle sympathetic nerve activity (MSNA) between FM patients and healthy controls in the recumbent position or during cold pressor stimulation, whereas the results of other studies indicate increased sympathetic activity on the grounds that a selective sympathetic blockade induced by guanethidine reduced pain and the number of tender points.[39] Studies based on power spectrum analyses of heart rate variability have shown increased sympathetic and decreased parasympathetic modulation,[40] and research by the National Cardiology Institute of Mexico suggests that dysautonomia is frequent in FM patients insofar as it was found that the sympathetic nervous system (SNS) is persistently hyperactive at base line (most apparently during the night), but hypoactive in response to stress.[41,42] The dysautonomia in FM patients can be characterized by unrelenting sympathetic hyperactivity throughout the day, associated with a deranged sympathetic response to different stressors.[42]

Sleep also greatly influences autonomic function, and so the increased sympathetic tone at night may be due to altered sleep or alterations in ANS regulation caused by sleep.

The results of studies aimed at quantifying possible changes in plasma and urinary catecholamine levels in FM patients are contradictory.[40–43]

We have recently tested the hypothesis that FM is characterized by sympathetic overactivity and alterations in the cardiovascular autonomic response to gravitational stimulus.[44] Sixteen FM patients and 16 healthy controls underwent ECG, finger blood pressure, respiration, and MSNA recordings at rest and during stepwise tilting up to 75°. Their autonomic profile was assessed on the basis of MSNA, plasma catecholamine levels, and the spectral indices of cardiac sympathetic (LF_{RR}) and vagal (HF_{RR}) modulation, and sympathetic vasomotor control (LF_{SAP}) computed by means of spectrum analysis of RR interval and systolic arterial pressure (SAP) variability. Arterial baroreflex function was evaluated on the basis of spontaneous SAP/RR sequences, index α, and the gain in the MSNA/diastolic pressure relationship during progressive tilting.

At rest, the FM patients had higher HR, MSNA, LF_{RR}, LF/HF, and LF_{SAP} values, and lower HF_{RR} values than the controls. The increase in tilting-induced MSNA was less in the FM patients (3.9 ± 2 bursts/min and 3.4 ± 2.4 bursts/100 beats vs. 15.9 ± 3.2 bursts/min and 14.1 ± 2.7 bursts/100 beats in the controls; $P < 0.05$), whereas the increases in the spectral indices of the cardiac autonomic profile (LF_{RR} and LF/HF) and plasma catecholamine level values were similar in the two groups; furthermore, the decrease in the index of cardiac vagal modulation (HF_{RR}) was less ($P < 0.05$) in the patients (-16.2 ± 3.7 n.u. and -139.6 ± 50.0 ms^2) than in the controls (-32.3 ± 4.6 n.u. and -901.4 ± 375.2 ms^2). These data and the excessive (44%) rate of syncope during tilting suggest a reduced ability to enhance the sympathetic activity to the vessels and withdraw the vagal modulation to the sino-atrial node. Baroreflex function was similar in both groups.

Patients with FM are characterized by an overall increase in resting cardiovascular sympathetic activity: the absence of an increased sympathetic discharge to the vessels and decreased cardiac vagal activity characterizes their autonomic profile during tilt, and may account for the excessive rate of syncope.

Assessing the autonomic profile of FM patients is clinically relevant, because the pharmacologic rebalancing of potentially altered cardiovascular neural regulation may have positive effects on both chronic pain and non-rheumatic symptoms, including orthostatic intolerance.[44]

The Interactions between the HPA Axis and the ANS

The HPA axis and the ANS interact at multiple sites. If an impaired neuroendocrine and ANS stress response is involved in the onset of FM, reduced stress responsiveness may provide one explanation for its greater prevalence among females, because their activation of many of the components of the neuroendocrine and ANS stress response is less than that of men.[11,7,45,46]

FM patients report a history of one or more forms of emotional or physical trauma, and the ability of stress to reduce the neuroendocrine and ANS stress response may explain the association between life stresses and the development of FM.[47]

It is possible that the reduced neuroendocrine and ANS stress responses represent a response to the chronic and acute stresses and symptoms associated with FM. Sleep disturbance, stress, and low levels of physical fitness are all variables that may affect ANS functioning in FM patients,[48,49] and various studies have demonstrated that stress reduction interventions, such as relaxation training and stress management training as well as exercise training cause a shift toward increased activity of the parasympathetic system and decreased activity of the SNS, as assessed by spectral analysis, resting heart rate, or circulating levels of catecholamines.[40–42,50,51] Pain may also explain the reduced neuroendocrine and ANS responsiveness, as FM patients have high cerebrospinal fluid levels of substance P, a potent inhibitor of CRH.[29]

In conclusion, decreased ANS activity and neuroendocrine function may contribute to the chronic pain and nonrheumatic symptoms (including orthostatic intolerance), but may also be a consequence of pain.

TREATMENT

Low β-blocker doses have been tried in selected cases of FM with prominent autonomic symptoms, such as palpitations and orthostatic tachycardia; however, their effects have not been reported.[10] It is not known whether it is possible (or even desirable) to try to treat SNS hyperactivity in the absence of prominent cardiovascular symptoms. Graded physical exercise, relaxation training, interventions aimed at improving sleep, and cognitive-behavioral interventions aimed at reducing stress may theoretically improve ANS functioning, but have not yet been evaluated. FM patients do not generally meet the clinical definitions of hormone deficiency; however, some of the symptoms of FM resemble those of endocrine disorders (e.g., hypothyroidism), and it would be prudent to treat individuals. Steroid treatment is not indicated for many reasons.[52] Despite the suggestion of relative GH deficiency in subjects with FM and reports of improvements after GH injections, the adverse effects, need for frequent injections, and economic costs have dampened the initial enthusiasm.[53]

CONCLUSIONS

Alterations in the HPA axis and the ANS are involved in pain-processing pathways and the multisystem features of FM. We have found that FM patients seem to be characterized by a global increase in central cardiovascular sympathetic activity while recumbent.[44] Their autonomic profile during gravitational stress is characterized by a blunted enhancement of sympathetic modulation to the vessels and impaired cardiac vagal withdrawal, which explain the excessive rate of syncope observed in the FM population.

REFERENCES

1. Clauw, D.J. 1995. The pathogenesis of chronic pain and fatigue syndromes, with special reference to fibromyalgia. Med. Hypotheses **44:** 369–378.

2. WOLFE, F., K. ROSS, J. ANDERSON & J.J. RUSSELL. 1995. The prevalence and characteristics of fibromyalgia in the general population. Arthritis Rheum. **38:** 19–28.
3. WOLFE, F., H. SMYTHE, M. YUNUS, *et al.* 1990. The American College of Rheumatology 1990 criteria for the classification of fibromyalgia: report of the multicenter criteria committee. Arthritis Rheum. **33:** 160–172.
4. GOLDENBERG, D.L. 1993. Do infections trigger fibromyalgia? Arthritis Rheum. **36:** 1489–1492.
5. BERGLUND, B., E.L. HARJU, E. KOSEK, *et al.* 2002. Quantitative and qualitative perceptual analysis of cold dysesthesia and hyperalgesia in fibromyalgia. Pain **96:** 177–187.
6. GRANGES, G. & G. LITTLEJOHN. 1993. Pressure pain threshold in pain-free subjects, in patients with chronic regional pain syndromes, and in patients with fibromyalgia syndrome. Arthritis Rheum. **36:** 642–646.
7. ADLER, G.K. & R. GEENEN. 2005. Hypothalamic-pituitary-adrenal and autonomic nervous system functioning in fibromyalgia. Rheum. Dis. Clin. North Am. **31:** 187–202.
8. JÄNIG, W. 1992. Pain and sympathetic nervous system: pathophysiological mechanism. *In* Autonomic Failure. A Textbook of Clinical Disorders of the Autonomic Nervous System. S.R. Bannister & C.J. Mathias, Eds. Oxford University Press, New York.
9. DESSEIN, P.H., E.A. SHIPTON, A.E. STANWIX, *et al.* 2000. Neuroendocrine deficiency-mediated development and persistence of pain in fibromyalgia: a promising paradigm? Pain **86:** 213–215.
10. MARTINEZ-LAVIN, M. 2002. Management of dysautonomia in fibromyalgia. Rheum. Dis. Clin. North Am. **28:** 379–387.
11. TSIGOS, C. & G.P. CHROUSOS. 2002. Hypothalamic-pituitary-adrenal axis, neuroendocrine factors and stress. J. Psychosom. Res. **53:** 865–871.
12. MAGIAKOU, M.A. & G.P. CHROUSOS. 1994. Corticosteroid therapy, nonendocrine disease, and corticosteroid withdrawal. Curr. Ther. Endocrinol. Metab. **5:** 120–124.
13. MILLER, W.L. & J.B. TYRRELL. 1995. The adrenal cortex. *In* Endocrinology and Metabolism. P. Felig, J.D. Baxter & L.A. Frohman, Eds.: 555–711. McGraw-Hill, Inc. New York.
14. LARIVIERE, W.R. & R. MELZACK. 2000. The role of corticotropin-releasing factor in pain and analgesia. Pain **84:** 1–12.
15. BRONNEGARD, M., S. WERNER & J.A. GUSTAFSSON.1986. Primary cortisol resistance associated with a thermolabile glucocorticoid receptor in a patient with fatigue as the only symptom. J. Clin. Invest. **78:** 1270–1278.
16. CHROUSOS, G.P., S.D. TERA-WADLEIGH & M. KARL. 1993. Syndromes of glucocorticoid resistance. Ann. Intern. Med. **119:** 1113–1124.
17. GRIEP, E.N., J.W. BOERSMA & E.R. DE KLOET. 1993. Altered reactivity of the hypothalamicpituitary-adrenal axis in the primary fibromyalgia syndrome. J. Rheumatol. **20:** 469–474.
18. WEIGENT, D.A., L.A. BRADLEY, J.E. BLALOCK, *et al.* 1998. Current concepts in the pathophysiology of abnormal pain perception in fibromyalgia. Am. J. Med. Sci. **315:** 405–412.
19. NEECK, G. 1992. Thyroid function in patients with fibromyalgia syndrome. J. Rheumatol. **19:** 1120–1122.

20. BAGGE, E., B.A. BENGTSSON, L. CARLSSON, *et al.* 1998. Low growth hormone secretion in patients with fibromyalgia—a preliminary report on 10 patients and 10 controls. J. Rheumatol. **25:** 145–148.
21. LANDIS, C.A., M.J. LENTZ, J. ROTHERMEL, *et al.* 2001. Decreased nocturnal levels of prolactin and growth hormone in women with fibromyalgia. J. Clin. Endocrinol. Metab. **86:** 1672–1678.
22. BENNETT, R.M., D.M. COOK, S.R. CLARK, *et al.* 1997. Hypothalamic-pituitary-insulin-like growth factor-I axis dysfunction in patients with fibromyalgia. J. Rheumatol. **24:** 1384–1389.
23. BENNETT, R.M., S.R. CLARK, S.M. CAMPBELL, *et al.* 1992. Low levels of somatomedin C in patients with the fibromyalgia syndrome: a possible link between sleep and muscle pain. Arthritis Rheum. **35:** 1113–1116.
24. WEHRENBERG, W.B., B.A. JANOWSKI, A.W. PIERING, *et al.* 1990. Glucocorticoids: potent inhibitors and stimulators of growth hormone secretion. Endocrinology **126:** 3200–3203.
25. MCCALL-HOSENFEL, J.S., D.L. GOLDENBERG, S. HURWITZ, *et al.* 2003. Growth hormone and insulin-like growth factor-1 concentrations in women with fibromyalgia. J. Rheumatol. **30:** 809–814.
26. KORSZUN, A., E.A. YOUNG, N.C. ENGLEBERG, *et al.* 2000. Follicular phase hypothalamic pituitary-gonadal axis function in women with fibromyalgia and chronic fatigue syndrome. J. Rheumatol. **27:** 1526–1530.
27. RUSSELL, I.J., J.E. MICHALEK, G.A. VIPRAIO, *et al.* 1992. Platelet H-imipramine uptake receptor density and serum serotonin levels in patients with fibromyalgia/fibrositis syndrome. J. Rheumatol. **19:** 104–109.
28. BUSKILA, D. & J. PRESS. 2001. Neuroendocrine mechanisms in fibromyalgia-chronic fatigue. Best Pract. Res. Clin. Rheumatol. **15:** 747–758.
29. RUSSELL, I.J., M.D. ORR, B. LITTMAN, *et al.* 1994. Elevated cerebrospinal fluid levels of substance P in patients with the fibromyalgia syndrome. Arthritis Rheum. **37:** 1593–1601.
30. DEMITRACK, M.A. & L.J. CROFFORD. 1998. Evidence for and pathophysiologic implications of hypothalamic-pituitary-adrenal axis dysregulation in fibromyalgia and chronic fatigue syndrome. Ann. N. Y. Acad. Sci. **840:** 684–697.
31. SCHOTT, G.D. 1992. Pain and the sympathetic nervous system. *In* Autonomic Failure, a Textbook of Clinical Disorders of the Autonomic Nervous System. S.R. Bannister & C.J. Mathias, Eds.: 904–916. Oxford University Press. Oxford.
32. BOU-HOLAIGAH, I., H. CALKINS, J.A. FLYNN, *et al.* 1997. Provocation of hypotension and pain during upright tilt table testing in adults with fibromyalgia. Clin. Exp. Rheumatol. **15:** 239–246.
33. EVANS, J.A. 1946. Reflex sympathetic dystrophy. Surg. Clin. North Am. **26:** 435–448.
34. BARON, R.M., J.D.M.P. LEVINE & H.M.P. FIELDS. 1999. Causalgia and reflex sympathetic dystrophy: does the sympathetic nervous system contribute to the generation of pain? Muscle Nerve **22:** 678–695.
35. NARKIEWICZ, K. & V.K. SOMERS. 1998. Chronic orthostatic intolerance: part of a spectrum of dysfunction in orthostatic cardiovascular homeostasis? Circulation **98:** 2105–2107.
36. FURLAN, R., G. JACOB, M. SNELL, *et al.* 1998. Chronic orthostatic intolerance: a disorder with discordant cardiac and vascular sympathetic control. Circulation **98:** 2154–2159.

37. Martinez-Lavin, M. 2004. Fibromyalgia as a sympathetically maintained pain syndrome. Curr. Pain Headache Rep. **8:** 385–389.
38. Elam, M., G. Johansson & B. Wallin. 1992. Do patients with primary fibromyalgia have an altered muscle sympathetic nerve activity? Pain **48:** 371–375.
39. Backman, E., A. Bengtsson, M. Bengtsson, *et al.* 1998. Skeletal muscle functions in primary fibromyalgia: effect of regional sympathetic blockade with guanethidine. Acta Neurol. Scand. **77:** 187–191.
40. Cohen, H., L. Neumann, M. Shore, *et al.* 2000. Autonomic dysfunction in patients with fibromyalgia: application of power spectral analysis of heart rate variability. Semin. Arthritis Rheum. **29:** 217–227.
41. Martinez-Lavin, M., A.G. Hermosillo, M. Rosas, *et al.* 1998. Circadian studies of autonomic nervous balance in patients with fibromyalgia: a heart rate variability analysis. Arthritis Rheum. **41:** 1966–1971.
42. Martinez-Lavin, M., A.G. Hermosillo, C. Mendoza, *et al.* 1997. Orthostatic sympathetic derangement in subjects with fibromyalgia. J. Rheumatol. **24:** 714–718.
43. Raj, S.R., D. Brouillard, C.S. Simpson, *et al.* 2000. Dysautonomia among patients with fibromyalgia: a noninvasive assessment. J. Rheumatol. **27:** 2660–2665.
44. Furlan, R., S. Colombo, F. Perego, *et al.* 2005. Abnormalities of cardiovascular neural control and reduced orthostatic tolerance in patients with primary fibromyalgia. J. Rheumatol. **32:** 1787–1793.
45. Davis S.N., P. Galassetti, D.H. Wasserman, *et al.* 2000. Effects of gender on neuroendocrine and metabolic counter regulatory responses to exercise in normal man. J. Clin. Endocrinol. Metab. **85:** 224–230.
46. Kirschbaum, C., B.M. Kudielka, J. Gaab, *et al.* 1999. Impact of gender, menstrual cycle phase, and oral contraceptives on the activity of the hypothalamus-pituitary-adrenal axis. Psychosom. Med. **61:** 154–162.
47. Van, H.B. & U.T. Egle. 2004. Fibromyalgia: a stress disorder? Piecing the biopsychosocial puzzle together. Psychother. Psychosom. **73:** 267–275.
48. Ako, M., T. Kawara, S. Uchida, *et al.* 2003. Correlation between electroencephalography and heart rate variability during sleep. Psychiatry Clin. Neurosci. **57:** 59–65.
49. Trinder, J., J. Kleiman, M. Carrington, *et al.* 2001. Autonomic activity during human sleep as a function of time and sleep stage. J. Sleep Res. **10:** 253–264.
50. Albright, G.L., J.L. Andreassi & A.L. Brockwell. 1991. Effects of stress management on blood pressure and other cardiovascular variables. Int. J. Psychophysiol. **11:** 213–217.
51. Goldsmith, R.L., D.M. Bloomfield & E.T. Rosenwinkel. 2000. Exercise and autonomic function. Coron. Artery Dis. **11:** 129–135.
52. Clark, S., E. Tindall & R.M. Bennett. 1985. A double blind crossover trial of prednisone versus placebo in the treatment of fibrositis. J. Rheumatol. **12:** 980–983.
53. Bennett, R.M., S.C. Clark & J. Walczyk. 1998. A randomized, double-blind, placebo-controlled study of growth hormone in the treatment of fibromyalgia. Am. J. Med. **104:** 227–231.

Anti-Endothelial Antibodies and Neuropsychiatric Systemic Lupus Erythematosus

GUIDO VALESINI, CRISTIANO ALESSANDRI, DOMENICO CELESTINO, AND FABRIZIO CONTI

Cattedra e Divisione di Reumatologia, Università La Sapienza, Rome, Italy

Abstract: The pathogenesis of neuropsychiatric systemic lupus erythematosus (NPSLE) has been attributed to autoantibody-mediated neural dysfunction, vasculopathy, and coagulopathy. Several autoantibodies specificities have been reported in serum and cerebrospinal fluid of NPSLE patients (i.e., antineuronal, antiribosomal P proteins, antiglial fibrillary acidic proteins, antiphospholipid, and anti-endothelial antibodies). We have recently demonstrated an association between serum anti-endothelial antibodies and psychosis or depression in patients with SLE. Subsequently, by screening a cDNA library from human umbilical artery endothelial cells with serum from a SLE patient with psychosis, one positive strongly reactive clone was identified encoding the C-terminal region (C-ter) of Nedd5, an intracytoplasmatic protein of the septin family. Anti-Nedd5 antibodies have been found significantly associated with psychiatric manifestations in SLE patients, strengthening the view of a possible implication of autoantibodies in the development of psychiatric disorders.

Keywords: NPSLE; neuropsychiatric; psychiatric; systemic lupus erythematosus; AECA; Nedd5; autoantibodies

INTRODUCTION

Systemic lupus erythematosus (SLE) is a chronic autoimmune disease characterized by multisystemic involvement with a broad spectrum of clinical manifestations.

Neuropsychiatric systemic lupus erythematosus (NPSLE) includes neurologic syndromes involving the central, peripheral, and autonomic nervous system as well as the psychiatric disorders observed in patients with SLE. These manifestations can precede the onset of SLE or occur at any time during

Address for correspondence: Prof. Guido Valesini, Dipartimento di Clinica e Terapia Medica Applicata, Cattedra di Reumatologia, Università "La Sapienza," V.le del Policlinico 155, 00161 Rome, Italy. Voice: +39 0649974631; fax: +39 0649974642.
e-mail: guido.valesini@uniroma1.it

Ann. N.Y. Acad. Sci. 1069: 118–128 (2006).
doi: 10.1196/annals.1351.010

the course of the disease. In 1999 the American College of Rheumatology nomenclature for NPSLE provided case definitions for 19 neuropsychiatric syndromes seen in SLE, with diagnostic criteria and methods for ascertainment.[1] None of the syndromes are specific for SLE and there is no reliable diagnostic test, and thus the diagnosis of NPSLE is difficult. Manifestations also vary in severity, ranging from mild headaches to life-threatening coma.

The pathogenesis of NPSLE has been attributed to autoantibody-mediated neural dysfunction, vasculopathy, and coagulopathy. It has been suggested that several autoantibody specificities may play a role in the pathogenesis of NPSLE. Among others, a potential pathogenic relevance has been attributed to antineuronal, antiribosomal P proteins, antiglial fibrillary acidic proteins (GFAPs), antiphospholipid, and more recently to anti-endothelial antibodies (AECA) (TABLE 1).[2,3] Nevertheless, the etio-pathogenic role of these autoantibodies, detected in serum and cerebrospinal fluid (CFS), in NPSLE remains unclear. Here, we analyzed briefly what is known about the role of these autoantibodies in the pathogenesis of NPSLE, in particular focusing on the new endothelial target antigens of AECA recently associated with NPSLE.

AUTOANTIBODIES AND NPSLE

A hypothetic role for antineuronal antibodies in the pathogenesis of NPSLE was first suggested by studies of Bresnihan and colleagues in 1979. In particular, a cross-reactivity between antilymphocyte IgG with antineuronal IgG was observed in sera of SLE patients with neuropsychiatric involvement[4,5] as well as in patients with cognitive impairment.[6] In another study CSF from patients with SLE and central nervous system manifestations was reactive with the

TABLE 1. Autoantibodies associated with neuropsychiatric systemic lupus erythematosus

Antibody Specificity	Reference
Anti-neuronal antibodies	Bresnihan *et al.*[4,5]; Bluestein *et al.*[7]; Denburg *et al.*[6]; How *et al.*[8]; Danon *et al.*[9]; Mevorach *et al.*[18]
Anti-ribosomal P protein antibodies	Bonfa *et al.*[26,27]; Isshi *et al.*[20]
Anti-glial fibrillary acidic protein antibodies	Sanna *et al.*[31]
Anti-DNA antibodies cross-reacting with NMDA	DeGiorgio *et al.*[39]
Antibodies to microtubule-associated protein 2	Williams *et al.*[40]
Anti-phospholipid antibodies	Harris *et al.*[41]; Asherson *et al.*[42]; Herranz *et al.*[43]
Anti-endothelial cell antibodies	Conti *et al.*[3]; Song *et al.*[56]; Meroni *et al.*[57]
Anti-NEDD5 antibodies	Margutti *et al.*[64];

cultured human neuronal cell line SK-N-SH as compared with patients without these manifestations, suggesting an intrathecal synthesis of these autoantibodies.[7] In addition, NPSLE patients with diffuse disease showed a higher titer of antibodies against neuroblastoma cell line in comparison to those with focal manifestations.[8] Interestingly, a similar reactivity was also observed in pediatric SLE patients with neuropsychiatric involvement.[9] In contrast, several other studies did not confirm the association between antineuronal antibodies and NPSLE in either pediatric or adult patients.[10–14] The differences among studies may be related to the selection and the number of enrolled patients as well as to the various assay systems used for autoantibody detection.

The mechanism by which antineuronal antibodies might play a role in the pathogenesis of NPSLE has not yet been established[15]; however, the evidence for binding of antineuronal antibodies in brains of NZB/W mice supports a direct pathogenic role.[16]

The impairment of the blood–brain barrier, frequently observed in NPSLE patients, might account for crossing of lymphocytotoxic antibodies or antibodies reactive against mycobacterial glycolipids, which showed a cross-reactivity also with anti-neuronal antibodies.[17] On the other hand, the higher reactivity of antineuronal antibodies, as well as other antibodies, in cerebrospinal fluid of patients with NPSLE supports an intrathecal synthesis.[7,18]

In summary, it is likely that several mechanisms are implicated in the pathogenesis of NPSLE and the question whether antineuronal antibodies might be the epiphenomenon of primary inflammation or be directly involved in triggering neurological injury is still matter of debate. Further studies are needed to clarify whether autoantibody detection, both in sera and in CSF of NPSLE patients could be a useful diagnostic and prognostic tool, as previously suggested.[19,20]

Antiribosomal P protein antibodies (anti-P) are directed to three phosphoproteins that are located on the larger 60S subunit of eukaryotic ribosomes (P0, P1, and P2). The prevalence of anti-P in SLE patients ranges from 6% to 36%, and shows ethnic differences.[21] Interestingly, the titers of anti-P antibodies were significantly higher in SLE sera positive for both anti-Sm and anti-dsDNA antibodies,[22,23] and correlated with SLE disease activity[24] and lupus nephritis.[25] Bonfa *et al.* first described a close association between lupus psychosis and the presence of anti-P antibodies,[26,27] which decreased after a successful treatment. Subsequently, other authors investigated the same relationship, reporting controversial findings. Schneebaum *et al.* observed the presence of a high titer of anti-P antibodies in about 19% of 269 patients with SLE, 88% of them presenting with major depression and 45% with lupus psychosis.[28] In contrast, Teh and co-workers reported a prevalence of anti-P antibodies in 16% of patients with SLE, without any significant associations with psychosis or depression.[29] Recently, Yoshio and colleagues demonstrated that the frequency of CSF anti-P in patients with NPSLE was significantly higher than in patients without NPSLE.[30] Therefore, the association between anti-P and lupus psychosis has not always been confirmed and still represents a matter of debate.[25–30] Recently, we have estimated a prevalence of 7.8% for anti-P antibodies in SLE patients without any association with psychiatric disturbances.[3] Remarkably, all patients with lupus psychosis were seronegative for this autoantibody specificity.[3] This high variability among different studies could be related either to differences in criteria used to define lupus psychosis or to the sensitivity of the assays used to detect autoantibodies.

With regard to antiglial fibrillary acidic protein antibodies (anti-GFAPs), Sanna *et al.* described a high positive predictive value for this antibody specificity in NPSLE.[31] The glial fibrillary acidic protein (GFAP) is a 50 kDa intracytoplasmic filamentous protein of the astrocytes and it is thought to stabilize the cytoskeleton and to maintain astrocyte cell shape through interaction with the nuclear and the plasma membrane.[32] GFAP has proved to be the most specific marker for cells of astrocytic origin under normal and pathological conditions. For instance, GFAP is upregulated in gliotic hypertrophy and perivascular inflammation of Alzheimer's disease and multiple sclerosis.[33–35] It is noteworthy that anti-GFAP antibodies were also described in these diseases.[33–35]

Recently, Trysberg and coworkers described increased levels of GFAP in the CSF of SLE patients with neuropsychiatric involvement, suggesting that GFAP might be a useful tool in the diagnosis and monitoring of NPSLE.[36] The increased level of this protein in the cerebrospinal fluid may account for an antigen-specific or polyclonal B cell response. We found an anti-GFAP prevalence of 15.7% in sera of our SLE patients, without any significant correlation with neurologic or psychiatric morbidity.[37] Nevertheless, anti-GFAP were described also in the CSF from one SLE patient with headache and anosmia.[38] Furthermore, the role of anti-GFAP antibodies in NPSLE should be clarified by prospective studies using both intrathecal and serum determination.

DeGiorgio *et al.* demonstrated *in vitro* that a subset of anti-DNA antibodies cross-reacts with the NMDA (*N*-methyl-D-aspartate) subtype of glutamate receptors and induces neuronal cell injury. Moreover, the results showed that such antibodies can be present in the CSF of patients with lupus.[39]

More recently, antibodies to microtubule-associated protein 2 (MAP-2), a cellular protein expressed almost exclusively in neurons, have been associated with neuropsychiatric symptoms (i.e., psychosis, seizure, neuropathy, and cerebritis) in SLE patients.[40]

The association between anti-phospholipid antibodies (aPLs) and CNS involvement in SLE, first reported in 1984, has now been confirmed, and thrombosis associated with these antibodies is considered the main pathogenic mechanism.[41–43] Moreover, aPLs may contribute to neurological damage by reacting with brain cells by means of β2-GPI interaction. In this context we previously demonstrated the expression of β2-GPI mRNA by astrocytes and neuronal and endothelial cells, suggesting that these cells can represent a target of autoantibodies in the APS.[44–45]

ANTI-ENDOTHELIAL CELL ANTIBODIES AND NPSLE

Anti-endothelial cell antibodies (AECAs) consist of a group of heterogeneous antibodies that react with different endothelial cell antigens that range from 10 to 200 kDa in molecular size in immunoblot analysis.[46] These autoantibodies have been detected in several autoimmune diseases and have been associated with nephritis and vasculitis in SLE patients.[47] Moreover, recent data suggest their implication in endothelial dysfunction and a pathogenic role of AECAs in SLE.[47–52] Interestingly, some *in vitro* and *in vivo* reports have demonstrated an increased expression of adhesion molecules on HUVEC, mediated by AECA IgG purified from sera of SLE patients.[53–55] Few data are available on AECA in NPSLE. Song and coworkers showed the clinical association of AECAs with disease activity in their cohort of 41 SLE patients.[56] Interestingly, they described the association of AECAs with neuropsychiatric lupus.[56] Meroni and co-workers found AECAs positivity in 5 of 14 SLE patients with involvement of the central nervous system.[57] We have recently reported an association between serum AECAs and psychosis or depression in patients with SLE, strengthening the view of a possible implication of AECAs in the development of psychiatric disorders in SLE.[3] In our study patients were categorized as either with (psychiatric group) or without (nonpsychiatric group) psychiatric disorders on the basis of the clinical psychiatric examination. We considered as patients with psychiatric manifestations only those with a more severe psychopathology, such as psychosis and mood disorders (recurrent major depressive disorder, dysthymyic disorder, and depressive disorder not otherwise specified). Anxiety and mild depression are frequently detected in SLE patients and it was suggested that these disorders are predominantly psychoreactive.[1,58–60] However, in a large retrospective study, SLE patients with depression presented CNS involvement more often than patients without, supporting the view that mood disorders are not merely a response to stress.[61] Data demonstrating the presence of serum AECAs in patients with depression support the hypothesis that depression in SLE could have a biological origin.

Ribosomal P antigens have been described on the surface of endothelial cells.[62] Moreover, purified IgG anti-P derived from patients with SLE activate human umbilical vein endothelial cells, as well as monocytes, resulting in the increase of interleukin 6 (IL-6) production.[30,63] Serum anti-P may bind to ribosomal P antigens on the endothelial surface in the brain and activate endothelial cells, leading to entry of serum anti-P into the CSF by disruption of the blood–brain barrier and the activation of intrathecal B lymphocytes by IL-6 production.

Looking for the target antigen(s) of AECAs detected in our series of NPSLE patients we evaluated anti-P antibodies by means of enzyme-linked immunosorbent assay (ELISA), but no significant associations were found between these autoantibodies and AECA reactivity.[3] In addition, it has been postulated that AECA reactivity may be due in part to the binding to a complex of β2-GPI with phospholipids on endothelial cells,[50–51] although we did not find any correlation between aPL/aβ2-GPI and AECA reactivity.[3]

In order to identify possible molecular target(s) of AECAs in an SLE patient with active psychosis, we used a molecular cloning strategy.[64] Our results provide evidence that the C-terminal region of Nedd5 is a novel autoantigen with a role in neuropsychiatric manifestations. Nedd5 is a mammalian septin known to associate with actin-based structures, such as the contractile ring and stress fibers.[65,66] The septins are a family of cytoskeletal GTPases that play an essential role in cytokinesis in yeast and mammalian cells.[67] Interestingly, Nedd5 is predominantly expressed in the nervous system and may contribute to the formation of neurofibrillary tangles as integral constituents of paired helical filaments in Alzheimer's disease.[68,69] Moreover, Nedd5 shows an intracellular redistribution on the cell surface during apoptosis, which may be in part responsible for its immunogenity.[64]

Although anti-Nedd5 autoantibodies are not specific to SLE, they are significantly associated with neuropsychiatric SLE and could be immunological markers of psychiatric manifestations in this disorder. Nevertheless, we found no significant correlation between AECAs and anti-Nedd5 antibodies in patients with SLE. This finding is not surprising, since the cell-surface ELISA on living cells used to detect AECAs reveals only plasma membrane antigens, whereas Nedd5, which is normally confined within the cytoplasm, becomes exposed on the cell surface after triggering apoptosis. Moreover, we cannot exclude the possibility that the autoimmune response we observed was generated against Nedd5 present in other cellular compartments, such as the nervous system. Remarkably, a higher titer of anti-Nedd5 was also detected in systemic sclerosis (SS), a disease characterized by endothelial damage. Thus, the unanswered question is whether anti-Nedd5 C-ter antibodies can cause damage, contributing to the pathogenesis of psychiatric manifestations in SLE, or they are merely an epiphenomenon. Further studies *in vivo* are in progress in order to clarify the effective role of anti-Nedd5 C-ter antibodies in SLE and SS patients.

In conclusion, a significant association between neuropsychiatric involvement in SLE patients and AECAs was reported. The target antigen of these autoantibodies is still under investigation. In this contest, recent studies suggest that specific antigens, such as ribosomal P protein,[62] Nedd5,[64] and Ro52/SS-A[70] may be expressed on the surface of ECs after apoptosis, being accessible to the immune system and supporting a direct pathogenic role of these autoantibodies in NPSLE.

REFERENCES

1. ACR AD HOC COMMITTEE ON NEUROPSYCHIATRIC LUPUS NOMENCLATURE. 1999. The American College of Rheumatology nomenclature and case definitions for neuropsychiatric lupus syndromes. Arthritis Rheum. **42:** 599–608.

2. GREENWOOD, D.L., V.M. GITLITS, F. ALDERUCCIO, *et al.* 2002. Autoantibodies in neuropsychiatric lupus. Autoimmunity **35:** 79–86.
3. CONTI, F., C. ALESSANDRI, D. BOMPANE, *et al.* 2004. Autoantibody profile in systemic lupus erythematosus with psychiatric manifestations: a role for anti-endothelial-cell antibodies. Arthritis Res. Ther. **6:** R366–R372.
4. BRESNIHAN, B., M. OLIVER, B. WILLIAMS, *et al.* 1979. An antineuronal antibody cross-reacting with erythrocytes and lymphocytes in systemic lupus erythematosus. Arthritis Rheum. **22:** 313–320.
5. BRESNIHAN, B., R. HOHMEISTER, J. CUTTING, *et al.* 1979. The neuropsychiatric disorder in systemic lupus erythematosus: evidence for both vascular and immune mechanisms. Ann. Rheum. Dis. **38:** 301–306.
6. DENBURG, J.A., R.M. CARBOTTE & S.D. DENBURG. 1987. Neuronal antibodies and cognitive function in systemic lupus erythematosus. Neurology **37:** 464–467.
7. BLUESTEIN, H.G., G.W. WILLIAMS & A.D. STEINBERG. 1981. Cerebrospinal fluid antibodies to neuronal cells: association with neuropsychiatric manifestations of systemic lupus erythematosus. Am. J. Med. **70:** 240–246.
8. HOW, A., P.B. DENT, S.K. LIAO, *et al.*1985. Antineuronal antibodies in neuropsychiatric systemic lupus erythematosus. Arthritis Rheum. **28:** 789–795.
9. DANON, Y.L. & B.Z. GARTY. 1986. Autoantibodies to neuroblastoma cell surface antigens in neuropsychiatric lupus. Neuropediatrics **17:** 23–27.
10. PAPERO, P.H., H.G. BLUESTEIN, P. WHITE, *et al.* 1990. Neuropsychologic deficits and antineuronal antibodies in pediatric systemic lupus erythematosus. Clin. Exp. Rheumatol. **8:** 417–424.
11. TISHLER, M., I. ALOSACHIE, Y. CHAPMAN, *et al.* 1995. Anti-neuronal antibodies in antiphospholipid syndrome with central nervous system involvement: the difference from systemic lupus erythematosus. Lupus **4:** 145–147.
12. HANLY, J.G., N.M. WALSH, J.D. FISK, *et al.* 1993. Cognitive impairment and autoantibodies in systemic lupus erythematosus. Br. J. Rheumatol. **32:** 291–296.
13. HANLY, J.G., N.M. WALSH & V. SANGALANG. 1992. Brain pathology in systemic lupus erythematosus. J. Rheumatol. **19:** 732–741.
14. SAILER, M., W. BURCHERT, C. EHRENHEIM, *et al.* 1987. Positron emission tomography and magnetic resonance imaging for cerebral involvement in patients with systemic lupus erythematosus. J. Neurol. **244:** 186–193.
15. HANLY, J.G. & C. HONG. 1993. Antibodies to brain integral membrane proteins in systemic lupus erythematosus. J. Immunol. Methods **161:** 107–118.
16. MOORE, P.M. 1992. Evidence for bound antineuronal antibodies in brains of NZB/W mice. J. Neuroimmunol. **38:** 147–154.
17. AVINOACH, I., H. AMITAL-TEPLIZKI, O. KUPERMAN, *et al.* 1990. Characteristics of antineuronal antibodies in systemic lupus erythematosus patients with and without central nervous system involvement: the role of mycobacterial cross-reacting antigens. Isr. J. Med. Sci. **26:** 367–373.
18. MEVORACH, D., E. RAZ & I. STEINER. 1994. Evidence for intrathecal synthesis of autoantibodies in systemic lupus erythematosus with neurological involvement. Lupus **3:** 117–121.
19. WEST, S.G., W. EMLEN, M.H. WENER, *et al.* 1995. Neuropsychiatric lupus erythematosus: a 10-year prospective study on the value of diagnostic tests. Am. J. Med. **99:** 153–163.
20. ISSHI, K. & S. HIROHATA. 1998. Differential roles of the anti-ribosomal P antibody and antineuronal antibody in the pathogenesis of central nervous system

involvement in systemic lupus erythematosus. Arthritis Rheum. **41:** 1819–1827.

21. ARNETT, F.C., J.D. REVEILLE, H.M. MOUTSOPOULOS, *et al.* 1996. Ribosomal P autoantibodies in systemic lupus erythematosus: frequencies in different ethnic groups and clinical and immunogenetic associations. Arthritis Rheum. **39:** 1833–1839.
22. ELKON, K.B., E. BONFA, R. LLOVET, *et al.* 1989. Association between anti-Sm and anti-ribosomal P protein autoantibodies in human systemic lupus erythematosus and MRL/lpr mice. J. Immunol. **143:** 1549–1554.
23. CHINDALORE, V., B. NEAS & M. REICHLIN. 1998. The association between anti-ribosomal P antibodies and active nephritis in systemic lupus erythematosus. Clin. Immunol. Immunopathol. **87:** 292–296.
24. SATO, T., T. UCHIUMI, T. OZAWA, *et al.* 1991. Autoantibodies against ribosomal proteins found with high frequency in patients with systemic lupus erythematosus with active disease. J. Rheumatol. **18:** 1681–1684.
25. MARTIN, A.L. & M. REICHLIN. 1996. Fluctuations of antibody to ribosomal P proteins correlate with appearance and remission of nephritis in SLE. Lupus **5:** 22–29.
26. BONFA, E. & K.B. ELKON. 1986. Clinical and serologic associations of the antiribosomal P protein antibody. Arthritis Rheum. **29:** 981–985.
27. BONFA, E., S.J. GOLOMBEK, L.D. KAUFMAN, *et al.* 1987. Association between lupus psychosis and antiribosomal P protein antibodies. N. Engl. J. Med. **317:** 265–271.
28. SCHNEEBAUM, A.B., J.D. SINGLETON, S.G. WEST, *et al.* 1991. Association of psychiatric manifestations with antibodies to ribosomal P proteins in systemic lupus erythematosus. Am. J. Med. **90:** 54–62.
29. THE, L.S., A.E. BEDWELL, D.A. ISENBERG, *et al.* 1992. Antibodies to protein P in SLE. Ann. Rheum. Dis. **51:** 489–494.
30. YOSHIO, T., D. HIRATA, K. ONDA, *et al.* 2005. Antiribosomal P protein antibodies in cerebrospinal fluid are associated with neuropsychiatric systemic lupus erythematosus. J. Rheumatol. **32:** 34–39.
31. SANNA, G., M. PIGA, J.W. TERRYBERRY, *et al.* 2000. Central nervous system involvement in systemic lupus erythematosus: cerebral imaging and serological profile in patients with and without overt neuropsychiatric manifestations. Lupus **9:** 573–583.
32. JACQUES, C.M., M. KUJAS & A. POREAU. 1981. GFAP and S100 protein levels as an index for malignancy in human gliomas and neurinomas. J. Natl. Cancer. Inst. **62:** 479–483.
33. KATO, S., T. GONDO, Y. HOSHII, *et al.* Confocal observation of senile plaques in Alzheimer's disease: senile plaque morphology and relationship between senile plaques and astrocytes. Pathol. Int. **48:** 332–340.
34. TANAKA, J., K. NAKAMURA, M. TAKEDA, *et al.* 1989. Enzyme-linked immunosorbent assay for human autoantibody to glial fibrillary acidic protein: higher titer of the antibody is detected in serum of patients with Alzheimer's disease. Acta Neurol. Scand. **80:** 554–560.
35. NEWCOMBE, J., S. GAHAN & M.L. CUZNER. 1985. Serum antibodies against central nervous system proteins in human demyelinating disease. Clin. Exp. Immunol. **59:** 383–390.
36. TRYSBERG, E., K. NYLEN, L.E. ROSENGREN, *et al.* 2003. Neuronal and astrocytic damage in systemic lupus erythematosus patients with central nervous system involvement. Arthritis Rheum. **48:** 2881–2887.

37. ALESSANDRI, C., F. CONTI & G. VALESINI. 2004. Role of anti-glial fibrillary acidic protein antibodies in the pathogenesis of neuropsychiatric systemic lupus erythematosus should be clarified: comment on the article by Trysberg *et al.* Arthritis Rheum. **50:** 1698–1699.
38. STUART, B.M. & N.A. GREGSON. 1998. Cerebral calcification in a patient with systemic lupus erythematosus and a monoclonal IgG reactive with glial fibrillary acidic protein. Br. J. Rheumatol. **37:** 1355–1357.
39. DEGIORGIO, L.A., K.N. KONSTANTINOV, S.C. LEE, *et al.* 2001. A subset of lupus anti-DNA antibodies cross-reacts with the NR2 glutamate receptor in systemic lupus erythematosus. Nat. Med. **7:** 1189–1193.
40. WILLIAMS JR., R.C., K. SUGIURA & E.M. TAN. 2004. Antibodies to microtubule-associated protein 2 in patients with neuropsychiatric systemic lupus erythematosus, Arthritis Rheum. **50:** 1239–1247.
41. HARRIS, E.N., A.E. GHARAVI, R.A. ASHERSON, *et al.* 1984. Cerebral infarction in systemic lupus erythematosus: association with anticardiolipin antibodies. Clin. Exp. Rheumatol. **2:** 47–51.
42. ASHERSON, R.A., M.A. KHAMASHTA, A. GIL, *et al.* 1989. Cerebrovascular disease and antiphospholipid antibody in systemic lupus erythematosus, lupus-like disease and the primary antiphospholipid syndrome. Am. J. Med. **86:** 391–399.
43. HERRANZ, M.T., G. RIVIER, M.A. KHAMASHTA, *et al.* 1994. Association between antiphospholipid antibodies and epilepsy in patients with systemic lupus erythematosus. Arthritis Rheum. **37:** 569–571.
44. CARONTI, B., C. CALDERARO, C. ALESSANDRI, *et al.*1998. Serum anti-beta2-glycoprotein I antibodies from patients with antiphospholipid antibody syndrome bind central nervous system cells. J. Autoimmun. **11:** 425–429.
45. CARONTI, B., C. CALDERARO & C. ALESSANDRI. 1999. Beta2-glycoprotein I (beta2-GPI) mRNA is expressed by several cell types involved in anti-phospholipid syndrome-related tissue damage. Clin. Exp. Immunol. **115:** 214–219.
46. DEL PAPA, N., G. CONFORTI, D. GAMBINI, *et al.* 1994. Characterization of the endothelial surface proteins recognized by anti-endothelial antibodies in primary and secondary autoimmune vasculitis. Clin. Immunol. Immunopathol. **70:** 211–216.
47. D'CRUZ, D.P., F.A. HOUSSIAU, G. RAMIREZ, *et al.* 1991. Antibodies to endothelial cells in systemic lupus erythematosus: a potential marker for nephritis and vasculitis. Clin. Exp. Immunol. **85:** 254–261.
48. CARVALHO, D., C.O.S. SAVAGE, C.M. BLACK, *et al.* 1996. IgG antiendothelial cell autoantibodies from scleroderma patients induce leukocyte adhesion to human vascular endothelial cells *in vitro*. J. Clin. Invest. **97:** 111–119.
49. BORDRON, A., M. DUEYMES, Y. LEVY, *et al.* 1999. The binding of some human antiendothelial cell antibodies induces endothelial cell apoptosis. J. Clin. Invest. **101:** 2029–2035.
50. DEL PAPA, N., L. GUIDALI, L. SPATOLA, *et al.* 1995. Relationship between anti-phospholipid and antiendothelial cell antibodies III: β 2 glycoprotein I mediates the antibody binding to endothelial membranes and induces the expression of adhesion molecules. Clin. Exp. Rheumatol. **13:** 179–185.
51. DEL PAPA, N., L. GUIDALI, A. SALA, *et al.* 1997. Endothelial cell as target for anti-phospholipid antibodies: human polyclonal and monoclonal anti-beta 2-glycoprotein I antibodies react in vitro with endothelial cells through adherent

beta 2-glycoprotein I and induce endothelial activation. Arthritis Rheum. **40:** 551–561.

52. DEL PAPA, N., E. RASCHI, G. MORONI, *et al.* 1999. Anti-endothelial cell IgG fractions from systemic lupus erythematosus patients bind to human endothelial cells and induce a pro-adhesive and a pro-inflammatory phenotype *in vitro*. Lupus **8:** 423–429.
53. KAPAHI, P., J.C. MASON, Y. LEBRANCHU, *et al.* 1993. Detection of a circulating form of vascular cell adhesion molecule-1: raised levels in rheumatoid arthritis and systemic lupus erythematosus. Clin. Exp. Immunol. **92:** 412–418.
54. BELMONT, H.M., J. BUYON, R. GIORNO, *et al.* 1994. Up-regulation of endothelial cell adhesion molecules characterizes disease activity in systemic lupus erythematosus. Arthritis Rheum. **3:** 376–383.
55. CARSON, C.W., L.D. BEALL, G.G. HUNDER, *et al.* 1993. Serum E-selection is increased in vasculitis, scleroderma, and systemic lupus erythematosus. J. Rheumatol. **20:** 809–814.
56. SONG, J., Y.B. PARK, W.K. LEE, *et al.* 2000. Clinical associations of anti-endothelial cell antibodies in patients with systemic lupus erythematosus. Rheumatol. Int. **20:** 1–7.
57. MERONI, P.L., A. TINCANI, N. SEPP, *et al.* 2003. Endothelium and the brain in CNS lupus. Lupus **12:** 919–928.
58. AINIALA, H., A. HIETAHARJU, J. LOUKKOLA, *et al.* 2001. Validity of the new American College of Rheumatology criteria for neuropsychiatric lupus syndromes: a population-based evaluation. Arthritis Rheum. **45:** 419–423.
59. LINDAL, E., S. THORLACIUS, K. STEINSSON, *et al.* 1995. Psychiatric disorders among subjects with systemic lupus erythematosus in an unselected population. Scand. J. Rheumatol. **24:** 346–351.
60. SHORTALL, E., D. ISENBERG & S.P. NEWMAN. Factors associated with mood and mood disorders in SLE. Lupus **4:** 272–279.
61. UTSET, T.O., M. GOLDEN, G. SIBERRY, *et al.* 1994. Depressive symptoms in patients with systemic lupus erythematosus: association with central nervous system lupus and Sjögren's syndrome. J. Rheumatol. **21:** 2039–2045.
62. YOSHIO, T., J. MASUYAMA & S. KANO. 1996 Antiribosomal P0 protein antibodies react with the surface of human umbilical vein endothelial cells. J. Rheumatol. **23:** 1311–1312.
63. NAGAI, T., Y. ARINUMA, T. YANAGIDA, *et al.* 2005. Anti-ribosomal P protein antibody in human systemic lupus erythematosus up-regulates the expression of proinflammatory cytokines by human peripheral blood monocytes. Arthritis Rheum. **52:** 847–855.
64. MARGUTTI, P., M. SORICE, F. CONTI, *et al.* 2005. Screening of an endothelial cDNA library identifies the C-terminal region of Nedd5 as a novel autoantigen in systemic lupus erythematosus with psychiatric manifestations. Arthritis Res. Ther. **7:** R896–R903.
65. VEGA, I.E. & S.C. HSU. 2003. The septin protein Nedd5 associates with both the exocyst complex and microtubules and disruption of its GTPase activity promotes aberrant neurite sprouting in PC12 cells. NeuroReport **14:** 31–37.
66. SURKA, M.C., C.W. TSANG & W.S. TRIMBLE. 2002. The mammalian septin MSF localizes with microtubules and is required for completion of cytokinesis. Mol. Biol. Cell **13:** 3532–3545.
67. MARTINEZ, C. & J. WARE. 2004. Mammalian septin function in hemostasis and beyond. Exp. Biol. Med. **229:** 1111–1119.

68. PENG, X.R., Z. JIA, Y. ZHANG, *et al.* 2002. The septin CDCrel-1 is dispensable for normal development and neurotransmitter release. Mol. Cell. Biol. **22:** 378–387.
69. KINOSHITA, A., M. KINOSHITA, H. AKIYAMA, *et al.* 1998. Identification of septins in neurofibrillary tangles in Alzheimer's disease. Am. J. Pathol. **153:** 1551–1560.
70. SHUSTA, E.V., J.Y. LI, R.J. BOADO, *et al.* 2003. The Ro52/SS-A autoantigen has elevated expression at the brain microvasculature. NeuroReport **14:** 1861–1865.

Neuroendocrine-Immune Interactions

The Role of Cortistatin/Somatostatin System

DIEGO FERONE,[a,b] MARA BOSCHETTI,[a] EUGENIA RESMINI,[a] MASSIMO GIUSTI,[a,b] VALERIA ALBANESE,[a] UMBERTO GOGLIA,[a] MANUELA ALBERTELLI,[a] LARA VERA,[a] FEDERICO BIANCHI,[a] AND FRANCESCO MINUTO[a,b]

[a]*Department of Endocrinological and Metabolic Sciences, and* [b]*Centre of Excellence for Biomedical Research, University of Genova, 16132 Genova, Italy*

ABSTRACT: **Hormones and neuropeptides may influence the activities of lymphoid organs and cells via endocrine and local autocrine/paracrine pathways. A paradigm of the interactions between the neuroendocrine and immune system is sophisticatedly represented in the thymus. Indeed, receptors for these molecules are heterogeneously expressed in all subsets of thymic cells, and the communications are tuned by feedback circuitries. Herein, we focus on somatostatin (SS), a ubiquitous peptide that regulates several physiological cell processes and acts via five specific receptor (SSR) subtypes (sst_{1-5}). Neuronal and accessory cells, so-called neuroendocrine cells, and immune cells, heterogeneously express SSRs. The functional characterization of SSRs *in vivo* by nuclear medicine techniques opened a complex scenario on the significance of SS/SSR pathway in immune system and related diseases. Several studies have established that SSR scintigraphy may benefit patients with chronic inflammatory and granulomatous diseases, as well as lymphoproliferative diseases. The results are sufficiently promising to warrant larger studies aimed at defining the exact role of these techniques. The development of SS analogs with antisecretory and antiproliferative effects has radically changed the management of neuroendocrine tumors. Moreover, very important recent findings, emerging from *in vitro* studies on SSR physiology in immune cells, will certainly expand the potential applications of SS analogs for *in vivo* diagnostic and therapeutic options. Indeed, the anti-inflammatory and analgesic effects of these drugs remain incompletely understood, but may prove useful in a number of autoimmune diseases. Because SS expression is absent in different immune tissues where SSRs are present, the existence of another ligand was hypothesized. In fact, it has been recently demonstrated that human lymphoid tissues and immune cells may express cortistatin (CST). CST is known to bind SSRs and shares many pharmacological and functional properties with SS.**

Address for correspondence: Diego Ferone, M.D., Ph.D., Department of Endocrinological and Metabolic Sciences, University of Genova, Viale Benedetto XV, 6, 16132 Genova, Italy. Voice: +39-010-3537946; fax: +39-010-3538977.
e-mail: ferone@unige.it

Ann. N.Y. Acad. Sci. 1069: 129–144 (2006).
doi: 10.1196/annals.1351.011

However, CST has also properties distinct from SS, and the higher expression of CST in immune cells supports the hypothesis that CST rather than SS may act as a potential endogenous ligand for SSRs in the human immune system.

KEYWORDS: somatostatin; cortistatin; immune cells; thymus; immune-related diseases

INTRODUCTION

Compelling data have been collected indicating that the cross-talk between the neuroendocrine and immune systems has a critical role in restraining and shaping immune responses, as well as in understanding the development of immune-mediated disorders.[1–3] These systems use similar ligands and receptors to establish a physiological intra- and intersystem communication circuitry that plays an important role in homeostasis. Hormones and neuropeptides, in particular gut and brain peptides, can be considered potent immunomodulators, participating in various aspects of immune system function, in both health and disease.[4] Receptors for various regulatory peptides are expressed by rat, mice, or human immune cells and various effects of these regulatory peptides have been reported *in vivo* or *in vitro* on several immunocyte activities.[1–4]

Neuroendocrine regulation of inflammatory and immune responses and diseases occurs at multiple levels: systemically, through the anti-inflammatory action of glucocorticoids released via hypothalamic-pituitary-adrenal axis stimulation; regionally, through local production of hormones and neuropetides in immune organs, such as the thymus; locally, at sites of inflammation, through release of proinflammatory neuropeptides and neurohormones from peripheral nerves.[4] Neural regulation of immune responses also occurs regionally through sympathetic nervous system activation and the effects of neurotransmitters on immune cells in spleen and lymph nodes.[4] Many other hormones also regulate immune responses, including growth hormone, prolactin, insulin-like growth factor-1, thyroid hormone,[5] and sexual steroids.[6]

Moreover, several investigations have described interactions between different regulatory peptides involved in immune functions, suggesting close topographical links between the various peptide systems. Among these, the attention has been focused on somatostatin (SS), a ubiquitous hormone involved in cell growth and other phenomena (FIG. 1). SS interacts with specific receptors (SSR) that are detectable *in vivo* by scintigraphy. SSR scintigraphy was used initially to detect neuroendocrine tumors and other tumors characterized by overexpression of SSRs. A role for SS and its receptors was then established in other cell types, including cells mediating inflammation and immune response. The recent development of new SS analogs (SSA) and the emerging novel findings on SSR physiology has opened a wide field of investigations aimed at developing new diagnostic tools and, perhaps, therapeutic approaches.

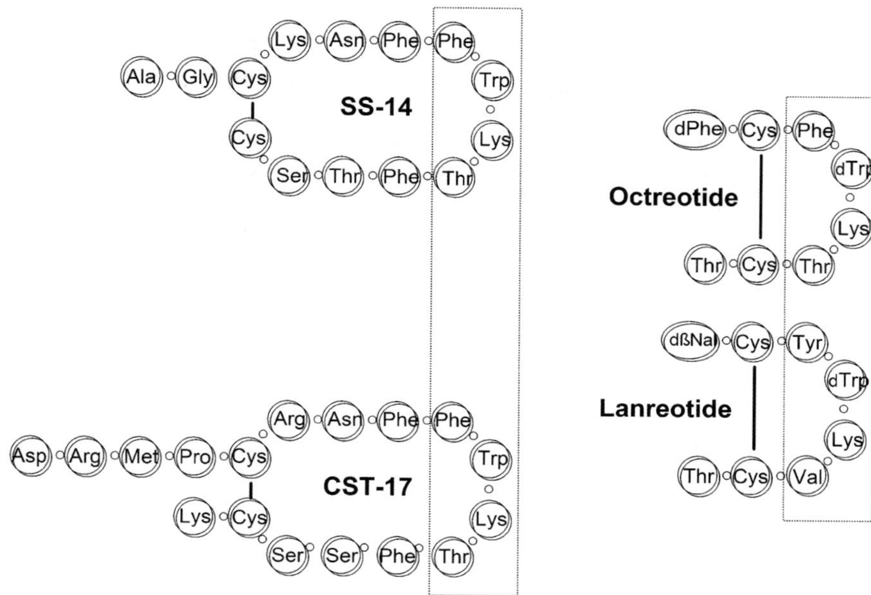

FIGURE 1. Amino acid sequences of native human somatostatin-14 (SS-14), cortistatin-17 (CST-17), and of the two synthetic stable octapeptide analogs, octreotide and lanreotide. The dotted boxes delimitate the amino acids essential for binding with the receptors.

SOMATOSTATIN AND SOMATOSTATIN RECEPTOR LIGANDS

SS is a widespread neuropeptide with generally inhibitory function on hormone release in the anterior pituitary and the gastrointestinal system, as well as with antiangiogenic, antiproliferative, and analgesic properties.[7–9] Within the nervous system, SS acts as a neuromodulator with physiological effects on neuroendocrine, motor, and cognitive functions.[7–9] SS biosynthesis involves the proteolytic processing of a single precursor molecule into the biologically active peptides SS-14 and SS-28. Recently, the complexity of the somatostatinergic system has been extended by the discovery of cortistatin (CST) (Fig. 1), a neuropeptide displaying strong structural similarity with SS.[10,11] Similar to SS, CST occurs in a short 14 (CST-14) or 17 amino acid form (CST-17) in rat, mouse, and human, respectively, and a longer one of 29 amino acids (CST-29) in rat and human. Although CST and SS are products of different genes, CST-14 shares 11 of the 14 amino acids with SS-14. In the central nervous system (CNS), CST mRNA expression is mainly restricted to the cerebral cortex and hippocampus. CST shares several functional properties with SS, however, some biological functions of CST are unique, such as the induction of slow-wave sleep and reduction of locomotor activity.[12]

SS mediates its biological functions via at least five receptor subtypes (sst_{1-5}), belonging to the family of seven transmembrane domain G protein–coupled receptors.[8] The genes encoding the five receptor subtypes are localized on different chromosomes (TABLE 1). Via alternative splicing, two protein isoforms of the sst_2 receptor can be generated, i.e., sst_{2A} and sst_{2B}.[8,9] The only difference between sst_{2A} and sst_{2B} is the length of their cytoplasmic tail, however, this latter is not greatly expressed in humans.[8,9] Natural ligands of the different SSRs are SS-14 and SS-28. However, CST is also capable of binding to all SSRs with high affinity, and a role as potential endogenous ligand of the sst_2 in the human immune system has recently been proposed (see below).[13,14]

Based on the finding of atypical pharmacological profiles in specific cell lines, as well as in certain normal and neoplastic cells and tissues,[8,15] the existence of at least a novel SSR subtype, which escaped molecular cloning, has been recurrently hypothesized. However, an alternative possible explanations for the unusual pharmacological profiles observed might include hetero-oligomerization between SSRs or between SSRs and other G protein–coupled receptors, such as dopamine receptors. Indeed, homo- and hetero-dimerization have been observed in transfected cell lines, leading in an alternative modulation of the properties of the involved receptors, including important changes in their pharmacological profile, membrane trafficking, and intracellular pathways activation.[16–19] Although the occurrence of this interesting phenomenon has not been clearly demonstrated in cells constitutively expressing these receptors, the discovering of dimerization forced to explore the properties of new compounds, potentially able to induce, or at least, to facilitate this process. In fact, an enhanced potency in controlling both cell secretion and proliferation has been recently demonstrated *in vitro* using chimeric molecules that combine structural elements of both SS and dopamine, and retain affinity for both the sst_2 and dopamine D_2 receptors.[20,21]

The signal transduction pathways coupled to activation of SSRs have been studied in transfected cell systems, as well as in normal and tumor cells constitutively expressing different SSR subtypes. Depending on the cell type, the various SSRs are coupled to a diversity of transduction systems. Binding of SSR ligands induces G-protein activation and signaling through various pathways: adenylyl cyclase, phosphotyrosine phosphatases (PTPases), mitogen-activated protein kinase (MAPK), or p53, and are modulated along with Na^+/H^+ exchanger and changes in the intracellular levels of calcium and potassium ions (TABLE 1).[8] In particular, the antiproliferative effects of SS and its analogs are thought to be due to the activation of a subclass of PTPases, or p53 for the induction of apoptosis.[8]

Because the half-life of SS is < 3 min, in the early 1980s the first octapeptide analogs of SS, octreotide and lanreotide, have been synthesized (FIG. 1). These analogs can be administered by multiple subcutaneous injections or by continuous infusion, as well as by the intravenous route. The

TABLE 1. Somatostatin receptor properties

Receptors	sst_1	sst_2	sst_3	sst_4	sst_5
Signaling					
G protein–coupling	+	+	+	+	+
Adenylyl cyclase activity	↓	↓	↓	↓	↓
PTPase activity	↑	↑	↑	↑↓	↑
MAP kinase activity	↑	↑↓	↑↓	↑	↑
K^+ channels	–	↑	↑	↑	↑
Ca^{2+} channels	↓	↓	–	–	–
Na^+/H^+ exchanger	↓	–	↓	↓	–
Phospholipase C/IP_3 activity	↑	↑	↑	↑	↑↓
Phospholipase A_2 activity	–	–	–	↑	–
Secretion					
GH	↓	↓	–	↓	↓
Insulin	–	↓	–	–	↓
Cell growth					
Proliferation	↓	↑↓	↓	↑↓	↓
Apoptosis	–	↑	↑	–	–
Specific properties					
Chromosome localization	14q13	17q24	22q13.1	20p11.2	16p13.3
Molecular weight	42.7	41.3	45.9	41.9	39.3
Expression	Brain, pituitary pancreas, stomach, liver, kidneys	Brain, pituitary pancreas, stomach, kidneys, immune cells	Brain, pituitary pancreas, stomach, T cells B cells	Brain, pancreas, stomach, lung, placenta	Pituitary pancreas, stomach

slow-release depot intramuscular formulation of octreotide (octreotide-LAR) has to be administered once every 4 weeks and that of lanreotide (lanreotide-SR) has to be administered once every 2 weeks. A new slow release depot preparation of lanreotide (Autogel, Ipsen, St. Jean D'Illac, France) has been more recently introduced and can be administered subcutaneously once every 4 weeks.[22–24] Both SS-14 and SS-28 bind with high affinity to all SSR subtypes. Octreotide and lanreotide have comparable binding profiles and bind with a high affinity to sst_2 and with relative lower affinity to sst_5 and sst_3. These analogs do not bind sst_1 and sst_4.[22,23]

The rationale for the diagnostic and therapeutic use of SSAs is essentially based on the expression of SSR in normal and tumor tissues.[15,25,26] SSRs are largely expressed within the CNS, whereas the periphery tissues that normally express SSRs include gastrointestinal and pancreatic tissues.[8,15,26] Most tumor tissues preferentially express sst_2 receptors, less frequently $sst_{1,3,5}$, whereas the sst_4 receptor is very rarely detected in humans.

In lymphoid tissues and immune cells, the expression of sst_1, sst_2, and sst_3 has been found, in both normal and pathologic conditions.[27–32] Although the interest on this emerging field is constantly growing, the possible relevance of SSR expression in the pathophysiology immune-mediated diseases and also the therapeutic implications remain to be elucidated (see below). In general, the knowledge of the receptor distribution in normal and cancer tissue is of primary importance. However, at the present, still conflicting data on the heterogeneity and quantity of individual receptor subtypes are available, and further studies are warranted for the potential therapeutic application of new subtype-specific, hybrid molecules or universal analogs in certain endocrine and nonendocrine indications.[7,20,21,33]

SIGNIFICANCE OF THE SOMATOSTIN/CORTISTATIN SYSTEM IN LYMPHOID ORGANS AND IMMUNE-MEDIATED DISEASES

In the peripheral nervous system, SS is present in sympathetic and sensory neurons innervating the lymphoid organs, and SSRs are located predominantly in lymphoid follicle germinal centers.[34] Additional non-neuronal sources of SS (such as granuloma cells within Schistosoma-induced liver granulomas, lymphocytes, macrophages, and thymic epithelial cells) have been described in both experimental and normal conditions.[27–32] The presence of binding sites for SS and the expression of mRNA for SSRs on lymphocytes and monocytes is established, although the expression of a particular SSR subtype on T lymphocytes seems to vary with species and with the origins of the T cells.[29–32] As in other cell systems or tissues, SS is generally inhibitory for diverse immune cell functions, including proliferation. Interestingly, in specific and complex local autocrine/paracrine circuitries of lymphoid organs, SS seems to antagonize the effects of other neuropeptides. For instance, it suppresses the production of IFN-γ from murine and human T lymphocytes, a finding that has deserved the most attention within the granulomatous inflammation induced by Schistosoma, where it generally antagonizes the stimulatory effects of substance P and vice versa.[35] However, stimulatory effects have been observed as well, especially in certain conditions.

Increasing evidence has placed the human thymus as a target for neuroendocrine control. We briefly focus on the pleiotropic effects of SS/CST system on this primary lymphoid organ, with emphasis on data derived from both *in vivo* evidences and *in vitro* experiments.[36]

The thymus plays a pivotal role in the control of the immune system and for the establishment of immunocompetence. Apart the local production of SS, three receptor subtypes, sst_1, sst_{2A}, and sst_3, have been found in the thymic tissue.[37] However, SSR expression in the human thymus is age-dependent, and the expression of the three SSR subtypes is heterogeneously distributed within the different cell subsets forming the complex architecture of this organ.[37,38] A selective expression of sst_1 and sst_{2A} has been detected in cultured thymic epithelial cells (TEC), whereas the whole population of isolated thymocytes express sst_{2A} and sst_3.[39,40] Interestingly, these two SSRs are expressed and regulated in thymocytes following a sort of developmental pathway. In fact, sst_{2A} seems selectively expressed in very early thymocytes, however, while this latter SSR is downregulated during thymocytes maturation, sst_3 is upregulated and appears predominantly, or even selectively, expressed in the mature subsets.[40] Conversely, thymic macrophages and dendritic cells maintain the selective expression of sst_{2A}.[39–41] In resting thymocytes, SS, but not octreotide, has been shown to increase apoptosis for the first time in cells constitutively expressing SSRs, suggesting a potential pathway possibly mediated by an endogenous ligand–sst_3 interaction.[40,41]

However, as already mentioned, SS is expressed in specific subset of TEC while not in thymocytes. Interestingly, in other human lymphoid tissues, such as spleen tissue, SSRs are heterogeneously expressed, again maintaining a preferential localization of sst_2 in cells of the monocyte–macrophage lineage, and of sst_3 in resting and activated lymphocytes.[42,43] Although the receptors are definitely expressed in these cell systems or tissues, SS is not present. Conversely, different levels of CST mRNA are constantly expressed in immune cells, lymphoid tissues, and bone marrow.[13,14] The expression of CST is also upregulated during differentiation of monocytes into macrophages and dendritic cells (FIG. 2), together with sst_2.[14] Moreover, by ligand-binding studies it has been also demonstrated that CST can displace [^{125}I-Tyr^3]octreotide binding with relatively high affinity on human thymic tissue and sst_2-expressing cells.[13] These studies firstly demonstrated that human lymphoid tissues and immune cells express different levels of CST, suggesting a role for CST as an endogenous ligand of at least the sst_2 in the human immune system, rather than SS itself. CST has a broader distribution in human body

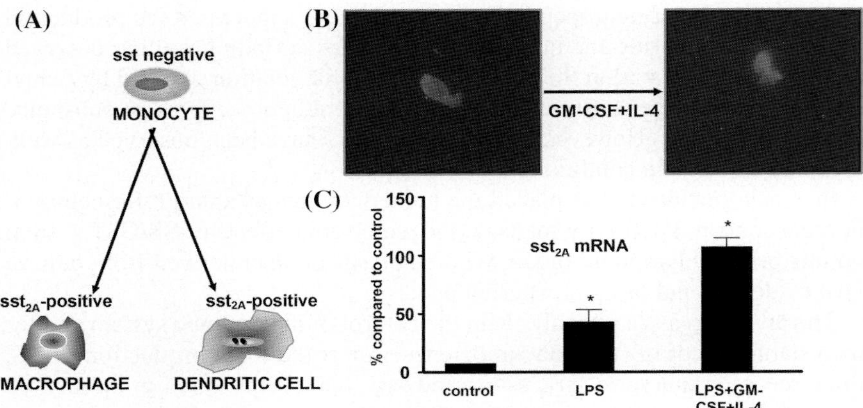

FIGURE 2. Potential differentiating pathways of monocytes and regulation of sst_{2A} expression in monocytes, macrophages, and dendritic cells. **(A)** Isolated peripheral blood monocytes (from healthy donors) can be induced to differentiate into macrophages and dendritic cells after activation with lipopolysaccharide (LPS) and stimulation with granulocyte macrophage colony-stimulating factor (GM-CSF) and interleukin-4 (IL-4). **(B)** Immunofluorescent detection of sst_{2A} on activated monocytes and dendritic cells. Monocytes were activated and allowed to differentiate into dendritic cells and were incubated for 24 h with GM-CSF and IL-4. **(C)** sst_{2A} mRNA expression in unstimulated (control), LPS-stimulated (LPS), GM-CSF plus IL-4 treated (GM-CSF+IL-4) cells. $^{*}P > 0.001$ compared with control.

than previously expected.[44] However, the functional significance of CST in peripheral tissues is under current investigation. SS plays important roles in regulating various processes in humans through its SSRs, and CST may act via these receptors as well, reason why we could expect that this neuropeptide might have comparable effects in the body with respect to regulation of cell proliferation and secretion. In preliminary studies, it has been demonstrated that CST inhibits proliferation of isolated human thymocytes suggesting that also CST may contribute to the development of mature T lymphocytes.[44] However, as already mentioned, in the human brain differences in effects of CST and SS have been described.[12] These differences may be explained by different postreceptor signaling pathways or the existence of a selective CST receptor. Recently, a novel receptor, the MrgX2 receptor, has been cloned.[45] CST is the peptide with the highest affinity to MrgX2, suggesting that this receptor could be the putative CST receptor, although further studies are warranted to support this hypothesis.

The initial descriptions of high *in vivo* uptake of [^{111}In-DTPA^{0}]octreotide during SSR scintigraphy in patients bearing thymoma or thymic carcinoid indicated a specific expression of SSRs in thymic-derived neoplasms.[46–48] Indeed, sst_1, sst_{2A}, and sst_3 have been demonstrated by immunohistochemistry and

RT-PCR in thymic tumor tissues.[49,50] Surprisingly, the *in vitro* evaluation of receptor subtype distribution within these tumors pointed out for the first time that the presence of sst_2 might not be essential for the visualization of SSR-positive tissues during [^{111}In-DTPA^0]octreotide scintigraphy. In fact, among tumors with similar volume and containing comparable levels of sst_{2A}, the highest [^{111}In-DTPA^0]octreotide uptake was observed in those cases with a higher expression of sst_3.[50] The hypothesis on the involvement of sst_3 in determining the uptake of [^{111}In-DTPA^0]octreotide has been recently confirmed by the evidence that pheocromocytomas lacking the expression of sst_2, but with relative high expression of sst_3, can be clearly visualized during SSR scintigraphy.[51] The heterogeneity and variability in SSR expression in thymic tumors may also explain the limited results obtained treating these diseases with the currently available SSAs, driving to search for the application in this disease of new compounds with different binding profile.[52–54]

SSR scintigraphy has been also used to visualize the site of disease in a large number of patients with both T and B non-Hodgkin lymphomas and Hodgkin disease.[55–60] We have recently reviewed the role of SSR scintigraphy for staging of lymphomas, observing that this technique, using the current available SSAs, does not seem to have a significant impact in patients with lymphomas for diagnostic purposes with few exceptions.[61] However, positron emission tomography (PET) will probably replace SSR scintigraphy for these hematological malignancies, as it detects tumor foci with greater sensitivity.[62] In contrast, studies demonstrating SSRs in plasma cells raise the possibility that SSR scintigraphy may be useful in patients with myeloma or plasmacytoma.[63–65] Studies targeted to clarify the exact cellular localization of SSRs in hematological and lymphoproliferative disorders, together with the new knowledge on receptor regulation mechanisms and on the potential role of CST, will probably expand the opportunities of diagnostic and therapeutic application of SSAs in this field.[66–68]

SSR scintigraphy has been proved useful in several chronic inflammatory diseases. Granulomas in sarcoidosis, tuberculosis, as well as Wegener's granulomatosis can be visualized with high sensitivity,[69,70] evidencing foci missed by conventional radiographic techniques in a subset of patients.[71] Similarly, patients with skeletal or extraskeletal histiocytosis may benefit of SSR scintigraphy.[72,73] The cellular expression of SSRs in granulomas has been evaluated with different techniques, however, immunohistochemistry firstly allowed the particular localization of different receptors on specific cells.[70,74] The *in vitro* studies have definitively contributed also to explain the *in vivo* evidences of receptor regulation during glucocorticoid therapy that can be useful for predicting the outcome of the disease.[69–71,74] In granulomatous diseases, the subtype distribution resembles the preferential expression of a given receptor on specific cell subsets already observed in lymphoproliferative disorders and in autoimmune diseases (see below).[70,74] In fact, sst_{2A} is expressed on cell of monocyte/macrophage lineage, whereas activated lymphocytes preferentially express sst_3. Preliminary results suggest that once again an SS/CST circuitry might be involved in the pathophysiology of immune-mediated diseases.[75]

SSR scintigraphy can visualize affected joints of patients with rheumatoid arthritis.[76] The uptake of radioactivity in the sites of disease was found to be correlated with the clinical activity.[76] However, scintigraphy failed in indicating whether the disease is erosive, which is the main determinant of the prognosis of rheumatoid arthritis. Subsequently, immunohistochemical and RT-PCR studies showed the presence of sst_{2A} receptors in endothelial cells and in cells of the monocyte/macrophage lineage, and sst_1 and sst_{2A} in rheumatoid synovial fibroblasts.[64,77,78] Although, uncontrolled studies suggested a potential role in the treatment of rheumatoid arthritis with currently available SSAs,[79,80] conflicting results have been obtained, and this might be related to the lack of expression of sst_2 on lymphocytes, which do express sst_3.[43] More recently, results of an experimental study demonstrated that a new SSA, with different properties compared with the current available compounds, exerted a potent anti-inflammatory and analgesic actions in the CFA-induced chronic arthritis model in the rat.[81] Moreover, in a patient with Sjögren's syndrome, SSA therapy produced the resolution of the symptoms.[82] This case is of particular interest given the lack of systemic treatments for this condition and recent evidence from a controlled trial that anti-TNF-α agents seem ineffective.[83] Similarly, in a patient with exudative enteropathy due to amyloidosis from ankylosing spondylitis, combined glucocorticoid and SSA therapy provided symptom relief.[84] Based on these findings, the recently developed long acting SSA, SOM-230, which binds to all SSRs except sst_4, might be a promising candidate for medical therapy in a larger spectrum of immune-mediated diseases.[33]

CONCLUSIONS

The SS/CST system represents a paradigm of neuroendocrine–immune interaction. In this setting, neuropeptides can be considered a functional equivalent of cytokines. The acquisition of immunomodulatory actions by neuropeptides in the course of evolution may probably represent an advantage selected in terms of the fine-tuning of the immune response to nonself antigens. SS, but perhaps even more CST, might play an important role in immune system, being involved in autocrine/paracrine circuitries within the complex cellular structure of lymphoid organs. However, further studies are warranted to elucidate the complex mechanisms of actions and the role of neuropeptides in pathophysiology of immune-related diseases.

The presence of SS first, and later of CST in lymphoid organs, together with the successful employment of SSR scintigraphy in the visualization of lymphoproliferative and immune-mediated diseases, provided the first evidences for the expression and for a potential importance of SSRs in immune cells. SSR scintigraphy might be considered as a complementary or alternative diagnostic tool in this field. It is a noninvasive and direct imaging technique and can provide additional information on the extent of the disease activity and also reflecting the response to treatments. This imaging technique may also identify previously unknown disease localizations. These properties may facilitate and improve the clinical assessment of patients with immune diseases leading to an earlier and more precise diagnosis.

Other possible relevance of SSR expression in the pathophysiology of lymphoproliferative and immune-mediated diseases and also therapeutic implications remain to be clarified. Based on the receptor pattern observed in normal and altered immune cells, controlled studies are warranted to investigate the efficacy of SSAs in the treatment of inflammatory, lymphoproliferative, and granulomatous diseases. Finally, the recent findings emerged from studies on SSR physiology, namely receptor dimerization as well as internalization, together with the availability of new compounds with a different affinity profile, will certainly expand the potential applications of SSAs for diagnostic and therapeutic purposes in this topic.

REFERENCES

1. Besedovsky, H. & A. Del Rey. 1996. Immune-neuro-endocrine interactions: facts and hypothesis. Endocr. Rev. **17:** 64–102.
2. van Hagen, P.M., L.J. Hofland, E.G.R. Lichtenauer-Kaligis, *et al.* 1999. Neuropeptides and their receptors in the immune system. Ann. Med. **31**(Suppl 2):15–22.
3. Ferone, D., L.J. Hofland, A. Colao, *et al.* 2001. Neuroendocrine aspects of immunolymphoproliferative diseases. Ann. Oncol. **12**(Suppl 2): S125–S130.
4. Webster, J.I., L. Tonelli & E.M. Sternberg. 2002. Neuroendocrine regulation of immunity. Annu. Rev. Immunol. **20:** 125–163.
5. Dorshkind, K. & N.D. Horseman. 2000. The roles of prolactin, growth hormone, insulin-like growth factor-I, and thyroid hormones in lymphocyte development and function: insights from genetic models of hormone and hormone receptor deficiency. Endocr. Rev. **21:** 292–312.
6. Kocar, I.H., Z. Yesilova, M. Ozata, *et al.* 2000. The effect of testosterone replacement treatment on immunological features of patients with Klinefelter's syndrome. Clin. Exp. Immunol. **121:** 448–452.
7. Weckbecker, G., I. Lewis, A. Albert, *et al.* 2003. Opportunities in somatostatin research: biological, chemical and therapeutic aspects. Nat. Rev. **2:** 999–1017.
8. Møller, L.N., C.E. Stidsen, B. Hartmann & J.J. Holst. 2003. Somatostatin receptors. Biochim. Biophys. Acta **1616:** 1–84.
9. Olias, G., C. Viollet, H. Kusserow, *et al.* 2004. Regulation and function of somatostatin receptors. J. Neurochem. **89:** 1057–1091.
10. de Lecea, L., J.R. Criado, O. Prospero-Garcia, *et al.* 1996. A cortical neuropeptide with neuronal depressant and sleep-modulating properties. Nature **381:** 242–245.

11. DE LECEA, L., J.A. DEL RIO, J.R. CRIADO, *et al.* 1997. Cortistatin is expressed in a distinct subset of cortical interneurons. J. Neurosci. **17:** 5868–5880.
12. SPIER, A.D. & L. DE LECEA. 2000. Cortistatin: a member of the somatostatin neuropeptide family with distinct physiological functions. Brain Res. Brain Res. Rev. **33:** 228–241.
13. DALM, V.A., P.M. VAN HAGEN, P.M. VAN KOETSVELD, *et al.* 2003. Cortistatin rather than somatostatin as a potential endogenous ligand for somatostatin receptors in the human immune system. J. Clin. Endocrinol. Metab. **88:** 270–276.
14. DALM, V.A., P.M. VAN HAGEN, P.M. VAN KOETSVELD, *et al.* 2003. Regulation of the expression of somatostatin, cortistatin and somatostatin receptors in human monocytes, macrophages and dendritic cells. Am. J. Physiol. Endocrinol. Metab. **285:** E344–E353.
15. REUBI, J.C., B. WASER, J.C. SCHAER & J.A. LAISSUE. 2001. Somatostatin receptor sst1-sst5 expression in normal and neoplastic human tissues using receptor autoradiography with subtype-selective ligands. Eur. J. Nucl. Med. **28:** 836–846.
16. ROCHEVILLE, M., D.C. LANGE, U. KUMAR, *et al.* 2000. Subtypes of the somatostatin receptor assemble as functional homo- and heterodimers. J. Biol. Chem. **17:** 7862–7869.
17. ROCHEVILLE, M., D.C. LANGE, U. KUMAR, *et al.* 2000. Receptors for dopamine and somatostatin: formation of hetero-oligomers with enhanced functional activity. Science **288:** 154–157.
18. PFEIFFER, M., T. KOCH, H. SCHRODER, *et al.* 2001. Homo- and heterodimerization of somatostatin receptor subtypes. Inactivation of sst(3) receptor function by heterodimerization with sst(2A). J. Biol. Chem. **276:** 14027–14036.
19. PFEIFFER, M., T. KOCH, H. SCHRODER, *et al.* 2002. Heterodimerization of somatostatin and opioid receptors cross-modulates phosphorylation, internalization, and desensitization. J. Biol. Chem. **277:** 19762–19772.
20. SAVEANU, A., E. LAVAQUE, G. GUNZ, *et al.* 2002. Demonstration of enhanced potency of a chimeric somatostatin-dopamine molecule, BIM-23A387, in suppressing growth hormone and prolactin secretion from human pituitary somatotroph adenoma cells. J. Clin. Endocrinol. Metab. **87:** 5545–5552.
21. FERONE, D., M. ARVIGO, C. SEMINO, *et al.* 2005. Somatostatin and dopamine receptor expression in lung carcinoma cells and effects of chimeric somatostatin-dopamine molecules on cell proliferation. Am. J. Physiol. Endocrinol. Metab. **289:** E1044–E1050.
22. DE HERDER, W.W. & S.W. LAMBERTS. 2002. Somatostatin and somatostatin analogues: diagnostic and therapeutic uses. Curr. Opin. Oncol. **14:** 53–57.
23. LAMBERTS, S.W., A.J. VAN DER LELY, W.W. DE HERDER & L.J. HOFLAND. 1996. Octreotide. N. Engl. J. Med. **334:** 246–254.
24. LAMBERTS, S.W.J., W.W. DE HERDER & L.J. HOFLAND. 2002. Somatostatin analogs in the diagnosis and treatment of cancer. Trends Endocrinol. Metab. 13: 451–457.
25. REUBI, J.C. & B. WASER. 2003. Concomitant expression of several peptide receptors in neuroendocrine tumours: molecular basis for in vivo multireceptor tumour targeting. Eur. J. Nucl. Med. Mol. Imaging **30:** 781–793.
26. HOFLAND, L.J. & S.W.J. LAMBERTS. 2003. The pathophysiological consequences of somatostatin receptor internalization and resistance. Endocrine Rev. **24:** 28–47.
27. VAN HAGEN, P.M., E.P. KRENNING, D.J. KWEKKEBOOM, *et al.* 1994. Somatostatin and the immune and haematopoetic system: a review. Eur. J. Clin. Invest. **24:** 91–99.

28. HOFLAND, L.J., P.M. VAN HAGEN, S.W. LAMBERTS. 1999. Functional role of somatostatin receptors in neuroendocrine and immune cells. Ann. Med. **31**(Suppl 2): 23–27.
29. TEN BOKUM, A.M., L.J. HOFLAND, P.M. VAN HAGEN. 2000. Somatostatin and somatostatin receptors in the immune system: a review. Eur. Cytokine. Netw. **11:** 161–176.
30. LICHTENAUER-KALIGIS, E.G., P.M. VAN HAGEN, S.W. LAMBERTS & L.J. HOFLAND. 2000. Somatostatin receptor subtypes in human immune cells. Eur. J. Endocrinol. **143**(Suppl 2): S21–S25.
31. FERONE, D., G. LOMBARDI & A. COLAO. 2001. Somatostatin receptors in immune system cells. Minerva Endocrinol. **26:** 165–173.
32. FERONE, D., P.M. VAN HAGEN, C. SEMINO, *et al.* 2004. Somatostatin receptor distribution and function in immune system. Dig. Liver Dis. **36**(Suppl 1): S68–S77.
33. VAN DER HOEK, J., L.J. HOFLAND & S.W. LAMBERTS. 2005. Novel subtype specific and universal somatostatin analogues: clinical potential and pitfalls [review]. Curr. Pharm. Des. **11:** 1573–1592.
34. REUBI, J.C., U. HORISBERGER, A. KAPPELER & J.A. LAISSUE. 1998. Localization of receptors for vasoactive intestinal peptide, somatostatin and substance P in distinct compartments of human lymphoid organs. Blood **92:** 191–197.
35. ELLIOTT, D.E., J.V. WEINSTOCK. 1996. Granulomas in murine schistosomiasis mansoni have a somatostatin immunoregulatory circuit. Metabolism **45**(Suppl 1): 88–90.
36. SAVINO, W. & M. DARDENNE. 2000. Neuroendocrine control of thymus physiology. Endocr. Rev. **21:** 412–443.
37. FERONE, D., P.M. VAN HAGEN, P.M. VAN KOETSVELD, *et al.* 1999. In vitro characterization of somatostatin receptors in the human thymus and effects of somatostatin and octreotide on cultured thymic epithelial cells. Endocrinology **140:** 373–380.
38. FERONE, D., R. PIVONELLO, P.M. VAN HAGEN, *et al.* 2000. Age-related decrease of somatostatin receptor number in the normal human thymus. Am. J. Physiol. Endocrinol. Metab. **279:** E791–E798.
39. FERONE, D., P.M. VAN HAGEN, A. COLAO, *et al.* 1999. Somatostatin receptors in the thymus. Ann. Med. **31**(Suppl 2): 28–33.
40. FERONE, D., R. PIVONELLO, P.M. VAN HAGEN, *et al.* 2002. Quantitative and functional expression of somatostatin receptor subtypes in human thymocytes. Am. J. Physiol. Endocrinol. Metab. **283:** E1056–E1066.
41. FERONE, D., P.M. VAN HAGEN, R. PIVONELLO, *et al.* 2000. Physiological and pathophysiological role of somatostatin receptors in the human thymus. Eur. J. Endocrinol. **143**(Suppl 1): S27–S34.
42. DALM, V.A., L.J. HOFLAND, D. FERONE, *et al.* 2003. The role of somatostatin and somatostatin analogs in the pathophysiology of the human immune system. J. Endocrinol. Invest. **26**(Suppl 8): 94–102.
43. LICHTENAUER-KALIGIS, E.G., V.A. DALM, S.P. OOMEN, *et al.* 2004. Differential expression of somatostatin receptor subtypes in human peripheral blood mononuclear cell subsets. Eur. J. Endocrinol. **150:** 565–577.
44. DALM, V.A., P.M. VAN HAGEN, R.R. DE KRIJGER, *et al.* 2004. Distribution pattern of somatostatin and cortistatin mRNA in human central and peripheral tissues. Clin. Endocrinol. **60:** 625–629.
45. ROBAS, N., E. MEAD & M. FIDOCK. 2003. MrgX2 is a high potency cortistatin receptor expressed in dorsal root ganglion. J. Biol. Chem. **278:** 44400–44404.

46. CADIGAN, D.G., P.D. HOLLETT, P.W. COLLINGWOOD & E. UR. 1996. Imaging of a mediastinal thymic carcinoid tumor with radiolabeled somatostatin analogue. Clin. Nucl. Med. **21:** 487–488.
47. LASTORIA, S., E. VERGARA, G. PALMIERI, *et al.* 1998. In vivo detection of malignant thymic masses by [111In-DTPA-D-Phe1]-Octreotide scintigraphy. J. Nucl. Med. **39:** 634–639.
48. LIN, K., B.D. NGUYEN, D.S. ETTINGER & B.B. CHIN. 1999. Somatostatin receptor scintigraphy and somatostatin therapy in the evaluation and treatment of malignant thymoma. Clin. Nucl. Med. **24:** 24–28.
49. FERONE, D., P.M. VAN HAGEN, D.J. KWEKKEBOOM, *et al.* 2000. Somatostatin receptor subtypes in human thymoma and inhibition of cell proliferation by octreotide in vitro. J. Clin. Endocrinol. Metab. **85:** 1719–1726.
50. FERONE, D., D.J. KWEKKEBOOM, R. PIVONELLO, *et al.* 2001. In vivo and in vitro expression of somatostatin receptors in two human thymomas with similar clinical presentation and different histological features. J. Endocrinol. Invest. **24:** 522–528.
51. MUNDSCHENK, J., N. UNGER, S. SCHULZ, *et al.* 2003. Somatostatin receptor subtypes in human pheochromocytoma: subcellular expression pattern and functional relevance for octreotide scintigraphy. J. Clin. Endocrinol. Metab. **88:** 5150–5177.
52. WITZIG, T.E., L. LETENDRE, J. GERSTNER, *et al.* 1995. Evaluation of a somatostatin analog in the treatment of lymphoproliferative disorders: results of a phase II North Central Cancer Treatment Group trial. J. Clin. Oncol. **13:** 2012–2015.
53. PALMIERI, G., S. LASTORIA, A. COLAO, *et al.* 1997. Successful treatment of a patient with thymoma and pure red-cell aplasia with octreotide and prednisone. N. Engl. J. Med. 336: 263–265.
54. PALMIERI, G., L. MONTELLA, A. MARTINETTI, *et al.* 2002. Somatostatin analogs and prednisone in advanced refractory thymic tumors. Cancer **94:** 1414–1420.
55. REUBI, J.C., B. WASER, P.M. VAN HAGEN, *et al.* 1992. In vivo and in vitro detection of somatostatin receptors in human malignant lymphomas. Int. J. Cancer **50:** 895–900.
56. LIPP, R.W., H. SILLY, G. RANNER, *et al.* 1995. Radiolabeled octreotide for the demonstration of somatostatin receptors in malignant lymphoma and lymphoadenopathy. J. Nucl. Med. **36:** 13–18.
57. VAN HAGEN, P.M. 1996. Somatostatin receptor expression in clinical immunology. Metabolism **45:** 96–97.
58. VAN DEN ANKER-LUGTENBURG, P.J., B. LÖWENBERG, S.W.J. LAMBERTS & E.P. KRENNING. 1996. The relevance of somatostatin receptor expression in malignant lymphomas. Metabolism **45:** 96–97.
59. LUGTENBURG, P.J., E.P. KRENNING, R. VALKEMA, *et al.* 2001. Somatostatin receptor scintigraphy useful in stage I–II Hodgkin's disease: more extended disease identified. Br. J. Haematol. **112:** 936–944.
60. LUGTENBURG, P.J., B. LOWENBERG, R. VALKEMA, *et al.* 2001. Somatostatin receptor scintigraphy in the initial staging of low-grade non-Hodgkin's lymphomas. J. Nucl. Med. **42:** 222–229.
61. FERONE, D., C. SEMINO, M. BOSCHETTI, *et al.* 2005. Initial staging of lymphoma with octreotide and other receptor imaging agents. Semin. Nucl. Med. **35:** 176–185.

62. BOURGUET, P. & S.O.R. GROUPE DE TRAVAIL. 2003. Standards, options and recommendations for the use of [18F]-FDG (PET-FDG) in cancerology. Bull. Cancer **90:** S88–S95.

63. GEORGII-HEMMING, P., T. STROMBERG, E.T. JANSON, *et al.* 1999. The somatostatin analog octreotide inhibits growth of interleukin-6 (IL-6)-dependent and IL-6-independent human multiple myeloma cell lines. Blood **93:** 1724–1731.

64. DUET, M. & F.F. LIOTÉ. 2004. Somatostatin and somatostatin analog scintigraphy: any benefits for rheumatology patients? Joint Bone Spine **71:** 530–535.

65. DUET, M., T.B. PATRICE, W. MICHEL & F. LIOTÉ. 2005. Plasma cell problems: case 3. Plasmacytoma mimicking a paraganglioma of the skull base: diagnostic value of somatostatin receptor scintigraphy. J. Clin. Oncol. **23:** 3143–3145.

66. FERONE, D., M. ARVIGO, C. SEMINO, *et al.* 2003. The role of somatostatin analogs in the management of immunoproliferative disease. J. Endocrinol. Invest. **26**(Suppl 8): 103–108.

67. KRANTIC, S., I. GODDARD, A. SAVEANU, *et al.* 2004. Novel modalities of somatostatin actions. Eur. J. Endocrinol. **151:** 643–655.

68. DALM, V.A., L.J. HOFLAND, C.M. MOOY, *et al.* 2004. Somatostatin receptors in malignant lymphomas: targets for radiotherapy? J. Nucl. Med. **45:** 8–16.

69. VAN HAGEN, P.M., E.P. KRENNING, J.C. REUBI, *et al.* 1994. Somatostatin analogue scintigraphy in granulomatous diseases. Eur. J. Nucl. Med. **21:** 497–502.

70. NEUMANN, I., S. MIRZAEI, R. BIRCK, *et al.* 2004. Expression of somatostatin receptors in inflammatory lesions and diagnostic value of somatostatin receptor scintigraphy in patients with ANCA-associated small vessel vasculitis. Rheumatology (Oxford) **43:** 195–201.

71. KWEKKEBOOM, D.J., E.P. KRENNING, G.S. KHO, *et al.* 1998. Somatostatin receptor imaging in patients with sarcoidosis. Eur. J. Nucl. Med. **25:** 1284–1292.

72. WEINMANN, P., B. CRESTANI, A. TAZI, *et al.* 2000. 111In-pentetreotide scintigraphy in patients with Langerhans' cell histiocytosis. J. Nucl. Med. **41:** 1808–1812.

73. LASTORIA, S., L. MONTELLA, L. CATALANO, *et al.* 2002. Functional imaging of Langerhans cell histiocytosis by (111)In-DTPA-D-Phe(1)-octreotide scintigraphy. Cancer **94:** 633–640.

74. TEN BOKUM, A.M., L.J. HOFLAND, G. DE JONG, *et al.* 1999. Immunohistochemical localization of somatostatin receptor sst2A in sarcoid granulomas. Eur. J. Clin. Invest. **29:** 630–636.

75. DALM, V.A., P.M. VAN HAGEN & E.P. KRENNING. 2003. The role of octreotide scintigraphy in rheumatoid arthritis and sarcoidosis. Q. J. Nucl. Med. **47:** 270–278.

76. VAN HAGEN, P.M., H.M. MARKUSSE, S.W. LAMBERTS, *et al.* 1994. Somatostatin receptor imaging. The presence of somatostatin receptors in rheumatoid arthritis. Arthritis Rheum. **37:** 1521–1527.

77. REUBI, J.C., B. WASER, H.M. MARKUSSE, *et al.* 1994. Vascular somatostatin receptors in synovium from patients with rheumatoid arthritis. Eur. J. Pharmacol. **271:** 371–378.

78. TEN BOKUM, A.M, M.J. MELIEF, A. SCHONBRUNN, *et al.* 1999. Immunohistochemical localization of somatostatin receptor sst2A in human rheumatoid synovium. J. Rheumatol. **26:** 532–535.

79. KOSEOGLU, F. & T. KOSEOGLU. 2002. Long acting somatostatin analogue for the treatment of refractory RA. Ann. Rheum. Dis. **61:** 573–574.

80. PARAN, D. & H. PARAN. 2003. Somatostatin analogs in rheumatoid arthritis and other inflammatory and immune-mediated conditions. Curr. Opin. Investig. Drugs **4:** 578–582.
81. HELYES, Z., A. SZABO, J. NEMETH, *et al.* 2004. Antiinflammatory and analgesic effects of somatostatin released from capsaicin-sensitive sensory nerve terminals in a Freund's adjuvant-induced chronic arthritis model in the rat. Arthritis Rheum. **50:** 1677–1685.
82. PHAN, T.G., T.P. GORDON, M.H. TATTERSALL & R.H. LOBLAY. 2002. Octreotide therapy for the Sjögren syndrome. Ann. Intern. Med. **137:** 777–778.
83. MARIETTE, X., P. RAVAUD, S. STEINFELD, *et al.* 2003. Absence of efficiency of infliximab in primary Sjögren's syndrome: preliminary results of the TRIPPS Study. Trial of Remicade® in primary Sjögren's syndrome. Ann. Rheum. Dis. **62**(Suppl 1): 66.
84. JEONG, Y.S., J.B. JUN, T.H. KIM, *et al.* 2000. Successful treatment of protein-losing enteropathy due to AA amyloidosis with somatostatin analogue and high dose steroid in ankylosing spondylitis. Clin. Exp. Rheumatol. **18:** 619–621.

Prolactin and Growth Hormone Responses to Hypoglycemia in Patients with Systemic Sclerosis and Psoriatic Arthritis

JOZEF ROVENSKY,[a] HELENA RAFFAYOVA,[a] RICHARD IMRICH,[b] ZOFIA RADIKOVA,[b] ADELA PENESOVA,[b] LADISLAV MACHO,[b] JOZEF LUKAC,[a] MARCO MATUCCI-CERINIC,[c] MILAN VIGAS[b]

[a]*National Institute of Rheumatic Diseases, 921 23 Piestany, Slovakia*

[b]*Institute of Experimental Endocrinology, Slovak Academy of Sciences, 83306 Bratislava, Slovakia*

[c]*Department of Medicine, Division of Rheumatology, University of Florence, 50139 Florence, Italy*

ABSTRACT: This study compared prolactin (PRL) and growth hormone (GH) responses to hypoglycemia in premenopausal females with systemic sclerosis (SSc) and psoriatic arthritis (PsA) with those in matched healthy controls. No differences were found in glucose and GH responses to hypoglycemia in both groups of patients compared to controls. SSc patients had lower PRL response ($P < 0.05$) to hypoglycemia compared to controls. PRL response tended to be lower also in PsA patients, however the difference did not reach level of statistical significance ($P = 0.11$). The present study showed decreased PRL response to hypoglycemia in premenopausal females with SSc.

KEYWORDS: prolactin; growth hormone; hypoglycemia; systemic sclerosis; psoriatic arthritis

INTRODUCTION

Prolactin (PRL) and growth hormone (GH) are pituitary hormones, which belong to the family of lactogenic and growth factors. Functional receptors and nonpituitary production of both PRL and GH have been identified in numerous tissue types including cells of the immune system. Several lines of evidence suggest an immunomodulating effect of PRL and GH.[1–3] Thus, the involvement of PRL and GH has been suggested in human diseases in which altered function

Address for correspondence: Prof. J. Rovensky, M.D., D.Sc., National Institute of Rheumatic Diseases, Nabr. I. Krasku 4, 921 23 Piestany, Slovakia. Voice: +421-33-7723508; fax: +421-33-7721192. e-mail: rovensky@nurch.sk

Ann. N.Y. Acad. Sci. 1069: 145–148 (2006). © 2006 New York Academy of Sciences.
doi: 10.1196/annals.1351.012

of the immune system plays important role. Considering an immunomodulatory role for PRL and GH, their dysregulated secretion has been believed to play an aggravating role in rheumatic diseases. Elevated baseline PRL levels were observed in about one-third of patients with rheumatoid arthritis (RA), systemic sclerosis (SSc), psoriatic arthritis (PsA), Sjögren's syndrome, or systemic lupus erythematosus.[4] Increased frequency of glucocorticoid treatment in hyperprolactinemic RA patients compared to normoprolactinemic patients was observed in our previous study.[5] Moreover suppression of PRL secretion by dopamine D2 receptor agonist bromocriptine was successfully used in experimental models of autoimmune disorders as well as in controlled human studies, further supporting possible involvement of PRL in rheumatic diseases.[4]

It has been suggested that the effect of PRL and GH on immune function *in vivo* may be more apparent when the organism is subjected to a stress challenge.[6] The authors of the latter review proposed a hypothesis that stress-related elevation of PRL and GH might compensate for the immunosuppressive effect of glucocorticoids on immune responses. Paradoxically, recent findings of our group indicate decreased stress-induced secretion of PRL in RA patients.[7,8] The present study was aimed at assessment of PRL and GH responses in patients with SSc and PsA.

SUBJECTS AND METHODS

In order to investigate the proportion of PRL and GH responses to stress stimulus, we performed insulin-induced hypoglycemia (0.1 IU/kg, Actrapid HM; Novo Nordisk, A/S Bagsvaerd, Denmark) in 16 SSc females (mean $\pm$ SEM, age $= 38.4 \pm 2.8$ years, body mass index $= 21.8 \pm 0.5$ kg/m^2), 15 PsA females (age $= 40.1 \pm 1.4$ years, body mass index $= 23.5 \pm 1.05$ kg/m^2), and in 18 healthy female controls (CN) (age $= 40.9 \pm 1.6$ years, body mass index $= 22.6 \pm 0.8$ kg/m^2). All patients were premenopausal and neither of them was treated with drugs known to affect PRL or GH levels. Concentrations of plasma glucose, PRL, and GH were measured before and 15, 30, 45, 60, and 90 min after insulin administration using immunoradiometric analysis (Immunotech a.s., Prague, Czech Republic). Plasma glucose concentrations were analyzed by glucose-oxidase method (Hitachi, Ibaraki, Japan).

Basal plasma glucose concentrations were similar in both groups of patients and controls. Insulin administration was followed by a significant fall in plasma glucose concentrations. The nadir occurred 30 min after insulin administration. Changes in plasma glucose concentrations did not differ in SSc and PsA patients compared to CN. No significant differences were observed in basal concentrations of PRL and GH in both groups of patients when compared to CN. SSc patients had lower PRL response ($P < 0.05$, General Linear Model for repeated measurements) compared to CN. PRL response did not significantly

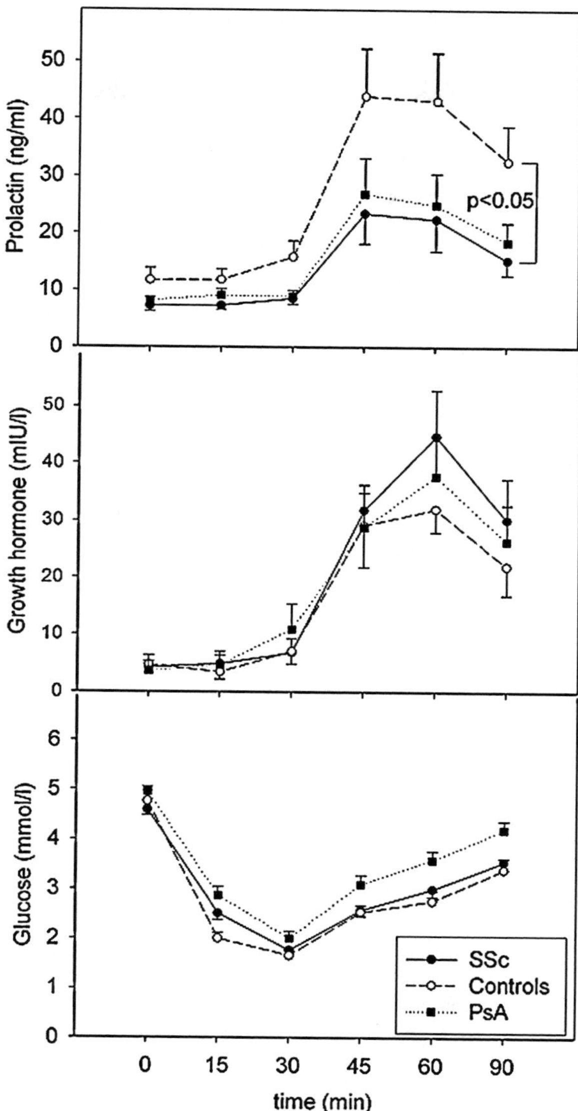

FIGURE 1. Concentrations of prolactin (top), growth hormone (middle), and glucose (bottom) during insulin-induced hypoglycemia in 16 SSc (black circles), 15 PsA arthritis female patients (black squares), and 18 healthy controls (white circles). Data are mean ± standard error. A statistically significant difference in PRL responses was found between SSc and healthy controls ($P < 0.05$) as assessed by General Linear Model for repeated measurements.

differ in PsA patients compared to CN ($P = 0.11$), however, tendency toward lower PRL response was found also in this group of patient. Neither SSc nor PsA patients did differ in their GH response when compared to CN (FIG. 1).

CONCLUSIONS

To our knowledge, this is the first study demonstrating hypoglycemia-induced PRL and GH responses in premenopausal females with SSc and PsA. In line with our previous findings in RA patients,[7,8] present results showed lower hypoglycemia-induced PRL response in SSc patients. In addition to this, a similar trend was also observed in PsA patients, however the difference did not reach level of statistical significance. Collectively, the findings are suggestive of downregulated lactotropic axis in patients with RA, SSc, and possibly with PsA. Elucidation of mechanisms responsible for the attenuated stress-stimulated response of PRL in those patients warrants further investigation.

ACKNOWLEDGMENT

This work was supported by Ministry of Health of Slovak Republic.

REFERENCES

1. KOOIJMAN, R., S. GERLO, A. COPPENS, *et al*. 2000. Growth hormone and prolactin expression in the immune system. Ann. N. Y. Acad. Sci. **917:** 534–540.
2. MATERA, L. 1996. Endocrine, paracrine and autocrine actions of prolactin on immune cells. Life Sci. **59:** 599–614.
3. SAITO, H., T. INOUE, K. FUKATSU, *et al*. 1996. Growth hormone and the immune response to bacterial infection. Horm. Res. **45:** 50–54.
4. WALKER, S.E. & J.D. JACOBSON. 2000. Roles of prolactin and gonadotropin-releasing hormone in rheumatic diseases. Rheum. Dis. Clin. North Am. **26:** 713–736.
5. ROVENSKY, J., J. BAKOSOVA, J. PAYER, *et al*. 2001. Increased demand for steroid therapy in hyperprolactinemic patients with rheumatoid arthritis. Int. J. Tissue React. **23:** 145–149.
6. DORSHKIND, K. & N.D. HORSEMAN. 2000. The roles of prolactin, growth hormone, insulin-like growth factor-I, and thyroid hormones in lymphocyte development and function: insights from genetic models of hormone and hormone receptor deficiency. Endocr. Rev. **21:** 292–312.
7. ROVENSKY, J., R. IMRICH, F. MALIS, *et al*. 2004. Prolactin and growth hormone responses to hypoglycemia in patients with rheumatoid arthritis and ankylosing spondylitis. J. Rheumatol. **31:** 2418–2421.
8. IMRICH, R., M. VIGAS & J. ROVENSKY. 2005. Different threshold for prolactin response to hypoglycaemia in patients with rheumatoid arthritis? Ann. Rheum. Dis. **64:** 515–516.

Innervation of the Joint and Role of Neuropeptides

YRJÖ T. KONTTINEN,[a,b,c] VELI-MATTI TIAINEN,[b] ENRIQUE GOMEZ-BARRENA,[d] MIKA HUKKANEN,[a] AND JARI SALO[a]

[a]*Department of Medicine and Department of Orthopaedics and Traumatology, Helsinki University Central Hospital, Helsinki, Finland*

[b]*ORTON Orthopaedic Hospital of the Invalid Foundation, Helsinki, Finland*

[c]*COXA Hospital for Joint Replacement, Tampere, Finland*

[d]*Servicio de Cirugía Ortopédica y Traumatología, Fundación "Jiminez Díaz," Madrid, Spain*

ABSTRACT: Rheumatoid arthritis is considered to represent a disease of the synovial membrane, osteoarthritis of the hyaline articular cartilage, and osteoporosis of the bone. It can be questioned to what extent this is true and to what extent these diseases could be considered to be due to extra-articular, extra-skeletal pathology related to the neuroendocrine system. Pain is the main symptom in arthritis. This is related to prostaglandin-mediated sensitization of the primary afferent nociceptive nerves. Accordingly, nonsteroidal anti-inflammatory drugs are used in symptomatic treatment, occasionally together with opioids and tricyclic antidepressants. The midline symmetry and involvement of the richly innervated, small peripheral joints in rheumatoid arthritis have raised speculation about the role of neurogenic inflammation and neuropeptides in its pathogenesis. In contrast to the free nerve endings, the role of the proprioceptive sensors is to provide information of our actual motor performance (the afferent copy of our movements) compared to the efferent motor program, which is activated by our will to move. These include proprioceptors in the skin (e.g., Meissner corpuscles), muscles (annulospiral and flower-spray endings of the muscle spindles), Golgi tendon organs, and Ruffini end organs and Pacinian corpuscles in the superficial and deep layers of the joint capsule. Elderly people may have slow reflexes, lax joints, joint incongruity, and loss of muscle power; obesity, alcohol and medicinal use, and joint pain can be combined with poor/nonexisting capacity for repair and remodeling of the musculoskeletal tissues. Impaired biomechanics contributes to increased joint tenderness, accumulation of minor trauma (secondary osteoarthritis), and falls (osteoporotic fractures). More attention needs to be paid to aging of proprioception, not only to the terminal disease target.

Address for correspondence: Yrjö T. Konttinen, Professor of Medicine, Biomedicum, PO Box 700, FIN-00029 HUS, Finland. Voice: +358-9-191 25210; fax: +358-9-191 25218.
e-mail: yrjo.konttinen@helsinki.fi

Ann. N.Y. Acad. Sci. 1069: 149–154 (2006). © 2006 New York Academy of Sciences.
doi: 10.1196/annals.1351.013

Keywords: osteoarthritis; cartilage; subchondral bone; proprioception; feed forward; feed back

PROPRIOCEPTORS

The nervous system forms an extravascular, intraneuronal system for the body's information technology including upstream- and downstream transport of neurotransmitters and neuropeptides.[1] Specialized nerve endings or proprioceptors provide information about the position and movement of the body in space at any given moment.[2] The particular form of energy or molecule to which a sensor is most sensitive is called its adequate stimulus. Because different sensory modalities can be perceived, it follows that there are different types of peripheral nerve endings and fibers responsible for different sensory modalities. Those of relevance to our joints are located in skin, muscles, tendons, and joint capsule (Table 1, Fig. 1).

ROLE OF THE PROPRIOCEPTORS

Input from these proprioceptive nerve terminals relays feedback information on motor performance, which in turn forms the afferent copy of the motor program (e.g., walking) being executed. It can be compared to the efferent feed-forward copy, which has been activated by an internal drive to move (Fig. 2). As far as discrepancies between the plan and its execution occur, corrections are made, all usually automatically at the subconscious level, so that the higher centers can, it is hoped, continue with their intellectual cognitive functions. In elderly people, this system malfunctions as a result of slow reflexes, lax joints, joint incongruity, loss of muscle power, obesity, alcohol and medicinal use, and joint pain. The cumulative microtrauma targeting avascular and aneural articular cartilage with minimal capacity for repair contributes to wear of the nondisposable cartilage tissue as well as to osteoporotic fractures. Pain associated with osteoarthritis of the knees increases the propensity to trip on an obstacle,[3] whereas aging impairs standing balance.

THE AFFERENT FUNCTION OF THE NOCICEPTIVE SYSTEM

The afferent feedback helps us avoid harmful stresses and strains of articular cartilage, and if trauma occurs in spite of all, the nociceptive system from sinovial membrane may indirectly provide a delayed warning. If the musculoskeletal tissues are already traumatized or diseased, local production of prostaglandins provides an effective stimulation able to sensitize the nerves to avoid any further damage.[1,5] Accordingly, arthritis is symptomatically treated with nonsteroidal anti-inflammatory drugs, which inhibit COX enzymes (PGH_2 synthetase), whereas the development of slow-acting, structure-modifying drugs of osteoarthritis has only progressed very slowly.[6]

TABLE 1. Proprioceptors

Ending	Principal location	Characteristics	Functional description	Information provided
Ruffini end organs* 6–9 μm fibers	Superficial layers of fibrous capsule	Low threshold, slowly adapted, unencapsuled, myelinated	Direction and speed of movement, regulate muscle tone	Statistic position of the joint, stretching of the tendon bundles
Pacinian corpuscles** 9–12 μm fibers	Deep layers of the fibrous capsule, muscle fascia	Low threshold, rapidly adapted, encapsulated, myelinated	Acceleration and deceleration of the joint movement and pressure	Quick changes of joint movement
Golgi tendon organs*** 13–17 μm fibers	Ligaments near the joint	Low threshold, slowly adapted, encapsulated, myelinated	Direction of movement, record tension	Muscle contraction or stretching during contraction
Annulospiral endings of muscle spindles	Centers of intrafusal muscle fibers	Encapsulated, thickly myelinated, 12–20 μm fibers	Stretch receptors	Length change of the muscle
Flower-spray endings	At one or both sides of annulospiral endings	Encapsulated, thinly myelinated, 5–12 μm fibers	Stretch receptors	Length of the muscle
Cutaneous SAI	Merkel's disc in dermis	Slowly adapted, small receptive fields, low threshold, unencapsulated	Spatial resolution, duration of skin indentation	Long-lasting mechanical stimulus on the surface of the skin
Cutaneous SAII	Ruffini endings[1]	Slowly adapted, large receptive fields, low threshold, unencapsulated	Stretching of the skin	Stretching the skin
Cutaneous RA	Meissner corpuscles[1]	Rapidly adapted, small receptive fields, low threshold, encapsulated	Sense velocity	Slight movement of a hair
Cutaneous PC	Pacinian corpuscles, subcutis	Very rapidly adapted, encapsulated	Acceleration or vibration	Discharges only when the velocity of skin deformation changes

Sensor dimenions (μm): *100 × 40, **280 × 120, and ***600 × 100; [1]hairy and glabrous skin.

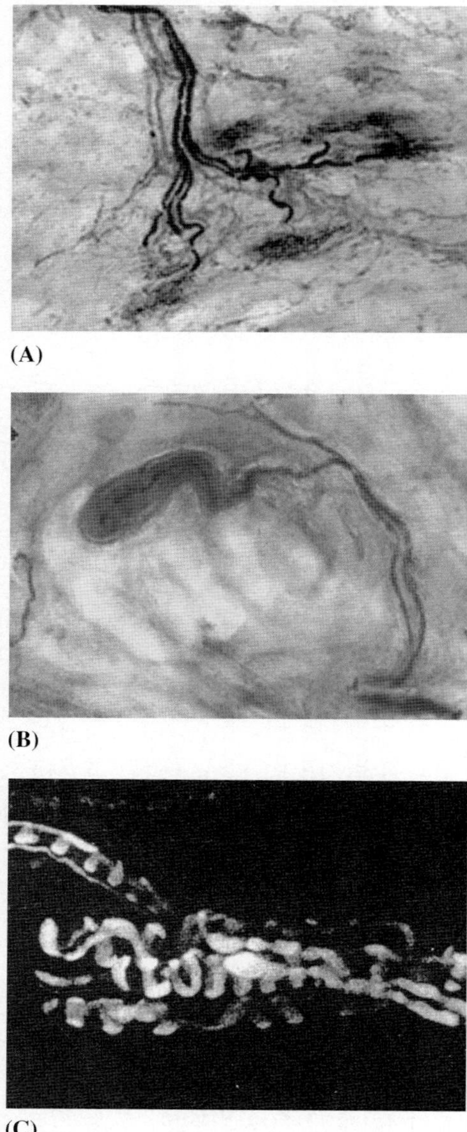

FIGURE 1. Panel A demonstrates Ruffini end organ in the superficial joint capsule and panel B Pacinian corpuscle in the deep joint capsule in gold chloride labeling (thick sections are good for morphometric counting of the proprioceptors) and panel C demonstrates annulospiral endings of a muscle spindle in a 3-D construct composed of several optical sections produced using laser scanning confocal microscopy (suitable for detailed structural studies of individual proprioceptors).

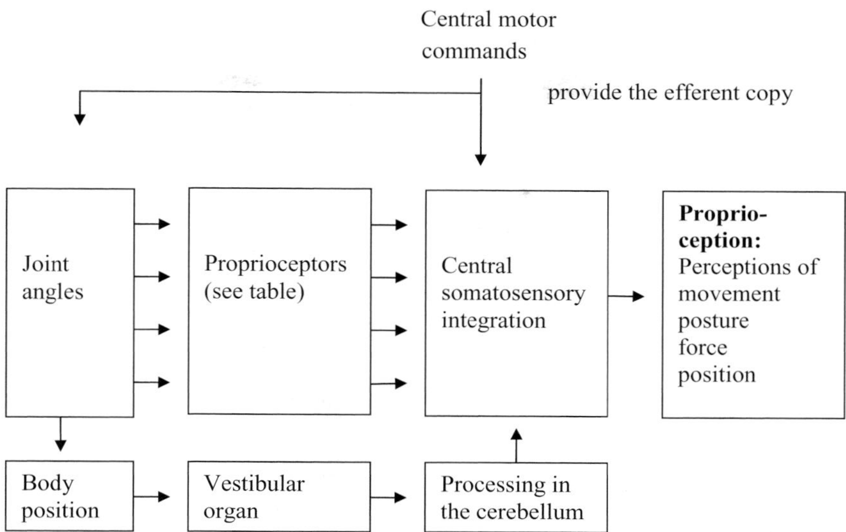

FIGURE 2. A ready made efferent copy of the motor program is fed forward to α-motorneurons and motor units, which move the body and joints. This is perceived by proprioceptors, which feed back an afferent copy of our actual motor performance. The efferent and afferent copies are compared in cerebellum and corrective movements performed when required.

THE EFFERENT FUNCTION OF THE NEUROPEPTIDE NERVES

The efferent function of the sensory nerves is exemplified by their neuropeptide content. Paradoxically, primary afferent nociceptive nerves seem to play a major role for this efferent function. At the moment, it is impossible to know whether perhaps the joint nerves play a primary role in arthritis pathology, but at least it is clear that the sensitization of the primary afferent nociceptive nerves leads to altered stimulus–response coupling. This leads to excessive and untimely release of potent neuropeptides in some areas and to depletion and lack of such release in other areas. Furthermore, responses are also more pronounced in areas of inflammation. Neuropeptides have powerful effects on cytokine production and release leading to a close correlation, for example, between bombesin/gastrin-releasing peptide and substance P, and interleukin-6 in arthritic synovial fluid.[7] Vasoactive intestinal peptide is a ubiquitous 28-amino acid. Amphipathic and pleiotropic mammalian neuropeptide seems to be effective not only in the treatment of arthritis, but also in some other diseases.[8] The activity of the sympathetic nervous system (e.g., NPY concentration) is elevated, but the response of the hypothalamus-pituitary-adrenal axis is decreased with all the systemic consequences thereof.[9] This scaled-down production of endogenous glucocorticosteroids might explain why patients with rheumatoid arthritis seem to be able to use small-dose prednisolon without adverse events. Study of the neuronal involvement in arthritis pain and inflammation has led to promising findings regarding possibility to hit back with the use of the same weapon.

REFERENCES

1. Konttinen, Y.T., P. Kemppinen, M. Segerberg, *et al.* 1994a. Peripheral and spinal neural mechanisms in arthritis, with particular reference to treatment of inflammation and pain. Arthritis Rheum. **37:** 965–982.
2. Konttinen, Y.T., H. Koski, S. Santavirta, *et al.* 1994b. Nociception, proprioception and neurotransmitters. *In* Disorders of the Cervical Spine. Diagnosis and Medical Management, 2nd ed. J.H. Bland, Ed.: 339–363. W.B. Saunders Company. Philadelphia.
3. Pandya, N.K., L.F. Draganich, A. Mauer, *et al.* 2005. Osteoarthritis of the knees increases the propensity to trip on an obstacle. Clin. Orthop. Relat. Res. **431:** 150-156.
4. Bennell, K.L. & R.S. Hinman. 2005. Effect of experimentally induced knee pain on standing balance in healthy older individuals. Rheumatology (Oxford) **44:** 378–381.
5. Konttinen, Y.T., M. Grönblad, M. Hukkanen, *et al.* 1989. Pain fibers in osteoarthritis—a review. Semin. Arthritis Rheum. **18**(Suppl 2): 35–40.
6. Steinmeyer, J. & Y.T. Konttinen. Oral treatment options for degenerative joint disease—presence and future. Adv. Drug Deliv. Rev. In press.
7. Green, P.G. 2005. Gastrin-releasing peptide, substance P and cytokines in rheumatoid arthritis. Arthritis Res. Ther. **7:** 111–113.
8. Delgado, M., C. Abad, C. Martinez, *et al.* 2001. Vasoactive intestinal peptide prevents experimental arthritis by downregulating both autoimmune and inflammatory components of the disease. Nat. Med. **7:** 563–568.
9. Harle, P., R.H. Straub, R. Wiest, *et al.* 2006. Increase of sympathetic outflow measured by NPY and decrease of the hypothalamic-pituitary-adrenal axis tone in patients with systemic lupus erythematosus and rhematoid arthritis—another example of uncoupling of response systems. Ann. Rheum. Dis. **65:** 51–56.

Neurogenic Inflammation and Arthritis

JON D. LEVINE,[a] SACHIA G. KHASAR,[b] AND PAUL G. GREEN[b]

[a]*Department of Medicine, NIH Pain Center, University of California, San Francisco, San Francisco, California 94143-0440, USA*

[b]*Oral and Maxillofacial Surgery, NIH Pain Center, University of California, San, Francisco, San Francisco, California 94143-0440, USA*

ABSTRACT: Inflammation and inflammatory diseases are sexually dimorphic, but the underlying causes for this observed sexual dimorphism are poorly understood. We discuss neural-immune mechanisms that underlie sexual dimorphism in three critical aspects of the inflammatory process—plasma extravasation, neutrophil function, and inflammatory hyperalgesia. Plasma extravasation and accumulation/activation of leukocytes into tissues are critical components in inflammation and are required for several other aspects of the inflammatory response. Pain (hyperalgesia) also markedly influences the magnitude of other components of the inflammatory response and induces a feedback control of plasma extravasation and neutrophil function. More important, this feedback control itself is powerfully modulated by vagal afferent activity and both the function of the primary afferent nociceptor and the modulation of inflammatory hyperalgesia by vagal afferent activity are highly sexually dimorphic.

KEYWORDS: nociception; pain; hyperalgesia; inflammation; inflammatory diseases; sympathoadrenal axis; adrenal medulla; hypothalamic-pituitary-adrenal axis; plasma extravasation; sex differences; 17β-estradiol; testosterone; chemotaxis; β-adrenergic receptor; polymorphonuclear leukocytes

INTRODUCTION

The adrenal medulla, probably via release of epinephrine, is required for the vagus-mediated modulation of nociceptive threshold, inflammatory mediator-induced hyperalgesia, and plasma extravasation; and the adrenal medulla may play a role in mediating the sex differences in the inflammatory response. Such sex-related differences may, in turn, have an impact on the severity of joint injury in arthritis, because pain itself provides an important signal from the inflammatory response to elicit a reflex modulation of the inflammatory

Address for correspondence: Jon D. Levine, NIH Pain Center, C522 Box 0440, UCSF, 521 Parnassus Avenue, San Francisco, CA 94143-0440, USA. Voice: +1-415-476-5108; fax: +1-415-476-6305. e-mail: Jon.Levine@ucsf.edu

Ann. N.Y. Acad. Sci. 1069: 155–167 (2006).
doi: 10.1196/annals.1351.014

response. We have recently shown that fasting is a natural, vagal-mediated stimulus that can potentiate formalin-induced nociception in female but not in male rats.

The sympathoadrenal axis and its modulation by vagal afferents, both of which are sexually dimorphic, can have a powerful impact on the inflammatory response, and may thus also be important in establishing sexual dimorphism in inflammatory diseases. An understanding of sex differences in the inflammatory response, including nociception, will provide the information necessary to understand differences in inflammatory diseases in women and men, answer fundamental questions regarding biology of sex differences, and assist in the rational development of new therapeutic modalities.

Inflammation is an extremely common reason for people to seek medical treatment. Current therapies for inflammatory diseases, primarily consisting of steroidal and nonsteroidal anti-inflammatory drugs, immunosuppressive agents, and recently, biologic therapies (e.g., anti-TNF-α) provide only temporary relief, only partially ameliorate the disease process, and have significant adverse effects. In order to find new targets for therapeutic interventions to treat inflammatory diseases, a better understanding of the mechanisms by which the inflammatory process is established and maintained is needed.

Interestingly, inflammation and inflammatory diseases are sexually dimorphic.[1–6] The underlying causes for the observed sexual dimorphism of inflammatory diseases are poorly understood. Elucidating them may provide new targets for therapies as we increase our understanding of critical components of the inflammatory process and the biology of sex differences. We discuss neural-immune mechanisms that underlie sexual dimorphism in three critical aspects of the inflammatory process—plasma extravasation, neutrophil function, and inflammatory hyperalgesia.

INFLAMMATION

Inflammation, which is characterized by redness, warmth, pain, and swelling, is usually a protective response to tissue injury, irritation, or infection. Redness and warmth are the results of increased blood flow; pain (hyperalgesia) is caused by the sensitization of neurons of the primary afferent nerve; and swelling is the result of increased vascular permeability, which causes the extravasation of plasma proteins. The attraction of neutrophils and other leukocytes to the site and their activation is also a critical component of the inflammatory process, especially when it occurs in the setting of inflammatory disease. A large number of mediators produced by the inflammatory response —for example, bradykinin, platelet-activating factor, adenosine, serotonin, prostaglandins, and leukotrienes—all act to promote plasma extravasation and/or attract neutrophils and other leukocytes to the site of an inflammatory response where they are activated. Plasma extravasation is a critical component in inflammation, because the increase in vascular permeability and subsequent extravasation of plasma that is initiated early in the inflammatory response is a first line of defense required for several other aspects of the inflammatory response, and is the principal determinant of the molecular environment of inflamed tissue.[7] The accumulation and activation of neutrophils and other leukocytes into tissues are also an essential component of the inflammatory response.[8,9] Chronic accumulation of leukocytes at sites of inflammation and production of neutrophil-derived reactive oxygen species contribute to the development of the tissue injury associated with a variety of inflammatory disease states.[10]

More important, available evidence supports plasma extravasation as a tissue-*protective* component of the inflammatory response, which limits damage to synovial joints; in fact, we have shown that the magnitude of bradykinin-induced plasma extravasation in the rat knee joint is *inversely* related to the severity of joint injury.[11–14] Specifically, we have shown in the rat that agents that inhibit bradykinin-induced knee joint plasma extravasation (viz., epinephrine, the β_2-agonist salbutamol, the α_2-antagonist yohimbine, and nicotine) exacerbate the radiological severity of joint injury in experimental arthritis, while agents that enhance bradykinin-induced plasma extravasation in the knee joint (viz., the β_2-antagonist ICI-118,551, the α_2-agonist, clonidine, ATP, and adenosine) reduce the severity of experimental arthritis. These results support the suggestion that plasma extravasation is a tissue-protective component of the inflammatory response in chronic arthritis—plasma extravasation may exert this effect by increasing the rate of removal of tissue-damaging products of the inflammatory response.[15,16] Importantly, there is evidence in the clinical literature for the dissociation between clinical signs of inflammation and the progression of joint destruction, supporting the suggestion that there is a differential contribution of different components of the inflammatory response to either tissue/joint injury or protection. Thus, in the setting of inflammatory diseases, some components of the inflammatory response still function to *protect* inflamed tissue from injury and destruction. This may help explain why therapies that markedly suppress the immune system, including immunosuppressive and cytotoxic drugs, and even total nodal radiation, more often than not fail to produce complete remission in patients with "inflammatory disease."[17–20] Components of the inflammatory response need to be analyzed independently to be able to understand their relative contribution to morbidity in an individual inflammatory disease, for example, plasma extravasation, recruitment and activation of neutrophils, and pain (which correlates with severity of experimental arthritis,[21] and is a predictor of severity of arthritis in humans).[22–24] It should be noted that bradykinin-induced plasma extravasation is powerfully affected by stress,[25] activity in the subdiaphragmatic vagus,[26] and by noxious stimulation.[27–30]

Inflammation is more than a product of an immune response; its severity is also powerfully controlled by the nervous and endocrine systems. An example of influence by the former is neurogenic inflammation, where activation of nociceptors triggers local release of substance P, calcitonin gene-related peptide, and other proinflammatory mediators.[31–33] Endocrine modulation of inflammation includes the release of glucocorticoid from the adrenal cortex and also the release of epinephrine and endogenous opioids from the adrenal medulla, both of which can decrease plasma extravasation in the rat knee joint.[34,35]

While the inflammatory response normally functions as a homeostatic reparative process, it becomes pathological when it does not subside, interfering with normal function and producing the tissue injury associated with inflammatory diseases.

HYPERALGESIA

Pain (hyperalgesia) is not only one of the defining components of inflammation (dolor), but it also markedly influences the magnitude of other components of the inflammatory response. We have shown that pain induces a feedback control of the other two components of the inflammatory response, plasma extravasation and neutrophil function.[25,27,36] More important, this feedback control of the inflammatory response is powerfully modulated by vagal afferent activity.[30] In addition, we have shown that both the function of the primary afferent nociceptor and the modulation of inflammatory hyperalgesia by vagal afferent activity are highly sexually dimorphic.[37,38]

At sites of tissue inflammation, normally nonnoxious stimuli produce pain and noxious stimuli produce enhanced pain, a phenomenon commonly referred to as inflammatory hyperalgesia. Inflammatory hyperalgesia in peripheral tissues results from the direct action of inflammatory mediators on primary afferent fibers.[39] Clinically important chemical mediators of primary hyperalgesia include the prostanoids—prostaglandins E_2, E_1, and I_2 (PGE_2, PGE_1, and PGI_2, respectively), as well as adenosine, serotonin, epinephrine, endothelin, and nerve growth factor. These mediators are thought to act directly, through G protein–coupled receptors or receptor tyrosine kinases, on the peripheral terminals of primary afferent nociceptors. Activation of these receptors triggers specific second-messenger cascades that ultimately alter the excitability of the nerve terminal by phosphorylating ion channels such as the sodium channel $Na_V1.8$, which contributes to the tetrodotoxin-resistant sodium current.[40]

In contrast to the hyperalgesia caused by agents acting directly on nociceptive nerve terminals, agents that act indirectly through other cells in inflamed tissue can also cause acute hyperalgesia. Bradykinin, which is generated from plasma kininogens at the site of an inflammatory response, is one such indirect-acting agent and it has been used extensively in our lab and by others to study additional mechanisms of inflammatory hyperalgesia. For example, bradykinin acts on sympathetic nerve terminals, which in turn release prostaglandins to act directly on nociceptors, and thus has a slower onset of action than the prostaglandins.[41] Inflammatory hyperalgesia caused by bradykinin is dependent on the sympathetic nervous system and can be modulated by activity in the vagus nerve[42] (see below). More important, we have found evidence that hyperalgesia induced by some direct- and indirect-acting agents is sexually dimorphic.[37,43,44]

While mechanisms underlying acute inflammatory hyperalgesia have been well characterized, the mechanisms underlying chronic inflammatory pain syndromes (e.g., arthritis) are less well understood. Such chronic inflammatory pain states often follow episodes of acute inflammation. We have established a long-term pain sensitization model in the rat, in which a single application of carrageenan produces a weeks-long hypersensitivity to subsequent exposure of hyperalgesic agents.[45] In this model of chronic inflammatory pain, prostaglandin E_2 and other direct-acting agents produce a markedly prolonged hyperalgesia (>24 hours as compared to 4 hours or less in naïve rats), when injected weeks after the initial response to carrageenan has resolved. Thus, carrageenan-induced hyperalgesic priming is dependent on the ε isoform of protein kinase C. While protein kinase A or protein kinase G inhibitors attenuated the initial carrageenan-induced hyperalgesia, these treatments do not prevent the subsequent priming, indicating that development of the primed state does not require actual hyperalgesia during the priming phase.[45] Because we have seen marked sex differences in the development of hyperalgesic priming,[46] this model is ideally suited for the study of sexual dimorphism in chronic inflammatory pain.

SEXUAL DIMORPHISM IN CLINICAL AND EXPERIMENTAL INFLAMMATORY PAIN

There is a marked female preponderance in the incidence of many inflammatory diseases and in the severity of experimental inflammation in animals.[1–4] The prevalence of rheumatoid arthritis is three times greater in females than in males, while that for systemic lupus erythematous is ten times greater.[5,47] An increased susceptibility to inflammatory rheumatic disease has also been observed in laboratory animals.[6] Such pronounced effects of sex on inflammatory diseases suggest that understanding the mechanism underlying this sexual dimorphism will profoundly influence our ability to treat patients with inflammatory diseases.

Although studies of sex differences in inflammatory pain in humans may be confounded by sex differences in magnitude of the inflammatory response, we have shown that postoperative inflammatory pain is worse in women than in men.[48] In support of a sexual dimorphism of pain perception in humans, numerous studies with experimental (noninflammatory) pain models indicate that women exhibit lower pain thresholds and less tolerance to noxious stimuli than do men.[49–61] Studies in rodents have shown that females exhibit greater sensitivity to a range of noxious stimuli and greater responsiveness in experimental nociceptive models.[62–65]

While the physiological basis of these sex differences is uncertain, sex hormones have been implicated. For example, the marked female predominance for inflammatory disease begins at menarche and continues up until menopause.[66] Sex differences in the development of experimental arthritis are abolished following castration in male rats,[3] and the principal female gonadal hormone, 17β-estradiol, can exacerbate experimental arthritis in intact males. Sensitivity to noxious mechanical stimulation has been shown to decrease prior to parturition,[67] while the severity of rheumatoid arthritis is markedly suppressed during pregnancy in both humans[68] and in animal models.[69] Rheumatoid arthritis is also suppressed in women taking oral contraceptive pills.[68] Despite this evidence for a role of gonadal hormones in the establishment of sex differences in inflammation and inflammatory diseases, where and how these hormones act in the systemic and intracellular signaling pathways for inflammation remains unclear.

An understanding of sex differences in the inflammatory response including nociception will provide the information necessary to understand differences in inflammatory diseases in women and men, answer fundamental questions regarding biology of sex differences, and assist in the rational development of new therapeutic modalities. We suggest that there are sex differences in responses to inflammatory mediators, such as plasma extravasation, leukocyte attraction, and inflammatory hyperalgesia that are mediated by sexually dimorphic mechanisms in adrenal medullary function, and that these differences are substantially attributable to the effects of sex steroids. Furthermore, we suggest that the adrenal medulla is central to many of the effects of vagal activity and stress on multiple components of the inflammatory response. Such sex-related differences may, in turn, have an impact on the severity of joint injury in arthritis, because, as discussed above, pain itself provides an important signal from the inflammatory response to elicit a reflex modulation of the inflammatory response.

MODULATION OF INFLAMMATION BY THE ADRENAL MEDULLA

The adrenal medulla, which is the effector organ of the sympathoadrenal neuroendocrine axis, is an important modulator of inflammation. We have shown that the adrenal medulla is required for the modulation of baseline nociceptive threshold and bradykinin-induced hyperalgesia by vagal afferent activity.[70] We have also shown that the adrenal medulla is required for the enhancement by subdiaphragmatic vagotomy of noxious-stimulus-induced depression of bradykinin-induced plasma extravasation[36]; it is to be noted that this particular effect of noxious stimulation is mediated by the hypothalamic-pituitary-adrenal axis.[29] Furthermore, we have recently shown that repeated nonhabituating sound stress (i.e., using a protocol that produces a sustained elevation in plasma epinephrine levels) produced an adrenal medulla-dependent inhibition of bradykinin-induced plasma extravasation[71].

Epinephrine, a key mediator released by the adrenal medulla, is involved in the control of inflammation.[72] For example, epinephrine has multiple effects on plasma levels of the pro- and anti-inflammatory cytokines.[73,74] In addition, epinephrine and norepinephrine act via β-adrenergic receptors to inhibit the production of macrophage inflammatory protein,[75] while β-adrenergic agonists also decrease the number of leukocytes expressing L-selectin.[76] L-selectin is needed for neutrophils to enter inflammatory sites, and we have shown that blocking L-selectin also inhibits bradykinin-induced plasma extravasation.[25] In addition, we have observed that a sexually dimorphic effect of isoproterenol, a β-adrenergic agonist, on neutrophil function and β-adrenergic receptor binding is less in females than in males.[77] Because of these many interactions of the sympathoadrenal axis with inflammatory pain, we suggest that the adrenal medulla, acting through release of epinephrine, plays a role in mediating the sex differences in the inflammatory response.

The role of the sympathoadrenal axis is of particular interest in inflammation research, because inflammatory diseases can cause chronic stress in patients, and stress can in turn influence many aspects of inflammation, including pain.[78–80] We have begun to elucidate sex differences in the interactions of the sympathoadrenal axis and inflammation. Thus, an adrenal medulla-dependent background inhibition of bradykinin-induced plasma extravasation occurs in normal female but not in male rats; it is enhanced by estrogen and suppressed by testosterone.[81] Furthermore, there are gender differences in the adrenal medulla–mediated stress response in the two sexes. In our most recent data on stress and sexual dimorphism, we show that repeated stress markedly *inhibits* bradykinin-induced plasma extravasation in males but markedly *enhances* it in females, while repeated stress did not affect lipopolysaccharide (LPS)-induced neutrophil recruitment in males but significantly inhibited it in females.[82] Finally, we have begun to elucidate sexually dimorphic aspects of β-adrenergic receptor signaling in human neutrophils, specifically co-administration of the β-adrenergic agonist, isoproterenol, which have significantly enhanced LPS-induced neutrophil recruitment in male but not in female rats.[82]

VAGAL MODULATION OF INFLAMMATION AND INFLAMMATORY HYPERALGESIA

The vagus nerve contains afferent fibers that innervate thoracic and abdominal viscera. Information conveyed by these afferents is important for the feedback modulation of homeostatic functions such as those in the circulatory, respiratory gastrointestinal, and neuroendocrine systems. The ability of activity in these afferents to also modulate the inflammatory process, including inflammatory hyperalgesia, is well known. Our work has helped delineate details of how vagal afferent activity affects components of the inflammatory response, and recently, we have detected sexual dimorphism in several aspects of this modulation.[83]

The modulatory effect of vagal activity is striking when observing the ability of peripheral noxious stimuli to inhibit inflammation. Thus, intraplantar capsaicin in a paw acts to modestly inhibit bradykinin-induced plasma extravasation in the knee joint of the rat, but when the vagus nerve is cut below the level of the diaphragm, this inhibition is markedly increased.[28] This suggests that ongoing activity in the subdiaphragmatic vagus nerve potently antagonizes the ability of noxious stimuli to inhibit inflammation. Work in our laboratory has revealed that the relevant signals are carried by the celiac and accessory celiac branches of the subdiaphragmatic vagus,[84] which primarily innervate the intestinal tract, and that removal of the duodenum or 48 hours of fasting mimics the effect of subdiaphragmatic vagotomy.[85] This system may be part of a general pattern of responses known as “illness symptoms,” which in this case would consist of a potentiation of the inflammatory response when duodenal afferents signal invasion by toxins or pathogens.

Vagal activity also has well-described effects on pain and inflammatory hyperalgesia. Stimulation of vagal afferents can raise or lower baseline nociceptive thresholds, depending on the strength of stimulation[86–88]; and lesioning the vagus nerve, at the subdiaphragmatic level, can either increase or decrease the magnitude of hyperalgesia produced by inflammatory mediators, depending on the agent.[42,89] Vagotomy in the rat causes a long-lasting decrease in the baseline paw withdrawal threshold as well as a potentiation of the hyperalgesia caused by the indirect-acting mediator bradykinin[42]; and both these effects are adrenal medulla–dependent.[70] In contrast, vagotomy decreases tonic inflammatory hyperalgesia (nociceptive behavior in phase 2 of the formalin test) in male but not in female rats,[83] but does not affect inflammatory hyperalgesia caused by PGE_2.[42] Recently, we have shown that a chronic elevation in plasma concentration of epinephrine induced by vagotomy is likely to mediate the effects of the adrenal medulla on pain signaling. Thus, chronic administration of the selective β_2-adrenergic receptor agonist, ICI 118,551, attenuated vagotomy-induced enhancement of bradykinin hyperalgesia, while chronic administration of epinephrine in normal animals, to produce plasma levels of epinephrine seen in vagotomized animals, enhanced bradykinin hyperalgesia.[90] We have also recently shown that fasting is a natural vagally mediated stimulus that can potentiate formalin-induced nociception in female but not in male rats.[91] In sum, the adrenal medulla plays a pivotal role in the vagal modulation of inflammation and inflammatory hyperalgesia.

In conclusion, inflammation is a ubiquitous clinical problem, yet its many forms are often intractable to currently available therapies. A distinctive characteristic of many inflammatory diseases is their greater incidence and severity in women versus men. Gonadal hormones modulate inflammation in order to suggest potential future therapies that target those endogenous modulatory pathways. We suggest that gonadal sex hormones differentially affect components of the inflammatory response in males and females through their regulation of neuroendocrine-immune circuits that strongly influence the inflammatory response. The sympathoadrenal axis and its modulation by vagal afferents, both of which are sexually dimorphic, can have a powerful impact on the inflammatory response, and may thus also be important in establishing sexual dimorphism in inflammatory diseases. We have discussed the roles of gonadal hormones, the sympathoadrenal axis, and control of the sympathoadrenal axis by stress and by vagal afferent activity in the sexually dimorphic modulation of three principal components of the inflammatory response: plasma extravasation, leukocyte neutrophil function, and hyperalgesia.

ACKNOWLEDGMENT

This work was supported by the National Institutes of Health.

REFERENCES

1. MacKenzie, A.R., P.R. Sibley & B.P. White. 1979. Resistance and susceptibility to the induction of rat adjuvant disease: diverging susceptibility and severity achieved by selective breeding. Br. J. Exp. Pathol. **60:** 507–512.
2. Wilder, R.L. *et al.* 1982. Strain and sex variation in the susceptibility to streptococcal cell wall-induced polyarthritis in the rat. Arthritis Rheum. **25:** 1064–1072.
3. Allen, J.B. *et al.* 1983. Sex hormonal effects on the severity of streptococcal cell wall-induced polyarthritis in the rat. Arthritis Rheum. **26:** 560–563.
4. Griffiths, M.M. *et al.* 1994. Exacerbation of collagen-induced arthritis in rats by rat cytomegalovirus is antigen-specific. Autoimmunity **18:** 177–187.
5. Da Silva, J.A. 1995. Sex hormones, glucocorticoids and autoimmunity: facts and hypotheses. Ann. Rheum. Dis. **54:** 6–16.
6. Holmdahl, R. 1995. Female preponderance for development of arthritis in rats is influenced by both sex chromosomes and sex steroids. Scand. J. Immunol. **42:** 104–109.
7. Greiff, L. *et al.* 2003. Airway microvascular extravasation and luminal entry of plasma. Clin. Physiol. Funct. Imaging **23:** 301–306.
8. Luster, A.D. 1998. Chemokines—chemotactic cytokines that mediate inflammation. N. Engl. J. Med. **338:** 436–445.
9. Eriksson, E.E. 2003. Leukocyte recruitment to atherosclerotic lesions, a complex web of dynamic cellular and molecular interactions. Curr. Drug. Targets Cardiovasc. Haematol. Disord. **3:** 309–325.
10. Fantone, J.C. & P.A. Ward. 1985. Polymorphonuclear leukocyte-mediated cell and tissue injury: oxygen metabolites and their relations to human disease. Hum. Pathol. **16:** 973–978.

11. CODERRE, T.J. *et al.* 1990. Epinephrine exacerbates arthritis by an action at presynaptic β2-adrenoceptors. Neuroscience **34:** 521–523.
12. CODERRE, T.J. *et al.* 1991. Increasing sympathetic nerve terminal-dependent plasma extravasation correlates with decreased arthritic joint injury in rats. Neuroscience **40:** 185–189.
13. GREEN, P.G. *et al.* 1991. Purinergic regulation of bradykinin-induced plasma extravasation and adjuvant-induced arthritis in the rat. Proc. Natl. Acad. Sci. USA **88:** 4162–4165.
14. MIAO, F.J. *et al.* 1992. Chronically administered nicotine attenuates bradykinin-induced plasma extravasation and aggravates arthritis-induced joint injury in the rat. Neuroscience **51:** 649–655.
15. BASBAUM, A.I. & J.D. LEVINE. 1991. The contribution of the nervous system to inflammation and inflammatory disease. Can. J. Physiol. Pharmacol. **69:** 647–651.
16. KOZIK, A. *et al.* 1998. A novel mechanism for bradykinin production at inflammatory sites: diverse effects of a mixture of neutrophil elastase and mast cell tryptase versus tissue and plasma kallikreins on native and oxidized kininogens. J. Biol. Chem. **273:** 33224–33229.
17. SIMON, J.A. 2001. Biologic therapy in rheumatoid arthritis. Rev. Invest. Clin. **53:** 452–459.
18. RACKOFF, P. & T. FELDMAN. 1997. Total lymphoid irradiation—not for rheumatoid arthritis. Lancet **350:** 752–753.
19. BINDER, A.I. *et al.* 1986. Intensive immunosuppression in intractable rheumatoid-arthritis. Br. J. Rheumatol. **25:** 380–383.
20. CROOK, P.R. *et al.* 1986. Lack of effect of total-body irradiation in rheumatoid-arthritis. Br. J. Rheumatol. **25:** 384–387.
21. DARDICK, S.J., A.I. BASBAUM & J.D. LEVINE. 1986. The contribution of pain to disability in experimentally induced arthritis. Arthritis Rheum. **29:** 1017–1022.
22. LAMONTAGNA, G. *et al.* 1997. Clinical pattern of pain in rheumatoid arthritis. Clin. Exp. Rheumatol. **15:** 481–485.
23. LA MONTAGNA, G. *et al.* 2000. The predictive value of attributes of pain to classify rheumatoid arthritis. Clin. Rheumatol. **19:** 258–261.
24. ROJKOVICH, B. & T. GIBSON. 1998. Day and night pain measurement in rheumatoid arthritis. Ann. Rheum. Dis. **57:** 434–436.
25. STRAUSBAUGH, H.J., M.F. DALLMAN & J.D. LEVINE. 1999. Repeated, but not acute, stress suppresses inflammatory plasma extravasation. Proc. Natl. Acad. Sci. USA **96:** 14629–14634.
26. MIAO, F.J. *et al.* 1994. Role of vagal afferents and spinal pathways modulating inhibition of bradykinin-induced plasma extravasation by intrathecal nicotine. J. Neurophysiol. **72:** 1199–1207.
27. GREEN, P.G., W. JANIG & J.D. LEVINE. 1997. Negative feedback neuroendocrine control of inflammatory response in the rat is dependent on the sympathetic postganglionic neuron. J. Neurosci. **17:** 3234–3238.
28. MIAO, F.J. *et al.* 1997. Inhibition of bradykinin-induced plasma extravasation produced by noxious cutaneous and visceral stimuli and its modulation by vagal activity. J. Neurophysiol. **78:** 1285–1292.
29. MIAO, F.J. & J.D. LEVINE. 1999. Neural and endocrine mechanisms mediating noxious stimulus-induced inhibition of bradykinin plasma extravasation in the rat. J. Pharmacol. Exp. Ther. **291:** 1028–1037.

30. MIAO, F.J. *et al.* 2001. Spino-bulbo-spinal pathway mediating vagal modulation of nociceptive-neuroendocrine control of inflammation in the rat. J. Physiol. **532:** 811–822.
31. WALLENGREN, J. 1997. Vasoactive peptides in the skin. J. Invest. Dermatol. Symp. Proc. **2:** 49–55.
32. MCMAHON, S.B. 1996. NGF as a mediator of inflammatory pain. Philos. Trans. R. Soc. Lond. B. Biol. Sci. **351:** 431–440.
33. SANN, H. & F.K. PIERAU. 1998. Efferent functions of C-fiber nociceptors. Z. Rheumatol. **57**(Suppl 2): 8–13.
34. GREEN, P.G. & J.D. LEVINE. 1992. Delta- and kappa-opioid agonists inhibit plasma extravasation induced by bradykinin in the knee joint of the rat. Neuroscience **49:** 129–133.
35. MIAO, F.J. *et al.* 1992. Sympathoadrenal contribution to nicotinic and muscarinic modulation of bradykinin-induced plasma extravasation in the knee joint of the rat. J. Pharmacol. Exp. Ther. **262:** 889–895.
36. MIAO, F.J., W. JANIG & J.D. LEVINE. 2000. Nociceptive neuroendocrine negative feedback control of neurogenic inflammation activated by capsaicin in the rat paw: role of the adrenal medulla. J. Physiol. **527:** 601–610.
37. DINA, O.A. *et al.* 2001. Sex hormones regulate the contribution of PKCepsilon and PKA signalling in inflammatory pain in the rat. Eur. J. Neurosci. **13:** 2227–2233.
38. KHASAR, S.G. *et al.* 2003. Vagal modulation of bradykinin-induced mechanical hyperalgesia in the female rat. J. Pain **4:** 278–283.
39. TREEDE, R.D. *et al.* 1992. Peripheral and central mechanisms of cutaneous hyperalgesia. Prog. Neurobiol. **38:** 397–421.
40. GOLD, M.S. *et al.* 1996. Hyperalgesic agents increase a tetrodotoxin-resistant Na+ current in nociceptors. Proc. Natl. Acad. Sci. USA **93:** 1108–1112.
41. TAIWO, Y.O., E.J. GOETZL & J.D. LEVINE. 1987. Hyperalgesia onset latency suggests a hierarchy of action. Brain Res. **423:** 333–337.
42. KHASAR, S.G. *et al.* 1998. Modulation of bradykinin-induced mechanical hyperalgesia in the rat by activity in abdominal vagal afferents. Eur. J. Neurosci. **10:** 435–444.
43. JOSEPH, E.K. & J.D. LEVINE. 2003. Sexual dimorphism in the contribution of protein kinase C isoforms to nociception in the streptozotocin diabetic rat. Neuroscience **120:** 907–913.
44. JOSEPH, E.K. & J.D. LEVINE. 2003. Sexual dimorphism for protein kinase C epsilon signaling in a rat model of vincristine-induced painful peripheral neuropathy. Neuroscience **119:** 831–838.
45. ALEY, K.O. *et al.* 2000. Chronic hypersensitivity for inflammatory nociceptor sensitization mediated by the epsilon isozyme of protein kinase C. J. Neurosci. **20:** 4680–4685.
46. JOSEPH, E.K., C.A. PARADA & J.D. LEVINE. 2003. Hyperalgesic priming in the rat demonstrates marked sexual dimorphism. Pain **105:** 143–150.
47. LAHITA, R.G. 1996. The connective tissue diseases and the overall influence of gender. Int. J. Fertil. Menopausal Stud. **41:** 156–165.
48. FAUCETT, J., N. GORDON & J. LEVINE. 1994. Differences in postoperative pain severity among four ethnic groups. J. Pain Symptom Manage. **9:** 383–389.
49. BRENNUM, J. *et al.* 1989. Measurements of human pressure-pain thresholds on fingers and toes. Pain **38:** 211–217.
50. BUCHANAN, H.M. & J.A. MIDGLEY. 1987. Evaluation of pain threshold using a simple pressure algometer. Clin. Rheumatol. **6:** 510–517.

51. FISCHER, A.A. 1987. Pressure algometry over normal muscles: standard values, validity and reproducibility of pressure threshold. Pain **30:** 115–126.
52. JENSEN, R. *et al.* 1992. Cephalic muscle tenderness and pressure pain threshold in a general population. Pain **48:** 197–203.
53. HALL, E.G. & S. DAVIES. 1991. Gender differences in perceived intensity and affect of pain between athletes and nonathletes. Percept. Mot. Skills **73:** 779–786.
54. MCCAUL, K.D. & C. HAUGTVEDT. 1982. Attention, distraction, and cold-pressor pain. J. Pers. Soc. Psychol. **43:** 154–162.
55. NOTERMANS, S.L. 1967. Measurement of the pain threshold determined by electrical stimulation and its clinical application II. Clinical application in neurological and neurosurgical patients. Neurology **17:** 58–73.
56. ROBIN, O. *et al.* 1987. Influence of sex and anxiety on pain threshold and tolerance. Funct. Neurol. **2:** 173–179.
57. COULTHARD, P. & J.P. ROOD. 1993. Anxiety measures during induced experimental pain. Anesth. Pain Control Dent. **2:** 150–153.
58. FRID, M., G. SINGER & C. RANA. 1979. Interactions between personal expectations and naloxone: effects on tolerance to ischemic pain. Psychopharmacology (Berl.) **65:** 225–231.
59. MAIXNER, W. & C. HUMPHREY. 1993. Gender differences in pain and cardiovascular responses to forearm ischemia. Clin. J. Pain **9:** 16–25.
60. LAUTENBACHER, S. & G.B. ROLLMAN. 1993. Sex differences in responsiveness to painful and nonpainful stimuli are dependent upon the stimulation method. Pain **53:** 255–264.
61. MEH, D. & M. DENISLIC. 1994. Quantitative assessment of thermal and pain sensitivity. J. Neurol. Sci. **127:** 164–169.
62. ALOISI, A.M., M.E. ALBONETTI & G. CARLI. 1994. Sex differences in the behavioral response to persistent pain in rats. Neurosci. Lett. **179:** 79–82.
63. COYLE, D.E., C.S. SEHLHORST & C. MASCARI. 1995. Female rats are more susceptible to the development of neuropathic pain using the partial sciatic nerve ligation (PSNL) model. Neurosci. Lett. **186:** 135–138.
64. KEPLER, K.L. & R.J. BODNAR. 1988. Yohimbine potentiates cold-water swim analgesia: re-evaluation of a noradrenergic role. Pharmacol. Biochem. Behav. **29:** 83–88.
65. ROMERO, M.T. *et al.* 1988. Gender-specific and gonadectomy-specific effects upon swim analgesia: role of steroid replacement therapy. Physiol. Behav. **44:** 257–265.
66. LAHITA, R.G. 1996. The basis for gender effects in the connective tissue diseases. Ann. Med. Interne (Paris) **147:** 241–247.
67. COGAN, R. & J.A. SPINNATO. 1986. Pain and discomfort thresholds in late pregnancy. Pain **27:** 63–68.
68. SPECTOR, T.D., E. ROMAN & A.J. SILMAN. 1990. The pill, parity, and rheumatoid arthritis. Arthritis Rheum. **33:** 782–789.
69. BRANDELY, M. *et al.* 1982. Adjuvant arthritis in rat during pregnancy and lactation. Biomed. Pharmacother. **36:** 308–313.
70. KHASAR, S.G. *et al.* 1998. Vagotomy-induced enhancement of mechanical hyperalgesia in the rat is sympathoadrenal-mediated. J. Neurosci. **18:** 3043–3049.
71. STRAUSBAUGH, H.J. *et al.* 2003. Repeated, nonhabituating stress suppresses inflammatory plasma extravasation by a novel, sympathoadrenal dependent mechanism. Eur. J. Neurosci. **17:** 805–812.

72. DERIJK, R.H. *et al.* 1994. Induction of plasma interleukin-6 by circulating adrenaline in the rat. Psychoneuroendocrinology **19:** 155–163.
73. VAN DER POLL, T. & S.F. LOWRY. 1997. Epinephrine inhibits endotoxin-induced IL-1 beta production: roles of tumor necrosis factor-alpha and IL-10. Am. J. Physiol. **273:** R1885–R1890.
74. VAN DER POLL, T. & S.F. LOWRY. 1997. Lipopolysaccharide-induced interleukin 8 production by human whole blood is enhanced by epinephrine and inhibited by hydrocortisone. Infect. Immun. **65:** 2378–2381.
75. HASKO, G. *et al.* 1998. Exogenous and endogenous catecholamines inhibit the production of macrophage inflammatory protein (MIP) 1 alpha via a beta adrenoceptor mediated mechanism. Br. J. Pharmacol. **125:** 1297–1303.
76. MILLS, P.J., R.S. KARNIK & E. DILLON. 1997. L-selectin expression affects T-cell circulation following isoproterenol infusion in humans. Brain Behav. Immun. **11:** 333–342.
77. DE COUPADE, C. *et al.* 2004. Beta 2-adrenergic receptor regulation of human neutrophil function is sexually dimorphic. Br. J. Pharmacol. **143:** 1033–1041.
78. BLACKBURN-MUNRO, G. & R.E. BLACKBURN-MUNRO. 2001. Chronic pain, chronic stress and depression: coincidence or consequence? J. Neuroendocrinol. **13:** 1009–1023.
79. KEEFE, F.J. *et al.* 2001. Pain and emotion: new research directions. J. Clin. Psychol. **57:** 587–607.
80. CHAPMAN, C.R. & J. GAVRIN. 1999. Suffering: the contributions of persistent pain. Lancet **353:** 2233–2237.
81. GREEN, P.G. *et al.* 2001. Role of adrenal medulla in development of sexual dimorphism in inflammation. Eur. J. Neurosci. **14:** 1436–1444.
82. BARKER, L.A. *et al.* 2005. Sympathoadrenal-dependent sexually dimorphic effect of nonhabituating stress on in vivo neutrophil recruitment in the rat. Br. J. Pharmacol. **145:** 872–879.
83. KHASAR, S.G. *et al.* 2001. Gender and gonadal hormone effects on vagal modulation of tonic nociception. J. Pain **2:** 91–100.
84. MIAO, F.J., W. JANIG & J.D. LEVINE. 1997. Vagal branches involved in inhibition of bradykinin-induced synovial plasma extravasation by intrathecal nicotine and noxious stimulation in the rat. J. Physiol. **498:** 473–481.
85. MIAO, F.J., P.G. GREEN & J.D. LEVINE. 2004. Mechanosensitive duodenal afferents contribute to vagal modulation of inflammation in the rat. J. Physiol. **554:** 227–235.
86. RANDICH, A. & G.F. GEBHART. 1992. Vagal afferent modulation of nociception. Brain Res. Rev. **17:** 77–99.
87. WATKINS, L.R. *et al.* 1995. Mechanisms of tumor necrosis factor-alpha (TNF-alpha) hyperalgesia. Brain Res. **692:** 244–250.
88. KIRCHNER, A. *et al.* 2000. Left vagus nerve stimulation suppresses experimentally induced pain. Neurology **55:** 1167–1171.
89. SAADE, N.E. *et al.* 1998. Involvement of capsaicin sensitive primary afferents in thymulin-induced hyperalgesia. J. Neuroimmunol. **91:** 171–179.
90. KHASAR, S.G. *et al.* 2003. Vagal modulation of nociception is mediated by adrenomedullary epinephrine in the rat. Eur. J. Neurosci. **17:** 909–915.
91. KHASAR, S.G. *et al.* 2003. Fasting is a physiological stimulus of vagus-mediated enhancement of nociception in the female rat. Neuroscience **119:** 215–221.

Effects of Testosterone, 17β-Estradiol, and Downstream Estrogens on Cytokine Secretion from Human Leukocytes in the Presence and Absence of Cortisol

DAVID JANELE,[a] THOMAS LANG,[a] SILVIA CAPELLINO,[a] MAURIZIO CUTOLO,[b] JOSE ANTONIO P. DA SILVA,[c] AND RAINER H. STRAUB[a]

[a]*Laboratory of Neuroendocrinoimmunology, Department of Internal Medicine I, University Hospital, 93042 Regensburg, Germany*

[b]*Division of Rheumatology, Department of Internal Medicine and Medical Specialities, University of Genova, Genova, Italy*

[c]*Department of Medicine III and Rheumatology, Coimbra University Hospital, Coimbra, Portugal*

ABSTRACT: Estrogens at physiological concentrations are thought to play an immune-stimulating role, whereas androgens have an anti-inflammatory impact. However, their role on cytokine secretion in the presence or absence of cortisol has not been investigated. Furthermore, the role of hydroxylated estrogens downstream of 17β-estradiol (E2) on secretion of tumor necrosis factor (TNF) is not known. In this study on peripheral blood leukocytes of healthy male subjects, we scrutinized the influence of prior sex hormones (for 24 h) with and without later addition of cortisol (for another 24 h) on stimulated secretion of TNF, IL-2, IL-4, IL-6, IL-10, and interferon-γ (IFN-γ). E2 stabilized or increased immune stimuli–induced secretion of TNF, IL-2, IL-4, IL-6, IL-10, and IFNγ in relation to testosterone. Testosterone, in contrast, inhibited (IL-2, IL-4, IL-10) or tended to inhibit stimulated secretion of these cytokines (TNF, IFNγ). This effect of E2 was pronounced at a concentration of 10^{-10} M (testosterone: 10^{-7} M) in the presence of cortisol. E2 (10^{-8} M, 10^{-10} M) and testosterone (10^{-7} M) did not change glucocorticoid receptor expression. The downstream estrogens 2OH-estradiol(one), 4OH-estradiol(one), and 16OH-estradiol(one) did not stimulate TNF secretion at 10^{-10} M, but even inhibited its secretion at 10^{-11} M. However, the combination of 16OH-estradiol(one) on one side and 2OH-estradiol(one) or 4OH-estradiol(one) on the other side markedly stimulated TNF secretion that was only observable in the presence of cortisol. In conclusion, at physiological concentrations, E2 and a combination of downstream estrogens

Address for correspondence: Rainer H. Straub, M.D., Laboratory of Neuroendocrinoimmunology, Department of Internal Medicine I, University Hospital, 93042 Regensburg, Germany. Voice: +49 941 944 7120; fax: +49 941 944 7121.

e-mail: rainer.straub@klinik.uni-regensburg.de

Ann. N.Y. Acad. Sci. 1069: 168–182 (2006).
doi: 10.1196/annals.1351.015

stabilized or increased immune stimuli–induced TNF secretion. These effects are dependent on the presence of physiological concentrations of cortisol. This study underlines the proinflammatory role of E2, which is probably dependent on conversion to a proinflammatory cocktail of downstream estrogens and the presence of cortisol.

KEYWORDS: **testosterone; 17β-estradiol; 2-hydroxyestrogens; 4-hydroxyestrogens; 16-hydroxyestrogens; cortisol; TNF; cytokines**

INTRODUCTION

The pro- and anti-inflammatory effects of 17β-estradiol (E2) and other estrogens on secretion of proinflammatory cytokines have been a matter of debate for two decades. Authors in the field of rheumatology investigated estrogens in the context of a strong proinflammatory microenvironment and came to the conclusion that estrogens most often exert a proinflammatory influence on chronic inflammatory diseases, whereas androgens are considered to be anti-inflammatory.[1,2] The proinflammatory influence of estrogens was regarded to be a major factor for the known female-to-male preponderance in autoimmune diseases.[1,3–5] On the other hand, researchers in the field of bone research demonstrated inhibitory effects of estrogens on cytokine secretion in a noninflamed microenvironment leading to osteoprotective effects.[6,7] This discrepancy probably depends on very different conversion of estrogens to downstream metabolites.

A proinflammatory microenvironment leads to conversion of androgens to E2 and downstream estrogens[8] that are further converted to 16-hydroxylated active estrogens but not to 2-hydroxylated endogenous anti-estrogens.[9,10] In contrast, in normal macrophages, conversion of androgens to estrogens is much less pronounced and 16-hydroxylated estrogens were not detected.[11] Furthermore, in osteopenic postmenopausal women without inflammation, 16-hydroxylated estrone levels are much lower and correlated positively with bone mineral density, whereas levels of 2-hydroxylated anti-estrogens showed a negative correlation with bone mineral density.[12,13] This indicates that the relation of 16-hydroxylated to 2-hydroxylated estrogens is completely different in chronic inflammatory diseases as compared to the situation in postmenopausal women with osteoporosis and without inflammation.

Breast cancer research revealed a mitogenic tumor growth-stimulating role of 16α-hydroxylated estrogens, which indicates the potent estrogenic activity of these hormones.[14] *In vivo* animal studies demonstrated a strong TNF-increasing role of 16-hydroxyestradiol (estriol).[15,16] Other conversion products of estrone and 17β-estradiol are the 2-hydroxylated estrogens, such as 2-hydroxyestrone and 2-hydroxyestradiol. In contrast to 16α-hydroxylated estrogens, the 2-hydroxylated forms inhibit growth-promoting effects of 17β-estradiol.[17] Furthermore, the estrogen metabolism pathway favoring

2-hydroxylation over 16α-hydroxylation is associated with a reduced risk of invasive breast cancer in premenopausal women.[18] We can summarize that 16α-hydroxylated estrogens are biologically active, proinflammatory, and proproliferative, whereas the 2-hydroxylated metabolites act as naturally occurring estrogen antagonists.

Apart from the very different metabolism of E2 to downstream estrogens under inflamed and noninflamed conditions, the presence of glucocorticoids may play an additional role for effects of sex hormones on proinflammatory cytokine secretion from peripheral blood leukocytes and local macrophages. At least on the level of the hypothalamus and pituitary gland, it has been demonstrated that females mount a stronger hypothalamic-pituitary-adrenal (HPA) axis response, and gonadectomy diminishes or abrogates this effect.[2,19] It was discussed that feedback inhibition by cortisol of the hypothalamus or the pituitary gland may be modulated by sex hormones.[2,19] The possibility that similar interactions between sex hormones and cortisol occur in peripheral leukocytes would have implications in understanding the known gender dimorphism of the immune and neuroendocrine system.

In this study, we focussed on the role of testosterone and E2 on cytokine secretion from human peripheral blood leukocytes in the presence and absence of cortisol. For this pilot study, we used blood leukocytes because of their availability in healthy subjects. Furthermore, we studied effects on cytokine secretion caused by downstream E2 metabolites: 16-hydroxylated estrogens, 2-hydroxylated estrogens, and 4-hydroxylated estrogens. In addition, we investigated whether or not E2 and testosterone modulate glucocorticoid receptor expression.

MATERIALS AND METHODS

Subjects and Blood Samples

For cytokine secretion studies, 9 (age 24–40 years) and, for analysis of glucocorticoid receptor expression, 15 (24–40 aged) healthy male subjects were recruited. All subjects were informed about the purpose of the experiments and gave informed consent for further use of blood samples. Blood was drawn in heparinized tubes between 9:00 and 10:00 AM and immediately processed.

Culture Conditions and Application of Sex Hormones and Cortisol

For cytokine secretion studies, a defined volume of whole blood was cultured in 48-well plates together with serum-free medium (whole blood assay in RPMI 1640 without phenol red, 0.57 mM ascorbic acid, Sigma Aldrich, Taufkirchen, Germany). Preliminary assays demonstrated optimal cytokine secretion when using 100 μL of whole blood (for IL-2, IL-4, IL-10, IFNγ, and

TNF) and 25 μL of whole blood (for IL-6) in an end volume of 1,250 μL (TABLE 1). During the first 24 h, cells were incubated with vehicle, testosterone (10^{-7} and 10^{-8} mol/L, Sigma Aldrich), E2 (10^{-8} and 10^{-10} mol/L, Sigma Aldrich), 2-hydroxyestradiol (10^{-10} and 10^{-11} mol/L, Steraloids, Newport, Rhode Island, USA), 2-hydroxyestrone (10^{-10} and 10^{-11} mol/L, Steraloids), 4-hydroxyestradiol (10^{-10} and 10^{-11} mol/L, Steraloids), 4-hydroxyestrone (10^{-10} and 10^{-11} mol/L, Steraloids), 16-hydroxyestradiol (10^{-10} and 10^{-11} mol/L, Steraloids), and 16-hydroxyestrone (10^{-10} and 10^{-11} mol/L, Steraloids). After 24 h, the culture medium was removed and substituted with new medium without sex hormones, carrying lipopolysaccharide (LPS for IL-6 stimulation, 0.5 ng/mL, Sigma Aldrich) or concanavalin A (100μg/mL, for stimulation of other cytokines, Sigma Aldrich), two strong immune stimuli, with or without cortisol (hydrocortisone, 10^{-6} mol/L, Pharmacia Upjohn, Karlsruhe, Germany). We used cortisol at 10^{-6} mol/L because in preceding whole blood assays with naturally available binding proteins this concentration yielded half-maximum inhibition of TNF secretion (without cortisol: 109.1 ± 9.7 pg TNF/mL [100%] vs. with cortisol: 79.4 ± 5.1 pg TNF/mL [73%]). These first assays also demonstrated that the observed decrease of about 27% reflects the half-maximum effect of cortisol. After 12 and 24 h, supernatants were taken and stored at −30°C. TABLE 1 summarizes applied conditions.

For analysis of the influence of sex hormones on glucocorticoid receptor expression, 30 mL of heparinized whole blood were cultured in 25 cm^2 culture flasks (70 mL) for 24 h with vehicle, testosterone (10^{-7} mol/L), or 17β-estradiol (10^{-8} and 10^{-10} mol/L, Sigma Aldrich). In these experiments, no cortisol was added. After 24 h, cultured cells were re-suspended, centrifuged, treated twice with distilled water to remove erythrocytes, and washed twice in phosphate-buffered saline (Sigma Aldrich). Then, leukocytes were lysed for 30 min in lysis buffer containing PMSF, SDS, NP-40, sodium deoxycholate, and a mixture of protein inhibitors ("complete" from Roche Diagnostics, Mannheim, Germany). After centrifuging, supernatants were stored at −30°C. Protein concentrations were measured using the BCA assay (reagents from Sigma Aldrich).

TABLE 1. Mode of stimulation, use of whole blood, and observation time for different cytokines

Cytokine	Volume of WB [μL]	Stimulation	Observation Time [h]
IL-2	100	ConA 100 μg/mL	24
IL-4	100	ConA 100 μg/mL	24
IL-6	25	LPS 0.5 ng/mL	12
IL-10	100	ConA 100 μg/mL	12
IFNγ	100	ConA 100 μg/mL	24
TNFα	100	ConA 100 μg/mL	12

Cytokine Determination in Supernatants

The cytokines IL-2, IL-4, IL-6, IL-10, IFNγ, and TNF were measured by immunometric enzyme immunoassays making use of antibody pairs (OptEIA^{TM}, BD Pharmingen, San Diego, CA). In our hands, intra- and inter-assay coefficients of variation were below 10%. The detection limit was approximately 4–20 pg/mL depending on the cytokine tested.

Western Blotting

Gels (Novex 8% Tris-Glycine, Invitrogen, Karlsruhe, Germany) were loaded with 25 μg of protein and, after electrophoretic processing, transferred to nitro-cellulose. Membranes were blocked in Tris-buffered saline (TBS) containing 2.5% of human serum protein and 2.5% of bovine serum albumin (Biomol, Hamburg, Germany). Blots were then incubated for 1 h at room temperature with primary antibodies against the human glucocorticoid receptor (1:500 in 5% nonfat dry milk in TBS, Affinity Bioreagents, Golden, Colorado, USA). Subsequently, membranes were washed in TBS and incubated with secondary antibodies (1:1000 in TBS, horseradish peroxidase–conjugated, Affinity Bioreagents). After another washing step, blots were developed using chemiluminescent reagents (ECL+, Amersham Biosciences, Amersham, UK) and then subjected to autoradiography. The films (Hyperfilm, Amersham, UK) were scanned and analyzed using a densitometric method (Molecular Dynamics, Amersham, UK).

Statistical Analysis and Data Presentation

Data are given as the mean $\pm$ SEM. Medians were compared by Mann–Whitney test (SPSS/PC for Windows 11.0, SPSS, Chicago, IL).

RESULTS

Influence of Testosterone and E2 on Cytokine Secretion in the Presence and Absence of Cortisol

In order to test the influence of testosterone and E2 on cytokine secretion, we used physiological concentrations of these hormones in a relatively natural microenvironment (whole blood). In the presence of cortisol, E2, in relation to testosterone, at concentrations of 10^{-8} and 10^{-10} mol/L stabilized secretion of TNF, IL-2, IFNγ, and IL-10 (FIGS. 1A, 1C, 1D, and 2B). For IL-6 and IL-4, only E2 at 10^{-10} mol/L exerts similar effects (FIGS. 1B and 2A). E2 at 10^{-10}

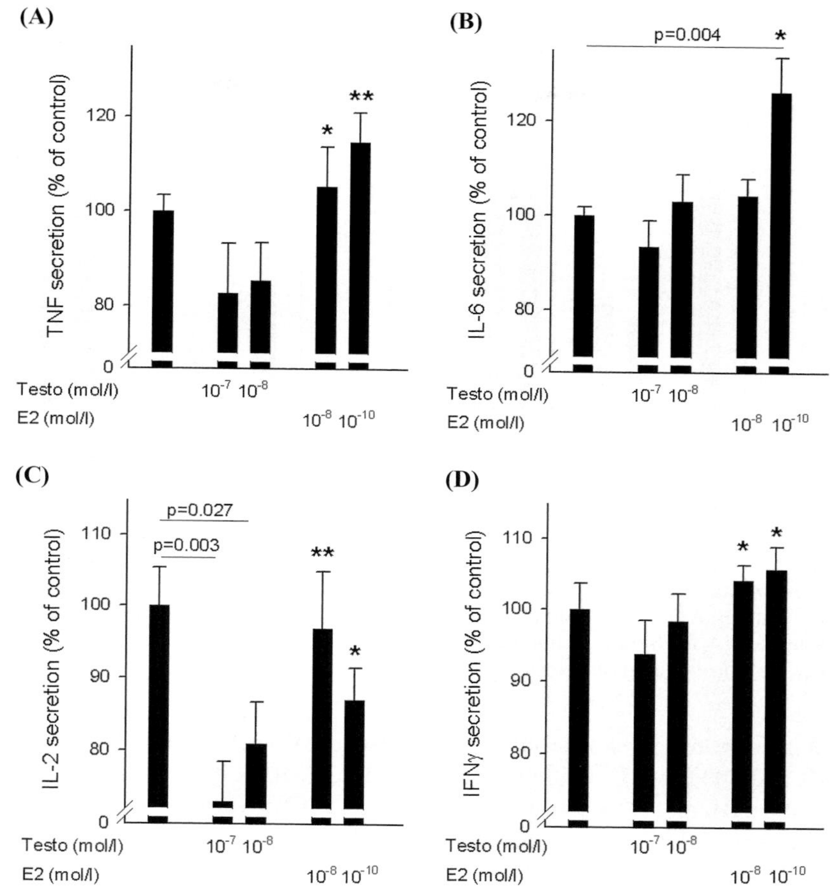

FIGURE 1. Modulation of cytokine secretion by 17β-estradiol (E2) and testosterone in the presence of cortisol. Whole blood of five healthy male subjects was incubated in triplicate with vehicle, testosterone, and E2 for 24 h at indicated concentrations. After 24 h, medium was replaced and cells were stimulated with 0.5 ng/mL LPS (IL-6) or 100 μg/mL concanavalin A (TNF, IL-2, IFNγ) for further 12 h (IL-6, TNF) or 24 h (IL-2, IFNγ) in the presence of 10^{-6} mol/L cortisol. Supernatants were removed and cytokines were measured by enzyme-linked immunosorbent assay (ELISA). Means ± SEM are shown for TNF (**A**: control = 79.4 ± 5.1 pg/mL), IL-6 (**B**: control = 857 ± 137 pg/mL), IL-2 (**C**: control = 289 ± 27 pg/mL), and IFNγ (**D**: control = 521 ± 49 pg/mL). $^{*}P < 0.05$, $^{**}P < 0.01$ versus the respective concentration of testosterone.

mol/L stimulated IL-6 secretion in relation to vehicle (FIG. 1B). With respect to other cytokines, E2 had no stimulating activity in relation to vehicle (FIGS. 1 and 2). In the absence of 10^{-6} mol/L cortisol, we observed very similar effects for IL-2, IL-4, IL-6, and IL-10 (data not shown).

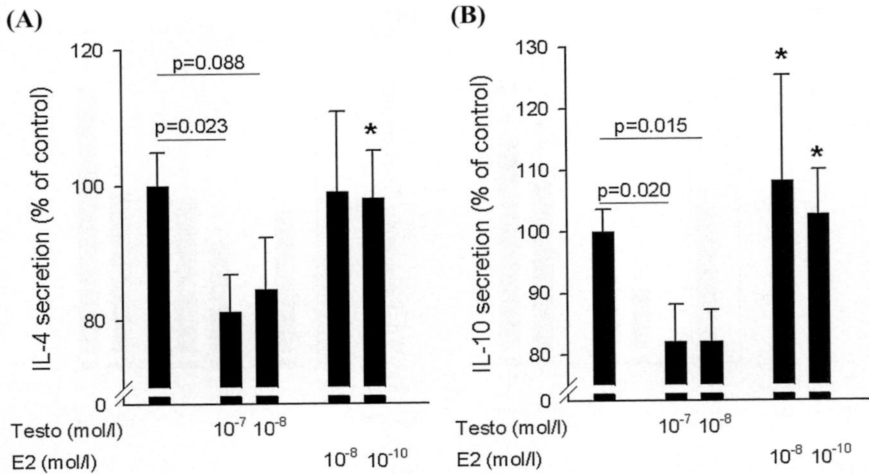

FIGURE 2. Modulation of cytokine secretion by 17β-estradiol (E2) and testosterone in the presence of cortisol. Means ± SEM are shown for IL-4 (**A**: control = 94.5 ± 13.5 pg/mL) and IL-10 (**B**: control = 127.1 ± 8.4 pg/mL). Whole blood of five healthy male subjects was incubated in triplicate with vehicle, testosterone, and E2 for 24 h at indicated concentrations. After 24 h, medium was replaced and cells were stimulated with 100 μg/mL concanavalin A for further 24 h in the presence of 10^{-6} mol/L cortisol. $^{*}P < 0.05$ versus respective concentration of testosterone.

With respect to testosterone, in the presence of cortisol, this hormone at 10^{-7} and 10^{-8} mol/L inhibited secretion of IL-2, IL-4, and IL-10 (FIGS. 1C, 2A, and 2B), and it tended to inhibit TNF and IFNγ (FIGS. 1A and 1D) but not IL-6 (FIG. 1B). Similar effects on IL-2, IL-4, and IL-10 were seen in the absence of cortisol (data not shown).

Influence of Testosterone and E2 on Glucocorticoid Receptor Expression

Neither testosterone at 10^{-7} mol/L nor E2 at 10^{-8} and 10^{-10} mol/L changed glucocorticoid receptor expression (FIG. 3).

Effects of Downstream Metabolites of E2 on TNF Secretion

Since metabolites of estrogens may modulate cytokine secretion, we investigated effects of various metabolites of E2 and their combinations on TNF secretion in the presence of cortisol. Metabolites were used in concentrations similar to those E2 (or lower) because their maximum concentration is expected to be equal to or lower than the concentration of the precursor E2. In the presence of

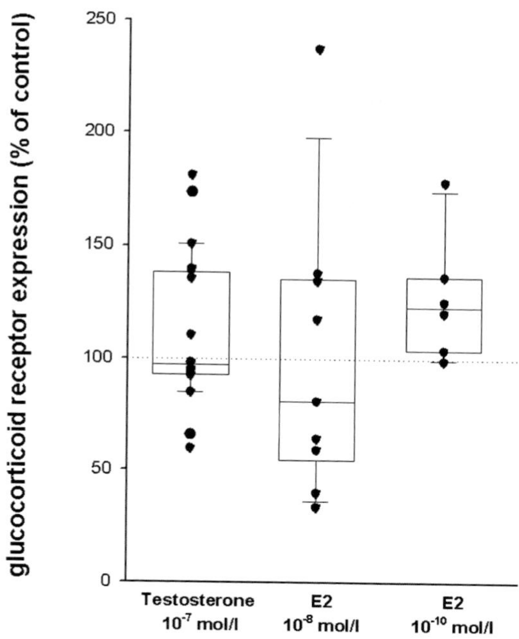

FIGURE 3. Influence of testosterone and 17β-estradiol (E2) on glucocorticoid receptor expression in peripheral blood leukocytes. The values are given in percent densitometric control, which is indicated by *dotted horizontal line*. The boundary of the box closest to zero indicates the 25th percentile, a line within the box marks the median, and the boundary of the box farthest from zero indicates the 75th percentile. Whiskers above and below the box indicate the 90th and 10th percentiles. *Black symbols* give the individual values of participating subjects (for T at 10^{-7} $M = 9$, for E2 at 10^{-8} $M = 9$, and for E2 at 10^{-10} $M = 6$).

cortisol, all investigated metabolites at 10^{-10} mol/L did not change TNF secretion (FIG. 4A). Thus, these effects were similar as compared to E2 (compare FIG. 1A). Interestingly, sole application of 2-hydroxyestradiol, 2-hydroxyestrone, 4-hydroxyestrone, or 16-hydroxyestradiol at 10^{-11} mol/L inhibited secretion of TNF (FIG. 4A). Similarly, sole application of 4-hydroxyestradiol or 16-hydroxyestrone tended to inhibit TNF secretion (FIG. 4A).

One molecule of E2 may be converted to different downstream metabolites. In order to further delineate effects of combinations of estrogens downstream of E2, 16-hydroxyestradiol and 16-hydroxyestrone at 10^{-10} mol/L were combined with the other metabolites. It is obvious that combinations of 16-hydroxyestradiol (16OHE2) at 10^{-10} mol/L and 2- and 4-hydroxylated estrogens at 10^{-11} mol/L markedly increased TNF secretion (FIG. 4B). Thus, a preponderance of 16-hydoxyestradiol over 2-/4-hydroxylated estrogens using a ratio of 10:1 increased TNF secretion. A similar increase was observed for the combination of 16-hydroxyestrone (16OHE1) and 4-hydroxylated

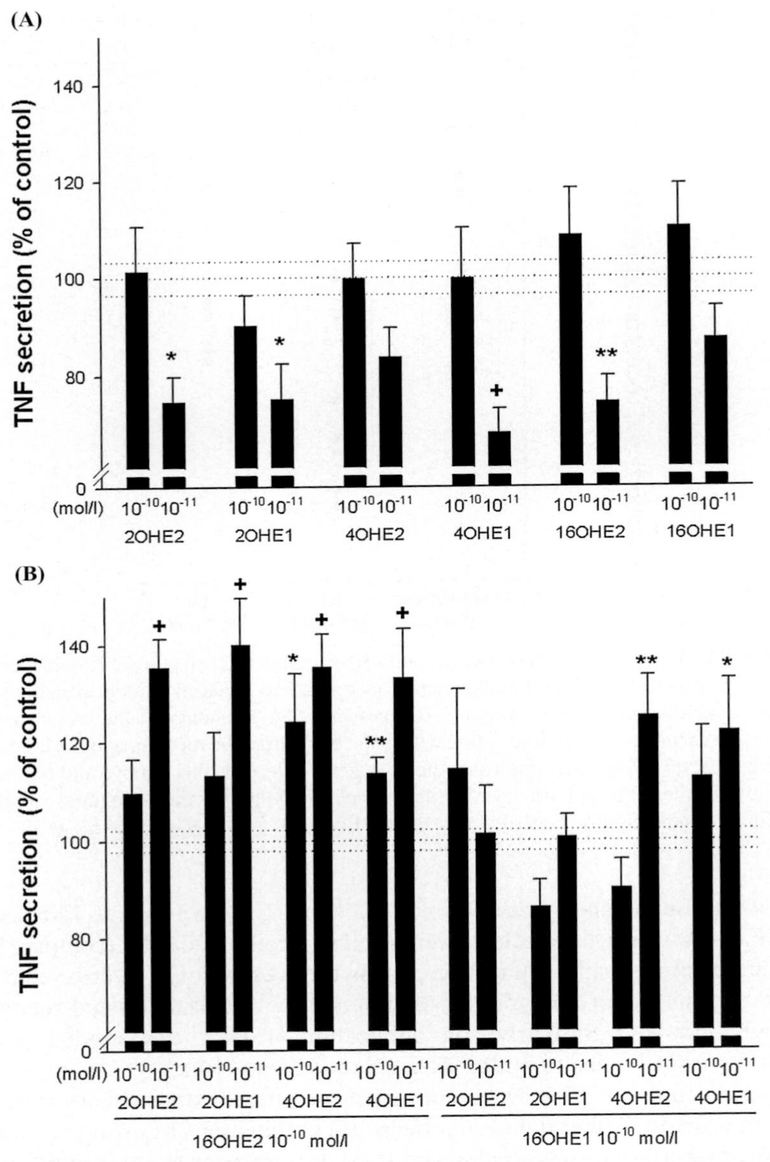

FIGURE 4. Influence of downstream metabolites of 17β-estradiol (E2) on secretion of TNF. **(A)** Influence of individual metabolites on TNF secretion. Control TNF was 54.1 ± 5.2 pg/mL. **(B)** Influence of combinations of metabolites on TNF secretion. Control TNF was 21.8 ± 2.1 pg/mL. For both panels: Data are given as means ± SEM in percent of control. $^{*}P < 0.05$, $^{**}P < 0.01$, $+P < 0.001$ versus control. Abbreviations: 2OHE2, 2-hydroxyestradiol; 2OHE1, 2-hydroxyestrone; 4OHE2, 4-hydroxyestradiol; 4OHE1, 4-hydroxyestrone; 16OHE2, 16-hydroxyestradiol; 16OHE1 (= estriol), 16-hydroxyestrone.

TABLE 2. Effect of the combination of 16-hydroxylated estrogens and 2-/4-hydroxylated estrogens on secretion of TNF in the absence of cortisol.

16-Hydroxylated Estrogen	2-/4-Hydroxylated Estrogen	TNF Secretion (% of Control)
–	–	Control: 100 ± 4.2
16OH-estradiol 10^{-10} mol/L	2OH-estradiol 10^{-11} mol/L	91.4 ± 10.9
	2OH-estrone 10^{-11} mol/L	77.7 ± 10.1
	4OH-estradiol 10^{-11} mol/L	100.8 ± 7.6
	4OH-estrone 10^{-11} mol/L	123.2 ± 16.5
16OH-estrone 10^{-10} mol/L	2OH-estradiol 10^{-11} mol/L	66.8 ± 5.7*
	2OH-estrone 10^{-11} mol/L	54.5 ± 6.8**
	4OH-estradiol 10^{-11} mol/L	104.1 ± 5.2
	4OH-estrone 10^{-11} mol/L	119.5 ± 24.7

Data are given as means ± SEM.
Control TNF = 55.0 ± 4.5 pg/mL. $^{*}P < 0.01$, $^{**}P < 0.001$ for the comparison versus control.

metabolites but not for 2-hydroxylated estrogens (FIG. 4B). Such a stimulatory effect of combinations of downstream metabolites was not observed in the absence of cortisol (TABLE 2). In contrast, in the absence of cortisol, the combination of 16-hydroxyestrone and 2-hydroxylated estrogens even inhibited TNF secretion (TABLE 2).

DISCUSSION

This study showed dichotomous effects of sex hormones: E2 and metabolites stabilized or increased cytokine secretion whereas testosterone inhibited this secretion. This dual role of estrogens and testosterone on cytokine secretion has been described in the literature and it was thought that this phenomenon could explain the well-known female-to-male preponderance in acquiring autoimmune diseases, particularly when TNF and IFNγ play a dominant disease-perpetuating role.[1,3–5] However, two aspects have not been studied so far.

First, the additional role of cortisol for sex hormone modulation of cytokines from peripheral blood leukocytes has been unclear. This can be important because these mechanisms may explain interactions of hormones on the level not only of the pituitary gland, but also in peripheral inflammation. We demonstrated that a stimulus of the HPA axis (injection of IL-1β, ether anesthesia, or granulomatous disease) led to stronger corticosterone responses in female than in male mice,[19] which corroborated a similar study in humans.[20] Evidence from the literature strongly supports the concept that estrogens enhance and androgens diminish the glucocorticoid response to a variety of inflammatory and noninflammatory stimuli. Although the mechanisms for these interactions are not fully elucidated, there is strong evidence that sex steroids affect the expression of glucocorticoid receptors in the central nervous system and modulate the negative feedback exerted by cortisol at the hypothalamus.[2,19] These observations led us to hypothesize that cortisol interacts with testosterone or estradiol on the cellular level, which can be studied in humans using peripheral blood leukocytes. This study demonstrates that E2 (in relation to testosterone) stimulated production of TNF, IL-6, IL-2, IFNγ, IL-4, and IL-10 caused by the proinflammatory influence of applied immune stimuli (LPS and Con A). The question arises as to how these findings may be linked to the estrogenic support of the HPA axis response.

It has been demonstrated that the pituitary folliculo-stellate cell is a macrophage type of cell located in the pituitary gland.[21,22] This type of cell, similar to peripheral blood monocytes/macrophages, can be stimulated by immune stimuli in order to produce proinflammatory cytokines locally.[23,24] Locally produced cytokines can act as secretagogues for ACTH and other pituitary hormones.[24] In this respect, the folliculo-stellate cell may be an important local linking element between immune stimuli and hormone production.[24] In this present study, we have shown that E2 stabilized (in relation to testosterone) or increased cytokine secretion induced by stimulatory agents in peripheral blood cells. A similar effect upon the folliculo-stellate cell might explain the facilitating effects of E2 on pituitary hormone secretion and the inhibitory effect of testosterone via an increase or decrease of locally produced cytokines, respectively.

The second open question that was addressed in this study is the role of downstream metabolites of E2 on stimulated TNF secretion. Our results demonstrate that the ratio of 16-hydroxylated estrogens in relation to 2-/4-hydroxylated estrogens is important for TNF secretion. We were able to describe that a ratio of 10:1 of 16-hydroxyestradiol in relation to 2-/4-hydroxylated estrogens markedly stimulated TNF secretion in the presence of cortisol. This effect was not observed in the absence of cortisol. Furthermore, in the absence of cortisol, the combination of 16-hydroxyestrone and 2-hydroxylated estrogens even strongly inhibited TNF secretion. These results delineate the importance of downstream estrogens in respective concentrations. Again, this may play a role not only on the pituitary level, but also in the peripheral immune response. As pointed out in the introduction to this article, in persons with chronic inflammatory diseases, we observe a large shift toward 16-hydroxylated estrogens in comparison to that measure in postmenopausal osteopenic women.[9,10,12,13] Authors in the field of rheumatology trust that estrogens exert proinflammatory effects in most rheumatic diseases, whereas authors in bone research believe that estrogens prevent osteoporosis through inhibition of cytokine secretion. We suggest the following model to find an answer for this obvious discrepancy (FIG. 5):

In the noninflammatory situation, an osteopenia-inducing milieu (FIG. 5, left panel) is characterized by increased levels of 2-hydroxylated estrogens and low levels of 16-hydroxylated estrogens.[12,13] This balance would diminish the basal secretion of TNF, IL-1, and IL-6 and, therefore, avoid bone loss

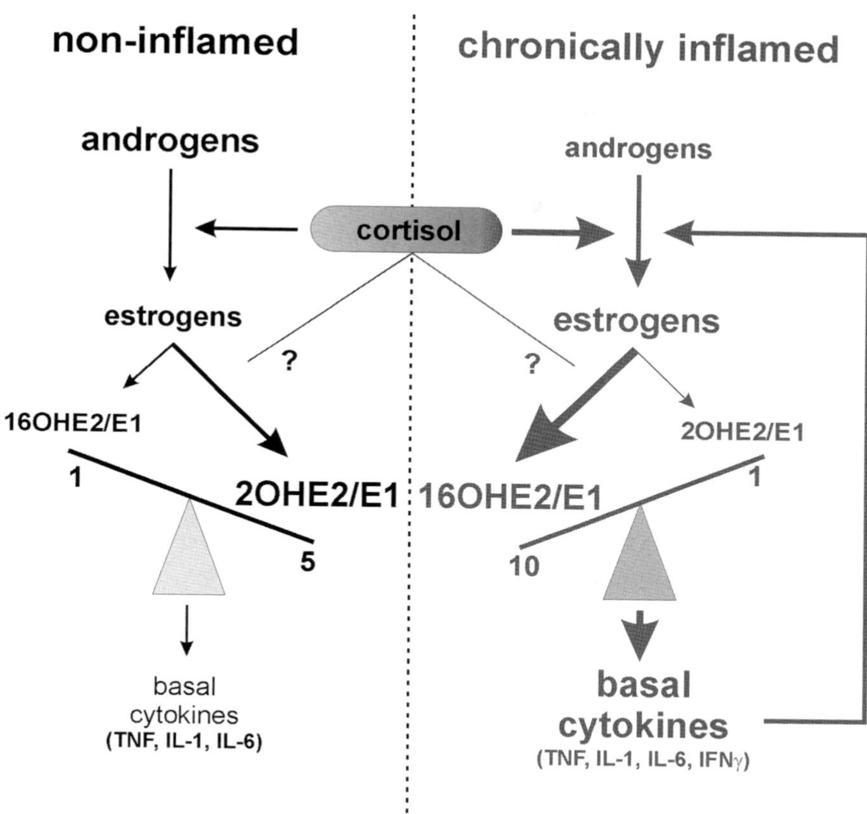

FIGURE 5. Model of the estrogen influence on secretion of proinflammatory cytokines in a noninflamed and chronically inflamed microenvironment. For abbreviation of estrogens see legend to FIGURE 4. *Left panel*: In the noninflamed situation, an osteopenia-inducing milieu is characterized by increased levels of 2OHE1/E2 and low levels of 16OHE1/E2. In this situation, basal secretion of TNF, IL-1, and IL-6 is osteoclastogenic. However, TNF, IL-1 and IL-6 are markedly lower than in chronically inflamed tissue. In such a situation, administration of therapeutic estrogens probably increases the 2OHE1/E2 because this particular pathway is switched on. This would be a negative signal for the osteoclastogenic TNF secretion. *Right panel*: In contrast, during chronic inflammation in the situation of rheumatic diseases, such as rheumatoid arthritis, the balance is switched to 16OHE1/E2. Under these conditions, one can assume that therapeutic administration of estrogens would enhance 16OHE1/E2 over 2OHE1/E2, which would support secretion of proinflammatory cytokines. Cortisol itself is a stimulator of aromatase, and somewhat elevated cortisol concentrations in the tissue, although inadequately low in relation to inflammation, would promote estrogen-induced secretion of proinflammatory TNF. Thus, under inflamed conditions estrogens appear as proinflammatory agents whereas under noninflamed conditions estrogens appear as anti-inflammatory.

(for review see Ref. 6). In chronic inflammation (FIG. 5, right panel), administration of therapeutic estrogens probably increases the 16-hydroxylated estrogens because this particular pathway is switched on. During estrogen therapy of postmenopausal women without inflammation, the 2-hydroxylated estrogens would appear in higher concentrations compared to 16-hydroxylated estrogens, which would be a negative signal for the osteoclastogenic TNF secretion (FIG. 5, left panel). In contrast, during chronic inflammation in the situation of rheumatic diseases, such as rheumatoid arthritis, the balance is switched to estrogens and particularly to 16-hydroxylated estrogens (FIG. 5, right panel). As shown in this study, a preponderance of 16-hydroxyestradiol versus 2-/4-hydroxylated estrogens in the presence of cortisol markedly increased TNF secretion. In this situation, one can assume that therapeutic administration of estrogens would enhance 16-hydroxylated estrogens over 2-/4-hydroxylated estrogens, which would support secretion of proinflammatory cytokines (FIG. 5, right panel). Cortisol itself promotes the conversion of androgens to estrogens.[25] Therefore, somewhat elevated cortisol concentrations in the tissue[26] would result in higher estrogen levels and, indirectly, increased secretion of proinflammatory TNF. Thus, under inflammatory conditions estrogens appear as proinflammatory agents.

In conclusion, this study on peripheral blood leukocytes demonstrated that E2 stabilized or increased and testosterone inhibited immune stimuli–induced secretion of proinflammatory cytokines, such as TNF and IFNγ. Furthermore, combined application of 16-hydroxylated estrogens and 2-/4-hydroxylated estrogens in a ratio of 10:1 increased TNF secretion only in the presence of cortisol. The findings of this study shed new light on the gender dimorphism of the neuroendocrine and immune systems. Furthermore, it demonstrated that distinct cocktails of downstream E2 metabolites may induce pro- or anti-inflammatory responses in blood leukocytes. Further studies in folliculostellate cells and synovial cells of patients with rheumatoid arthritis are needed in order to further elucidate the importance of these findings on the local level.

ACKNOWLEDGMENT

This study was supported by a grant from the Deutsche Forschungsgemeinschaft (Str 511/10 – 1).

REFERENCES

1. CUTOLO, M. & R. WILDER. 2000. Different roles for androgens and estrogens in the susceptibility to autoimmune rheumatic diseases. Rheum. Dis. Clin. North Am. **26:** 825–839.
2. DA SILVA, J.A. 1995. Sex hormones, glucocorticoids and autoimmunity: facts and hypotheses. Ann. Rheum. Dis. **54:** 6–16.

inflammation (for review, see Ref. 1). However, COX is not the only (and possibly not even the rate-limiting) enzyme of the PGE_2-synthesizing cascade (FIG. 1).

While studying the expression of multiple enzymes involved in PGE_2 synthesis during the febrile response of rats to a low dose of bacterial LPS,[6] we have noticed several remarkable features of another enzyme, microsomal PGE synthase (mPGES)-1. Identified by Jakobsson *et al.*,[7] mPGES-1 is a 16-kDa member of the so-called MAPEG (*m*embrane-*a*ssociated *p*roteins involved in *e*icosanoid and *g*lutathione metabolism) family. This enzyme catalyzes the final step of PGE_2 synthesis: a nonoxidative rearrangement of the COX product PGH_2 into PGE_2 (FIG. 1). Not only does mPGES-1 occupy the most terminal position in the PGE_2-synthesizing cascade, but it also preferentially couples with bad COX, COX-2.[8,9] In our study,[6] the febrile response of rats to LPS was accompanied by strong transcriptional upregulation of the *Ptges* gene (which encodes mPGES-1) in peripheral LPS-processing organs (liver and lung) and in the brain. This upregulation occurred very early after LPS challenge, at the so-called *Phase 1* of LPS fever (for more information on febrile phases, see Refs. 10–12). The upregulation of mPGES-1 was dramatic in its magnitude (more than 1,200-fold in the liver and more than 30-fold in the lung and hypothalamus) and had a long duration (several hours after a single injection of LPS). Even when COX-2 expression had returned to base line, mPGES-1 remained overexpressed. The revealed unique features of the response of this enzyme to LPS, as well as its downstream position within the PGE_2-synthesizing cascade, allowed us to speculate that mPGES-1 is an attractive, selective target for antipyretic and anti-inflammatory therapy in systemic inflammation.[6] We have further developed this speculation in later publications.[1,13] Undisputable evidence for the crucial involvement of mPGES-1 in LPS fever was obtained by Engblom *et al.*[14] and Saha *et al.*[15] by using mice with deletion of the *Ptges* gene.[16,17]

While studying mPGES-1 expression and being focused on systemic inflammation and fever, we thought little about local inflammation or arthritic diseases. Concurrently, cytokine-induced upregulation of mPGES-1 was reported to occur in synovial cells from patients with RA.[18,19] These reports were promptly followed by studies that addressed the role of mPGES-1 in arthritis by utilizing a variety of models, techniques, and approaches.[20–25] Importantly, it was shown that arthritis has a much milder course in mice genetically deficient in mPGES-1, as several arthritic symptoms, including pannus formation and joint erosion, are attenuated in these knockout mice in collagen-induced[17] and collagen antibody-induced[26] models of RA. Within a couple of years, several reviews on the role of mPGES-1 in the pathogenesis of RA were published, and a unanimous guilty verdict against mPGES-1 was reached.[27–29] Looking back, one could have fed our[6] and our predecessors'[9,30–32] data on systemic inflammation into the "criminal profiles" of arthritic diseases and arrived at the conclusion that mPGES-1 is a primary suspect in arthritis. Can new

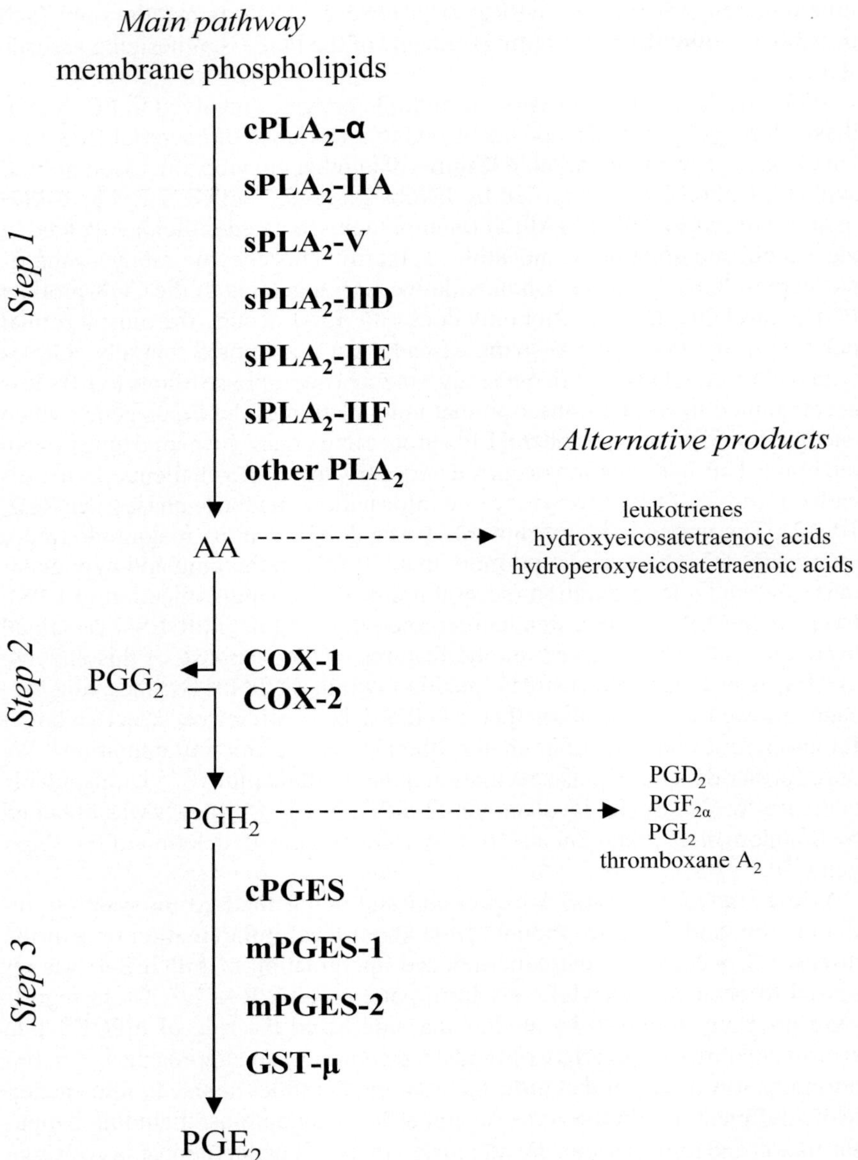

FIGURE 1. The PGE_2-synthesizing cascade. Substrates and products are shown in regular font, enzymes in bold, and explanatory signs in italics. AA = arachidonic acid; c = cytosolic (as in $cPLA_2$ or cPGES); COX = cyclooxygenase; GST = glutathione-*S*-transferase; m = microsomal (as in mPGES); PG = prostaglandin; PGES = PGE synthase; PL = phospholipase; s = secretory (as in $sPLA_2$). (From Ivanov *et al.*[6] Reproduced with permission.)

information about mediators of systemic inflammation be combined with the profiling technique to make predictions?

IDENTIFYING NEW SUSPECTS: EPHRINS AND EPHRIN KINASES

In a recent study,[33] we used differential mRNA display to hunt genes overexpressed in response to a low dose of bacterial LPS *in vivo*. Of the thousands of genes studied, only seven were consistently upregulated in the liver of LPS-treated rats compared to saline-treated controls. One of them appeared to be ephrin-A1, formerly known as B61 protein (FIG. 2, enlarged band), which directed our attention toward ephrins and their receptors, ephrin kinases (Eph kinases, or Eph). Eph (from *e*rythropoietin-*p*roducing *h*epatocellular) receptor kinases constitute the largest family of receptor tyrosine kinases (RTKs). Based on their structure, Eph kinases are divided into two subclasses, A and B, which are composed of 10 (EphA1–EphA10) and 6 (EphB1–EphB6) members, respectively.[34] Corresponding to the two subclasses of receptors, there are also two subclasses of ephrins, A and B. All five ephrins of the A subclass (viz., A1–A5) activate all ten EphA receptors, whereas all three ephrins-B (B1–B3) interact with all six EphB receptors.[34,35] Since all Eph receptors and their ligands are predominantly membrane-associated proteins, direct cell-to-cell contact is required for receptor activation. Such activation usually induces repulsion of the cells involved.[34,36] Eph-ephrin–mediated cell-to-cell interactions play prominent roles in the formation of tissue boundaries, neural crest cell migration, axon guidance, and angiogenesis.[35–37]

In our study,[33] we have shown that LPS fever in rats is characterized by robust transcriptional upregulation (up to 16-fold) and downregulation (up to 21-fold) of several ephrins and Eph receptors in the liver and lung. Expressional changes of Eph receptors were also recorded at the protein level. Typical for Eph receptors and ephrins, their expressional regulation was affected in a counter-directed manner: downregulation of EphB3 occurred simultaneously with upregulation of ephrin-B2 in the liver (*Phase 2* of LPS fever); upregulation of EphA2 coincided with downregulation of ephrin-A1 in the liver and lung (*Phase 2*); and downregulation of EphA1 and EphA3 co-developed with upregulation of ephrin-A1 and ephrin-A3 in the liver (*Phase 3*). Although a small number of mostly *in vitro* studies reported that LPS or proinflammatory cytokines induce changes in the expression of some ephrins and Eph receptors in various models,[38–43] this was the first observation of altered expressional regulation of multiple ephrins and Eph receptors in an *in vivo* model of systemic inflammation.

The adhesion of blood leukocytes to the vascular endothelium with their subsequent extravasation and tissue transmigration is a classic example of a cellular event in systemic inflammation.[44,45] There are several lines of evidence

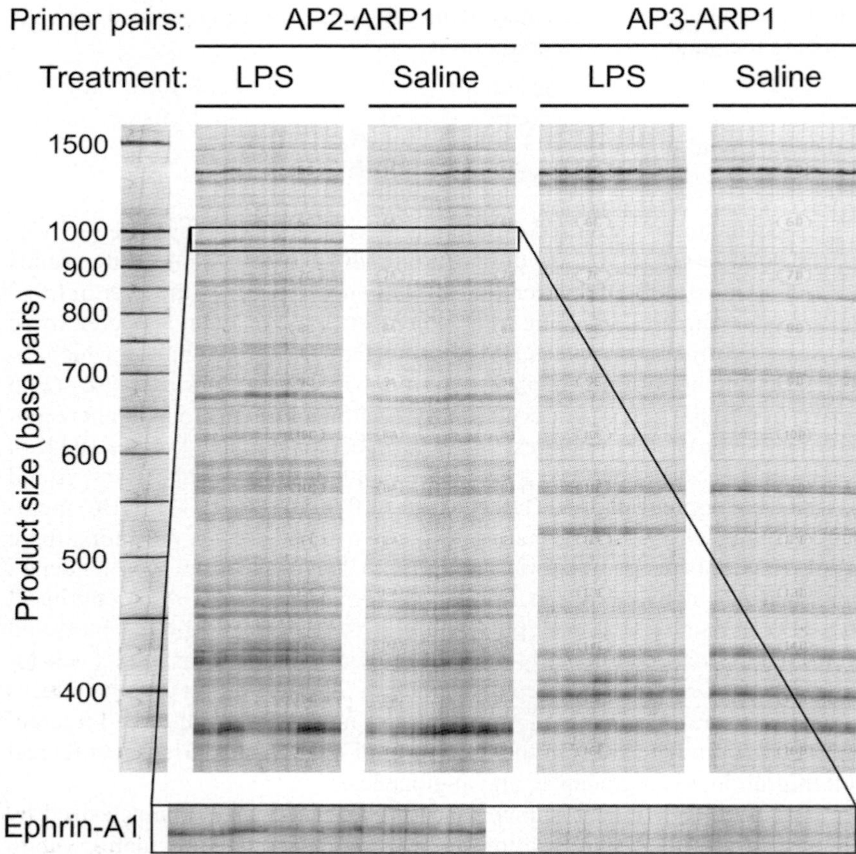

FIGURE 2. Differential display of mRNA amplified from the liver of Wistar Kyoto rats injected intravenously with either LPS (50 μg/kg) or saline (1 mL/kg) 6 h before harvesting the samples. RT-PCR was performed on total liver RNA using two different "anchored" primer (AP)–"arbitrary" primer (ARP) pairs. For each pair of primers shown, the area marked as LPS corresponds to samples from three LPS-treated rats loaded in duplicate (6 wells in total); the area marked as saline corresponds to samples from three saline-treated rats loaded in duplicate (6 wells in total). The enlarged band shows the upregulation of the ephrin-A1 amplicon in the samples from LPS-treated rats. (From Ivanov *et al.*[33] Reproduced with permission.)

suggesting the involvement of Eph receptors and ephrins in inflammatory trafficking of leukocytes. First, Eph receptors and ephrins are expressed on both cell types involved: leukocytes[46,47] and endotheliocytes.[38,43,48,49] Second, adhesion and transmigration of leukocytes require activation of their surface-adhesive molecules, integrins.[50,51] Signaling through several Eph receptors has

42. YUAN, K., Y.T. JIN & M.T. LIN. 2000. Expression of Tie-2, angiopoietin-1, angiopoietin-2, ephrinB2 and EphB4 in pyogenic granuloma of human gingiva implicates their roles in inflammatory angiogenesis. J. Periodontal Res. **35:** 165–171.
43. CHENG, N. & J. CHEN. 2001. Tumor necrosis factor-α induction of endothelial ephrin A1 expression is mediated by a p38 MAPK- and SAPK/JNK-dependent but nuclear factor-κB-independent mechanism. J. Biol. Chem. **276:** 13771–13777.
44. LUSTER, A.D. 1998. Chemokines—chemotactic cytokines that mediate inflammation. N. Engl. J. Med. **338:** 436–445.
45. MCINTYRE, T.M. *et al.* 2003. Cell–cell interactions: leukocyte-endothelial interactions. Curr. Opin. Hematol. **10:** 150–158.
46. AASHEIM, H.C., L.W. TERSTAPPEN & T. LOGTENBERG. 1997. Regulated expression of the Eph-related receptor tyrosine kinase Hek11 in early human B lymphopoiesis. Blood **90:** 3613–3622.
47. YU, G. *et al.* 2003. Ephrin B2 induces T cell costimulation. J. Immunol. **171:** 106–114.
48. OIKE, Y. *et al.* 2002. Regulation of vasculogenesis and angiogenesis by EphB/ephrin-B2 signaling between endothelial cells and surrounding mesenchymal cells. Blood **100:** 1326–1333.
49. WU, J. & H. LUO. 2005. Recent advances on T-cell regulation by receptor tyrosine kinases. Curr. Opin. Hematol. **12:** 292–297.
50. WORTHYLAKE, R.A. & K. BURRIDGE. 2001. Leukocyte transendothelial migration: orchestrating the underlying molecular machinery. Curr. Opin. Cell Biol. **13:** 569–577.
51. LINDBOM, L. & J. WERR. 2002. Integrin-dependent neutrophil migration in extravascular tissue. Semin. Immunol. **14:** 115–121.
52. ZOU, J.X. *et al.* 1999. An Eph receptor regulates integrin activity through R-Ras. Proc. Natl. Acad. Sci. USA **96:** 13813–13818.
53. MIAO, H. *et al.* 2000. Activation of EphA2 kinase suppresses integrin function and causes focal-adhesion kinase dephosphorylation. Nat. Cell Biol. **2:** 62–69.
54. SHARFE, N. *et al.* 2002. Ephrin stimulation modulates T cell chemotaxis. Eur. J. Immunol. **32:** 3745–3755.
55. TAKEUCHI, T. & T. ABE. 1998. Tyrosine phosphorylated proteins in synovial cells of rheumatoid arthritis. Int. Rev. Immunol. **17:** 365–381.
56. SWEENEY, S.E. & G.S. FIRESTEIN. 2004. Signal transduction in rheumatoid arthritis. Curr. Opin. Rheumatol. **16:** 231–237.
57. WONG, B.R. *et al.* 2004. Targeting Syk as a treatment for allergic and autoimmune disorders. Expert Opin. Investig. Drugs **13:** 743–762.
58. JUURIKIVI, A. *et al.* 2005. Inhibition of c-kit tyrosine kinase by imatinib mesylate induces apoptosis in mast cells in rheumatoid synovia: a potential approach to the treatment of arthritis. Ann. Rheum. Dis. **64:** 1126–1131.
59. GROSIOS, K. *et al.* 2004. Angiogenesis inhibition by the novel VEGF receptor tyrosine kinase inhibitor, PTK787/ZK222854, causes significant anti-arthritic effects in models of rheumatoid arthritis. Inflamm. Res. **53:** 133–142.
60. CLAVEL, G., N. BESSIS & M.C. BOISSIER. 2003. Recent data on the role for angiogenesis in rheumatoid arthritis. Joint Bone Spine **70:** 321–326.
61. SZEKANECZ, Z., L. GASPAR & A.E. KOCH. 2005. Angiogenesis in rheumatoid arthritis. Front. Biosci. **10:** 1739–1753.

62. TAYLOR, P.C. & B. SIVAKUMAR. 2005. Hypoxia and angiogenesis in rheumatoid arthritis. Curr. Opin. Rheumatol. **17:** 293–298.
63. LU, J. *et al*. 2000. Vascular endothelial growth factor expression and regulation of murine collagen-induced arthritis. J. Immunol. **164:** 5922–5927.
64. MIOTLA, J. *et al*. 2000. Treatment with soluble VEGF receptor reduces disease severity in murine collagen-induced arthritis. Lab. Invest. **80:** 1195–1205.
65. SONE, H. *et al*. 2001. Neutralization of vascular endothelial growth factor prevents collagen-induced arthritis and ameliorates established disease in mice. Biochem. Biophys. Res. Commun. **281:** 562–568.
66. DE BANDT, M. *et al*. 2000. Suppression of arthritis and protection from bone destruction by treatment with TNP-470/AGM-1470 in a transgenic mouse model of rheumatoid arthritis. Arthritis Rheum. **43:** 2056–2063.
67. ROGERS, M.S. *et al*. 2004. Genetic loci that control the angiogenic response to basic fibroblast growth factor. FASEB J. **18:** 1050–1059.
68. YUAN, K. *et al*. 2004. Syndecan-1 up-regulated by ephrinB2/EphB4 plays dual roles in inflammatory angiogenesis. Blood **104:** 1025–1033.
69. OLIGINO, T.J. & S.A. DALRYMPLE. 2003. Targeting B cells for the treatment of rheumatoid arthritis. Arthritis Res. Ther. **4** (Suppl 5): S7–S11.
70. FIRESTEIN, G.S. 2004. The T cell cometh: interplay between adaptive immunity and cytokine network in rheumatoid arthritis. J. Clin. Invest. **114:** 471–474.

Sympathetic Nervous System Influence on the Innate Immune Response

GEORGES J.M. MAESTRONI

Center for Experimental Pathology, Cantonal Institute of Pathology, 6601 Locarno, Switzerland

ABSTRACT: Our studies focused on the sympathetic nervous system (SNS) influence on dendritic cells (DCs), which play a crucial role in the innate immune response. We found that DCs express a variety of adrenergic receptors (ARs) with α1-ARs playing a stimulatory and β2-ARs an inhibitory effect on DCs migration. β2-ARs in skin and bone marrow-derived DCs when stimulated by bacterial toll-like receptors (TLRs) agonists respond to norepinephrine (NE) by decreased interleukin-12 (IL-12) and increased IL-10 production which in turn downregulates inflammatory cytokine production and CCR7 expression and thus their migration ability leading to reduced T helper-1 (Th1) priming.[1,2] We also found that contact sensitizers that may induce a predominant Th1 response, do so by inhibiting the local NE turnover in the skin.[3] The SNS seems therefore to contribute in shaping the information conveyed by DCs to T cells and thus in inducing the appropriate adaptive immune response. In this sense, the SNS physiological influence may allow Th2 priming to fight infections sustained by extracellular pathogens and limit the risk for organ-specific autoimmune reactions associated with excessive Th1 priming and inhibition of T regulatory cell functions. More recently, we found that preconditioning of the skin by β-adrenergic antagonist and the TLR2 agonist S. Aureus peptidoglycan (PGN) may instruct a Th1 adaptive response to a soluble protein antigen. On the contrary, when the TLR4 agonist E. Coli lipopolysaccharide was used, the presence of the β-adrenergic antagonist was not effective. These effects were consonant with the pattern of TLRs expression shown by epidermal keratinocytes (EKs) but not by skin DCs. As β-ARs signaling defects[4–6] together with S. Aureus infections[7] are thought to serve as initiation and/or persistence factors for numerous Th1-sustained autoimmune inflammatory skin diseases, we might have disclosed at least part of the relevant pathogenetic mechanism.

KEYWORDS: sympathetic nervous system; dendritic cells; epidermal keratinocytes; innate immunity; adaptive immunity; toll-like receptors; adrenergic receptors; T cell priming; $CD4^+$; $CD25^+$; regulatory T cells; autoimmune diseases

Address for correspondence: Georges J.M. Maestroni, Center for Experimental Pathology, Cantonal Institute of Pathology, PO Box, 6601 Locarno, Switzerland. Voice: 41-91-816-07-91; fax: 41-91-816-07-99.

e-mail: georges.maestroni@ti.ch

Ann. N.Y. Acad. Sci. 1069: 195–207 (2006). © 2006 New York Academy of Sciences.
doi: 10.1196/annals.1351.017

INTRODUCTION

The innate immune system is endowed with a highly sophisticated ability to discriminate between self-antigens and foreign pathogens. This discrimination relies on a family of receptors, known as toll-like receptors (TLRs) that play a crucial role in early host defense mechanisms. The TLRs-dependent activation of innate immunity is necessary for the induction of acquired immunity, in particular for T helper-1 (Th1) priming. TLRs differ from each other in ligand specificities, expression pattern, and presumably in the target genes they can affect. To date, 11 TLRs are known.

The TLRs-mediated control of adaptive immune responses relies mainly on dendritic cells (DC) functions. After TLRs activation and antigen internalization DCs leave the tissues interfacing with the external environment and enter the lymphatic vessels to reach the lymphoid organs and undergo maturation.[8–10] While still immature, the primary function of DC is to capture and process antigens, then to present the antigenic peptides, and activate specific T cells.[8,9] Activation of naive Th cells also results in their polarization toward the Th1 and/or Th2 type, which orchestrates the immune effector mechanism that is more appropriate for the invading pathogen. Th1 cells promote cellular immunity, protecting against intracellular infection and cancer but carry the risk of organ-specific autoimmunity. Th2 cells promote humoral immunity, are highly effective against extracellular pathogens, and are involved in tolerance mechanisms and allergic diseases. Priming of Th1 cells is strictly dependent on cytokines, such as interleukin-12 (IL-12) and interferon-γ (INF-γ) while that of Th2 cells is promoted by IL-4, Il-5, and IL-10.[11,12] Interestingly, DCs are uniquely able to either induce immune responses or to maintain the state of self-tolerance. Recent evidence has shown that the ability of DCs to induce tolerance in the steady state is critical to the prevention of the autoimmune response. Similarly, DCs have been shown to induce several types of regulatory T cells, depending on the maturation state of the DCs and the local microenvironment. DCs have been shown to have therapeutic value in models of allograft rejection and autoimmunity.

SYMPATHETIC NERVOUS REGULATION OF DC'S FUNCTIONS

The type of Th priming determines whether an infection is efficiently cleared, however, the decision-making mechanisms linking the innate recognition of the pathogen and the type of Th priming are still poorly understood. Besides the type of invading pathogen and its route of entry into the organism, other local microenvironmental factors seem to play a role.[13,14]

The sympathetic nervous system (SNS) that innervates all parts of the body, constitutes the largest and most versatile component of the autonomic nervous system. Nerve activity results in the release of catecholamines that act on adrenergic receptors (ARs). In the periphery, the sympathetic neurotransmitter norepinephrine (NE) is released nonsynaptically, that is, from varicose axon terminals, without synaptic contacts. Thus, ARs on immune cells are targets of remote control, and NE, may act as a modulator of the sympathetic–immune interface. The ARs mediate the functional effects of epinephrine and NE by coupling to several of the major signaling pathways modulated by G proteins. In our studies we found that immature bone marrow-derived murine DCs express the mRNA coding for the α1b-, β2-, β1-, α-2B, and α2C-ARs.[15,16] Murine epidermal Langerhans cells (LCs) mobilization was inhibited by local treatment with the specific α1-AR antagonist, prazosin. Consistently, NE enhanced spontaneous emigration of DCs from ear skin explants, and prazosin inhibited this effect. In addition, local treatment with prazosin during sensitization with fluorescein isothiocyanate (FITC) inhibited the contact hypersensitivity (CHS) response 6 days later. *In vitro*, bone marrow-derived immature, but not CD40-stimulated mature DCs migrated in response to NE, and this effect was neutralized by prazosin. NE seems, therefore, to exert both a chemotactic and chemokinetic activity on immature DCs influencing their antigen-presenting capacity.[15] Furthermore, we found that short-term exposure of bone marrow-derived DCs to NE at the beginning of lipopolysaccharide (LPS) stimulation hampered IL-12 production and increased IL-10 release. The capacity of NE-exposed DCs to produce IL-12 upon CD40 cross-linking as well as to stimulate allogeneic Th lymphocytes was reduced. Noteworthy, the ganglionic blocker, pentolinium, administered in mice before skin sensitization with FITC could increase the Th1-type response in the draining lymph nodes.[17] More recently, we detailed that the inhibition of IL-12 was on account of activation of both β2-and α2A-ARs while stimulation of IL-10 was a β2-AR phenomenon only. IL-10, in turn, inhibited DCs migration in response to the homeostatic chemokines, CCL21 and CCL19, reducing their Th1 priming ability.[16] As we have shown that NE may enhance DCs migration via α1-ARs[15] and others have confirmed the expression of via α1-ARs in LCs,[18] the latter finding was seemingly in contrast with our previous study. A reasonable explanation is that, physiologically, the final NE effect on LCs migration results from two opposing effects: chemotaxis/chemokinesis mediated by α1-ARs and inhibition mediated by β2-ARs (IL-10). The selective blockade of these two ARs results, in fact, in divergent effects on both LCs migration and Th priming.

Other authors have also recently shown that catecholamines inhibit the antigen-presenting ability of epidermal LCs via β2-ARs.[18]

The overall effect of the sympathetic neurotransmitter NE in innate immunity seems thus that of modulating DCs migration and Th1 priming. Thus the role of the DCs ARs would be to limit the inflammatory response to a given pathogen and to modulate the type and strength of the adaptive response. Consistently, recent reports show that NE depletion decreased the resistance to Pseudomonas

TABLE 1. Effect of NE on inflammatory cytokine production in bone marrow-derived DCs stimulated by a TLR2 agonist

	TNF-α (pg/mL)	IL-6 (pg/mL)
MEDIUM	169 ± 35	35 ± 9
LTA	4104 ± 263	19848 ± 810
LTA + NE	721 ± 188 [a]	8269 ± 562 [a]
LTA + NE + a-IL-10	2870 ± 344	15082 ± 513
LTA + NE + mAb isotype	653 ± 196	5356 ± 145

Murine bone marrow-derived DCs were cultured in the presence of GM–CSF, purified by magnetic cell sorting and stimulated with the TLR2 agonist LTA (10 μg/mL) in the presence or absence of NE (1 μM). Anti-IL-10 mAb (a-IL-10) or a relative unspecific Ab isotype were also added. The experiments were in triplicates and the data reported represent the mean concentration of TNF-α and IL-6 in the supernatants from three experiments after 6-h incubation. The cytokine concentration was assessed by ELISA.

[a]$P < 0.01$ (ANOVA).

aeruginosa and Listeria monocytogenes.[19–21] Most interestingly, we also found that oxazolone that induces a predominant Th1-type CHS response, but not FITC that induces a prevailing Th2-type response, inhibits the local NE turnover in the skin of mice during the first 8 h of sensitization. Oxazolone also induced higher expression of the inflammatory cytokines IL-1 and IL-6 mRNA in the skin. Furthermore, FITC but not oxazolone sensitization in presence of the specific β2-AR antagonist ICI 118,551 enhanced the consequent response as well as the production of Th1 cytokines in draining lymph nodes; conversely Th2 cytokines were not affected. Thus, the extent of Th1 priming in the adaptive response to a sensitizing agent seems to depend also on its ability to modulate the local sympathetic nervous activity during the innate immune response.[3]

More recently, we reasoned that if the local sympathetic nervous activity played a role in determining the type of innate and adaptive response to a pathogen, activation of different TLRs should result in different NE effects on cytokine production in DCs. When DCs were stimulated by TLR agonists, activation of TLR2 and TLR4 allowed NE to induce large amounts of IL-10, while upon activation of TLR3 and TLR9 the effect of NE was much smaller (Maestroni, unpublished results).

ADRENERGIC MODULATION OF THE DCs—CD4$^+$,CD25$^+$ T REGULATORY CELLS INTERACTION

CD4$^+$,CD25$^+$ T regulatory (Treg) cells constitute a cell population that plays a crucial role in dampening exaggerated immune responses, as well as in the maintenance of immune tolerance to self or innocuous exogenous antigens. Part of their immunosuppressive effect depends on the ability to inhibit DCs maturation and antigen presentation.[22] Recent reports have indicated that regulatory T cells might traffic to the skin in a way much similar to that used

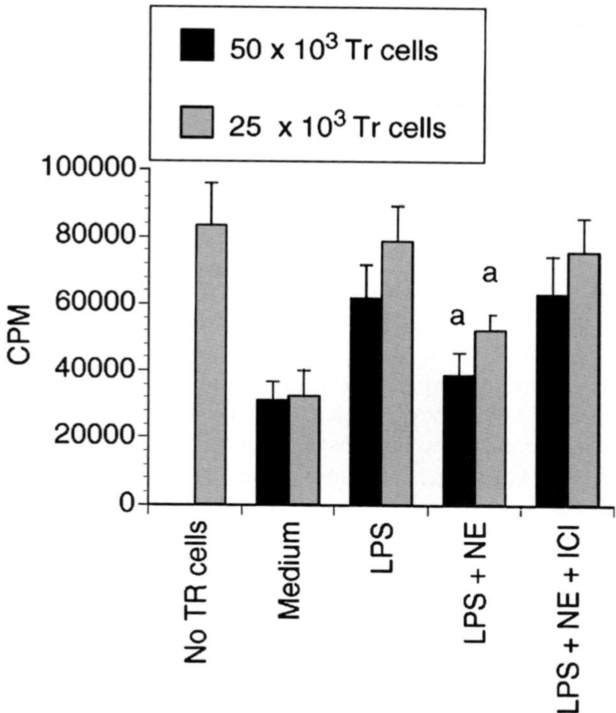

FIGURE 1. NE counteracts the inhibitory effect of TLR-activated DCs on the suppressive function of regulatory T cells. $CD4^+$, $CD25^-$ Th cells were incubated with murine bone marrow-derived DCs, anti-CD3 mAb, and indicated numbers of $CD4^+$, $CD25^+$ Treg cells in the presence or absence of LPS (TLR4 agonist) for 60 h in the presence or absence of NE (1 μM) and/or the β2-AR antagonist ICI 118,551 (1 μM). Proliferation of Th cells was assessed by ^{3}H-thymidine incorporation in the last 12–16 h of incubation. The results are reported as mean cpm from four different experiments. a: $P < 0.01$ (ANOVA).

by effector T cells.[23] However, TLRs stimulation by microbial product in DCs results in production of inflammatory cytokines, such as IL-6 that has been involved in decreasing the $CD4^+$, $CD25^-$ Th cell sensitivity to the suppressive action of Treg cells.[24] This effect has been suggested to promote autoimmune reactions during microbial infections. In fact, Treg cell number and function have been shown to be impaired in autoimmune prone animals.[25,26] We investigated whether the β2-AR-dependent IL-10 stimulation could also inhibit TNF-α and IL-6 production in TLR-stimulated DCs. TABLE 1 shows that addition of NE in DCs cultures stimulated by the TLR2 agonist lipoteichoic acid (LTA) resulted in decreased IL-6 and TNF-α and that anti-IL-10 mAb prevented the NE-dependent inhibition of these cytokines. We then set up a Treg cell assay (as described in Ref. 24) in order to study whether the increase of IL-10 and the inhibition of IL-6 production would allow antigen-specific

Treg cells to exert their suppressive action even in presence of a TLR agonist. Indeed, when NE was present in the Treg assay the suppressive effect on $CD4^+$, Th proliferation was maintained even in the presence of TLR4 agonist LPS (FIG. 1). Thus, besides shaping the appropriate immune response to the invading pathogen, NE (i.e., the SNS activity) might decrease the probability of autoimmune reactions by allowing the suppressive function of Treg cells during a microbial infection.

THE SNS INFLUENCE ON THE CUTANEOUS IMMUNE RESPONSE

The skin is the largest organ of the body and plays a central role in host defense. Epidermal keratinocytes (EKs) are important albeit underappreciated players in cutaneous immune responses. They express TLRs[27,28] and produce large quantity and variety of cytokines in response to infectious agents, kinetic and thermal trauma, and ultraviolet radiation.[29,30] These products have various effects on resident immune cells in the skin, such as LCs, DCs, mast cells, and macrophages resulting in stimulation of the expression of other inducible mediators and costimulatory molecules. The resulting inflammatory reaction activates LCs and dermal DCs, which emigrate to the draining lymph nodes carrying antigen for presentation to naive and memory T cells. It has also been reported that EKs express β2-ARs and may synthesize and release catecholamines.[31–33] The importance of this system has been studied in skin disorders. In vitiligo, there is a dysregulation of catecholamine biosynthesis with increased plasma and epidermal NE levels associated with high numbers of β2-ARs in differentiating keratinocytes and with a defective calcium uptake in both keratinocytes and melanocytes. In atopic eczema, a point mutation in the β-AR gene could alter the structure and function of the receptor, thereby leading to a low density of receptors on both keratinocytes and peripheral blood lymphocytes.[6] In psoriasis, β-ARs are downregulated and, interestingly, β-AR blockers may cause this inflammatory autoimmune skin disease.[4,5,34] Thus, on one hand, the evidence of an important participation of EKs in cutaneous immune responses, whose regulation is deranged in inflammatory skin disorders and possibly skin tumors, is rather clear.[7] On the other hand, various reports show alterations of catecholamine biosynthesis and β-ARs expression in EKs in the same inflammatory skin diseases. What is clearly missing is a study relating the two systems.

In the attempt to fill this gap, we first investigated the constitutive TLR2 and TLR4 mRNA expression in EKs with that of skin LCs and bone marrow-derived murine DCs. The analysis was performed by real time reverse transcriptase polymerase chain reaction (RT-PCR) taking bone marrow-derived DCs as reference. The results obtained indicate that the constitutive expression of TLR2 and TLR4 mRNA was similar in LCs and bone marrow-derived

influence might be exerted directly on the resident DCs. Alternatively, the adrenergic regulation of DCs might be of some relevance only in the tolerogenic function of these cells, that is, self-antigens presentation in the absence of co-stimulatory molecules upregulation and/or modulation of Treg function.

ACKNOWLEDGMENTS

The skillful technical assistance of Mrs. Elisabeth Hertens and Mrs. Paola Galli is acknowledged. These studies were supported by the Swiss National Science Foundation, grant no. 310000-107524/1.

REFERENCES

1. MAESTRONI, G.J.M. 2000. Dendritic cells migration controlled by α1b-adrenergic receptors. J. Immunol. **165:** 6743–6747.
2. MAESTRONI, G.J.M. 2002. Short exposure of antigen-stimulated dendritic cells to norepinephrine: impact on kinetic of cytokine production and Th polarization. J. Neuroimmunol. **129:** 106–114.
3. MAESTRONI, G.J.M. 2004. Modulation of skin norepinephrine turnover by allergen sensitization: impact on contact hypersensitivity and Th priming. J. Invest. Dermatol. **122:** 119–124.
4. STEINKRAUS, V. *et al.* 1993. Beta-adrenergic receptors in psoriasis: evidence for down-regulation in lesional skin. Arch. Dermatol. Res. **285:** 300–304.
5. HALEVY, S. & E. LIVNI. 1993. Beta-adrenergic blocking drugs and psoriasis: the role of an immunologic mechanism. J. Am. Acad. Dermatol. **29:** 504–505.
6. SCHALLREUTER, K.U. 1997. Epidermal adrenergic signal transduction as part of the neuronal network in the human epidermis. J. Investig. Dermatol. Symp. Proc. **2:** 37–40.
7. KUPPER, T.S. & R.C. FUHLBRIGGE. 2004. Immune surveillance in the skin: mechanisms and clinical consequences. Nat. Rev. Immunol. **4:** 211–222.
8. SHORTMAN, K. & C. CAUX. 1997. Dendritic cell development: multiple pathways to nature's adjuvants. Stem Cells **15:** 409–419.
9. SALLGALLER, M.L. & P.A. LODGE. 1998. Use of cellular and cytokine adjuvants in the immunotherapy of cancer. J. Surg. Oncol. **68:** 122–138.
10. WEINLICH, G. *et al.* 1998. Entry into lymphatics and maturation in situ of migrating murine cutaneous dendritic cells. J. Invest. Dermatol. **110:** 441–448.
11. BANCHERAU, J. & R.M. STEINMAN. 1998. Dendritic cells and the control of immunity. Nature **392:** 245–252.
12. SCHNARE, M. *et al.* 2001. Toll-like receptors control activation of adaptive immune responses. Nat. Immunol. **2:** 947–950.
13. KALINSKI, P. *et al.* 1999. T-cell priming by type-1 and type-2 polarized dendritic cells: the concept of a third signal. Immunol. Today **20:** 561–567.
14. PULENDRAN, B., K. PALUCKA & J. BANCHEREAU. 2001. Sensing pathogens and tuning immune responses. Science **293:** 253–256.
15. MAESTRONI, G.J. 2000. Dendritic cell migration controlled by alpha 1b-adrenergic receptors. J. Immunol. **165:** 6743–6747.

16. MAESTRONI, G.J. & P. MAZZOLA. 2003. Langerhans cells beta 2-adrenoceptors: role in migration, cytokine production, Th priming and contact hypersensitivity. J. Neuroimmunol. **144:** 91–99.
17. MAESTRONI, G.J. 2002. Short exposure of maturing, bone marrow-derived dendritic cells to norepinephrine: impact on kinetics of cytokine production and Th development. J. Neuroimmunol. **129:** 106–114.
18. SEIFFERT, C. *et al.* 2002. Catecholamines inhibit the antigen-presenting capability of epidermal Langerhans cells. J. Immunol. **168:** 6128–6135.
19. STRAUB, R.H. *et al.* 2000. A bacteria-induced switch of sympathetic effector mechanisms augments local inhibition of TNF-alpha and IL-6 secretion in the spleen. FASEB J. **14:** 1380–1388.
20. RICE, P.A. *et al.* 2001. Chemical sympathectomy increases the innate immune response and decreases the specific immune response in the spleen to infection with Listeria monocytogenes. J. Neuroimmunol. **114:** 19–27.
21. MIURA, K. *et al.* 2001. Effect of 6-hydroxydopamine on host resistance against Listeria monocytogenes infection. Infect. Immun. **69:** 7234–7241.
22. MISRA, N. *et al.* 2004. Cutting edge: human CD4+CD25+ T cells restrain the maturation and antigen-presenting function of dendritic cells. J. Immunol. **172:** 4676–4680.
23. COLANTONIO, L. *et al.* 2002. Skin-homing CLA+ T cells and regulatory CD25+ T cells represent major subsets of human peripheral blood memory T cells migrating in response to CCL1/I-309. Eur. J. Immunol. **32:** 3506–3514.
24. PASARE, C. & R. MEDZHITOV. 2003. Toll pathway-dependent blockade of CD4+CD25+ T cell-mediated suppression by dendritic cells. Science **299:** 1033–1036.
25. SALOMON, B. *et al.* 2000. B7/CD28 costimulation is essential for the homeostasis of the CD4+CD25+ immunoregulatory T cells that control autoimmune diabetes. Immunity **12:** 431–440.
26. WU, A.J. *et al.* 2002. Tumor necrosis factor-alpha regulation of CD4+CD25+ T cell levels in NOD mice. Proc. Natl. Acad. Sci. USA **99:** 12287–12292.
27. MEDZHITOV, R. 2001. Toll-like receptors and innate immunity. Nature Rev. Immunol. **1:** 135–145.
28. TAKEDA, K., T. KAISHO & S. AKIRA. 2003. Toll-like receptors. Annu. Rev. Immunol. **21:** 335–376.
29. KUPPER, T.S. & R.W. GROVES. 1995. The interleukin-1 axis and cutaneous inflammation. J. Invest. Dermatol. **105:** 62S–66S.
30. GRONE, A. 2002. Keratinocytes and cytokines. Vet. Immunol. Immunopathol. **88:** 1–12.
31. SCHALLREUTER, K.U. *et al.* 1995. Catecholamines in human keratinocyte differentiation. J. Invest. Dermatol. **104:** 953–957.
32. CHEN, J., B.B. HOFFMAN & R.R. ISSEROFF. 2002. Beta-adrenergic receptor activation inhibits keratinocyte migration via a cyclic adenosine monophosphate-independent mechanism. J. Invest. Dermatol. **119:** 1261–1268.
33. PULLAR, C.E., J. CHEN & R.R. ISSEROFF. 2003. PP2A activation by beta2-adrenergic receptor agonists: novel regulatory mechanism of keratinocyte migration. J. Biol. Chem. **278:** 22555–22562.
34. YILMAZ, M.B. *et al.* 2002. Beta-blocker-induced psoriasis: a rare side effect—a case report. Angiology **53:** 737–739.

35. BAKER, B.S. *et al.* 2003. Normal keratinocytes express toll-like receptors (TLRs) 1, 2 and 5: modulation of TLR expression in chronic plaque psoriasis. Br. J. Dermatol. **148:** 670–679.
36. MEMPEL, M. *et al.* 2003. Toll-like receptor expression in human keratinocytes: nuclear factor kappaB controlled gene activation by Staphylococcus aureus is toll-like receptor 2 but not toll-like receptor 4 or platelet activating factor receptor dependent. J. Invest. Dermatol. **121:** 1389–1396.
37. KRUEGER, J.G. & A. BOWCOCK. 2005. Psoriasis pathophysiology: current concepts of pathogenesis. Ann. Rheum. Dis. **64:** ii30–ii36.
38. MITTERMANN, I. *et al.* 2004. Autoimmunity and atopic dermatitis. Curr. Opin. Allergy Clin. Immunol. **4:** 367–371.
39. OU, L.S. *et al.* 2004. T regulatory cells in atopic dermatitis and subversion of their activity by superantigens. J. Allergy Clin. Immunol. **113:** 756–763.
40. GRACA, L. *et al.* 2004. Donor-specific transplantation tolerance: the paradoxical behavior of CD4+CD25+ T cells. Proc. Natl. Acad. Sci. USA **101:** 10122–10126.
41. SAINT-MEZARD, P. *et al.* 2004. The role of CD4+ and CD8+ T cells in contact hypersensitivity and allergic contact dermatitis. Eur. J. Dermatol. **14:** 131–138.
42. MCELWEE, K.J. *et al.* 2003. Alopecia areata susceptibility in rodent models. J. Investig. Dermatol. Symp. Proc. **8:** 182–187.

Alexithymia and Neuroendocrine-Immune Response in Patients with Autoimmune Diseases

Preliminary Results on Relationship between Alexithymic Construct and TNF-α Levels

R. BRUNI,[a] F.M. SERINO,[b] S. GALLUZZO,[c] G. COPPOLINO,[c]
F. CACCIAPAGLIA,[c] M. VADACCA,[c] S. NILO,[c] N. TERMINIO,[a]
AND A. AFELTRA[c]

[a]*Department of Psychiatry,* [b]*Department of Immunology and Clinical Medicine,* [c]*Department of Geriatrics, University "Campus Bio-Medico," Rome, Italy*

ABSTRACT: Alexithymia is conceptualized as a disorder of emotion regulation mechanisms, which involves a dissociation of emotional and physic responses to life events and bodily sensations. Our results might suggest a possible relationship between the alexithymic construct and TNF levels in RA patients. These preliminary findings corroborate the integrated bidirectional interactions between neuropsychological mechanisms and the neuroendocrine-immune system in patients affected by autoimmune diseases and contribute to finding a common biological pathway linking alexithymia and autoimmune-inflammatory diseases.

KEYWORDS: Alexithymia; rheumatoid arthritis; neuroendocrine immune system; TNF-α

Alexithymia is conceptualized as a disorder of emotion-regulation mechanisms[1] that involves a dissociation of emotional and physical responses to life events and bodily sensations. Disturbance of affect regulation (dysregulation model) is linked to failure in psychological self-regulation and deficit in experiencing emotional life. Although the alexithymia construct was formulated to identify affective and cognitive characteristics of patients with psychosomatic diseases, previous empirical studies have shown some evidence that alexithymia may be associated more strongly with functional somatic symptoms than with psychosomatic disorders.[2] Connective tissue diseases are

Address for correspondence: Dr. R. Bruni, Dipartimento di Informatica e Sistemistica "A. Ruberti" Università degli Studi di Roma "La Sapienza", Via M. Buonarroti, 12-00185 Roma, Italy. Voice: +39 06 482 99 213; fax: +39 06 478 25 618.
e-mail: bruni@dis.uniroma1.it

Ann. N.Y. Acad. Sci. 1069: 208–211 (2006).
doi: 10.1196/annals.1351.018

chronic inflammatory conditions, the more representative among them being rheumatoid arthritis (RA) and systemic lupus erythematosus (SLE). Patients affected by RA and SLE are subject to physical and/or psychological stress.[3] Usually, homeostasis is maintained by the action of the neuroendocrine immune system, which works to count mental and physical stresses.[4] The stress-response system is made up of psychological and neuroendocrine components that are activated by a variety of physical and mental stressors. It is believed that activation of the HPA axis by cytokines allows regulation of the immune response by the neuroendocrine system through a long-loop feedback mechanism. In addition, cognitive signals perceived as threatening to physiologic equilibrium and homeostasis may modify normal immune functions.[5]

OBJECTIVE

The purpose of the study was to investigate the possible interactions between alexithymia and the neuroendocrine immune response.

METHODS

We studied 81 patients: (*a*) 27 female patients (mean age: 6.74 ± 12.66 yr; disease duration: 11.41 ± 10.91 yr) with RA diagnosed according to the 1987 revised ARA criteria; (*b*) 27 female patients (mean age: 45.33 ± 10.94; disease duration: 11.53 ± 9.8) with SLE diagnosed according to the 1997 revised ARA criteria; and (*c*) a comparable group of healthy controls. All patients underwent a semi-structured interview and completed several questionnaires, including the Italian translation of the Toronto Alexithymia Scale, 20-item version (TAS-20).[6] TAS-20 score ≥51 was considered as an indicator of high alexithymia. Serum concentrations of: GH, PRL, and TNF-α were determined by ELISA using commercially available kits. SLE activity was assessed by the SLE Disease Activity Index (SLEDAI) score and RA activity was evaluated using the Disease Activity Score (DAS). ANOVA-Bonferroni test was used for statistical analysis (significant values: $P < 0.05$).

RESULTS

GH plasma concentrations were lower in patients affected by SLE (1.63 ± 2.2 μIU/mL) compared with RA (2.4 ± 3.5 μIU/mL) and the control group (2.4 ± 3.8 μIU/mL), but no statistical difference was found. Conversely, prolactin concentrations in the SLE group (22.03 ± 9.7 ng/mL) were statistically higher than in the RA (16.3 ± 8.3 ng/mL) and control groups (14.2 ± 5.9 ng/mL) ($P < 0.05$). TNF-α serum levels (4.9 ± 12.8 pg/mL in SLE group, 28 ± 33.5 in RA group, 2.4 ± 3.8 μIU/mL in control group) were significantly higher in RA than in the SLE and control groups ($P < 0.01$). Furthermore, in patients with high disease activity RA (DAS > 3.7) the TNF-α average serum concentrations were increased compared to those with DAS < 3.7 (68.46 ± 119 pg/mL vs. 45.2 ± pg/mL, P = NS). Both the RA and SLE populations were separated in two groups depending on the level of alexithymia, with discriminatory value established at score 51: a high-level alexithymia group (HA) with score ≥51 and a low-level alexithymia group (LA) with score <50. HA prevalence was, respectively, 61.53% in RA and 50% in SLE. The HA RA group showed mean TAS-20 values of 61.84 ± 12.90 while the HA SLE scored 54.46 ± 17.95. In RA patients, we observed a significant correlation between high alexithymia and TNF-α concentrations (27.03 ± 15.06 vs 13.03 ± 11.08, $P < 0.05$).

DISCUSSION

TNF-α exerts a wide variety of relevant immunoregulatory functions on a multiplicity of cells of the innate and adaptive immune system. This cytokine exerts a significant influence on B cells by virtue of its capacity to induce IL-6 or via T helper type 1 and T helper type 2 cells. Contrasting evidence has been reported in the literature about TNF-α role in SLE, supporting its capacity as a prime immune modulator or its role as a proinflammatory mediator. Our results demonstrated TNF-α serum levels significantly higher in the RA group than in the SLE and control groups. Furthermore, TNF-α concentrations correlate positively with disease activity in RA patients. Moreover, in the same group, we observed a significant positive correlation between degree of alexithymia and TNF-α concentrations. Our study confirms the importance of TNF-α as a key mediator of inflammation and tissue destruction in RA. Some authors reported that alexithymia is related to impaired immune response.[7] Our results suggest a possible relationship between the alexithymic construct and TNF-α levels in RA patients. These preliminary findings corroborate the integrated bidirectionally interactions between neuropsychological mechanisms and the neuroendocrine immune system in patients affected by autoimmune diseases, and contribute to find a common biological pathway linking alexithymia and autoimmune inflammatory diseases.

REFERENCES

1. Sifneos, P.E. 1973. The prevalence of "alexithymic" characteristics in psychosomatic patients. Psychother. Psychosom. **22:** 255–262.
2. Taylor, G.J. *et al.* 2000. An overview of the alexithymia construct. *In* Handbook of Emotional Intelligence. R. Bar-On & J.D.A. Parker, Eds.: 301–319. Jossey-Bass. San Francisco.

3. CUTOLO, M. *et al.* 1999. Is stress a factor in the pathogenesis of autoimmune rheumatic diseases? Clin. Exp. Rheumatol. **17:** 515–518.
4. BIJLSMA, J.W. *et al.* 2005. Clinical aspects of immune neuroendocrine mechanisms in rheumatic diseases. Rheum. Dis. Clin. North. Am. **31:** 13–14.
5. ADER, R., N. COHEN & D. FELTON. 1995. Psychoneuroimmunology: interactions between the nervous system and the immune system. Lancet **345:** 99–103.
6. BRESSI, C. *et al.* 1996. Cross validation of the factor structure of the 20-item Toronto Alexithmia Scale: an Italian multicenter study. J. Psychosom. Res. **41:** 551–559.
7. GUILBAUD, O. *et al.* 2003. Is there a psychoneuroimmunological pathway between alexithymia and immunity? Immune and physiological correlates of alexithymia. Biomed. Pharmacother. **57:** 292–295.

Epidemiological Aspects of Rheumatoid Arthritis

The Sex Ratio

TORE K. KVIEN, TILL UHLIG, SIGRID ØDEGÅRD, AND MARTE S. HEIBERG

Department of Rheumatology Diakonhjemmet Hospital, N-0319 Oslo, Norway

ABSTRACT: Many rheumatic diseases, including rheumatoid arthrits (RA) are more frequent in females than males. The objective of this article was to examine the female versus male perspective regarding prevalence/incidence, etiological factors, disease severity/outcomes, access to therapy and therapeutic responses. We also present results from some new analyses from the patient registers in Oslo to supplement existing literature in this area. We found that the prevalence of RA is higher in females than males, the incidence is 4–5 times higher below the age of 50, but above 60–70 years the female/male ratio is only about 2. Smoking is a consistent predictor of RA in males, but findings have been more inconsistent in females. We could not confirm that health status is worse in females than males when corrections were made for different disease duration and for the underlying tendency of healthy females to report worse subjective health status than males. Some studies and data presented here indicate that females have less access to health services. We also found that female sex reduces the likelihood of achiving treatment response with methotrexate and anti-tumor necrosis factor (anti-TNF) drugs by 30–50%. More research is needed to fully describe the differences between males and females regarding epidemiological data.

KEYWORDS: rheumatoid arthritis; incidence; prevalence; health status; outcomes; mortality; work disability; ani-TNF drugs; methotrexate; EULAR response; remission

INTRODUCTION

Rheumatoid arthritis (RA) is a heterogeneous inflammatory disease, with a natural history that often includes a disabling outcome and reduced life expectancy. Epidemiological studies in Scandinavia have revealed an annual

Address for correspondence: Tore K. Kvien, Department of Rheumatology, Diakonhjemmet Hospital, Box 23 Vinderen, N-0319 Oslo, Norway. Voice: +47 22 45 1500; fax: +47 22 47 1778.
e-mail: t.k.kvien@medisin.uio.no

Ann. N.Y. Acad. Sci. 1069: 212–222 (2006). © 2006 New York Academy of Sciences.
doi: 10.1196/annals.1351.019

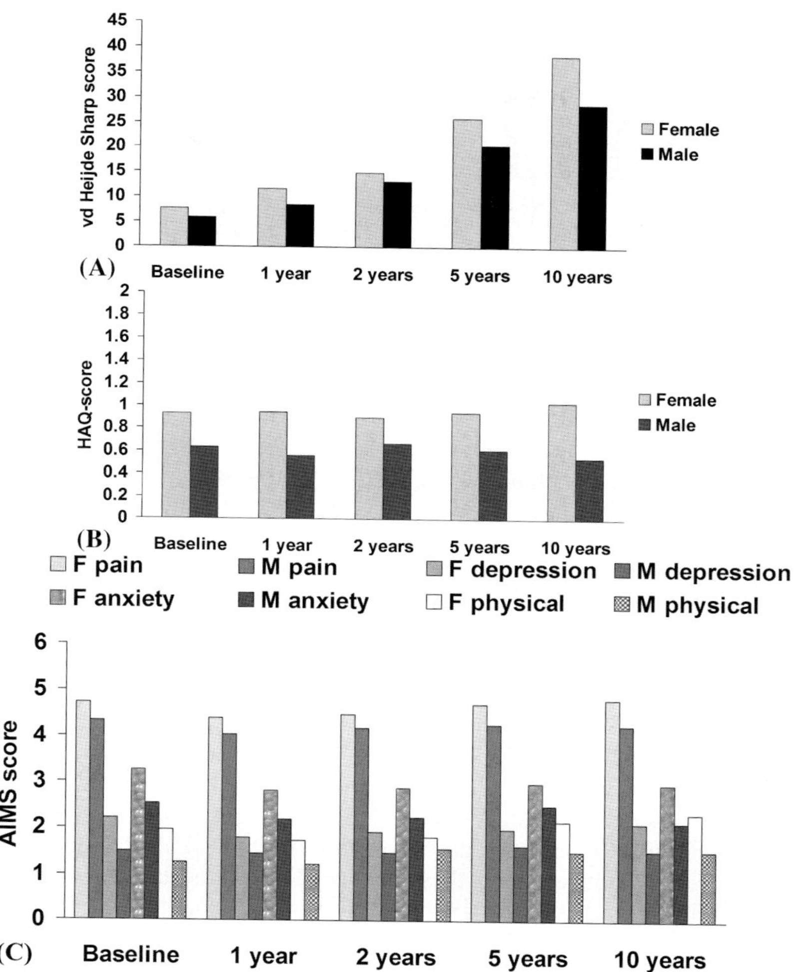

FIGURE 2. Longitudinal data from 149 patients with RA comparing outcomes between females and males. (**A**) Modified van der Heijde/ Sharp radiographic damage score. (**B**) Physical disability measured by HAQ. (**C**) Health status including psychological measures assessed by AIMS.

at the baseline examination. The progression rate was similar across sexes. Measures of health-related quality of life were consistently worse in females than males at baseline, both for physical disability (HAQ and AIMS) as well as pain, depression, and anxiety scores (FIG. 2B and C). However, the average changes over time seemed to be similar (FIG. 2B and C).

Healthy females report worse health status scores than healthy males. In the population data from Norway, Loge *et al.*[24] reported that the SF-36

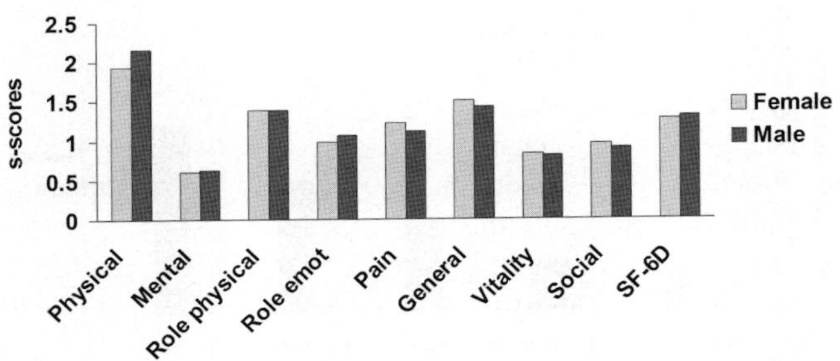

FIGURE 3. S-scores to describe the difference between female and male RA patients and the healthy population across the dimensions of SF-36.

physical functioning score was 89.8 in males and 84.8 in females. Score for males/females in some other dimesions were 80.0 and 77.6 for mental health, 77.2 and 73.0 for bodily pain, and 63.2 and 56.9 for vitality, respectively. Thus, comparison of health status in patients across sexes should ideally adjust for this underlying difference in reporting subjective health. One approach, which is only possible for generic health status measures, is to calculate s-scores, which represent the difference between patients and healthy controls (e.g., by the use of SF-36) divided by the standard deviations of the healthy controls. We had the opportunity to compare s-scores for patients in the Oslo RA register. FIGURE 3 shows that the s-scores differed across dimensions of health, but we could not observe any consistent difference between males and females.

Other important outcomes are work disability and mortality. Ødegård *et al.*[25] found that females with RA have an independent threefold increased risk of work disability during 7-year follow-up compared to males. RA is associated with an increased overall risk of mortality[26] and also cardiovascular mortality.[27,28] Results regarding the influence of sex on mortality have been inconsistent. Early studies by Wolfe *et al.*[26] suggested that male sex was an independent predictor of reduced survival, whereas Gabriel and co-workers[29] found that excess mortality among women was more pronounced than among men, with standardized mortality rates of 1.41 and 1.08, respectively.

ACCESS TO THERAPY AND CARE

Lard *et al.*[30] examined whether sex differences in referral exist in patients with RA. General practitioners (GPs) were encouraged to refer patients with joint complaints to an early arthritis clinic. The delays in patient's first encounter with a general practitioner for both sexes were comparable. However, a significant difference in the GP's delay in referring female patients with RA to the early arthritis clinic in comparison with male patients was observed (median of 93 days versus 58 days; $P = 0.008$).[30] A recent Norwegian study also demonstrated a delay in the referral of female patients to rheumatologist.[31]

The Norwegian NOR-DMARD study includes consecutive patients with inflammatory arthropathies starting with DMARD regimens in five Norwegian rheumatology departments, covering a population of about 1.2 million.[32,33] The selections of DMARD regimen is based on clinical judgment supported by current recommendations of selecting anti-TNF therapies.[34] We know that the prescription pattern of anti-TNF drugs is similar in Denmark and Norway, and that the disease activity and severity of patients starting with biological agents are similar.[35] The current analysis was focusing on 1754 RA patients who started either anti-TNF drugs or methotrexate (MTX). Of these 1754 patients, 39.0% of the females and 38.9% of the males had received anti-TNF drugs ($P = 0.96$). However, the female patients had more active and severe disease, e.g., the average disease activity score was 5.32 in females and 4.93 in males ($P < 0.001$) and the average number of previous DMARD regimens was 2.32 versus 1.86 ($P = 0.001$). Thus, a larger proportion of female than male patients should presumably have received anti-TNF treatment. In a logistic regression analyses, adjusting for age, disease duration, level of education, presence of erosive disease and rheumatoid factor, baseline disease activity score, and the number of previous DMARD regimens, we found that the likelihood ratio of receiving anti-TNF versus MTX in females compared to males was 0.56 (95% CI 0.42, 0.75, $P < 0.001$)

TREATMENT EFFECT

Few studies have addressed whether sex is a predictor of clinical response in randomized controlled clinical trials. For extrapolation to clinical practice, predictors of responses identified through real life observational studies may be even more important. We examined data from the Norwegian NOR-DMARD study[32,33] to explore whether sex is a predictor of treatment response in RA patients starting with MTX or anti-TNF drugs. The proportions of male and

TABLE 2. Proportions of females and males achieving EULAR good response and remission after real life treatment with MTX and anti-TNF drugs

	MTX		Anti-TNF	
	Female ($n = 553$)	Male ($n = 217$)	Female ($n = 325$)	Male ($n = 123$)
EULAR good response				
3 months	18.4	23.0	21.8	27.6
6 months	23.4	32.2	21.8	35.3
12 months	26.3	34.2	22.5	32.4
Remission				
3 months	15.1	21.6	11.4	24.2
6 months	15.9	29.4	11.7	28.3
12 months	21.4	32.8	12.5	27.0

female patients who achieved European league against rheumatism (EULAR) good response and remission were compared. TABLE 2 shows that response rates were lower in females than males, and these differences were consistent both in MTX and anti-TNF-treated patients. Since the female patients overall had a more severe and active disease than the male patients, we also performed logistic regression analyses adjusting for age, disease duration, presence of erosive disease and rheumatoid factor, baseline disease activity score, and the number of previous DMARD regimens. The likelihood of achieving responses remained to be between 30% and 50% lower for females than males after these adjustments (data not shown).

CONCLUSIONS

We have in this article, supplemented with new analyses from patient registers in Norway, shown that the incidence of RA is declining, that this decreased incidence is especially seen in females, and that there may be a shift in the incidence toward higher age. The general perception that females have a more severe disease than males was not confirmed if adjustments are made for disease duration and the underlying tendency of worse health status reporting by the female versus male population. Some studies indicate that female RA patients have less access to health care than males, and we show that response rates with DMARDs, including anti-TNF drugs are lower in females than males.

REFERENCES

1. UHLIG, T., T.K. KVIEN, A. GLENNAS, *et al.* 1998. The incidence and severity of rheumatoid arthritis, results from a county register in Oslo, Norway. J. Rheumatol. **25:** 1078–1084.
2. KVIEN, T.K., A. GLENNAS, O.G. KNUDSROD, *et al.* 1997. The prevalence and severity of rheumatoid arthritis in Oslo. Results from a county register and a population survey. Scand. J. Rheumatol. **26:** 412–418.
3. BUCKWALTER, J.A. & D.R. LAPPIN. 2000. The disproportionate impact of chronic arthralgia and arthritis among women. Clin. Orthop. Relat. Res. **372:** 159–168.
4. SYMMONS, D.P., E.M. BARRETT, C.R. BANKHEAD, *et al.* 1994. The incidence of rheumatoid arthritis in the United Kingdom: results from the Norfolk Arthritis Register. Br. J. Rheumatol. **33:** 735–739.
5. SODERLIN, M.K., O. BORJESSON, H. KAUTIAINEN, *et al.* 2002. Annual incidence of inflammatory joint diseases in a population based study in southern Sweden. Ann. Rheum. Dis. **61:** 911–915.
6. UHLIG, T. & T.K. KVIEN. 2005. Is rheumatoid arthritis disappearing? Ann. Rheum. Dis. **64:** 7–10.
7. SHICHIKAWA, K., K. INOUE, *et al.* 1999. Changes in the incidence and prevalence of rheumatoid arthritis in Kamitonda, Wakayama, Japan, 1965–1996. Ann. Rheum. Dis. **58:** 751–756.

8. DORAN, M.F., G.R. POND, C.S. CROWSON, *et al.* 2002. Trends in incidence and mortality in rheumatoid arthritis in Rochester, Minnesota, over a forty-year period. Arthritis Rheum. **46:** 625–631.
9. JACOBSSON, L.T., R.L. HANSON, W.C. KNOWLER, *et al.* 1994. Decreasing incidence and prevalence of rheumatoid arthritis in Pima Indians over a twenty-five-year period. Arthritis Rheum. **37:** 1158–1165.
10. ENZER, I., G. DUNN, L. JACOBSSON, *et al.* 2002. An epidemiologic study of trends in prevalence of rheumatoid factor seropositivity in Pima Indians: evidence of a decline due to both secular and birth-cohort influences. Arthritis Rheum. **46:** 1729–1734.
11. KAIPIAINEN-SEPPANEN, O., K. AHO, H. ISOMAKI, *et al.* 1996. Incidence of rheumatoid arthritis in Finland during 1980–1990. Ann. Rheum. Dis. **55:** 608–611.
12. DORAN, M.F., C.S. CROWSON, W.M. O'FALLON, *et al.* 2004. The effect of oral contraceptives and estrogen replacement therapy on the risk of rheumatoid arthritis: a population based study. J. Rheumatol. **31:** 207–213.
13. KAIPIAINEN-SEPPANEN, O., K. AHO, H. ISOMAKI, *et al.* 1996. Shift in the incidence of rheumatoid arthritis toward elderly patients in Finland during 1975–1990. Clin. Exp. Rheumatol. **14:** 537–542.
14. KRISHNAN, E. 2003. Smoking, gender and rheumatoid arthritis-epidemiological clues to etiology. Results from the behavioral risk factor surveillance system. Joint Bone Spine **70:** 496–502.
15. KRISHNAN, E., T. SOKKA & P. HANNONEN. 2003. Smoking-gender interaction and risk for rheumatoid arthritis. Arthritis Res. Ther. **5:** R158–R162.
16. UHLIG, T., K.B. HAGEN & T.K. KVIEN. 1999. Current tobacco smoking, formal education, and the risk of rheumatoid arthritis. J. Rheumatol. **26:** 47–54.
17. DE VRIES, N., P.P. TAK, H. TIJSSEN, *et al.* 2003. Female sex increases risk for rheumatoid arthritis only in individuals encoding low-risk HLA-DRB1 alleles. Arthritis Rheum. **48:** 1762–1763.
18. SCHUNA, A.A. 2002. Autoimmune rheumatic diseases in women. J. Am. Pharm. Assoc. (Wash.) **42:** 623–624.
19. GOSSEC, L., J. BARO-RIBA, M.C. BOZONNAT, *et al.* 2005. Influence of sex on disease severity in patients with rheumatoid arthritis. J. Rheumatol. **32:** 1448–1451.
20. WEYAND, C.M., D. SCHMIDT, U. WAGNER, *et al.* 1998. The influence of sex on the phenotype of rheumatoid arthritis. Arthritis Rheum. **41:** 817–822.
21. KVIEN, T.K. & T. UHLIG. 2003. The Oslo experience with arthritis registries. Clin. Exp. Rheumatol. **21:** S118–S122.
22. DOWDY, S.W., K.A. DWYER, C.A. SMITH, *et al.* Gender and psychological well-being of persons with rheumatoid arthritis. Arthritis. Care. Res. **9:** 449–456.
23. ØDEGÅRD, S., R.B.M. LANDEWE, D. VAN DER HEIJDE, *et al.* 2006. Radiographic damage predicts physical disability in rheumatoid arthritis: a 10-year longitudinal observational study of 238 patients. Arthritis Rheum. **54:** 68–75.
24. LOGE, J.H. & S. KAASA. 1998. Short form 36 (SF-36) health survey: normative data from the general Norwegian population. Scand. J. Soc. Med. **26:** 250–258.
25. ØDEGÅRD, S., T.K. KVIEN, A. FINSET, *et al.* 2005. Physical and psychological predictors for work disability over seven years in patients with rheumatoid arthritis. Scand. J. Rheumatol. **34:** 441–447.
26. WOLFE, F., D.M. MITCHELL, J.T. SIBLEY, *et al.* 1994. The mortality of rheumatoid arthritis. Arthritis Rheum. **37:** 481–494.

27. Douglas, K.M., A.V. Pace, G.J. Treharne, *et al.* 2006. Excess recurrent cardiac events in rheumatoid arthritis patients with acute coronary syndrome. Ann. Rheum. Dis. **65:** 348–353.
28. Wolfe, F., B. Freundlich & W.L. Straus. 2003. Increase in cardiovascular and cerebrovascular disease prevalence in rheumatoid arthritis. J. Rheumatol. **30:** 36–40.
29. Gabriel, S.E., C.S. Crowson, H.M. Kremers, *et al.* 2003. Survival in rheumatoid arthritis: a population-based analysis of trends over 40 years. Arthritis Rheum. **48:** 54–58.
30. Lard, L.R., T.W. Huizinga, J.M. Hazes, *et al.* 2001. Delayed referral of female patients with rheumatoid arthritis. J. Rheumatol. **28:** 2190–2192.
31. Palm, Ø. & E. Purinszky. 2005. Women with early rheumatoid arthritis are referred later than men. Ann. Rheum. Dis. **64:** 1227–1228.
32. Heiberg, M.S., B.Y. Nordvag, K. Mikkelsen, *et al.* 2005. The comparative effectiveness of tumor necrosis factor-blocking agents in patients with rheumatoid arthritis and patients with ankylosing spondylitis: a six-month, longitudinal, observational, multicenter study. Arthritis Rheum. **52:** 2506–2512.
33. Kvien, T.K., M.S. Heiberg, E. Lie, *et al.* 2005. A Norwegian DMARD register: prescriptions of DMARDs and biological agents to patients with inflammatory rheumatic diseases. Clin. Exp. Rheumatol. **23**(Suppl 39): 5188–5194.
34. Furst, D.E., F.C. Breedveld, J.R. Kalden, *et al.* 2004. Updated consensus statement on biological agents, specifically tumour necrosis factor alpha (TNFalpha) blocking agents and interleukin-1 receptor antagonist (IL-1ra), for the treatment of rheumatic diseases, 2004. Ann. Rheum. Dis. **63:** ii2–ii12.
35. Hjardem, E., M.L. Hetland, M. Ostergaard, *et al.* 2005. Prescription practice of biological drugs in rheumatoid arthritis during the first 3 years of post-marketing use in Denmark and Norway: criteria are becoming less stringent. Ann. Rheum. Dis. **64:** 1220–1223.

Sex Hormones and Risks of Rheumatoid Arthritis and Developmental or Environmental Influences

ALFONSE T. MASI,[a] JEAN C. ALDAG,[b] AND ROBERT T. CHATTERTON[c]

[a]*Department of Medicine, University of Illinois College of Medicine at Peoria (UICOMP), Illinois, USA*

[b]*Department of Medicine and Clinical Pharmacology, University of Illinois College of Medicine at Peoria (UICOMP), Illinois, USA*

[c]*Departments of OB/GYN and Physiology, Feinberg School of Medicine, Northwestern University, Chicago, Illinois, USA*

ABSTRACT: Sex hormone relationships for onset risks of rheumatoid arthritis (RA) were analyzed in a nested case–control study, derived from a large community-based prospective cohort. A self-reported history of RA in a first-degree relative, heavy cigarette smoking, and positive rheumatoid factor (RF) were confirmed predictors of subsequent RA onset in this data set. In the 11 premenopausal onset cases, lower serum dehydroepiandrosterone sulfate levels were observed as was an imbalance in serum IL-1β to IL-1ra levels; the latter was not observed in the 43 controls (CNs). In the 18 male cases, significantly higher serum cortisol was observed in the six cases with positive family history versus the 12 with a negative history. To the contrary, a small minority of the male cases had combined low serum cortisol and testosterone, which was not observed in the 72 CNs. Significant gender dimorphism was observed between the sex hormones and serum log RF titers as well as in the correlations of serum log testosterone and estradiol. Principal component analysis of multiply-imputed data sets extracted four uncorrelated components, which provided concordant neuroendocrine immune relationships to the previously investigated univariate and multivariate analyses. The literature on developmental and environmental influences on sex hormones and risks of RA was reviewed.

KEYWORDS: rheumatoid arthritis; neuroendocrine; immune; sex hormones; risk factors; familial predisposition; cigarette smoking; environmental hazards

Address for correspondence: Alfonse T. Masi, M.D., Department of Medicine, University of Illinois College of Medicine at Peoria (UICOMP), One Illini Drive, Peoria IL 61605. Voice: 309 671-8428; fax: 309 671-8528.

e-mail: amasi@uic.edu

Ann. N.Y. Acad. Sci. 1069: 223–235 (2006). © 2006 New York Academy of Sciences.
doi: 10.1196/annals.1351.020

INTRODUCTION

The relationship of sex hormones to the risk of developing rheumatoid arthritis (RA) is outlined in this article, and additional attention is given to the possible influences of developmental factors or environmental exposures. The physiopathogenesis of RA is unknown. However, it is believed to importantly involve neuroendocrine immune (NEI) dysregulation and microvascular endothelial activation pathways.[1–6] The long-term evolution of RA is complex and its disease expression is heterogeneous.[7,8] The clinically recognized, inflammatory phase involves varied course patterns and outcomes. Such heterogeneity is believed to result from host differences in immunological responsiveness, for example, rheumatoid factor (RF) production[7–9] and familial or genetic susceptibility factors.[3,7–10] Additional risk factors for RA include aging and female gender.[3] The largest ratio of female-to-male (F:M) age-specific incidence of RA, that is, approx. 5:1, occurs at the age of 20–50 years.[3,11] This important epidemiological finding indicates major roles of sex hormones or other gender-specific determinants in the risk of RA.[3–11] Furthermore, particular behavioral or environmental influences, for example, sufficient duration and intensity of cigarette smoking, have been documented to increase the risk of RA developing in both men and women.[6,12]

The first part of this review summarizes our earlier and newer findings on sex hormones in relation to risks of developing RA. The second section outlines a review of the literature related to developmental and environmental influences on the sex hormones. The background of the latter review as well as the literature retrieval methods, results, and interpretations from the literature are included in the second section.

CLINICAL-EPIDEMIOLOGICAL PERSPECTIVES ON INVESTIGATING THE COMPLEXITIES OF RA RISKS

The proposed model for onset of RA is a cumulative, multifactorial process, involving many risk factors, as mentioned above.[3,5–7] Since 1993, our research unit has been engaged in integrative analyses of data on baseline serum NEI factors, reports of familial disease occurrence and of the subject's cigarette smoking status as well as other demographic variables that may predict the subsequent outcome of RA. Our integrated results were recently summarized,[6] and support a model of RA which incorporates a multiyear *presymptomatic* (pre-RA) phase.[3–6] Although this concept is relatively new, it has been proposed previously by others and ourselves, as was recently reviewed.[6]

We have additionally proposed[6] that an early, dysregulated *physiological* phase can seamlessly or spontaneously transform into the symptomatic inflammatory phase,[7–9] which then becomes clinically evident. Currently, it is unknown whether or not particular immunological stimulation by specific antigenic peptide(s) may be required to initiate or "trigger" the enhanced clinical inflammatory phase.[6,9] We have emphasized prospective analyses in our research in order to attempt to decipher complex issues of sequential physiopathogenetic processes, as recently reviewed.[5,6]

Sex hormones have been included in the prospective analyses because of their demonstrated clinical and experimental effects upon immunological and inflammatory pathways related to RA.[10,13–16] However, discrimination of male versus female gender *per se* from sex hormone effects is challenging.[17–20] As indicated, age and sex are strong risk factors for the incident occurrence of RA.[11] Although these host-specific determinants are not well understood, we have accepted them in order to focus more precisely upon related NEI biomarkers and other personal factors. Accordingly, our research design analyzes data on age- and sex- matched pre-RA cases versus matched controls (CNs). Base-line data were obtained on pre-RA subjects enrolled in a large community-based cohort in 1974.[6] Following entry to the prospective study, 18 male and 36 female patients had developed onset of ACR criteria positive[21] for clinical RA after 3–20 years (mean of 12 years). Four CN subjects from the cohort were selected to match each pre-RA case on age (±2 years), sex, and race, all being caucasian.[6] Among multiple NEI factors, adrenal androgens and sex hormones have been studied in our Rheumatoid Arthritis Precursors Study (RAPS) data set.[6]

PREVIOUSLY IDENTIFIED NEI PREDICTORS FOR ONSET OF RA

A self-reported clinical history of RA in a first-degree relative (FDR), heavier cigarette smoking, and RF positivity are the major base-line predictive factors identified for the subsequent outcome of RA.[6] Pre-RA women with premenopausal onset of disease had lower levels of serum dehydroepiandrosterone sulphate (DHEAS) than their matched CNs,[6] as was also recently reported for clinical cases.[22] Six of the 11 patients with premenopausal onset also had an elevated base-line inflammatory cytokine (IL-1β, IL-6, or TNF-α) serum level *without* elevation of the respective immunological antagonist (IL-1ra) or the assayed receptors (sIL-2Rα and sTNF-R1), which was considered to be a "free" cytokine level.[3,6] None of the 43 CNs were observed to have such cytokine dysregulation ($P < 0.001$), which was mainly due to the IL-1β and IL-1ra imbalance.[6]

In multivariate analyses, men who had combined low baseline serum cortisol (<140 nmol/L) and low total testosterone (<10 nmol/L) had significant ($P < 0.01$) risk for RA outcome.[3,6] In partial correlation analysis with age adjustment,[23] low cortisol and relatively low testosterone (<15 nmol/L) were significantly ($P = 0.026$) correlated ($r = 0.536$).

TABLE 1. Spearman's correlations of IL-1β and TNF-α with luteinizing hormone (LH), androstenedione, and cortisol in female and male pre-symptomatic RA patients vs. Controls (CNs)

Sex and Subject Groups	LH		Adione		Cortisol	
	IL-1	TNF	IL-1	TNF	IL-1	TNF
Female CN (n = 82)	−0.319**	0.034	−0.100	−0.191[a]	−0.100	−0.071
Female RA (n = 15)	−0.518**[b]	−0.098[c]	0.024[d]	−0.227	0.012	0.170
Male CN (n = 60)	−0.055	−0.125[c]	0.020[f]	0.351**[a]	−0.036[g]	0.081
Male RA (n = 15)	0.338[b]	0.827***[c,e]	0.784***[d,f]	0.376	0.557*[g]	0.005

$^*P < 0.05$, $^{**}P < 0.010$, $^{***}P < 0.001$.
[a]TNF & adione- female vs. male CN, $P = 0.001$.
[b]IL-1 & LH-female vs. male RA, $P = 0.008$.
[c]TNF & LH- female vs. male RA, $P < 0.001$.
[d]IL-1 & adione-female vs. male RA, $P = 0.004$.
[e]TNF & LH-CN vs. RA males, $P < 0.001$.
[f]IL-1 & adione- CN vs. RA males, $P < 0.001$.
[g]IL-1 & cortisol- CN vs. RA males, $P = 0.030$.

In male cases, significant correlation was observed between a history of RA in FDR and serum cortisol levels, the mean level being higher ($P = 0.013$) in those with a positive history.[5,6] In addition, serum IL-1β positively correlated with androstenedione (adione) and cortisol levels in this male pre-RA group (TABLE 1). Two significant differences in correlations of baseline serum IL-1β versus TNF-α levels were observed with luteinizing hormone (LH), as also shown in TABLE 1. In 15 male patients with RA, a stronger ($P = 0.039$) correlation was observed of TNF-α ($r = 0.827$) than IL-1β ($r = 0.338$) with LH. In the larger sample of 82 female CNs, the negative correlation of IL-1β with LH ($r = -0.319$) was stronger ($P = 0.022$) than the TNF correlation ($r = 0.034$). However, a greater number of strong differences were observed in the particular cytokine correlations between sex and study groups with LH, adione, and cortisol (TABLE 1). For example, IL-1β showed a significant negative correlation with LH in RA females ($r = -0.518$), whereas a positive correlation was observed in RA males ($r = 0.338$), the difference being significant ($P = 0.008$) (TABLE 1). The gender differences may suggest effects of sex hormones on NEI regulation.

In males, adione levels may be a surrogate marker for cortisol responsiveness in hypothalamic-pituitary-adrenal (HPA) axis stimulation. This relation was not seen in females, who have the alternate ovarian source for this hormone.[5] A previous report[5] proposes that pre-RA males may have an increased HPA drive, which is correlated with IL-1β (TABLE 1). The relationship was particularly observed in those males with RA in FDR. However, a small minority of pre-RA males, (2 [11%] of 18) had evidence of low cortisol and testosterone,[3]

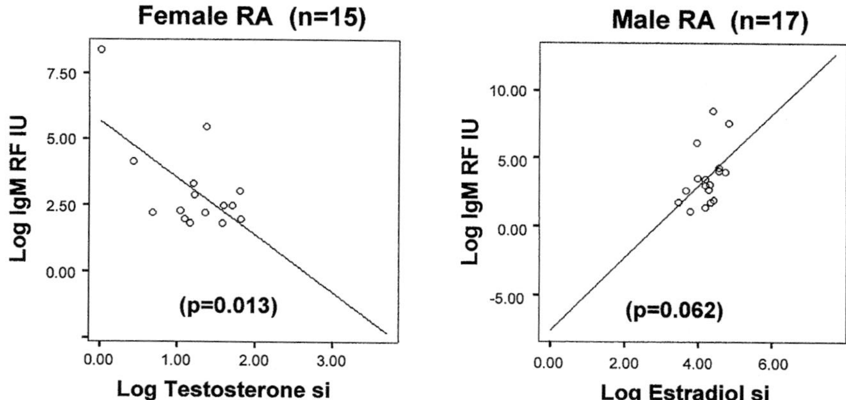

FIGURE 1. Correlations of log IgM RF IU with log serum estradiol (LN E2 SI) in pre-symptomatic male RA and log total testosterone (LN Test SI) in female RA cases.*$P = 0.002$, difference in the sex hormone correlations, which does not change on age adjustment.

as mentioned above. In a small subgroup of males, such relative hormonal deficiency may be analogous to a markedly low serum DHEAS in a minority of premenopausal onset cases (3 [27%] of 11).[3,6]

Sex hormones may be operating over prolonged intervals to gradually enhance or suppress immunological reactivity. In 15 female patients with RA, a negative correlation ($r = -0.624$, $P = 0.013$) was found between serum log T levels and their assayed log IgM RF titers (enzyme-linked immunosorbent assay [ELISA], TheraTest), as seen in FIGURE 1. Comparably strong negative correlations were found in the pre-RA females with T and IgA RF ($r = -0.670$, $n = 15$, $P = 0.006$), and in a smaller sample with log IgG RF ($r = -0.671$, $n = 8$, $P = 0.069$) assays. On the contrary, in male patients with RA, a positive correlation ($r = 0.462$, $P = 0.062$) was found between log estradiol (E2) levels and log IgM RF titers. No suggestive RF correlation was observed with serum E2 in female RA, nor with serum T in male RA. Also, no significant RF correlation was observed in CN subjects with either sex hormone levels.

The IgM RF titers (ELISA, TheraTest) correlated strongly with separate nephelometric assays (Behring, SLI) of total RF, performed in another referral laboratory in both males ($r = 0.873$, $n = 16$, $P < 0.001$) and females ($r = 0.888$, $n = 8$, $P = 0.003$). The concordance of RF titers of different isotypes and by alternative assay techniques implies validity for those immunological data and relations.

As yet, unexplained differences were found in the correlations of log T and log E2 levels between the total females versus males. Significant negative correlations were seen in both female RA ($r = -0.461$, $P = 0.016$) and CN ($r = -0.293$, $P = 0.004$) subjects, whereas the males had positive, but not significant correlations (FIG. 2). Gender differences in correlations were significant in both the CN ($P < 0.001$) and RA ($P = 0.032$) groups.

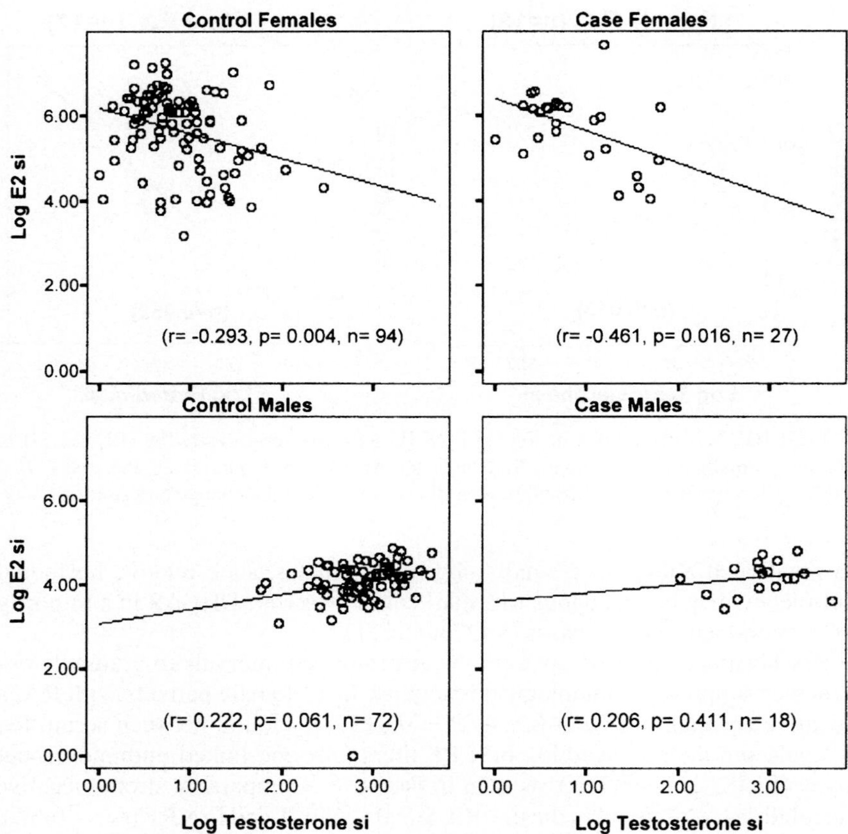

FIGURE 2. Regression of log serum estradiol (E2) and testosterone by gender and study subjects status.

In the female pre-RA cases, log Il-1β levels correlated significantly with serum log T ($r = 0.630$, $n = 25$, $P = 0.001$) and log DHEA ($r = 0.456$, $n = 24$, $P = 0.025$). In male cases, the corresponding correlations were also positive, but not significant ($r = 0.383$, $n = 16$, $P = 0.144$ and $r = 0.385$, $n = 16$, $P = 0.141$). The IL-1β correlations with E2 were significantly different ($P = 0.041$) between the male cases, which were positive ($r = 0.544$, $n = 16$, $P = 0.062$), and female cases, which were negative ($r = -0.208$, $n = 23$, $P = 0.341$).

PRELIMINARY PRINCIPAL COMPONENT ANALYSES OF THE DATA SET (6)

Donated sera were insufficient to conduct the full battery of all the tests that we have analyzed.[6] Accordingly, the technique of multiple imputation[24–27] was employed to incorporate acceptable values of those 13 main NEI variables that were missing at random, as recently described.[6] The multiple imputation data sets were subsequently analyzed using principal component analysis (PCA) and the results were combined. The PCA method is one of the statistical algorithms of factor analysis, which extracts the largest amount of variance from the variables, to explain the pattern of correlations.[28] Inspection of the 13 variable loadings on the uncorrelated and rotated components permits us to explore concepts underlying variables in the analysis (TABLE 2).

The first extracted component (C1) was labeled *sex-related*. As such, it explained the largest proportion of variance (27.2%) in the data set, as may be expected (TABLE 2). Its mean scores based upon individual subjects showed no difference between or within pre-RA and the matched CN subjects. These C1 findings are preliminary, but would seem to suggest similar overall sex hormone relations in the subject groups. The interaction of a history of RA in FDR with the mean C1 scores is being explored in male and female cases. However, conclusions cannot yet be drawn concerning this relationship.

The PCA extracted a second component (C2), which is *cytokine-related*, as is evident by its loadings (TABLE 2). This component accounted for 12.1% of the variance. Interestingly, sTNF-R1 loaded mainly on C1, rather than C2, because of its significantly higher levels in males than females.[29]

The third component (C3) extracted is labeled *youthful-related*, which explained 11.5% of the variance in the data set. Interestingly, its mean score was lower ($P = 0.015$) in female patients with RA versus CNs, as seen in FIGURE 3. The difference probably reflects adrenal androgens, since the pre-RA and CN subjects were matched and statistically adjusted for age. As expected, C3 was most heavily loaded by the chronological age of subjects at entry to study, but in a negative direction (−0.76). Accordingly, positive loadings on

TABLE 2. Four principal components extracted from a database matrix of 13 NEI variables and the main loadings of the individual variables on the four components

Component 1[a]		Component 2[b]		Component 3[c]		Component 4[d]	
Name of Variable	Loading	Name of Variable	Loading	Name of Variable	Loading	Name of Variable	Loading
Sex	0.92	IL-1ra	0.78	Age	−0.76	RAinFDR	0.80
T	0.86	TNF-α	0.68	Adione	0.65	Cig30+	0.61
STNF-R1	0.75	IL-1β	0.61	DHEAS	0.45		
DHEAS	0.71						
E_2	−0.71						
Adione	−0.48						

NOTE: Refer to Ref. 6 for definitions of the abbreviations and additional loadings.
[a]Sex-related component 1.
[b]Cytokine-related component 2.
[c]Youthful (vs. older)-related component 3.
[d]RA risk-related component 4.

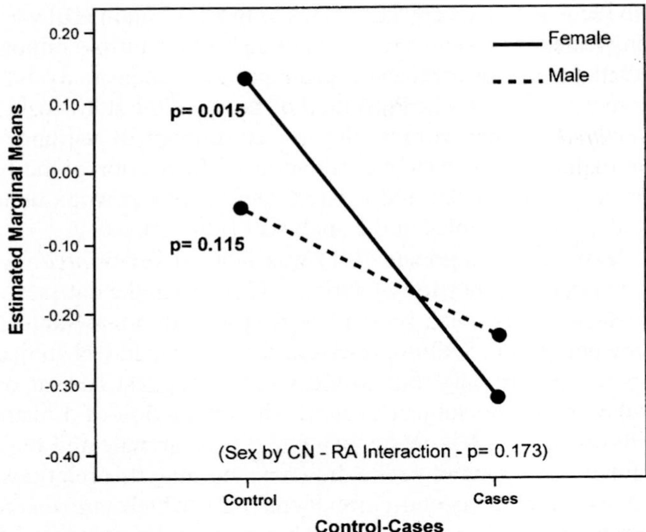

FIGURE 3. Estimated marginal means of component 3, adjusted for age, in female and male pre-RA versus CN subjects.

this component are *youthful-related*. The next strongest loadings on C3 were the adrenal androgens, adione (0.65), and DHEAS (0.45). These serum levels impressively diminish with aging.

The PCA also extracted the fourth and last component (C4), which may be interpreted as *RA-risk related*, by virtue of its loadings (TABLE 2). The extracted C4 accounted for 9.3% of the variance, making a total of 60% of the variance in the data set explained by the four components.[6] It is important to note that a designation of the subject's study status (*CN–RA*) was *not* entered into the PCA data matrix. The two main factor loadings on the RA risk-related C4 were the occurrence of RA in FDR and heavy cigarette smoking, that is, 30 or more daily (30+ cigarettes/d). Both of these risk factors were more frequent in the male versus female pre-RA cases.

Among the total subjects, RF also loaded weakly (0.17) on this C4, as did IL-1β (0.16). However, when this C4 score was analyzed only in the 54 RA cases, correlations increased meaningfully for RF (0.29) and IL-1β (0.48). In fact, among male patients with RA, IgG RF titers highly ($P = 0.002$) correlated ($r = 0.879, n = 9$) with C4. Thus, C4 may be considered an objective reflection of correlation patterns within the data set that are related to RA risk. Neither TNF-α, testosterone, nor estradiol levels loaded impressively on this C4 among all subjects combined.

In logistic regression analysis with RA versus CN status as the *outcome* variable and with adjustment for chronologic age, the *youthful-related* C3 was a significant predictor of outcome in females ($P = 0.007$), but not in males ($P = 0.405$). Thus, as-yet-unidentified biological factors related to a component of youthful versus aging status in females, possibly like adrenal androgens, were found to predict RA outcome. In addition, the somewhat stronger ($P = 0.002$) *RA-related* component 4 (C4) also predicted RA outcome in females, as well as in males.

DEVELOPMENTAL AND ENVIRONMENTAL FACTORS AND SEX HORMONES

Background

In embryogenesis, sequences of transcription factors control the differentiation of specific cell lines as well as their growth, in association with various growth factors.[30–33] Mutational errors in the relevant genes result in evident pathological abnormalities.[30–33] In normal development, growth and maturation progress under control of central (hypothalamic) pacemakers and growth factors.[34] In aging, various declines occur in multiple pacemakers, various hormones, and anabolic growth factors.[35]

Within such a paradigm, little attention has been given to *normal* polymorphic variabilities in the *trophic* status of individuals, i.e., the number of cells, their size, and competencies within tissues and organs.[10] Somatic effects of growth factor mediators (e.g., insulin, IGF-1) have been described for androgen synthesis in ovarian theca-interstitial cells.[36–38] However, the major focus has been on the stimulatory (or inhibitory) mechanisms of *tropic* factors (e.g., ACTH) and their regulatory systems.[30–33] Polycystic ovary syndrome (PCOS), which affects 5–10% of adolescent and younger women, is also described as a complex, heterogeneous, polygenic metabolic disorder influenced by environmental factors.[37–39]

Methods

Recent texts in endocrinology[30–33,37] and environmental sciences,[40–41] and indexed literature (PubMed) were reviewed with respect to developmental, genetic, and toxic environmental influences upon sex hormones, as well as possible relevance to RA.

Results

Literature review suggested potential genetic pathways by which polymorphic *trophic* variability may occur among normal individuals in their constitutional adrenal and gonadal organ competencies, as previously reviewed.[5] Modulation of genetic interactions between the nuclear receptors, SF-1 (steroidogenic factor-1), and DAX-1 (dosage-sensitive sex reversal, adrenal hypoplasia congenita, X-chromosome factor) might contribute to such polymorphic *trophic* variability.[5,30–33] Also, differences in growth factor (insulin/IGF-1) physiology may further influence the individual's somatic variability in adrenal cortical and gonadal development.[37,38] PCOS, which affects about 5–10% of menstruating younger women,[39] may be such a model of excessive *trophic* organogenesis and functional hyperandrogenicity.[10] The risk of RA in menstruating PCOS women is not known, and deserves further study.[39]

Unlike PCOS, hypoandrogenicity syndromes, in both females and males, are not well defined.[5,39] Great individual variability occurs in serum levels of anabolic hormones, particularly among younger persons of both sexes, as is fully documented with DHEAS.[10]

Regarding environmental factors, cigarette smoking complexly influences both the HPA and hypothalamic-pituitary-gonadal axes, tending to stimulate both systems, without clearly activating immunological activity.[6,30–33,40] Heavy smoking is a known risk factor for RA in males and females by unknown mechanisms.[6,12] It independently increases risk, aside from RF, C-reactive protein, prolactin, and family history, as recently reviewed.[6]

Chronic ethanol abuse is a documented gonadal toxin in males, but data are limited in females.[30–33,40,41] In males, ethanol damages Leydig cells and impairs the production and secretion of T, contributing to hypogonadism.[30–33,40,41] Also, it is toxic to germ cells, resulting in testicular atrophy. In chronic alcoholism, pituitary function is blunted, both in males and females.[30–33,40,41] Few data are available on the risks of developing RA from chronic alcoholism, which deserves further study.

Chronic cannabis (hashish, marijuana) usage may lower LH and T levels in males.[30–33,40,41] Acutely, however, it can increase serum cortisol levels, as does i.v. cocaine. Data on hormonal effects of these drugs in females are limited, as are risks of developing RA among abusers of such compounds.

Lead is an example of a heavy metal toxin which affects the testes, leading to reduced T production and increased LH, and may decrease sperm count.[30–33,40,41] Similar effects result from the pesticide DBCP (banned in 1979), and similar halogenated hydrocarbons.[30–33,40,41] However, their relation to risks of acquiring RA is not documented and needs further study.

SUMMARY OF RECENT RESEARCH AND LITERATURE REVIEW

A new model of the physiopathogenesis of RA was previously proposed.[2–6] Within this concept, a long-term, pre-symptomatic phase was described by others and ourselves.[6] A new model of sex hormone physiology was also proposed,[10] which incorporates influences of *trophic* cellular productive capacity in physiology, besides the classic *tropic* stimulatory (inhibitory) model.

Additionally, the individual's innate immunological system may be modeled over a long course by the polymorphic neuroendocrine system, that is, its *tropic* and *trophic* dynamics.[4–6,10]

NEI counterregulations may be transforming over many years in RA susceptibles, and would not be likely identified in a single base-line sample. In this regard, the above-described gender dimorphic correlations of serum log total T and E2 levels with log IgM RF titers (FIG. 1) are of relevance in implying that sex hormones can differentially affect immunological responsiveness.

Dysregulations of such developmental and longitudinal counter-regulatory dynamics may spontaneously transform, after many years, into the self-perpetuating inflammatory phase of RA.[4–6] Better understanding of NEI interactions in the normal population and in those exposed to the outlined behavioral and environmental exposures will clarify the respective risks for developing RA. The research challenges are exceedingly complex, due to the multiplicity of interacting factors. However, collaborative, integrative approaches over the course of the long physiopathogenic and inflammatory phases of RA promise to reveal fundamental mechanisms in this disease.

ACKNOWLEDGMENTS

Support for this project was provided by the Department of Medicine, University of Illinois College of Medicine at Peoria, and by a grant from the MTM Foundation. The invaluable technical assistance of Brooke Buchanan and Susan Jenkins is most gratefully recognized. This research was made possible by the generous donation of sera on the study subjects by Operation CLUE.[6] Doug Goessman kindly provided the graphics.

REFERENCES

1. CHROUSOS, G.P. 1995. The hypothalamic-pituitary-adrenal axis and immune-mediated inflammation. N. Engl. J. Med. **332:** 1351–1362.
2. MASI, A.T., J.W.J. BIJLSMA, I.C. CHIKANZA, *et al.* 1999. Neuroendocrine, immunologic, and microvascular systems interactions in rheumatoid arthritis: physiopathogenetic and therapeutic perspectives. Semin. Arthritis Rheum. **29:** 65–81.
3. MASI, A.T. 2000. Hormonal and immunologic risk factors for the development of rheumatoid arthritis: an integrative physiopathogenetic perspective. Rheum. Dis. Clin. North Am. **26:** 775–803.
4. STRAUB, R.H. & H.O. BESEDOVSKY. 2003. Integrated evolutionary, immunological, and neuroendocrine framework for the pathogenesis of chronic disabling inflammatory diseases. FASEB J. **7:** 2176–2183.
5. MASI, A.T., J.C. ALDAG & J.W.G. JACOBS 2005. Rheumatoid arthritis: neuroendocrine immune integrated physiopathogenetic perspectives and therapy. Rheum. Dis. Clin. North Am. **31:** 131–160.

6. MASI, A.T. & J.C. ALDAG. 2005. Integrated neuroendocrine immune risk factor relations to rheumatoid arthritis: should rheumatologists now adopt a model of a multi-year, pre-symptomatic phase? Scand. J. Rheumatol. **34:** 342–352.
7. HARRIS, E.D. Jr. 1997. Rheumatoid Arthritis. WB Saunders, Philadelphia.
8. ST. CLAIR, E.W., D.S. PISETSKY & B.F. HAYNES, Eds. 2004. Rheumatoid Arthritis. Lippincott Williams & Wilkins. Philadelphia.
9. CHOY, E.H.S. & G.S. PANAYI. 2001. Mechanisms of disease: cytokine pathways and joint inflammation in rheumatoid arthritis. N. Engl. J. Med. **344:** 907–916.
10. MASI, A.T., J.A.P. DASILVA & M. CUTOLO, 1996. Perturbations of hypothalamic-pituitary-gonadal (HPG) axis and adrenal androgen (AA) functions in rheumatoid arthritis. Baillieres Clin. Rheumatol. **10:** 295–332.
11. MASI, A.T., 1994. Incidence of rheumatoid arthritis: do the observed age-sex interaction patterns support a role of androgenic-anabolic steroid deficiency in its pathogenesis? Br. J. Rheumatol. **33:** 697–699.
12. MASI, A.T. & H.J. CHANG. 1999. Cigarette smoking and other acquired risk factors for rheumatoid arthritis. *In* Rheumatic Diseases and the Environment. L.D. Kaufman & J. Varga, Eds.: 111–127. Chapman & Hall. New York.
13. CUTOLO, M., B. VILLAGGIO, L. FOPPIANI, *et al.* 2000. The hypothalamic-pituitary-adrenal and gonadal axes in rheumatoid arthritis. Ann. N. Y. Acad. Sci. **917:** 835–843.
14. STRAUB, R.H. & M. CUTOLO. 2001. Involvement of the hypothalamic-pituitary-adrenal/gonadal axis and the peripheral nervous system in rheumatoid arthritis: viewpoint based on a systemic pathogenetic role. Arthritis Rheum. **44:** 493–507.
15. CUTOLO, M., B. VILLAGGIO, C. CRAVIOTTO, *et al.* 2002. Sex hormones and rheumatoid arthritis. Autoimmun. Rev. **1:** 284–289.
16. STRAUB, R.H., J. SCHOLMERICH & M. CUTOLO, 2003. The multiple facets of premature aging in rheumatoid arthritis. Arthritis Rheum. **48:** 2713–2721.
17. TOOGOOD, A.A., N.F. TAYLOR, S.M. SHALET, *et al.* 2000. Sexual dimorphism of cortisol metabolism is maintained in elderly subjects and is not oestrogen dependent. Clin. Endocrinol. (Oxf.). **52:** 61–66.
18. LAUGHLIN, G.A. & E. BARRETT-CONNOR, 2000. Sexual dimorphism in the influence of advanced aging on adrenal hormone levels: the Rancho Bernardo Study. J. Clin. Endocrinol. Metab. **85:** 3561–3568.
19. PUDER, J.J., P.U. FREDA, R.S. GOLAND, *et al.* 2001. Estrogen modulates the hypothalamic-pituitary-adrenal and inflammatory cytokine responses to endotoxin in women. J. Clin. Endocrinol. Metab. **87:** 3509.
20. REHMAN, K.S. & B.R. CARR. 2004. Sex differences in adrenal androgens. Semin. Reprod. Med. **22:** 349–360.
21. ARNETT, F.C., S.M. EDWORTHY, D.A. BLOCH, *et al*: The American Rheumatism Association 1987 revised criteria for the classification of rheumatoid arthritis. Arthritis Rheum. **31:** 315–324.
22. IMRICH, R., J. ROVENSKY, F. MALIS, *et al.* 2005. Low levels of dehydroepiandrosterone sulphate in plasma, and reduced sympathoadrenal response to hypoglycemia in premenopausal women with rheumatoid arthritis. Ann. Rheum. Dis. **64:** 202–206.
23. MASI, A.T., R.T. CHATTERTON, J.C. ALDAG, *et al.* 2002. Perspectives on the relationship of adrenal steroids to rheumatoid arthritis. Ann. N.Y. Acad. Sci. **996:** 1–12.
24. SCHAFER, J.L.. 1997. Imputation of missing covariates under a general linear mixed model. Technical report, Department of Statistics, Penn State University.

25. SCHAFER, J.L.. 1997. Analysis of Incomplete Multivariate Data. Chapman & Hall. London.
26. SCHAFER, J.L.. 1999. Multiple imputation: a primer. Stat. Methods Med. Res. **8:** 3–5.
27. DEMIRTAS, H.. 2004. Simulation driven inferences for multiply imputated longitudinal datasets. Stat. Neerl. **58:** 466–482.
28. SPSS Inc. 2004. SPSS (V13, 0) for Windows, Chicago, SPSS Inc.
29. MASI, A.T., J.C. ALDAG, R.T. CHATTERTON, *et al.* 2005. Gender dimorphisms in serum levels of soluble tumor necrosis factor receptor type 1 (sTNF-R1) observed in susceptibles to rheumatoid (RA) before clinical onset (pre-RA) and in matched cohort controls (CN). Arthritis Rheum. **52:** S654.
30. KACSOH, B.. 2000. Endocrine Physiology. McGraw-Hill. New York.
31. BECKER, K.L., J.P. BILEZIKIAN, W.J. BREMNER, *et al.* Eds. 2001. Principles and Practice of Endocrinology and Metabolism. 3rd ed. Lippincott Williams and Wilkins. Philadelphia.
32. BESSER, G.M. & M.O. THORNER. 2002. Comprehensive Clinical Endocrinology. 3rd ed. Mosby. St. Louis.
33. LARSEN, P.R., H.M. KRONENBERG, S. MELMED, *et al.*, Eds. 2003. Williams Textbook of Endocrinology. 10th ed. Saunders. Philadelphia.
34. HANDA, R.J., S. HAYASKI, E. TERASAWA, *et al.* 2002. Neuroplasticity, Development, and Steroid Hormone Action. CRC Press. Boca Raton.
35. LAMBERS, S.W.J., A.W. VAN DEN BELD & A.J. VAN DER LELY. 1997. The endocrinology of aging. Science **278:** 419–424.
36. CARA, J.F. & R.L. ROSENFIELD. 1988. Insulin-like growth factor I and insulin potentiate luteinizing hormone-induced androgen synthesis by rat ovarian theca-interstitial cells. Endocrinology **123:** 733–739.
37. WASS, J.A.H. & S.M. SHALET. 2002. Oxford Textbook of Endocrinology and Diabetes. Oxford University Press. Oxford, UK.
38. ROLDAN, B., SAN MILLIAN, J.L. & H.D. ESCOBAR-MORREALE. 2004. Genetic basis of metabolic abnormalities in polycystic ovary syndrome: implications for therapy. Am. J. Pharmacogenomics **4:** 93–107.
39. MASI, A.T. & G.P. CHROUSOS. 2003. Polycystic ovarian syndrome and rheumatoid arthritis: possible physiopathogenetic clues to hormonal influences on chronic inflammation. Semin. Arthritis Rheum. **33:** 67–71.
40. PAUL, M., Ed. 1993. Occupational and Environmental Reproductive Hazards. Williams and Wilkins. Baltimore, MD.
41. SCHETTLER, T.. 1999. Generations at Risk: Reproductive Health and the Environment. MIT Press, Cambridge, MA.

Inflammation and Sex Hormone Metabolism

MARTIN SCHMIDT,[a] HEIDRUN NAUMANN,[a] CLAUDIA WEIDLER,[b] MARTINA SCHELLENBERG,[a] SVEN ANDERS,[c] AND RAINER H. STRAUB[b]

[a]*Institute of Biochemistry II, Hospital of the Friedrich-Schiller-University, 07740 Jena, Germany*

[b]*Department of Internal Medicine I, University Hospital Regensburg, 93042 Regensburg, Germany*

[c]*Department of Orthopedic Surgery, University Regensburg, Bavarian Red Cross Hospital, 93077 Bad Abbach, Germany*

ABSTRACT: The incidence of autoimmune diseases is higher in females than in males. In both sexes, adrenal hormones, that is, glucocorticoids, dehydroepiandrosterone (DHEA), and androgens, are inadequately low in patients when compared to healthy controls. Hormonally active androgens are anti-inflammatory, whereas estrogens are pro-inflammatory. Therefore, the mechanisms responsible for the alterations of steroid profiles in inflammation are of major interest. The local metabolism of androgens and estrogens may determine whether a given steroid profile found in a subject's blood results in suppression or promotion of inflammation. The steroid metabolism in mixed synovial cells, fibroblasts, macrophages, and monocytes was assessed. Major focus was on cells from patients with rheumatoid arthritis (RA), while cells from patients with osteoarthritis served as controls. Enzymes directly or indirectly involved in local sex steroid metabolism in RA are: DHEA-sulfatase, 3β-hydroxysteroid dehydrogenase, 17β-hydroxysteroid dehydrogenase, and aromatase (CYP19), which are required for the synthesis of sex steroids from precursors, 5α-reductase and 16α-hydroxylase, which can be involved either in the generation of more active steroids or in the pathways leading to depletion of active hormones, and 3α-reductase and 7α-hydroxylase (CYP7B), which unidirectionally are involved in the depletion of active hormones. Androgens inhibit aromatization in synovial cells when their concentration is sufficiently high. As large amounts of estrogens are formed in synovial tissue, there may be a relative lack of androgens. Production of 5α-reduced androgens should increase the local anti-inflammatory activity; however, it also opens a pathway for the inactivation of androgens. The data discussed here suggest that therapy

Address for correspondence: Dr. Martin Schmidt, Institute of Biochemistry II, Hospital of the Friedrich-Schiller-University, 07740 Jena, Germany. Voice: +49-3641-938-683; fax: +49-3641-938-682.

e-mail: Schmidt@mti.uni-jena.de

Ann. N.Y. Acad. Sci. 1069: 236–246 (2006).
doi: 10.1196/annals.1351.021

of RA patients may benefit from the use of nonaromatizable androgens and/or the use of aromatase inhibitors.

KEYWORDS: **steroid metabolism; synovial cell; rheumatoid arthritis; testosterone; estradiol; DHEA; 7α-hydroxy-DHEA; dihydrotestosterone; androsterone**

INTRODUCTION

The incidence of autoimmune diseases is higher in females than in males. Although other factors may be involved, there is ample evidence that at least significant portions of these differences are causally related to the gender-specific differences in the serum levels of sex hormones and their metabolism.[1–3] In both sexes, adrenal hormones, that is, glucocorticoids, dehydroepiandrosterone (DHEA), and androgens are inadequately low in patients when compared to healthy controls.[4,5] A causal relationship between these altered steroid profiles in the blood and the autoimmune diseases is strongly suggested by the properties of the hormonally active sex steroids: androgens are anti-inflammatory, whereas estrogens are proinflammatory.[4,6,7] Therefore, it is of major interest to identify the mechanisms that are responsible for the alterations of steroid profiles in inflammation. As the low serum levels of adrenal androgens do not result from increased renal clearance,[8] decreased adrenal production of DHEA and androgens may explain some of the alterations observed in chronic inflammation. However, the local metabolism of androgens and estrogens may determine whether a given steroid profile found in the blood of a subject results in suppression or promotion of inflammation.

Here, data from some recent studies focusing on synovial cells from patients with rheumatoid arthritis (RA) and several experimental models are discussed. Functional data are mainly from *in vitro* studies with isolated, mixed synovial cells in the primary culture. For most of the experiments reviewed, cells from patients with osteoarthritis (OA) served as controls.

CONVERSION OF DHEA INTO ANDROGENS AND ESTROGENS

Within the scope of this contribution, the term "sex hormone" is used as a synonym for androgens and estrogens. However, analysis of sex hormone metabolism must take into account the fact that the generation of androgens is dependent on the availability of suitable precursors. There is experimental evidence that *de novo* synthesis of sex steroids from cholesterol or progesterone is almost undetectable in synovial cells (M. Schmidt, unpublished results). Therefore, these cells depend on available precursors, which can be converted into androgens by the enzymes expressed in these cells. The precursor most abundant in the blood is DHEA-sulfate, which indeed is a source for DHEA in cultured synovial cells. The enzyme responsible, steroid sulfatase, is expressed in synovial fibroblasts and macrophages, and is inhibited by the tumor necrosis factor.[9] These findings suggest that the local generation of free DHEA at the site of inflammation is diminished, resulting in an even pronounced dependence of the synovial tissue on free DHEA derived from the blood.

DHEA is converted into androgens and estrogens by mixed synovial cells, as summarized in FIGURE 1.[10] It is evident that the action of two enzymes is necessary for the synthesis of testosterone, the hormonally active androgen: a 3β-hydroxysteroid dehydrogenase (3β-HSD) shifting the double bond to the A-ring of the sterane backbone and a 17β-hydroxysteroid dehydrogenase (17β-HSD) acting as a reductase. The activity of the latter enzyme is not limited to

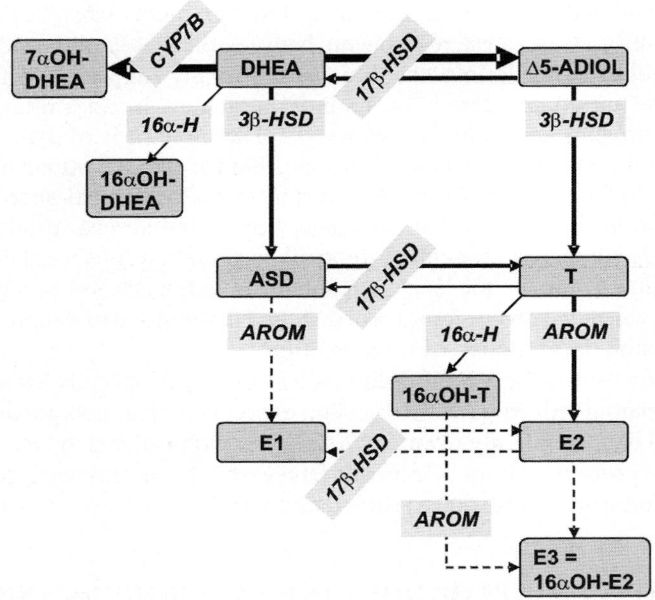

FIGURE 1. DHEA metabolism in synovial cells. Mixed synovial cells were isolated, cultured, and metabolism of radiolabeled DHEA was analyzed by thin-layer chromatography and high-performance liquid chromatography, as described previously.[10] The thickness of the arrows shall be seen as a rough measure of the amount of steroid conversion along the respective path. *Dashed arrows* indicate spurious or undetectable conversion. The meanings of the symbols and abbreviations are: ASD = androstenedione; AROM = cytochrome P-450 aromatase (CYP19); CYP7B = cytochrome P-450 7B; DHEA = dehydroepiandrosterone; E1 = estrone; E2 = estradiol; E3 = estriol; T = testosterone; 16α-H = 16α-hydroxylase; 16/7αOH-DHEA = 16/7α-hydroxy-DHEA; 16αOH-T = 16αOH-testosterone; 17β-HSD = 17β-hydroxysteroid dehydrogenase; 3β-HSD = 3β-hydroxysteroid dehydrogenase; Δ5-ADIOL = Δ5-androstenediol.

testosterone synthesis, as the most abundant product generated from DHEA is Δ5-androstenediol (Δ5-ADIOL).[10] Therefore, the rate-limiting enzyme for androgen synthesis in mixed synovial cells is the 3β-HSD.

While starting from DHEA, it takes two enzymes to generate the anti-inflammatory testosterone; only the cytochrome P-450 enzyme, CYP7B, is necessary for the synthesis of the other major metabolite of DHEA in synovial cells, 7α-hydroxy-DHEA (7αOH-DHEA).[10] This metabolite is the dominant product of DHEA conversion in synovial fibroblasts,[11] and CYP7B-activity correlates with the severity of collagen-induced arthritis in a mouse model.[12] In the synovial tissue, both pathways compete for DHEA. In addition, androgens are converted by the aromatase cytochrome P-450 (CYP19) into estrogens, mainly estradiol (FIG. 1),[10] further augmenting a local proinflammatory steroid environment.

With the exception of 7αOH-DHEA, all the products formed by mixed synoviocytes are also formed by *in vitro* differentiated human macrophages,[13] suggesting that the local synthesis of sex steroids occurs in synovial macrophages. In line with this conclusion is the fact that in both experimental systems, the amount of androgens formed exceed the amount of estrogens roughly by a factor of 10. However, there are also some differences between synoviocytes and isolated macrophages: mixed synoviocytes have much less capacity for 16α-hydroxylation as compared to macrophages, whereas macrophages have no CYP7B-activity.

ANDROGENS ARE CONVERTED MAINLY INTO MORE POTENT 5α-REDUCED ANDROGENS

Whereas there was no difference in steroids generated from DHEA by mixed synoviocytes from patients with OA and RA, respectively, there was a striking difference in product formation from androgens: synoviocytes produce large amounts of 5α-reduced androgens, with cells from RA patients producing significantly more than synoviocytes from OA patients (FIG. 2).[10] This is quite unexpected, as the 5α-reduction of testosterone yields 5α-dihydro-testosterone (5αDH-T), which is roughly three times as efficient at the androgen receptor as testosterone itself.[14] One theoretical explanation for the increase of 5α-reductase activity in RA might be that this enzyme could be involved in some kind of regulatory feedback mechanism, which would be defective in RA. Indeed, there is evidence that expression/activity of 5α-reductase is inhibited by androgens in various tissues.[15,16] Therefore, a testable hypothesis would be that in RA androgen receptor signaling is defective to some extent—which would have implications far beyond the regulation of the 5α-reductase.

Starting from testosterone, synoviocytes produce also large amounts of 6β-hydroxy-testosterone. Although not a biologically active hormone, it indicates the presence of additional members of the cytochrome P-450-family of monoxygenases in the cells.

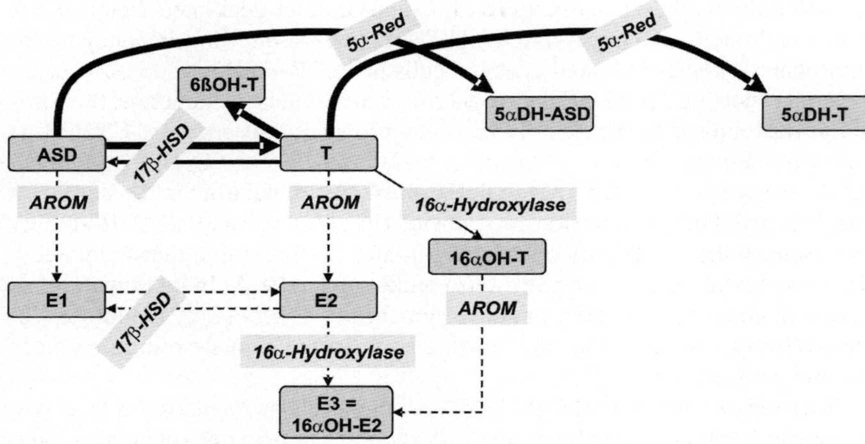

FIGURE 2. Androgen metabolism in synovial cells. Experimental procedures were as given in the legend to FIG. 1, except the substrates used, which were radiolabeled androstenedione and testosterone, respectively. The meanings of the symbols and abbreviations are as given for FIG. 1, with the addition of: 5αDH-ASD = 5α-dihydro-androstenedione; 5α DH-T = 5α-dihydro-testosterone; 5α-Red = 5α-reductase; 6βOH-T = 6β-hydroxy-testosterone; the testosterone-6β-hydroxylase is not indicated separately.

Synovial cells convert DHEA into androgens and estradiol plus some estriol; therefore, one would expect to obtain even more estrogens, if androgens were the substrates available to the cells. On the contrary, the amounts of estrogens produced by mixed synovial cells declined significantly, when androstenedione and testosterone, respectively, were used as substrates (TABLE 1).[10] As the amounts of testosterone produced from androstenedione were in the same range as the amounts of Δ5-ADIOL produced from DHEA, there is no evidence that the presence of androgens could have compromised the viability of the cultures.

TABLE 1. Estradiol production from various precursors by mixed synoviocytes

Precursor	Picomol estradiol produced per million cells in 2 days (means ± SD) by mixed synoviocytes from patients with: OA	RA
DHEA	1.39 ± 2.19 ($n = 24$)	1.13 ± 1.49 ($n = 23$)
Androstenedione	0.60 ± 1.64 ($n = 23$)	0.17 ± 0.36* ($n = 19$)
Testosterone	0.07 ± 0.19 ($n = 10$)	0.0 ± 0.0* ($n = 9$)

*Difference significant versus the amount of estradiol produced from DHEA (Mann-Whitney rank sum test, $P < 0.01$).

ANDROGENS MAY INHIBIT LOCAL AROMATIZATION

Testosterone is the substrate that is converted directly into estradiol by aromatase, whereas additional enzyme activities are necessary for estradiol synthesis when androstenedione (17β-HSD) or DHEA (17β-HSD and 3β-HSD) are the precursors. Aromatase and 3β-HSD are unidirectional, and 17β-HSD clearly works as a reductase in synoviocytes, which means that there is no way for "degradation" of estrogens in the experimental system. In addition, aromatase is regulated at the level of transcription.[17] Therefore, the most plausible explanation for the results summarized in TABLE 1 is: the expression of aromatase in synoviocytes may be inhibited by hormonally active androgens. Whereas androgens are known to induce aromatase in certain regions of the brain, it was clearly shown that aromatase expression can be inhibited by testosterone in skin fibroblasts.[18] The key to this kind of tissue-specific action of signaling molecules is the complex structure of the aromatase promoter regions.[17]

From a study of DHEA metabolism in *in vitro* differentiated macrophages,[13] it is known that aromatase expression is almost undetectable in monocytes, but is strongly induced in the course of macrophage differentiation. This suggests that macrophages are the cells responsible for estrogen synthesis in the synovial cell preparations. In the same study, aromatase activity in the macrophages could be inhibited by 35% upon treatment with DHEA. In mixed synovial cells, the formation of testosterone from DHEA was significantly augmented when the cells were treated with the nonaromatizable androgen 5αDH-T.[10] Concomitantly, the rate of estrogen formation tended to decrease; however, this effect did not reach statistical significance.

Taken together, these results suggest that the capacity of synovial cells (macrophages) for estrogen synthesis is dependent on the available amounts of androgens: if the concentrations of androgens are low, then aromatase is expressed, but if the concentrations of androgens are sufficiently high so to activate the androgen receptor, aromatase is repressed. In other words, if enough androgens are available, there is no local estrogen synthesis in the synovial tissue, and androgens are accumulated. If there is a short supply of androgens, these may be further depleted by conversion to estrogens.

EVIDENCE FOR RELATIVE ANDROGEN DEPLETION IN SYNOVIAL TISSUE

Immunohistochemical analysis of aromatase expression in synovial tissue from patients with OA and RA, respectively, revealed no difference in the number of aromatase-positive cells.[10] In addition, the concentrations of estradiol, estriol, and testosterone found in the effluate from superfused slices of synovial tissue were almost identical in those samples, indicating that there is no difference in aromatase activity between OA and RA. However, the molar ratio of estriol versus testosterone (375:1) was extremely high in both groups of samples, when compared to the normal ratios found in the sera of men (20:1) and women (200:1). In another study,[19] a significant increase of the ratio of synovial fluid levels of estrogens versus androgens in samples from RA patients was found when compared with the ratio of controls with traumatic lesions. Under the assumption that synovial fluid levels of steroids are proportional to tissue concentrations, it can be concluded that there is no difference between OA and RA. Macrophages from both groups of patients may be equally activated, at least with respect to estrogen synthesis.

Moreover, the above-mentioned experimental evidence strongly suggests that there is a relative lack of androgens in both conditions, OA as well as RA. This lack of androgens itself would permit local aromatization and relative accumulation of estrogens, thus establishing an estrogenic proinflammatory state.

A POSSIBLE ROLE FOR MONOCYTES

When the data from mixed synovial cells are compared to the data obtained for DHEA-conversion by the two major cell types found in synovial tissue, fibroblasts and macrophages, as discussed above, it is evident that the localization of the 5α-reductase is not clear. In monocytic cell lines we found that conversion of DHEA to downstream sex hormones was more restricted than in mixed synoviocytes (M. Schellenberg, H. Naumann, and M. Schmidt, unpublished results). Interestingly, the predominant pathway for conversion of androstenedione in monocytes is via 5α-reductase yielding 5α-androstan-3,17-dione (FIG. 3). Moreover, monocytes have high 3α-reductase activity, which results in large amounts of produced 4-androsten-3α-ol-17-one. Consequently, the action of both enzymes also results in the accumulation of androsterone (FIG. 4). In an earlier study with cultured synovial macrophages treated with cyclosporin A, it was shown that testosterone was similarly converted to downstream metabolites.[20]

Whereas these androgen metabolites are hormonally inactive, they are effectively excreted via the kidney, in part in their conjugated forms. Although the urinary concentrations of these inactive androgen metabolites are lower in patients with RA when compared with healthy controls,[21] this pathway represents an additional alternative for the depletion of synovial tissue from active androgens.

CONCLUSIONS

There are various enzymes involved in steroid metabolism expressed in synovial cells, as summarized in FIGURE 4. The balance between the

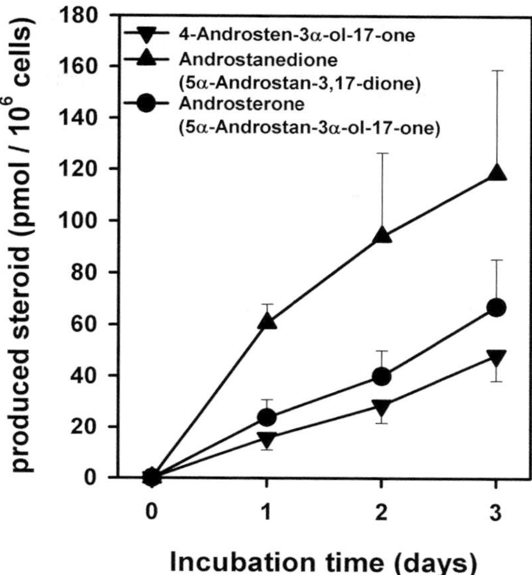

FIGURE 3. 3α-reductase and 5α-reductase in monocytes. Experimental procedures were essentially as given in the legend to FIGURE 1. The monocytic cell-line used was U937; the substrate was radiolabeled androstenedione.

anti-inflammatory androgens and the proinflammatory estrogens depends on several factors: (1) the expression levels of the enzymes, (2) the amounts of substrates available locally, and (3) the cell-type distribution within the synovial tissue. As the first two points were discussed in some detail above, the third will be briefly discussed here. Given that the number of fibroblasts is high in the synovial tissue, one could expect massive use of DHEA for 7α-hydroxylation. Less production of sex steroids would be the consequence. If the number of monocytes is high, effective inactivation of androgens, either locally generated from DHEA or delivered by the blood, could be expected. Finally, if macrophages predominate, local androgen synthesis is possible.

However, all available data strongly suggest that there is a lack of active androgens also within synovial tissue in inflammation. This local androgen deficiency causes local estrogen excess, and thus generates a predominantly proinflammatory steroid environment, which maintains itself.

This proinflammatory environment may be further consolidated by the action of additional enzymes involved in modification of estrogens, not discussed in detail here. One pathway is via 16α-hydroxylases, leading to the proinflammatory 16α-hydroxy-estrone.

The clinical relevance of the discussed experimental evidence is at least in part already proven: androgen supplementation improves clinical outcome in male and female patients with RA.[22,23] From the data discussed here, another

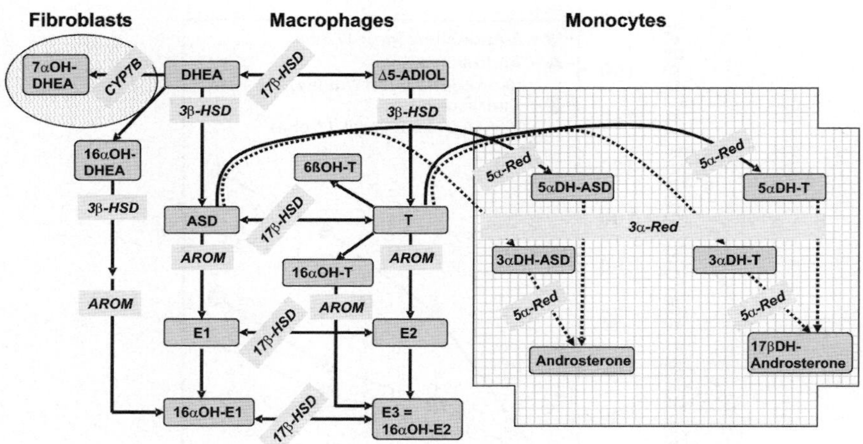

FIGURE 4. Steroid metabolism in synovial cells. Overview of the compartments and possible pathways of steroid metabolism in synovial cells. The meanings of the symbols and abbreviations are as given for FIGURES 1 and 2, with the addition of: 3αDH-ASD = 3α-dihydro-androstenedione; 3αDH-T = 3α-dihydro-testosterone; 3α-Red = 3α-reductase. The circled and boxed areas indicate enzymes expressed preferentially in fibroblasts and monocytic cells, respectively, and the steroids produced by these cell types.

suggestion can be derived: therapy of RA patients may benefit from the use of nonaromatizable androgens and/or the use of aromatase inhibitors.

ACKNOWLEDGMENT

Part of this work was funded by grants from the Deutsche Forschungsgemeinschaft (Schm 1611/1-1,2, Str 511/10-1,2) and by the respective institutions.

REFERENCES

1. MASI, A.T., S.L. FEIGENBAUM & R.T. CHATTERTON. 1995. Hormonal and pregnancy relationships to rheumatoid arthritis: convergent effects with immunologic and microvascular systems. Semin. Arthritis Rheum. **25:** 1–27.
2. MASI, A.T. 1995. Sex hormones and rheumatoid arthritis: cause or effect relationships in a complex pathophysiology? Clin. Exp. Rheumatol. **13:** 227–240.
3. SULLIVAN, D.A., A. BELANGER, J.M. CERMAK, *et al.* 2003. Are women with Sjogren's syndrome androgen-deficient? J. Rheumatol. **30:** 2413–2419.
4. STRAUB, R.H. & M. CUTOLO. 2001. Involvement of the hypothalamic-pituitary-adrenal/gonadal axis and the peripheral nervous system in rheumatoid arthritis: viewpoint based on a systemic pathogenetic role Arthritis Rheum. **44:** 493–507.

5. MASI, A.T., J.W. BIJLSMA, I.C. CHIKANZA, *et al.* 1999. Neuroendocrine, immunologic, and microvascular systems interactions in rheumatoid arthritis: physiopathogenetic and therapeutic perspectives. Semin. Arthritis Rheum. **29:** 65–81.
6. STRAUB, R.H., L. KONECNA, S. HRACH, *et al.* 1998. Serum dehydroepiandrosterone (DHEA) and DHEA sulfate are negatively correlated with serum interleukin-6 (IL-6), and DHEA inhibits IL-6 secretion from mononuclear cells in man *in vitro*: possible link between endocrinosenescence and immunosenescence. J. Clin. Endocrinol. Metab. **83:** 2012–2017.
7. CUTOLO, M., S. CAPELLINO, P. MONTAGNA, *et al.* 2005. Sex hormone modulation of cell growth and apoptosis of the human monocytic/macrophage cell line. Arthritis Res. Ther. **7:** R1124–R1132.
8. STRAUB, R.H., C. WEIDLER, B. DEMMEL, *et al.* 2004. Renal clearance and daily excretion of cortisol and adrenal androgens in patients with rheumatoid arthritis and systemic lupus erythematosus. Ann. Rheum. Dis. **63:** 961–968.
9. WEIDLER, C., S. STRUHAROVA, M. SCHMIDT, *et al.* 2005. Tumor necrosis factor inhibits conversion of dehydroepiandrosterone sulfate (DHEAS) to DHEA in rheumatoid arthritis synovial cells: a prerequisite for local androgen deficiency. Arthritis Rheum. **52:** 1721–1729.
10. SCHMIDT, M., C. WEIDLER, H. NAUMANN, *et al.* 2005. Androgen conversion in osteoarthritis and rheumatoid arthritis synoviocytes—androstenedione and testosterone inhibit estrogen formation and favor production of more potent 5-alpha-reduced androgens. Arthritis Res. Ther. **7:** R938–R948.
11. DULOS, J., M.A. VAN DER VLEUTEN, A. KAVELAARS, *et al.* 2005. CYP7B expression and activity in fibroblast-like synoviocytes from patients with rheumatoid arthritis: regulation by proinflammatory cytokines. Arthritis Rheum. **52:** 770–778.
12. DULOS, J., E. VERBRAAK, W.M. BAGCHUS, *et al.* 2004. Severity of murine collagen-induced arthritis correlates with increased CYP7B activity: enhancement of dehydroepiandrosterone metabolism by interleukin-1beta. Arthritis Rheum. **50:** 3346–3353.
13. SCHMIDT, M., M. KREUTZ, G. LOFFLER, *et al.* 2000. Conversion of dehydroepiandrosterone to downstream steroid hormones in macrophages. J. Endocrinol. **164:** 161–169.
14. KEMPPAINEN, J.A., E. LANGLEY, C.I. WONG, *et al.* 1999. Distinguishing androgen receptor agonists and antagonists: distinct mechanisms of activation by medroxyprogesterone acetate and dihydrotestosterone. Mol. Endocrinol. **13:** 440–454.
15. TORRES, J.M. & E. ORTEGA. 2003. Differential regulation of steroid 5-alpha-reductase isozymes expression by androgens in the adult rat brain. FASEB J. **17:** 1428–1433.
16. PRATIS, K., L. O'DONNELL, G.T. OOI, *et al.* 2003. Differential regulation of rat testicular 5alpha-reductase type 1 and 2 isoforms by testosterone and FSH. J. Endocrinol. **176:** 393–403.
17. SIMPSON, E.R. 2004. Aromatase: biologic relevance of tissue-specific expression. Semin. Reprod. Med. **22:** 11–23.
18. BERKOVITZ, G.D., K.M. CARTER, T.R. BROWN & C.J. MIGEON. 1990. Testosterone lowers aromatase activity in cultured human genital skin fibroblasts. Mol. Cell Endocrinol. **69:** 187–197.
19. CASTAGNETTA, L.A., G. CARRUBA, O.M. GRANATA, *et al.* 2003. Increased estrogen formation and estrogen to androgen ratio in the synovial fluid of patients with rheumatoid arthritis. J. Rheumatol. **30:** 2597–2605.

20. CUTOLO, M., M. GIUSTI, B. VILLAGGIO, *et al.* 1997. Testosterone metabolism and cyclosporin A treatment in rheumatoid arthritis. Br. J. Rheumatol. **36:** 433–439.
21. MASI, A.T., D.B. JOSIPOVIC & W.E. JEFFERSON. 1984. Low adrenal androgenic-anabolic steroids in women with rheumatoid arthritis (RA): gas-liquid chromatographic studies of RA patients and matched normal control women indicating decreased 11-deoxy-17-ketosteroid excretion. Semin. Arthritis Rheum. **14:** 1–23.
22. CUTOLO, M., E. BALLEARI, M. GIUSTI, *et al.* 1991. Androgen replacement therapy in male patients with rheumatoid arthritis. Arthritis Rheum. **34:** 1–5.
23. BOOJI, A., C.M. BIEWENGA-BOOJI, O. HUBER-BRUNING, *et al.* 1996. Androgens as adjuvant treatment in postmenopausal female patients with rheumatoid arthritis. Ann. Rheum. Dis. **55:** 811–815.

Estrogens in Pregnancy and Systemic Lupus Erythematosus

ANDREA DORIA,[a] LUCA IACCARINO,[a] PIERCARLO SARZI-PUTTINI,[b] ANNA GHIRARDELLO,[a] SANDRA ZAMPIERI,[a] SILVIA ARIENTI,[a] MAURIZIO CUTOLO,[c] AND SILVANO TODESCO[a]

[a]*Division of Rheumatology, Department of Clinical and Experimental Medicine, University of Padova, Italy*

[b]*Rheumatology Unit, L. Sacco Hospital, University of Milan, Italy*

[c]*Division of Rheumatology, Department of Internal Medicine, University of Genova, Italy*

ABSTRACT: Successful pregnancy depends on an adaptation of the maternal immune system that becomes tolerant to fetal antigens of paternal origin. The altered immune regulation induced by pregnancy occurs predominantly at the maternal–fetal interface, but it has also been observed in the maternal circulation. Th1/Th2 shift is one of the most important immunologic changes during gestation. It is due to the progressive increase of estrogens, which reach peak level in the third trimester of pregnancy. At these high levels, estrogens suppress the Th1-mediated responses and stimulate Th2-mediated immunologic responses. For this reason Th1-mediated diseases, such as rheumatoid arthritis, tend to improve, while Th2-mediated diseases, such as systemic lupus erythematosus (SLE) tend to worsen during pregnancy. However, in some recent studies SLE flare-ups were less frequently observed in the third trimester of gestation in comparison to the second trimester and postpartum period. These data are apparently in contrast to the Th2 immune-response polarization expected during pregnancy due to the progressive increase of estrogens. Some further data suggest that in SLE patients estradiol serum levels are surprisingly lower than expected during the third trimester of pregnancy, probably due to a placental compromise. This occurrence could lead to a lower-than-expected increase of IL-6, accounting for the low humoral immune response and the low disease activity observed in the third trimester of pregnancy in such patients.

KEYWORDS: estrogens; cytokines; pregnancy; systemic lupus erythematosus; steroid hormones; placenta

Address for correspondence: Andrea Doria, M.D., Division of Rheumatology, University of Padova, Via Giustiniani, 2, 35128 Padova, Italy. Voice: +39-049-8212190; fax: +39-049-8212191. e-mail: adoria@unipd.it

Ann. N.Y. Acad. Sci. 1069: 247–256 (2006). © 2006 New York Academy of Sciences. doi: 10.1196/annals.1351.022

INTRODUCTION

During normal pregnancy, the fetus shows both maternal and paternal human leukocyte antigens; therefore, from the mother's perspective it can be considered as a semiallogeneic transplant.[1]

Despite this, the maternal immune system does not reject the fetus. A possible explanation for this phenomenon is that the feto-maternal interface is located in an immunologically privileged site characterized by a mechanical barrier that reduces the interactions between fetal tissue and maternal lymphocytes[2] and/or functionally alters the maternal immune response.[3]

However, the maternal immune system remains systemically immunocompetent. In fact, in healthy subjects the response to passive and active immunization is normal and the frequency of infection and transplant rejection is not increased during pregnancy.[4,5]

ENDOCRINE AND CYTOKINE NETWORKS AT THE FETO-PLACENTAL INTERFACE

Feto-maternal unit organization starts with the invasion of maternal decidua by trophoblast. The maternal immune system does allow trophoblast invasion anchoring the placenta to the uterus.[6–9]

In the initial phases, the progesterone produced by the corpus luteum induces the differentiation of Th0 to Th2 lymphocytes.[10] Th2 cells inhibit Th1 by the production of IL-4, IL-10, IL-13 as well as by antigen-presenting cell (APC) activity secreting IL-4, IL-6, and IL-10 (FIG. 1). At the feto-maternal interface, APCs are almost all represented by dendritic cells.

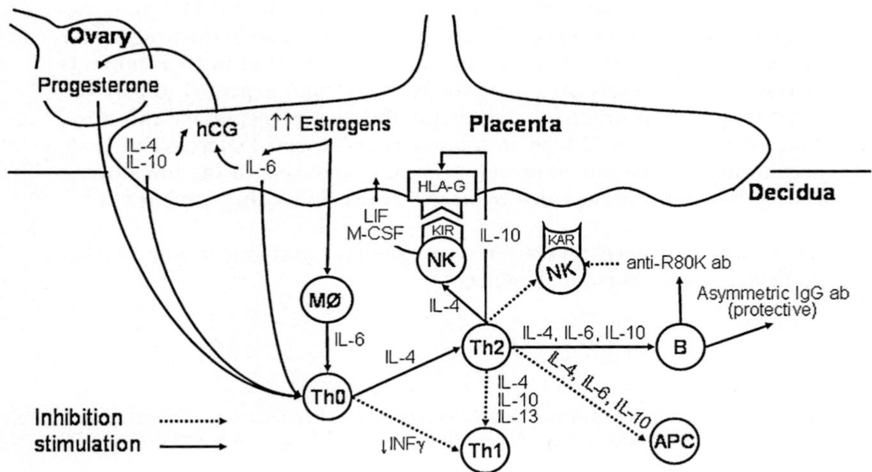

FIGURE 1. Cytokine and endocrine networks at the feto-maternal interface.

Th2 lymphocytes producing IL-4, IL-6, and IL-10 also stimulate differentiation of B cells to plasma cells and, in particular, they stimulate the synthesis of some trophoblast-protecting antibodies, such as asymmetric IgG and anti-R80K antibodies.[11–14] IL-4 produced by Th2 lymphocytes inhibits NK cells expressing the "killer activator receptor" (KAR). These cells are also inhibited by anti-R80K antibodies.

On the contrary, IL-4 stimulates "killer inhibitor receptor" (KIR)–expressing NK cells. This receptor forms a complex with HLA-G molecules expressed by the trophoblast[15] and this interaction blocks the killer activity of NK lymphocytes on trophoblastic cells.[16,17] NK cells start to produce LIF and M-CSF (monocyte-stimulating growth factor), which regulate the invasion of trophoblastic tissue.[18–20]

Th2 cytokines are produced not only by immune cells, but also by the placenta.[6–9] In particular, IL-4, IL-6, and IL-10 stimulate hCG secretion by the placenta,[6,9,21] which in turn stimulates the ovarium to produce progesterone. The same cytokines produced by the placenta can directly stimulate the differentiation of Th0 to Th2 lymphocytes.

Estrogens at high levels, such as those produced by the placenta during the second and third trimester of pregnancy,[22] can stimulate IL-6 production by the placenta itself or by macrophages. This cytokine plays a very important role during the differentiation of Th0 to Th2 lymphocytes.[23]

Therefore, at the feto-maternal interface, a Th1/Th2 shift plays a crucial role: Th1 cytokine reduction results in inhibition of the cellular immune response, and the Th2 increment results in stimulation of the humoral immune response.[24,25] If the Th1/Th2 balance does not shift, abortion can occur.

This shift is mainly modulated by progesterone and estrogens.[23,26] Progesterone participates in the first phase of pregnancy and estrogens seem to be more important during the second period of pregnancy, when they are produced in large amounts by the placenta.

ENDOCRINE AND CYTOKINE NETWORK IN PERIPHERY DURING PREGNANCY

Hormonal modifications during pregnancy are regulated by the feto-placental unit and depend on the interactions between mother and fetus.[27]

Progesterone has a placental origin, since it is secreted by the corpus luteum during the first 6–8 weeks of gestation. During physiological pregnancy progesterone levels are 4–6 times higher than those not during gestation.

Progesterone is the fundamental hormone during the first part of pregnancy and the precursor of some fetal hormones, and it also has other functions, some of which are still partially unknown.

Deoxicorticosterone, one of its metabolites, is found in a concentration 1000 times higher than that in the nonpregnant state, but the physiological role of this hormone is still not known.[27]

Estrogen concentration is also significantly increased during pregnancy, reaching levels 3–8 times higher compared to normal levels.[27] This increase results from a unique interchange between mother and fetus: The fetus uses the pregnenolone produced by the placenta, in order to produce adrenal dehydroepiandrosterone and dehydroepiandrosterone sulfate. These hormones are metabolized to androstenedione and testosterone at the level of the placenta. Finally, they are rapidly converted to estrose and estradiol and are released into the maternal circulation.[27]

The metabolite of dehydroepiandrosterone, which is 16α idroxilate, is converted to estriol in the fetal liver through the same pathways.

One of the main side effects of elevated levels of estrogens during pregnancy is the increased protein synthesis in maternal liver, thus increasing the concentrations of several proteins in the maternal circulation.[27] This phenomenon makes it difficult to explain the slight reduction in circulating levels of complement. An increase of several coagulation proteins has also been shown, which is probably responsible for the hypercoagulability state observed during pregnancy.

The feto-placental hormones, in particular progesterone, estrogens, and placental lactogenic hormone, are responsible for the altered metabolism of carbohydrates observed during gestation. In fact, during the second part of pregnancy, the mother develops a slight peripheral resistance to insulin, thus inducing an increased production and release of insulin by the pancreas.[27] Because of glucose tolerance–induced physiological stress, almost 5% of pregnant women develop gestational diabetes during the second part of pregnancy. The concomitant corticosteroid therapy might predispose to this condition.[27]

Pregnancy and the postpartum period represent a paradigm of how the modification of steroid hormone concentration can influence immune and inflammatory responses in women, as well as being able to modify the concentrations of immunoregulatory molecules (i.e., cytokines) and thereafter the expression of autoimmune diseases.

The physiological increase of cortisol, progesterone, estradiol, and testosterone during the third trimester of pregnancy seems to lead to Th2 cytokine polarization, both at the systemic level and at the feto-maternal interface.[28]

In fact, elevated levels of Th2 cytokines, such as IL-10, have been found in the placenta and amniotic fluid during the third trimester of pregnancy.[29] Therefore, the suppression of the immune response mediated by Th1 cytokines seems to be fundamental for fetal survival.

It has been suggested that some autoimmune diseases, such as SLE, which are mediated mainly by Th2 cytokines and humoral immune response, tend to develop or recrudesce during pregnancy,[30] whereas Th1-mediated diseases, such as rheumatoid arthritis, tend to remit. In both cases a flare-up or onset of disease occurs post partum, when the anti-inflammatory Th2 cytokines collapse.

During normal pregnancy IL-10 production by peripheral lymphocytes progressively increases.[31,32] It has also been demonstrated that during pregnancy IL-6 serum levels gradually increase in maternal circulation and even more during labor.[33] TNF-α serum levels do not vary during pregnancy, whereas those of the TNF-α soluble receptors increase, probably in order to protect the fetus from the dangerous effects of TNF-α.[34,35]

It is known that glucocorticoids inhibit IL-1, TNF-α, IFN-γ, and IL-2 production and that they stimulate IL-10, IL-4, and IL-13 synthesis confirming a modulatory effect on the balance between anti-inflammatory/immunosuppressive responses during pregnancy.[36] At a physiological concentration progesterone stimulates IL-4 (Th2 cytokine) synthesis, whereas estradiol stimulates TNF-α production (Th1 cytokine). On the contrary, at pharmacological levels, such as those observed during the second part of pregnancy, progesterone inhibits TNF-α secretion and stimulates IL-10 production in T lymphocyte clones, leading to an increased humoral immune response.[37,38]

Increased concentration of prolactin is associated with a worsening of renal involvement in animal studies, and that has been found both in SLE males and females. A study carried out to detect serum autoantibodies in women during the premenopausal period has shown that in 20% of these women the prolactin levels were found to be increased and high levels of anti-DNA antibodies were present at the same time. However, the levels of antinuclear antibodies (ANA) were not increased in many women with hyperprolactinemia, not diagnosed as having SLE, and followed at the Endocrinological Center.[39]

CYTOKINE NETWORK IN NONPREGNANT SLE PATIENTS

The cytokine profile has been widely investigated in SLE. An insufficient production of IL-2 *in vitro* by T lymphocytes from SLE patients was observed. This is probably due to several factors including downregulation of some Th2 cytokines.

The recent finding of the role of IL-10 in the pathogenesis of SLE supports this hypothesis. IL-10 is a Th2 cytokine that strongly stimulates B lymphocyte proliferation and differentiation, possibly playing a role as mediator of B cell polyclonal activation in SLE. Recent studies have demonstrated that spontaneous IL-10 production by B lymphocytes and peripheral blood mononuclear cells is significantly more elevated in SLE patients compared to controls.[40,41] In addition, IL-10 concentration in serum was found higher in SLE patients and correlated with clinical and serological activity of the disease, as well as with anti-DNA antibodies.[42–44] Increased production of IL-10 may be caused by a reduced Th1 *in vitro* response of T cells in SLE. This phenomenon has been suggested in a study showing that the addition of IL-10 blocking antibodies significantly increased the proliferative response of peripheral blood mononuclear cells.[45]

IL-12 cytokine is a heterodimer produced by B lymphocytes, macrophages, and dendritic cells,[46] which promotes cell-mediated immune response and has some inhibitory activity on humoral immune response.[47] It has been shown that IL-12 is insufficiently produced by peripheral blood mononuclear cells in SLE patients.[47,48] The deficit of IL-12 production is probably characteristic of monocytes, rather than B lymphocytes.[49] On the contrary, addition of IL-12 to SLE peripheral blood mononuclear cells significantly inhibits both spontaneous and IL-10-stimulated production of immunoglobulins and anti-DNA antibodies.[50] Therefore, the altered regulation of IL-10/IL-12 balance plays a crucial role in the inadequate cellular immune response observed in SLE patients.

IMMUNOENDOCRINE MODIFICATIONS IN SLE PATIENTS DURING PREGNANCY

In healthy subjects, the altered immunoregulation induced by pregnancy is manifested mainly at the feto-maternal interface, whereas systemic effects are negligible. The situation is different in patients affected by autoimmune rheumatic diseases (ARDs) during pregnancy. ARDs are already characterized by an altered immunoregulation and in these patients maternal immune system modifications can influence the course of disease.

One of the most important modifications is the Th1/Th2 shift. It occurs both at feto-placental barrier and in maternal circulation and is driven by the physiological increase of progesterone and estrogens, which occurs progressively throughout pregnancy, the maximal peak occurring during the third trimester of gestation. In particular, progesterone plays an important role in the first part of pregnancy and estrogens play a role in the second part.

In physiological conditions, it seems that estrogens stimulate both humoral and cellular immune responses (Th1 and Th2 cytokines). Nevertheless, at higher than physiological concentrations, such as those reached during pregnancy, it seems that estrogens inhibit cell-mediated immune response (Th1 cytokines), whereas they induce antibody production (Th2 cytokines). The polarization of the Th2 response may explain why the conditions of patients affected by rheumatoid arthritis generally improve during pregnancy whereas those with SLE worsen.

In SLE patients, pregnancy has always been considered a risk both for the mother and fetus since the relapse into disease is frequent during gestation. As a consequence, fetal loss, prematurity, and underweight babies are more common in women with SLE than in healthy subjects.

Nevertheless, in recent years, the number of successful pregnancies has increased, although disease relapse still remains a frequent event during both gestation and post partum.

Recently, a reduced frequency of relapse during the third trimester of pregnancy has been reported compared to those occurring in the second trimester and post partum.

It has been shown that serum levels of some hormones are lower in SLE patients compared to healthy controls.[51] In particular, the concentration of estradiol and progesterone in the serum is unexpectedly low in the second and most of the third trimester of pregnancy, periods during which these hormones are secreted mainly by the placenta. The reduced concentration of estradiol and progesterone may be due to the compromised placental activities, responsible for a lower activation of humoral response and leading to lower disease activity during the third trimester of pregnancy in SLE patients.[51]

The effects of steroid hormones on disease activity during pregnancy seem to be mediated by Th2 cytokines. IL-10 strongly stimulates B lymphocytes and anti-DNA production in SLE. In healthy subjects IL-10 progressively increases during pregnancy, whereas in SLE patients IL-10 serum levels persist at an elevated level before and after pregnancy in the case of both active and inactive disease. These effects support the hypothesis that IL-10 is constitutively hyperproduced in SLE rather than modulated by gonadal hormones (steroids).[52]

On the other hand, it is known that IL-6 is involved in Th0/Th2 shift.[53] The production of IL-6 seems to be correlated with disease activity. In healthy subjects during pregnancy, IL-6 progressively increases in maternal circulation and even more so during delivery. In SLE patients the peak of IL-6 during the third trimester seems to be lacking.[52] The modulation of estrogens on IL-6 production seems to be dose-dependent; at physiological levels estrogens inhibit IL-6, but at pharmacologic levels, such as those reached at the end of pregnancy in physiological conditions, estrogens inhibit IL-6 production.[54] The low levels of IL-6 observed during the third trimester of pregnancy in SLE may depend on the low levels of estrogens observed during the same period of gestation and may explain the lower frequency of relapse reported in the same period.[52]

REFERENCES

1. Abbas, A.K., A.H. Lichtman & J.S. Pober. 1994. Cellular and molecular immunology, 2nd ed. W. B. Saunders Co. Philadelphia.
2. Chaouat, G., J. Kolb & T.G. Wegmann. 1983. The murine placenta as an immunological barrier between the mother and the fetus. Immunol. Rev. **75:** 31–57.
3. Sargent, I.L. 1993. Maternal and fetal immune responses during pregnancy. Exp. Clin. Immunogenet. **10:** 85–97.
4. Falkoff, R. 1998. Maternal immune function during pregnancy. *In* Asthma and Immunological Diseases in Pregnancy and Early Infancy: 73–99. Marcel Dekker. New York.

5. First, M.R., A. Combs, P. Weiskittel, *et al.* 1995. Lack of effect of pregnancy on renal allograft survival or function. Transplantation **59:** 472–476.
6. Nishino, E., N. Matsuzaki, K. Masuhiro, *et al.* 1990. Trophoblast derived IL-6 regulates hCG release through IL-6 receptor on human trophoblasts. J. Clin. Endocrinol. Metab. **74:** 184–190.
7. De Moraes Pinto, M.L., G.S. Vince, B.F. Flanagan, *et al.* 1996. Localization of Il-4 and IL-4 receptors in the human term placenta, deciduas and amniochorionic membranes. Immunology **90:** 87–94.
8. Roth, I., D.B. Corry, R.M. Locksley, *et al.* 1996. Human placental cytotrophoblasts produce the immunosupressive cytokine interleukin 10. J. Exp. Med. **184:** 539–548.
9. Saito, S., N. Harada, N. Ishii, *et al.* 1997. Functional expression on human trophoblasts of interleukin 4 and interleukin 7 receptor complexes with common γ chain. Biochem. Res. Commum. **231:** 429–434.
10. Piccinni, M.P., M.G. Guidizi, R. Biagiotti, *et al.* 1995. Progesterone favors the development of human T helper cell producing Th-2 type cytokines and promotes both IL-4 production and membrane CD expression in established Th1 cell clones. J. Immunol. **155:** 128–133.
11. Margni, R.A. & R.A. Binaghi. 1988. Nonprecipitating asymmetric antibodies. Annu. Rev. Immunol. **6:** 535–554.
12. Margni, R.A. & I. Malan Borel. 1998. Paradoxical behaviour of asymmetric antibodies. Immunol. Rev. **163:** 77–87.
13. Malan Borel, I., T. Gentile, J. Angelucci, *et al.* 1991. IgG asymmetric molecules with anti-paternal activity isolated from sera and placenta of pregnant human. J. Reprod. Immunol. **20:** 129–140.
14. Margni, R.A. & I. Malan Borel. 1999. Role of asymmetric IgG antibodies in fetal maintenance. Curr. Trends Immunol. **2:** 153–163.
15. Carosella, E.D., P. Paul, P. Moreau, *et al.* 2000. HLA-G and HLA-E: fundamental and pathophysiological aspects. Immunol. Today **21:** 532–533.
16. Münz, C., N. Holmes, A. King, *et al.* 1997. Human histocompatibility leukocyte antigen (HLA)-G molecules inhibit NKAT3 expressing natural killer cells. J. Exp. Med. **185:** 385–391.
17. Davis, M.M. & Y.H. Chien. 1995. Issues concerning the nature of antigen recognition by alpha beta and gamma delta T-cell receptors. Immunol. Today **16:** 316–318.
18. Baines, M.G., A.J. Duclos, E. Antecka, *et al.* 1997. Decidual infiltration and activation of macrophages leads to early embryo loss. Am. J. Reprod. Immunol. **37:** 471–477.
19. Coulam, C.B., C. Goodman, R.G. Roussev, *et al.* 1995. Systemic CD56+ cells can predict pregnancy outcome. Am. J. Reprod. Immunol. **33:** 40–46.
20. Haddad, E.K., A.J. Duclos, W.S. Lapp, *et al.* 1997. Early embryo loss is associated with prior expression of macrophage activation markers in the decidua. J. Immunol. **158:** 4886–4892.
21. Sawai, K., N. Matsuzaki, T. Kameda, *et al.* 1995. Leukemia inhibitory factor produced at the fetomaternal interface stimulates chorionic gonadotropin production: its possible implication during pregnancy, including implantation period. J. Clin. Endocrinol. Metab. **80:** 1449–1456.
22. Piccinni, M.P., C. Scaletti, E. Maggi, *et al.* 2000. Role of hormone-controlled Th1- and Th2-type cytokines in successful pregnancy. J. Neuroimmunol. **109:** 30–33.

23. TUTOLO, M., A. SULLI, B. SERIOLO, *et al.* 1995. Estrogens, the immune response and autoimmunity. Clin. Exp. Rheumatol. **13:** 217–226.
24. WEGMANN, T.G., H. LIN, L. GUILBERT, *et al.* 1993. Bidirectional cytokine interactions in the maternal-fetal relationship: is successful pregnancy a Th2 phenomenon? Immunol. Today **14:** 353–356.
25. KRISHAN, L., L.J. GUILBERT, T.G. WEGMANN, *et al.* 1996. T helper response against *Leishmania major* in pregnant C57BL/6 mice increases implantation failure and fetal reabsorptions: correlation with increased IFNγ and TNF and reduced Il-10 production by placental cells. J. Immunol. **156:** 653–662.
26. SZEKERES-BARTHO, J. & T.G. WEGMANN. 1996. A progesterone-dependent immunomodulatory protein alters the Th1/Th2 balance. J. Reprod. Immunol. **31:** 81–95.
27. MARZI, M., A. VIGANO, D. TRABATTONI, *et al.* 1996. Characterization of type 1 and type 2 cytokine production profile in physiologic and pathologic human pregnancy. Clin. Exp. Immunol. **106:** 127–133.
28. MUNOZ-VALLE, J.F., M. VAZQUEZ-DEL MERCADO, T. GARCIA-IGLESIAS, *et al.* 2003. T(H)1/T(H)2 cytokine profile, metalloprotease-9 activity and hormonal status in pregnant rheumatoid arthritis and systemic lupus erythematosus patients. Clin. Exp. Immunol. **131:** 377–384.
29. OPSJØN, S.L., N.C. WETHER, S. TINGLSTAD, *et al.* 1993. Tumor necrosis factor, interleukin-1, and interleukin-6 in normal human pregnancy. Am. J. Obstet. Gynecol. **169:** 397–404.
30. ELENKOV, I.J., J. HOFFMANN & R.L. WILDER. 1997. Does differential neuroendocrine control of cytokine production govern the expression of autoimmune diseases in pregnancy and the postpartum period? Mol. Med. Today **3:** 379–383.
31. RUSSEL, A.S., C. JOHNSTON, C. CHEW, *et al.* 1997. Evidence for reduced Th1 function in normal pregnancy: a hypothesis for the remission of rheumatoid arthritis. J. Rheumatol. **24:** 1045–1050.
32. KUPFERMINE, M.J., A.M. PEACEMAN, D. ADERKA, *et al.* 1995. Soluble tumor necrosis factor receptors in maternal plasma and second-trimester amniotic fluid. Am. J. Obstet. Gynecol. **173:** 900–905.
33. BRANCH, D.W. 1992. Physiologic adaptation of pregnancy. Am. J. Reprod. Immunol. **28:** 120–112.
34. LIN, H., T.R. MOSMAN, L. GUILBERT, *et al.* 1993. Synthesis of T helper-2-cytokines at the maternal-fetal interface. J. Immunol. **151:** 4562–4573.
35. GREIG, P.C., W.N. HERBERT, B.L. ROBINETTE, *et al.* 1995. Amniotic fluid interleukin-10 concentrations increase through pregnancy and are elevated in patients with preterm labor associated with intrauterine infection. Am. J. Obstet. Gynecol. **173:** 1223–1227.
36. RAMIREZ, F., D.J. FOWELL, M. PUKLAVEC, *et al.* 1996. Glucocorticoids promote a Th2 cytokine response by CD4+ T cells *in vitro*. J. Immunol. **156:** 2406–2412.
37. PICCINNI, M.P., M.G. GIUDIZI, R. BIAGIOTTI, *et al.* 1995. Progesterone favors the development of human T helper cells producing Th2-type cytokines and promotes both IL-4 production and membrane CD30 expression in established Th1 cell clones. J. Immunol. **155:** 128–133.
38. CUTOLO, M., A. SULLI, B. SERIOLO, *et al.* 1995. Estrogens, the immune response and autoimmunity. Clin. Exp. Rheumatol. **13:** 217–226.
39. LAHITA, R.G. 1999. The role of sex hormones in systemic lupus erythematosus. Curr. Opin. Rheum. **11:** 352–356.

40. LLORENTE, L., Y. RICHAUD-PATIN, J. WIJDENES, *et al.* 1993. Spontaneous production of interleukin-10 by B-lymphocytes and monocytes in systemic lupus erythematosus. Eur. Cytokine Netw. **4:** 421–427.
41. LLORENTE, L., Y. RICHAUD-PATIN, R. FIOR, *et al.* 1994. In vivo production of interleukin-10 by non-T cells in rheumatoid arthritis, Sjögren's syndrome, and systemic lupus erythematosus. A potential mechanism of B lymphocyte hyperactivity and autoimmunity. Arthritis Rheum. **37:** 1647–1655.
42. HOUSSIAU, F.A., C. LEFEBVRE, M. VANDEN BERGHE, *et al.* 1995. Serum interleukin 10 titers in systemic lupus erythematosus reflect disease activity. Lupus **4:** 393–395.
43. PARK, Y.B., S.K. LEE, D.S. KIM, *et al.* 1998. Elevated interleukin-10 levels correlated with disease activity in systemic lupus erythematosus. Clin. Exp. Rheumatol. **16:** 283–288.
44. GRONDAL, G., I. GUNNARSON, J. RONNELID, *et al.* 2000. Cytokine production, serum levels and disease activity in systemic lupus erythematosus. Clin. Exp. Rheumatol. **18:** 565–570.
45. LAUWERYS, B.R., N. GAROT, J.C. RENAULD, *et al.* 2000. Interleukin-10 blockade corrects impaired in vitro cellular immune responses of systemic lupus erythematosus patients. Arthritis Rheum. **43:** 1976–1681.
46. TRINCHIERI, G. 1994. Interleukin-12: a cytokine produced by antigen-presenting cells with immunoregulatory functions in the generation of T-helper cells type 1 and cytotoxic lymphocytes. Blood **84:** 4008–4027.
47. HOROWITZ, D.A., J.D. GRAY, S.C. BEHRENDSEN, *et al.* 1998. Decreased production of interleukin-12 and other Th1-type cytokines in patients with recent-onset systemic lupus erythematosus. Arthritis Rheum. **41:** 838–844.
48. LIU, T.F. & B.M. JONES. 1998. Impaired production of IL-12 in systemic lupus erythematosus. I. Excessive production of IL-10 suppresses production of IL-12 by monocytes. Cytokine **10:** 140–147.
49. LIU, T.F. & B.M. JONES. 1997. Impairment of IL-12 production in SLE is due to defective monocytes, not B cells. Immuol. Lett. **56:** 314.
50. HOUSSIAU, F.A., F. MASCART-LEMONE, M. STEVENS, *et al.* 1997. IL-12 inhibits in vitro immunoglobulin production by human lupus peripheral blood mononuclear cells (PBMC). Clin. Exp. Immunol. **108:** 375–380.
51. DORIA, A., M. CUTOLO, A. GHIRARDELLO, *et al.* 2002. Steroid hormones and disease activity during pregnancy in systemic lupus eythematosus. Arthritis Rheum. **47:** 202–209.
52. DORIA, A., A. GHIRARDELLO, L. IACCARINO, *et al.* 2004. Pregnancy, cytokines and disease activity in systemic lupus erythematosus. Arthritis Rheum. **51:** 989–995.
53. DIEHL, S. & M. RINCON. 2002. The two faces of IL-6 on Th1/Th2 differentiation. Mol. Immunol. **39:** 531–536.
54. KOVACS, E.J., K.A. MESSINGHAM & M.S. GREGORY. 2002. Estrogen regulation of immune responses after injury. Mol. Cell. Endocrinol. **193:** 129–135.

Androgen and Prolactin (Prl) Levels in Systemic Sclerosis (SSc)

Relationship to Disease Severity

LUISA MIRONE,[a] ANGELA BARINI,[b] AND ANTONELLA BARINI[c]

[a]*U.O.C. Reumatologia – Cattedra di Reumatologia, Catholic University, Rome, Italy*

[b]*Istituto di Biochimica e Biochimica Clinica – Catholic University, Rome, Italy*

[c]*Complesso Integrato Columbus, Rome, Italy*

ABSTRACT: **Testosterone (T), sex hormone-binding globulin, (SHBG), dehydroepiandrosterone sulfate (DHEAS), and prolactin (Prl) serum levels were measured by electrochemiluminescense immunoassay (ECLIA) in 39 patients with systemic sclerosis (SSc) and compared with serum hormonal levels in control subjects matched for sex and reproductive status. A possible relationship with disease duration and disease severity was examined. Our data show an altered androgen and prolactin (Prl) status in SSc patients, in most cases related to disease duration and disease severity score. We can hypothesize that hormonal dysregulation is a consequence of the chronicity of the disease. The altered hormonal status could result in relative immunological hyperactivity contributing to enhance tissue damage and disease severity.**

KEYWORDS: **testosterone; dehydroepiandrosterone sulfate; prolactin, systemic sclerosis**

INTRODUCTION

Prolactin (Prl), adrenal androgens, and sex steroids seem to have multiple immunomodulatory functions and a number of observations suggest that the hormonal status may play a role in the pathogenesis, the onset, or the clinical course of autoimmune disorders, such as systemic sclerosis (SSc). SSc is a T cell–mediated connective tissue disease occurring more frequently in women than in men, women in childbearing (CB) age being at peak risk.[1,2] SSc is characterized by inflammatory and immunological abnormalities and activation or dysfunction of the endothelial cells with vascular lesions. Both Prl and

Address for correspondence: Dr. Luisa Mirone, U.O.C. Reumatologia – Cattedra di Reumatologia, Università Cattolica del Sacro Cuore c/o Complesso Integrato Columbus via G. Moscati 31 00168 Roma Italia. Voice: 06- 3503429; fax: 06- 35451740.
e-mail: luisa.mirone@rm.unicatt.it

Ann. N.Y. Acad. Sci. 1069: 257–262 (2006).
doi: 10.1196/annals.1351.023

the adrenal androgen DHEAS modulate the cell–mediated immune functions upregulating the T helper 1–mediated responses,[3–5] whereas T enhances suppressor/cytotoxic $CD4^-$ $CD8^+$ T cell activity.[6] Only a few clinical studies have dealt with serum Prl and DHEAS levels in patients with SSc, while no data are available to our knowledge on testosterone levels in SSc patients, except for one clinical study on impotence in male SSc patients.[7] The purpose of this study was to investigate the serum levels of Prl, DHEAS, and testosterone in SSc patients and to examine the possible correlation with disease severity and disease duration.

PATIENTS AND METHODS

Thirty-nine SSc patients, 34 women and 5 men, were examined. All patients entered the study consecutively without prior selection. The disease duration for each SSc patient was assessed at history and was calculated from either the appearance of Raynaud's phenomenon or the onset of the first symptom ascribable to SSc. Clinical and epidemiological data concerning SSc patients are illustrated in TABLE 1. A clinical evaluation was carried out and disease severity was assessed in each SSc patient using the preliminary nine organ/system severity scale proposed by Medsger *et al.* General peripheral vascular, skin, joint/tendon, muscle, gastrointestinal tract, lung, heart, and kidney involvement was detected and assigned a severity grade ranging from 0 (normal) to 4 (end stage). An autoantibody profile was assessed in each SSc patient. Corticosteroid use was taken into account in female SSc patients (methylprednisolone

TABLE 1. Epidemiological and clinical features of SSc patients

Systemic sclerosis	34F/5M
Age (years ± SD)	F: 48.5 ± 12.6/ M: 51.4 ± 13.6
Disease duration (years ± SD)	F: 7.8 ± 7.5/ M: 6.4 ± 3.4
Childbearing aged women	12 cases
Age (years ± SD)	35.3 ± 5.2
Disease duration (years ± SD)	5.1 ± 5.6
Postmenopausal women	22 cases
Age (years ± SD)	55.7 ± 8.9
Disease duration (years ± SD)	9.3 ± 8.2
Clinical subset of SSc	
Limited	19 cases
Diffuse	20 cases
Autoantibody profile	
ACA-positive	14 cases
Anti-Scl70-positive	14 cases
ANA others	11 cases

F: female; M: male; ACA: anticentromere.

≤8 mg/day). No patient was pregnant or breast feeding. No patient was on treatment with estrogen oral contraceptives or drugs known to influence Prl, DHEAS, or T serum levels. Serum levels of T, sex hormone-binding globulin (SHBG), DHEAS, and Prl were measured by electrochemiluminescense immunoassay (ECLIA) in each SSc patient and in 43 control subjects matched for sex and reproductive status. Data were analyzed using the Statistical Package for the Social Science (SPSS) version 11.5 for Windows. Values were expressed as the mean ± standard deviation (SD). Mann–Whitney U test and the Spearman's rank correlation test were used. The level of significance was $P < 0.05$.

RESULTS

Results concerning hormonal serum levels in SSc patients and controls are shown in TABLES 2 and 3.

When the correlation analysis was performed, we found that in all SSc patients ERS and PCR values positively correlated ($r = 0.498$; $P = 0.001$). The organ/system severity score positively correlated with ESR ($r = 0.38$; $P = 0.009$), PCR ($r = 0.27$; $P = 0.045$) and disease duration ($r = 0.404$; $P = 0.005$). Serum T and DHEAS levels negatively correlated with ESR ($r = -0.278$; $P = 0.044$ and $r = -0.304$; $P = 0.030$, respectively) and PCR ($r =$

TABLE 2. Hormonal serum levels in SSc patients of childbearing age, postmenopausal SSc patients, male SSc patients, and controls

	CB age women		
	SSc (12)	Controls (14)	P*
Testosterone (ng/mL)	0.24 ± 0.19	0.44 ± 0.12	0.005
SHBG (ng/mL)	53.05 ± 20.46	41.8 ± 17.5	ns
DHEAS (ng/mL)	990.83 ± 773.39	2095.73 ± 726.43	0.001
Prl (ng/mL)	24.88 ± 11.79	15.81 ± 3.6	0.019
		Post M women	
	SSc (22)	Controls (23)	P*
Testosterone (ng/mL)	0.16 ± 0.09	0.26 ± 0.16	0.03
SHBG (ng/mL)	41.49 ± 20.44	45.95 ± 21.66	ns
DHEAS (ng/mL)	668.63 ± 351.5	625.65 ± 269.3	ns
Prl (ng/mL)	22.88 ± 9.5	14.34 ± 3.8	0.001
		Males	
	SSc (5)	Controls (8)	P*
Testosterone (ng/mL)	4.4 ± 1.39	5.12 ± 1.2	ns
SHBG (ng/mL)	37.5 ± 19.6	43.21 ± 18.42	ns
DHEAS (ng/mL)	633 ± 511.78	1973 ± 600.7	0.005
Prl (ng/mL)	16.6 ± 7.56	11.37 ± 5.04	ns

CB age: childbearing age; post-M: postmenopausal.
The number of cases is shown between parentheses.
*Mann–Whitney U test.

TABLE 3. Hormonal serum levels in SSc women on steroids and those not on steroids

	CB age SSc women (12)		
	Steroid users (4)	Steroid nonusers (8)	P^*
Testosterone (ng/mL)	0.1 ± 0.13	0.3 ± 0.19	ns
SHBG (ng/mL)	60.85 ± 25.2	49.15 ± 18.24	ns
DHEAS (ng/mL)	519.75 ± 529.2	1226.37 ± 793.5	ns
Prl (ng/mL)	24.75 ± 10.34	24.87 ± 13.1	ns
	Post-M SSc women (22)		
	Steroid users (5)	Steroid nonusers (17)	P^*
Testosterone (ng/mL)	0.15 ± 0.11	0.16 ± 0.09	ns
SHBG (ng/mL)	34.5 ± 14.6	43.55 ± 21.81	ns
DHEAS (ng/mL)	879.6 ± 434.38	606.58 ± 311.46	ns
Prl (ng/mL)	23.8 ± 10.1	32.6 ± 9.6	ns

CB age: childbearing age; post-M: postmenopausal.
The number of cases is shown between parentheses.
*Mann–Whitney U test.

−0.281; $P = 0.042$ and $r = -0.380$; $P = 0.009$, respectively). Furthermore, serum DHEAS levels were negatively correlated with disease duration ($r = -0.381$; $P = 0.008$). Serum T and DHEAS levels were positively correlated ($r = 0.438$; $P = 0.003$). Similar results with regards to ESR, PCR, organ/system severity, and disease duration were found when only female SSc patients were considered. In female SSc patients serum T levels correlated with PCR ($r = -0.357$; $P = 0.019$) and disease duration ($r = 0.338$; $P = 0.025$) while serum DHEAS levels correlated with ESR ($r = -0.454$; $P = 0.003$), PCR ($r = -0.479$; $P = 0.002$), organ/system severity score ($r = 0.33$; $P = 0.028$), and disease duration ($r = -0.445$; $P = 0.004$). T and DHEAS serum levels strongly positively correlated ($r = 0.682$; $P = 0.0001$). Only when the 25 female SSc patients not on corticosteroid therapy were considered, the organ/system severity score correlated with ESR ($r = 0.386$; $P = 0.028$) and disease duration ($r = 0.338$; $P = 0.049$). T levels correlated with ESR ($r = -0.405$; $P = 0.022$) and disease duration ($r = -0.392$: $P = 0.026$). DHEAS levels correlated with ESR ($r = -0.585$; $P = 0.001$), PCR ($r = -0.485$; $P = 0.007$), and disease duration ($r = -0.414$; $P = 0.02$), while serum testosterone and DHEAS levels positively correlated ($r = 0.52$; $P = 0.004$).

DISCUSSION

This study shows an altered hormonal status in SSc patients. SSc is a T cell–mediated connective tissue disease occurring more frequently in women of childbearing age. The clinical hallmark of the disease is a progressive fibrosis of the skin and various internal organs. Inflammatory and immunological abnormalities and vascular lesions characterize the disease. Due to injury or dysfunction of the dermal microvascular endothelial cells, an activated expression of certain adhesion molecules (CAMs) seems to occur in SSc.[8] Sex steroids are known to affect the endothelial expression of CAMs, influence the immune system, and have immunomodulatory effects on both peripheral T cell and B cell subsets in adult life.[9] Data in the literature suggest that androgen steroids may play a protective anti-inflammatory/immunosuppressive role and exert a favorable effect on autoimmune diseases.[10] According to other authors we found a reduction in serum DHEAS levels in our female CB age and male SSc patients[11,12] and a reduction in serum T levels in female SSc patients, both in CB age and in postmenopausal status, in most cases related to disease duration and disease severity score. We can infer that hormonal dysregulation is a consequence of the chronicity of the disease. The altered hormonal status could result in relative immunological hyperactivity contributing to alter the functions of vascular cells and fibroblasts, resulting in the accumulation of collagen and other extracellular matrix constituents[13] and to enhance disease severity. Prl is a natural immune enhancer. The hormone upregulates the T helper 1–mediated responses, induces sIL-2R on lymphocytes, is an important intracellular prerequisite for T cell proliferation, and is thought to be a second messenger for IL-2 effects.[3,4] According to other studies,[11,14] we found a mild hyperprolactinemia in our SSc patients, which might have an exacerbating effect in the disease. However, because of the lack of association with laboratory and clinical disease severity in SSc, the implication of mild hyperprolactinemia in this disease should be investigated further. As in SLE and RA, Prl and DHEAS have shown contrasting serum levels in SSc patients, while under conditions other than aging or the presence of immune diseases, DHEAS and Prl have a positive feedback regulation. The dysregulation of adrenal (DHEAS) and hypothalamic-pituitary function (Prl) is a characteristic feature of immune diseases. Whether high Prl secretion is involved in the primary pathogenetic defect in patients with SSc cannot be answered by means of our study, but elevated levels of this hormone are probably linked to high T lymphocyte activity and enhanced lymphocyte adhesion via VCAM, while the reduced adrenocortical and/or gonadal steroidogenesis could favor the immunostimulatory effect of Prl.

REFERENCES

1. Smith E.A. & E.C. LeRoy. 1997. Connective tissue diseases—systemic sclerosis: etiology and pathogenesis. *In* J. Klippel, P.A. Dieppe, Eds.: Rheumatology, second edition. London: Mosby Yearbook Europe.
2. White B. 1996. Immunopathogenesis of systemic sclerosis. Rheum. Dis. Clin. North. Am. **22:** 695–708.
3. Viselli, S.M., E.M. Stanek, P. Mukherjee, *et al.* 1991. Prolactin-induced mitogenesis of lymphocytes from ovariectomized rats. Endocrinology **129:** 983–990.

4. Clevenger, C.V., S.W. Altmann & M.B. Prytowsky. 1991. Requirement of nuclear prolactin for interleukin-2-stimulated proliferation of T cells. Science **53:** 77–79.
5. Suzuki T., N. Suzuki, R.A. Daynes & E.G. Engeleman. 1991. Dehydroepiandrosterone enhances IL2 production and cytotoxic effector function of human T cells. Clin. Immunol. Imunopathol. **61:** 202–211.
6. Olsen, N.J. & W.J. Kovacs. 2001. Effects of androgens on T and B lymphocyte development. Immunol. Res. **23:** 281–288.
7. Nowlin, N.S., J.E. Brick, D.J. Weaver, *et al.* 1986. Impotence in scleroderma. Ann. Int. Med. **104:** 794–798.
8. Luscinskas, F.W. & M.A. Jr Gimbrone. 1996. Endothelial-dependent mechanisms in chronic inflammatory leukocyte recruitment. Annu. Rev. Med. **47:** 413–421.
9. Van Vollenhoven, R.F. 1995. Adhesion molecules, sex steroids and the pathogenesis of vasculitis syndromes. Curr. Opin. Rheumatol. **7:** 4–10.
10. Tanriverdi F., L.F.G. Silveira, G.S. MacColl & P.M.G. Bouloux. 2003. The hypothalamic-pituitary-gonadal axis. J. Endocrinol. **176:** 293–304.
11. La Montagna G., A. Baruffo, G. Buono, & G. Valentini. 2001. Dehydroepiandrosterone sulphate serum levels in systemic sclerosis. Clin. Exp. Rheumatol. **19:** 21–26.
12. Straub, R.H., M. Zeuner, G. Lock, *et al.* 1997. High prolactin and low dehydroepiandrosterone sulphate serum levels in patients with severe systemic sclerosis. Br. J. Rheumatol. **36:** 426–432.
13. Jimenez, S.A., E. Hitraya & J. Varga. 1996. Pathogenesis of scleroderma: collagen. Rheum. Dis. Clin. North Am. **22:** 647–674.
14. Hilty C., P. Bruhlmann, H. Sprott, *et al.* 2000. Altered diurnal rhythm of prolactin in systemic sclerosis. J. Rheumatol. **27:** 2160–2165.

Role of Estrogens in Inflammatory Response

Expression of Estrogen Receptors in Peritoneal Fluid Macrophages from Endometriosis

SILVIA CAPELLINO,[a] PAOLA MONTAGNA,[a] BARBARA VILLAGGIO,[a] ALBERTO SULLI,[a] STEFANO SOLDANO,[a] SIMONE FERRERO,[b] VALENTINO REMORGIDA,[b] AND MAURIZIO CUTOLO[a]

[a]*Research Laboratory and Division of Rheumatology, Department of Internal Medicine, San Martino Hospital, University of Genoa, 16126 Genoa, Italy*

[b]*Department of Obstetrics and Gynecology, San Martino Hospital, University of Genoa, 16126 Genoa, Italy*

ABSTRACT: Estrogens are involved in the immune response, and macrophages express estrogen receptors (ER). Moreover, macrophages are the predominant cell type in the peritoneal fluid from endometriosis patients. On this basis, the aim of our study was to evaluate the expression of ER on peritoneal macrophages from endometriosis patients and to compare these results with what is already known about ER and macrophages in RA. After macrophage extraction from peritoneal fluids we performed the immunohistochemical localization of ERα and ERβ and then the image analysis. We found that both ERs were significantly overexpressed in macrophages of women with endometriosis compared with controls. These results suggest that estrogens, through their functional receptors, might modulate the immune response at least on macrophages. Therefore, estrogens seem to play an important role in the immune response, independently from the pathology.

KEYWORDS: endometriosis; rheumatoid arthritis; estrogens; estrogen receptors; macrophages

INTRODUCTION

It is well known that estrogens play a key role in the immune response, following their binding to specific receptors. Estrogen receptors α (ERα) and

Address for correspondence: Silvia Capellino, Laboratory of Neuroendocrinoimmunology, Department of Internal Medicine I, University Hospital Regensburg, 93042 Regensburg, Germany. Voice: +49-941-944-7116; fax: +49-941-944-7121.
e-mail: silvia.capellino@klinik.uni-regensburg.de

**Ann. N.Y. Acad. Sci. 1069: 263–267 (2006). © 2006 New York Academy of Sciences.
doi: 10.1196/annals.1351.024**

β (ERβ) are nuclear receptors that directly interact with estrogen-regulated genes. Interestingly, the ERs could have various effects depending on the cell type.[1] It is demonstrated that macrophages express functional sex hormone receptors, such as ER. Through these receptors, estrogens can effect inflammatory mediator production by macrophages and play a role in monocyte differentiation.[2,3]

Furthermore, it is already demonstrated that estrogens play a key role in the immune-inflammatory response in most inflammatory rheumatic diseases, such as rheumatoid arthritis (RA),[4] and that synovial macrophages from RA patients overexpress ER.[5] Similarly, endometriosis is defined like a common, benign, *estrogen-dependent*, chronic gynecological disorder associated with pelvic pain and infertility,[6] and it has been observed that macrophages are the predominant nucleated cells in the peritoneal fluid of these patients.[7]

Therefore, the aim of this study was to evaluate the expression of ER on peritoneal macrophages from patients with endometriosis and to compare these results with what is already known about ER and macrophages in RA, in order to understand whether the effects of estrogens on macrophage response are disease related or not.

MATERIALS AND METHODS

Peritoneal Fluid Collection

Peritoneal fluid samples were obtained from 30 patients with endometriosis and 22 controls (infertility, $n = 12$; pelvic pain, $n = 10$) (TABLE 1). Only women in the reproductive age with a menstrual cycle length between 21 and 35 days were included in the study. At the time of surgery, all the patients were undergoing exclusively nonsteroidal anti-inflammatory treatments for at least 3 months. None had received any corticosteroid therapy nor was using oral contraceptive pills or GnRH analogs.

Macrophage Extraction from Peritoneal Fluids

Peritoneal fluids were centrifuged and the contaminant erythrocytes were eliminated from the cellular pellet by osmotic lysis. Vitality of freshly isolated macrophages was determined by trypan blue dye exclusion. The macrophages were resuspended in Dulbecco's Phosphate Buffered Saline (DPBS) at 3×10^5 cells/mL, placed on glass slides, incubated for 40 min at 4°C, fixed in cold acetone and stored at –20°C until analysis.

Immunohistochemistry (IHC)

Immunohistochemical localization of ERα and ERβ was performed by using a mouse monoclonal and a rabbit polyclonal antibody, respectively (Affinity Bioreagents, CO). Immunohistochemical staining was performed with the biotin-streptavidin-peroxidase method.

Image Analysis

The image analysis was performed by using the Leica Q500 MC image analysis system (Leica, Cambridge, UK) that allows measurement of the percentage of positive stained area of each cell; for the digital image analysis, about 100 cells were evaluated for each condition.

Statistical analysis was carried out using analysis of variance (ANOVA) or, if necessary, the nonparametric Mann–Whitney *U*-test. A probability (P) value ≤ 0.05 was considered statistically significant.

RESULTS

Both the isoforms of ER were expressed by macrophages of patients affected by endometriosis and also by macrophages of control subjects. However, ERα and ERβ were significantly overexpressed in macrophages of women with endometriosis compared with controls (ERα: 20.15 $\pm$ 1.85% of positive stained area in endometriosis and 5.4 $\pm$ 1.3% in the control group, $P < 0.001$, ERβ: 19 $\pm$ 2.5% of positive stained area in endometriosis and 6.15 $\pm$ 2% in the control group, $P < 0.005$) (FIGS. 1 and 2). No significant differences concerning macrophage ER expression were found between women in the follicular or in the luteal phase of menstrual cycle. Interestingly, the expression of ER in

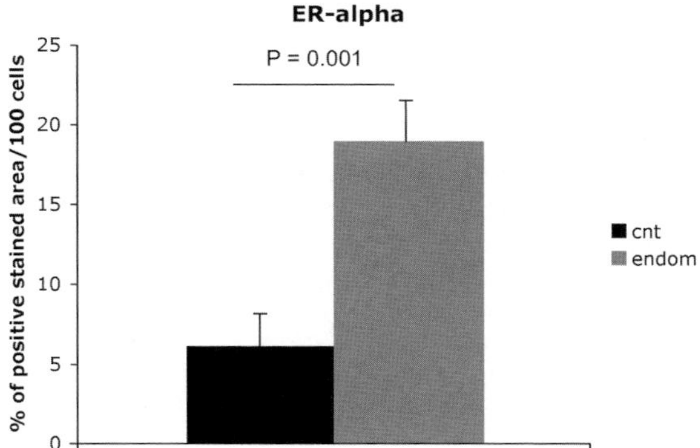

FIGURE 1. Expression of ERα on peritoneal macrophages from control subjects (dark column) and endometriosis patients (gray column). The results are obtained by using the Leica Q500 MC image analysis system that allows measurement of the percentage of positive stained area of each cell; for the digital image analysis about 100 cells were evaluated for each condition.

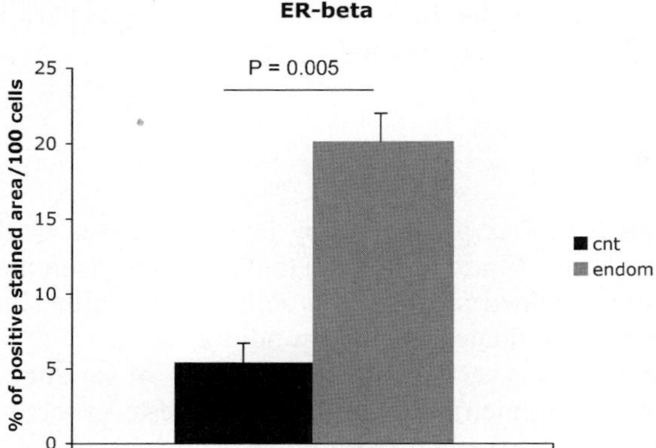

FIGURE 2. Expression of ERβ on peritoneal macrophages from control subjects (dark column) and endometriosis patients (gray column). The results are obtained by using the Leica Q500 MC image analysis system that allows measurement of the percentage of positive stained area of each cell; for the digital image analysis about 100 cells were evaluated for each condition.

endometriosis seems to be positively correlated to the expression of inflammatory cytokines and markers of macrophage differentiation (data not shown).

DISCUSSION

RA and endometriosis are two different pathologies; however, both diseases are characterized by a strong immune-inflammatory reaction, and in particular macrophages are strongly involved in this immune-inflammatory response. Interestingly, the influence of estrogens on macrophages seems to be common in both conditions. In fact, our data suggest that estrogens, through their functional receptors, might modulate the immune response at least on monocytes/macrophages, and that their expression seems to be related with the inflammatory reaction. Therefore, estrogens seem to play an important role in the immune response, independently from the pathology.

REFERENCES

1. LANG, T.J. 2004. Estrogen as an immunomodulator. Clin. Immunol. **113:** 224–230.
2. CARRUBA, G. *et al.* 2003. Estrogen regulates cytokine production and apoptosis in PMA-differentiated macrophage-like U937 cells. J. Cell. Biochem. **90:** 187–196.
3. MOR, G. *et al.* 2003. Interaction of the estrogen receptors with the Fas ligand promoter in human monocytes. J. Immunol. **170:** 114–122.

4. CUTOLO, M. *et al.* 1995. Estrogens, the immune response and autoimmunity. Clin. Exp. Rheumatol. **13:** 217–226.
5. CUTOLO, M. *et al.* 1996. Androgen and estrogen receptors are present in primary cultures of human synovial macrophages. J. Clin. Endocrinol. Metab. **81:**820–827.
6. GIUDICE, L. & L.C. KAO. 2004. Endometriosis. Lancet **364:** 1789–1799.
7. BECKER, J.L. *et al.* 1995. Human peritoneal macrophage and T lymphocyte populations in mild and severe endometriosis. Am. J. Reprod. Immunol. **34:** 179–187.

Are Glucocorticoids DMARDs?

JOHANNES W.J. BIJLSMA, JOS N. HOES, AMALIA A. VAN EVERDINGEN, SUZAN M.M. VERSTAPPEN, AND JOHANNES W.G. JACOBS

Department of Rheumatology and Clinical Immunology, University Medical Center Utrecht, 3508 GA Utrecht, The Netherlands

ABSTRACT: Disease modifying antirheumatic drugs (DMARDs) are drugs used in rheumatoid arthritis (RA) to control the disease and to limit joint damage and improve long-term outcome. The last decade evidence has accumulated that suggests that low dosages of glucocorticoids are indeed able to control the disease and limit the destruction. This role is especially present in early disease and in combination with other drugs. The evidence is carefully evaluated and discussed. The ultimate conclusion is that indeed glucocorticoids are DMARDs and are especially useful in early RA.

KEYWORDS: glucocorticoids; DMARDs; rheumatoid arthritis; erosions; prednisone

INTRODUCTION

Drugs for the management of rheumatoid arthritis (RA) have been traditionally, but imperfectly, divided into two groups: those used primarily for the control of joint pain and swelling, and those intended to, in addition, limit joint damage and improve long-term outcome. Drugs that are used principally to control the disease and to limit joint damage have been called disease modifying antirheumatic drugs, or DMARDs. These include traditional drugs, such as intramuscular gold (iAU), hydroxychloroquine (HC), sulphasalazine (SSZ), methotrexate (MTX), and biologic response modifiers with actions targeted against specific cytokines, such as tumor necrosis factor-α (TNF-α). As treatment of RA becomes more effective and more complex, more attention is given to drugs, which are able to control disease and induce remission and retard or even halt joint destruction. In this respect, there has been a revival of the role of glucocorticoids in the treatment of RA.[1]

Address for correspondence: Prof. J.W.J. Bijlsma, Department of Rheumatology and Clinical Immunology, University Medical Center Utrecht, Box 85 500, 3508 GA Utrecht, The Netherlands. Voice: +31-30-250-7357; fax: +31-30-252-3741.
e-mail: j.w.j.bijlsma@umcutrecht.nl

Ann. N.Y. Acad. Sci. 1069: 268–274 (2006). © 2006 New York Academy of Sciences.
doi: 10.1196/annals.1351.025

Mechanisms of Joint Destruction

Joint destruction in RA involves articular cartilage, ligaments, tendons, and bone. Several mechanisms contribute to this tissue destruction process. Inflammatory mediators and enzymes in the synovial fluid have a direct effect on articular cartilage. Focal bone erosions develop at the margin between bone and cartilage that is invaded by the proliferating synovial membrane, also referred to as pannus. One of the first steps in focal bone erosions is the recruitment and differentiation of cells into an osteoclast phenotype. T cells and fibroblast-like cells in rheumatoid synovium produce osteoclast differentiation factor.

Chondrocytes and osteoclasts actively participate in the loss of extracellular matrix.[2] Synovial tissue cells produce many chemoattractants and cytokines. Classic chemoattractants present in the joint include the complement factor C5a, which has been activated as a consequence of immune complex formation, and the leukotriene B4. The presence of cytokines and phagocytosis of soluble immune complexes by neutrophils, result in prostaglandin and leukotriene production, neutrophil degranulation and respiratory burst, facilitating accumulation of a critical concentration of active proteinases and oxygen metabolites. The tissue-destructive properties of pannus are closely related to the production of metalloproteinases and other proteinases, which are able to degrade collagen and proteoglycans. The production of these proteinases is controlled by a number of different cytokines, including interleukin-1, TNF-α, and T-cell growth factor beta (TGF-β). Chondrocytes respond to these cytokines with a decrease in collagen and proteoglycan synthesis, while simultaneously increasing synthesis of collagenase and stromelysin, which degrade type II collagen and proteoglycans of the cartilage.

Nearly all single steps described in this cascade of events can be blocked by glucocorticoids. Recently this was clearly shown in a study on the effects of oral prednisone on biomarkers in synovial tissue, showing among others a marked reduction in macrophage infiltration of the synovial tissue.[3] Therefore, there is a strong theoretical basis for the suggestion that glucocorticoids may act as DMARDs, slowing down the process of joint damage.

CLINICAL STUDIES

Glucocorticoids as Mono Therapy

In the mid 1950s, the Medical Research Council (MRC) was the first to conduct a trial of 122 patients with early RA, comparing the effect of cortisone 80 mg/day (equivalent to prednisone 16 mg/day) with that of aspirin 4.5 mg/day. After 2 years, the glucocorticoid-treated group had some better clinical results, but radiological deterioration had still occurred.[4] After this initial study, the MRC compared the effectiveness of prednisone 12 mg/day during the first year and 10 mg/day during the second year with aspirin and other nonsteroidal anti-inflammatory drugs (NSAIDs) in 77 patients. After 2 years, there was a statistically significant reduction of progression of erosions in the prednisone-treated group.[5] The same group was evaluated up to 7 years later, and at that time still a statistically significant radiological difference was noted in favor of the prednisone-treated patients. A similar study of 100 patients, performed by the Empire Rheumatism Council, compared the effect of cortisone 75 mg/day (equivalent to prednisone 15 mg/day) with that of aspirin 3.3 mg/day for 3 years. No clinical or radiological differences between these two treatment groups were found at 2 and 3 years.[6] However, interpretation of the results in these studies is difficult, because of the heterogeneity of the patient groups and long duration of disease in some of the groups at the start of the studies, confounding by indication as well as multiple, often suboptimal, concomitant therapies.

In 2002, we published the results of a randomized placebo-controlled trial on the effects of prednisolone in DMARD-naïve patients with early RA. Ten mg of prednisolone daily in these patients, who only got DMARD therapy as a rescue, clearly inhibited the progression of radiological joint damage (FIG. 1). Apart from this positive effect on the radiological joint damage, in this study a 40% decreased need for intra-articular glucocorticoid injections, 49% decreased need for acetaminophen use and, importantly, a 55% decreased need for NSAID use was found in the prednisolone group compared to the placebo group.[7,8] It is of great clinical importance to note that even 3 years after concluding the 2-year treatment strategy, the differences in the

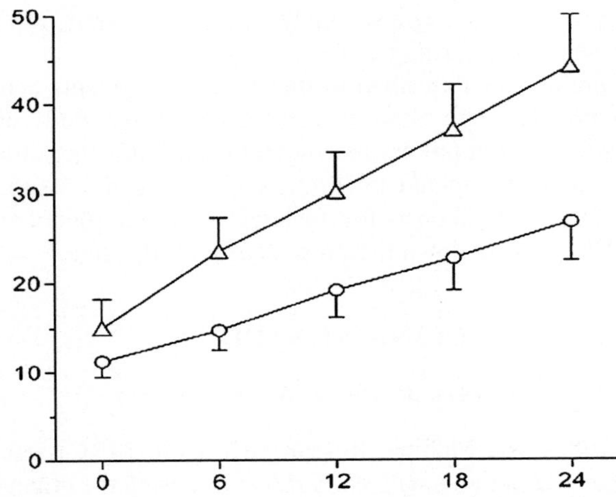

FIGURE 1. Radiological scores (y-axis, modified Sharp scores) of 40 patients, randomized to prednisone therapy (circles) and 41 patients, randomized to placebo (triangles) in time (x-axis, months); means and standard errors.* Differences between groups at 12, 18, and 24 months statistically significant.

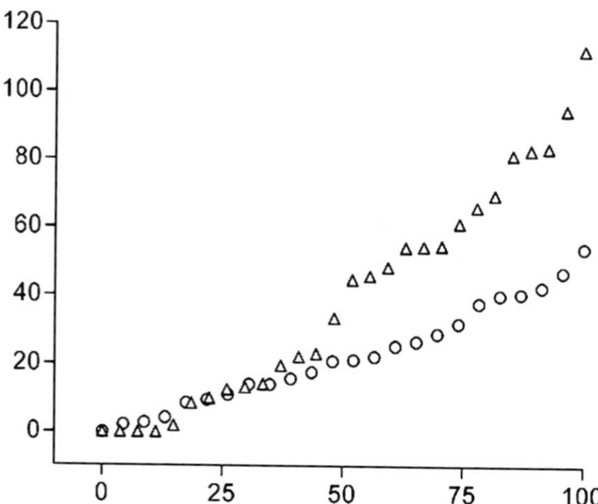

FIGURE 2. Cumulative probability plots of radiological progression during 3 years since the end of the 2-year study. Y-axis: radiological score (modified Sharp score); x-axis: cumulative probability. Circles indicate the scores of 24 patients, (originally) randomized to prednisone therapy and triangles those of 28 patients, (originally) randomized to placebo.

total joint damage and in the erosion score persisted statistically significantly (see FIG. 2).[9]

Glucocorticoids as Adjuvant Treatment

Kirwan performed in the United Kingdom a randomized, placebo-controlled study looking at the effect of 7.5-mg prednisone on joint damage. Either prednisolone or placebo was given for 2 years as adjuvant treatment to 128 patients with early RA, in addition to NSAIDs in 95% of the patients, and traditional DMARDs in 71% of patients. After 2 years, the number of patients with erosions and the total number of new erosions were significantly lower in the prednisolone-treated group.[10] The group of RA patients participating in this trial was heterogeneous, not only with respect to disease duration, but also to stages of the disease and the dosage schedules of DMARDs. In a follow-up of this cohort, it was shown that joint destruction resumed after tapering and discontinuation of the glucocorticoids.[11]

In the COBRA trial, published in 1997, patients with early RA were randomized to either step-down therapy with 2 DMARDs (SSZ and MTX) and prednisolone (start 60 mg/day tapered in 6 weekly steps to 7.5 mg/day and stopped at 28 weeks) or SSZ alone. In the combined drug strategy group, a statistically significant and clinically relevant effect in retarding joint damage was shown, compared to the effect of SSZ alone.[12] In an extension of the study, long-term (4–5 years) benefits were also shown with regard to radiological damage following the combination strategy.[13]

In a German study, a lower dose of prednisolone, i.e., 5-mg daily, was evaluated in 192 patients with early RA treated with either iAU or MTX. In this double-blind, placebo-controlled trial, 5-mg prednisolone proved to be more effective in reducing radiological progression of erosions, confirming the data in above-mentioned studies.[14]

In a Danish study, 102 patients with active longstanding RA were randomly allocated to treatment with DMARD alone or DMARD and prednisolone in a 1-year follow-up study. Dosage of prednisolone depended on disease activity of the individual patient.[15] Disease activity, Larsen score, and bone mineral density were measured. No firm conclusions could be drawn: disease activity was not well controlled; prednisolone was not able to retard progression of erosions significantly, but the effect on bone loss in the hand and distal forearm was protective.

Different results were reported by Scottish clinicians who performed a double-blind, placebo-controlled trial in 167 patients with RA with a slightly longer disease duration (< 3 years). All patients were started on the DMARD SSZ and in addition allocated by stratified randomization to prednisolone 7 mg/day or placebo. Only 112 patients completed the study after 2 years, with more patients in the prednisolone-treated group than in the placebo prednisolone-treated group: 61 versus 53. Though the progression of joint damage was comparable in both groups, the number of patients that had no erosions at the start but developed new erosions during the study period was 6 in the placebo-treated group and only 2 in the prednisolone-treated group.[16]

CONCLUSIONS

From the different studies, it has become clear that glucocorticoids are indeed able to reduce the progression of joint damage. It seems that the earlier in the disease glucocorticoids are given, the more they are effective in doing so. This is illustrated, e.g., in the differences between the Utrecht study and the Scottish study: in the Utrecht study patients had disease symptoms < 1 year and in the Scottish study < 3 years. The results were much better in the Utrecht study. In addition, it seems that when glucocorticoids are given early in the disease, the effect holds for a more prolonged period of time: in the studies on patients with early RA (< 1 year duration), there was still a clinically relevant and statistically significant difference in radiological damage after 4–5 years after the start of the treatment between the originally prednisolone-treated and the originally placebo-treated patients,[9,11] while this difference was not maintained in patients with a longer duration of the disease at the start of the treatment.[11] This is in line with other studies looking at the window of opportunity: the earlier treatment starts, the more effective this is. This seems especially to hold for treatment with glucocorticoids. For example, in the 5-years experience from the FIN-RACo study,[17] it was clearly shown that early and aggressive treatment with DMARDs is able to retard joint damage. In this study, the aggressive treatment included prednisolone in 100% of the patients, but the less intensive treatment also included 82% of patients adjuvantly treated with prednisolone. Due to the high number of prednisolone-treated patients in this total study population, it was not possible to discriminate the specific effects of glucocorticoids in this study.

It now seems realistic to consider glucocorticoids as DMARDs, and in some of the recent recommendations on treatment of early RA, glucocorticoids have now been included.[18] However, dose schedules of and guidelines on glucocorticoid use in RA have still to be refined and respectively developed.

REFERENCES

1. BIJLSMA, J.W.J., M. BOERS, K.G. SAAG & D.E. FURST. 2003. Glucocorticoids in the treatment of early and late RA. Ann. Rheum. Dis. **62:** 1033–1037.
2. KLIPPEL, J.H. 2001. Primer on the Rheumatic Diseases. Edition 12. Arthritis Foundation. Atlanta, GA.
3. GERLAG, D.M., J.J. HARINGMAN, T.J.M. SMEETS, *et al.* 2004. Effects of oral prednisolone on biomarkers in synovial tissue and clinical improvement in RA. Arthritis Rheum. **50:** 3783–3791.
4. MEDICAL RESEARCH COUNCIL AND NUFFIELD FOUNDATION. 1954. A comparison of cortisone and aspirin in the treatment of early cases of rheumatoid arthritis. Br. Med. J. **29:** 1223–1227.
5. MEDICAL RESEARCH COUNCIL AND NUFFIELD FOUNDATION. 1959. A comparison of prednisolone with aspirin or other analgesics in the treatment of RA. Ann. Rheum. Dis. **18:** 173–187.
6. EMPIRE RHEUMATISM COUNCIL. 1957. Multicentre controlled trial comparing cortisone acetate and acetylsalicylic acid in the long-term treatment of rheumatoid arthritis. Ann. Rheum. Dis. **16:** 277–289.
7. VAN EVERDINGEN, A.A., J.W. JACOBS, D.R. SIEWERTSZ VAN REESEMA & J.W.J. BIJLSMA. 2002. Low dose prednisone therapy for patients with early active rheumatoid arthritis: clinical efficacy, disease modifying properties and side effects. A double blind placebo controlled clinical trial. Ann. Intern. Med. **136:** 1–12.
8. VAN EVERDINGEN, A.A., D.R. SIEWERTSZ VAN REESEMA, J.W.G. JACOBS & J.W.J. BIJLSMA. 2004. The clinical effect of glucocorticoids in patients with rheumatoid arthritis may be masked by decreased use of additional therapies. Arthritis Rheum. **51:** 233–238.
9. JACOBS, J.W.G., A.A. VAN EVERDINGEN, S.M.M. VERSTAPPEN & J.W.J. BIJLSMA. 2006. Followup radiographic data on patients with rheumatoid arthritis who participated in a two-year trial of prednisone therapy or placebo. Arthritis Rheum. **54:** 1422–1428.
10. KIRWAN, J.R. ARTHRITIS AND RHEUMATISM COUNCIL. LOW-DOSE GLUCOCORTICOID STUDY GROUP. 1995. The effect of glucocorticosteroids on joint destruction in rheumatoid arthritis. N. Engl. J. Med. **333:** 142–146.
11. HICKLING, P. *et al.* 1998. Joint destruction after glucocorticoids is withdrawn in early RA. Br. J. Rheumatol. **37:** 930–936.

12. Boers, M. *et al.* 1997. Randomised comparison of combined step-down predisolone, methotrexate and sulphasalazine alone in early rheumatoid arthritis. Lancet **350:** 309–318.
13. Landewé, R.B., M. Boers, A.C. Verhoeven, *et al.* 2002. COBRA combination therapy in patients with early RA: long-term structural benefits of a brief intervention. Arthritis Rheum. **46:** 347–356.
14. Wassenberg, S., R. Rau, P. Steinfeld & H. Zeidler. 2005. Very low-dose prednisolone in early rheumatoid arthritis retards radiographic progression over two years: a multicenter, double-blind, placebo-controlled trial. Arthritis Rheum. **52**: 3371–3380.
15. Hansen, M., J. Podenphant, A. Florescu, *et al.* 1999. A randomised trial of differentiated prednisolone treatment in active rheumatoid arthritis: clinical benefits and skeletal side effects. Ann. Rheum. Dis. **58:** 713–718.
16. Capell, A.A., R. Nedhok, J.A. Hunter, *et al.* 2004. Lack of radiological and clinical benefit over 2 years of low dose prednisolone for rheumatoid arthritis: results of randomised trial. Ann. Rheum. Dis. **63:** 797–803.
17. Korpela, M., L. La Asonen, P. Hanonnen, *et al.* 2004. Retardation of joint damage in patients with early rheumatoid arthritis by initial aggressive treatment with disease modifying antirheumatic drugs. Arthritis Rheum. **50:** 2072–2081.
18. Combe, B. & R. Landewé. 2005. EULAR recommendations for management of early arthritis. Ann. Rheum. Dis. **64**(Suppl III): 19.

Revisiting the Toxicity of Low-Dose Glucocorticoids

Risks and Fears

JOSÉ A. P. DA SILVA,[a] JOHANNES W. G. JACOBS,[b] AND JOHANNES W. J. BIJLSMA[b]

[a]*Reumatologia, Hospitais da Universidade de Coimbra, Coimbra, Portugal*

[b]*Department of Rheumatology and Clinical Immunology, University Medical Center Utrecht, Utrecht the Netherlands*

ABSTRACT: We have recently participated in a careful literature search and critical evaluation of glucocorticoids, and we have revised the side-effects data of four recent controlled trials of low-dose glucocorticoids (GCs) in rheumatoid arthritis. The toxicity profile stands out as remarkably more benign than expected from most textbook recommendations. Data regarding low-dose therapy are scarce and of low quality, as no controlled trials have been designed to specifically address toxicity. Common fears of GC toxicity seem to originate from an excessive weight on anecdotal data and observations with high doses, as in organ transplantation. There is now evidence that mechanisms of action of GCs vary considerably according to the dose, thus allowing the possibility of a different toxicity profile. Data from recent controlled trials are quite reassuring, overall. Certainly, risks and benefits of GCs need to be carefully weighed in every patient. But we need to make a clear distinction between established risks and unchecked fears while trying to get the best result for our patient. Clearly, there is a need for studies that are appropriately designed to address the toxicity of GCs and to avoid the risk of "throwing out the baby with the bath water."

KEYWORDS: glucocorticoids; low dose; toxicity; safety; adverse effects; side effects; corticosteroids; steroids; prednisone; prednisolone; review

INTRODUCTION

Glucocorticoids (GCs) have a central role in the practical management of a large variety of conditions. Recent studies suggest, for instance, that 45–75% of all patients with rheumatoid arthritis (RA) in the United States receive GCs.[1] This is clearly in excess of what could be expected on the basis of

Address for correspondence: José A. P. Da Silva, M.D., Ph.D., Reumatologia, Hospitais da Universidade, 3000-075 Coimbra, Portugal. Voice: 351 230400554; fax: 351 239401045.
e-mail: jdasilva@ci.uc.pt

**Ann. N.Y. Acad. Sci. 1069: 275–288 (2006). © 2006 New York Academy of Sciences.
doi: 10.1196/annals.1351.026**

the portrayed toxicity and the conservative recommendations of textbooks and review papers. The fear of a wide and serious toxicity spectrum is well engraved in the international medical culture, but there are reasons to believe that this is strongly influenced by observations of high doses of GCs.

We have recently participated in a cooperative effort to perform a systematic search and critical appraisal of the literature related to GC side effects.[2] Unpublished toxicity data from four randomized control trials of low-dose ($\leq$10 mg prednisolone equivalent per day) GCs in RA were carefully revised and presented.[3–6] The strongest conclusion of this work is the recognition of the remarkable fragility of evidence available to support sound judgment on low-dose GC toxicity.

All trials of GCs were designed to look at efficacy and not at toxicity. Toxicity data were not collected (or reported) in a systematic way. A large number of references are based on observational or retrospective data. Doses, duration, and regime vary enormously, as do the underlying diseases and their potential influence upon toxicity. This precludes the application of the rules of systematic literature review, from quality analysis (present quality criteria would not be valid when assessing toxicity in an efficacy trial) to outcome selection and odds-ratio calculations. These limitations are highlighted by a recent review of the literature designed to estimate the costs associated with GC side effects.[7] These considerations especially apply to the literature search, but are also relevant regarding recent RA trials in which toxicity data were reviewed.

The fear of GC toxicity is probably excessively influenced by extrapolation from observations with high-dose therapy. The balance of risks and benefits of low-dose therapy clearly differs from that of medium- and high-dose therapy, of which the mechanisms of action of GCs may be different.[8] The literature and the recent trial results suggest that toxicity of low-dose GC therapy is much lower than anticipated. On the basis of existing evidence, monitoring or taking preventive measures for patients on low-dose GCs is not currently justifiable or cost effective, with the exception of osteoporosis. Glucose control, cataracts and glaucoma, growth retardation in children, weight gain and cutaneous side effects all merit clinical attention, especially in patients with additional risk factors (e.g., obesity, hypertension, family history of diabetes or glaucoma). These represent demonstrated risks, side effects that can be expected, even with low-dose therapy, in specific conditions. However, several common fears associated with GC use have no support in the literature as far as low-dose regimens are concerned.

ESTABLISHED RISKS

Osteoporosis

The impact of GCs upon bone metabolism with increased risk of osteoporosis and fractures merits no doubt. Although these effects are time- and dose-dependent, there seems to be no "safe" dose.[9,10]

Although some studies suggest that doses of 7.5 mg of prednisone per day or less are relatively safe and may even prevent bone loss in early RA,[11] a longitudinal study observed an average loss of 9.5% from spinal trabecular bone over 20 weeks in patients exposed to 7.5 mg of prednisolone per day.[12–14] Therapy with pulse of methylprednisolone is also associated with significant bone loss.[15]

A recent literature search for all prospective studies of bone mass during GC treatment for any disease includes almost 1,200 patients.[16] At a mean dose of almost 9 mg prednisone equivalent per day, the best estimate of bone loss overall in spine and hip (without bisphosphonate therapy) is 1.5% per year. Important factors predicting bone loss include GC starting dose, chronic usage, and lack of vitamin D supplementation. Alternate-day GC regimens have not been demonstrated to reduce bone loss.[17,18] Studies conflict as to whether cumulative GC dose is[14,19] or is not[20,21] associated with the degree of bone loss.

This bone mass loss has important consequences upon fracture risk. In a recent retrospective cohort study using the General Practice Research Database of the United Kingdom, it was shown that the rate of clinical vertebral fractures increased by 55% for a dose of prednisolone of less than 2.5 mg/day, and by more than 400% if the dose exceeded 7.5 mg/day.[21] It is quite likely that fractures occur at less-decreased bone mineral density (BMD) levels in GC-treated patients than in patients not treated with GC,[22,23] probably caused by a negative effect of GC also on bone structure. A useful score for the estimation of absolute risk of fracture in patients on oral GCs was recently published.[10]

BMD loss during 2 years of low-dose prednisone was not significantly different from placebo effects in the four reviewed trials of low-dose GCs in RA.[2] The incidence of osteoporotic fractures was not significantly increased by prednisolone, but this may be due to the small numbers of patients (type-II error).

Osteoporosis is probably the most common adverse effect of chronic low-dose GCs, but effective strategies for the prevention and treatment of GC-induced osteoporosis are well established and have been the object of recent extensive reviews,[24,25] and authoritative guidelines.[26–28]

Hyperglycemia and Diabetes

GC-related hyperglycemia is dose-dependent. Clearly, however, low-dose GCs are not devoid of this effect. According to a case–control study, patients receiving 0.25–2.5 mg prednisone equivalent per day have an increased risk (odds ratio 1.8) for needing antihyperglycemic drugs.[29] Hyperglycemia can also be observed after intra-articular administration of GCs.[30] It is likely that subjects with risk factors for the development of diabetes mellitus, such as a family history of this disease, increasing age, obesity, and previous gestational diabetes mellitus, are at increased risk to develop new-onset hyperglycemia during GC therapy.[31] Hyperglycemia is rapidly reversed upon GC cessation, but some patients develop persistent diabetes.[32]

A relevant and detailed discussion of glucose control under GC treatment has been published.[33] There are no preventive measures apart from the use of lower doses of GC. Alternate-day therapy is associated with alternate-day hyperglycemia.[34]

Data from the four RA trials revealed no cases of new-onset diabetes. The Utrecht trial[5] found the least favorable results: a significant increase in mean (SD) fasting glucose was seen in the prednisone group (from 5.1 [0.6] at base line to 5.9 [1.9] mmol/L at 2 years, $P = 0.01$). However, even in this study, hyperglycemia, as defined by the World Health Organization, developed in only two patients in the prednisone group ($n = 40$) and one in the placebo group ($n = 41$).

Cataract and Glaucoma

Reports on the frequency of cataract with long-term, low-dose systemic GC therapy are scarce. In a group of RA patients treated with 5–15 mg/day of prednisone, for a mean of 6 (SD: 5) years, 15% had cataracts, compared with 4.5% of matched RA controls.[35]

Cataract formation is considered to be irreversible. We could find no evidence regarding the possibility of halting progression with dose reduction or treatment interruption. There is no evidence that alternate-day therapy reduces the risk.[36]

The prevalence of glaucoma is associated with GC use in a dose-dependent manner, even in patients on long-term, low-dose GCs.[37] However, the occurrence and magnitude of elevation of intraocular pressure with GC administration are highly variable between individuals. Patients with diabetes mellitus, high grades of myopia and relatives of those with open-angle glaucoma (especially if related to GCs) are reported to be more vulnerable to GC-induced glaucoma.[38,39] Patients with preexisting glaucoma merit special attention, as this condition will be aggravated in 45% to 90% of them, if exposed to GCs.[38,40]

Elevation of intraocular pressure with exogenous GCs is generally reversible upon cessation. Glaucoma medications retain their efficacy under concomitant GCs.[41] Routine checks are not usually indicated for patients on low-dose GC therapy and no additional risk factors for glaucoma, but seem recommendable for patients on high-dose, long-term systemic treatment, especially for those with associated risk factors for this condition.

Only two of the four reviewed trials on low-dose GC treatment in RA included a regular ophthalmologic check in a significant number of patients: no excess of cataracts was found, but numbers suggest an increased risk of glaucoma.

Growth Retardation in Children

Pharmacologic doses of GCs inhibit linear growth.[42] This effect is generally considered to be dose dependent, but evidence for this is weak. Alternate-day therapy has been shown to have a smaller, perhaps negligible, effect upon growth even if GCs have been started before 5 years of age.[43] According to some retrospective studies, continuous GCs in children for less than 1 year have no effect upon final adult height.[44] If therapy is stopped before skeletal maturation is complete, around 70% of patients will benefit from "catch-up growth," although it is insufficient to allow normal adult height.[45]

Prevention should include consideration of the dose, type, and regimen of GC used. Chronic administration of human growth hormone can counteract the effects of GCs upon growth and body composition.[45,46]

Cutaneous Side Effects

Clinically relevant adverse effects on the skin include iatrogenic Cushing's syndrome, catabolic effects (skin atrophy, purpura, striae, easy bruisability, and impaired wound healing), steroid acne, and effects on hair.[47]

Cutaneous adverse effects are frequently a major concern for the patient and must be acknowledged. Available data suggest that these effects are relatively uncommon and of minor clinical relevance with low-dose GC treatment, although data on incidence are scarce. Cushingoid phenotype and skin atrophy are observed in over 5% of the patients exposed to $\geq$5 mg prednisone equivalent for $\geq$1 year.[48–50] Wound healing impairment seems uncommon at low dose, but there are no exact data on prevalence. There are no data on incidence of steroid acne and hair effects like hirsutism and scalp hair loss, but they are more frequent with long-term treatment with moderate to high doses of GCs, as after organ transplantation.[47]

There is no strong evidence to support the claim that use of the lowest possible dose and alternate-day therapy may fully prevent these adverse effects from occurring.

Fat Redistribution and Body Weight

Centripetal fat accumulation with sparing of the extremities is a characteristic feature of patients exposed to long-term, high GC dose. It is seen even with long-term, low-dose GC. Our own review of toxicity data from the four RA prospective trials shows that low-dose prednisone is associated with an increase of mean body weight over 2 years in the range of 4–8%. In two of these trials, this weight gain was significantly higher than in the placebo group.[4,5]

UNSUBSTANTIATED FEARS

Peptic Ulcer Disease

The association between GC use and the risk of peptic ulcer disease has been the subject of extensive debate and contradictory evidence. Piper *et al.* performed a nested-control study including 1,415 patients admitted to the hospital for gastroduodenal ulcer or hemorrhage and 7,063 randomly selected controls from Medicaid.[51] Patients receiving only GCs had no significant increase in risk: 1.1 (95% CI: 0.5–2.1), but those co-medicated with non-steroidal anti-inflammatory drugs (NSAIDs) had a relative risk of 4.4 (95% CI: 2.0–9.7). In large-scale studies based on the UK General Practice Research Database,[52] the relative risk of upper GI complications was 1.8 (95% CI: 1.3–2.4) for users of GCs as compared to nonusers. The risk was shown to be more than 12 times higher for concomitant users of both GCs and NSAIDs, compared with nonusers of either drug.

Data from the four RA prospective trials show no increased incidence of upper GI ulcers and bleeding, but these events are relatively uncommon and may not be detected in these clinical trials with relatively low numbers of participating patients.

Therefore, GC use without concomitant NSAIDs does not represent, *per se*, an indication for gastroprotective agents.

Hypertension

Induction of hypertension is a well-established effect of exogenous GCs,[53] but is rarely associated with low-dose therapy. A retrospective study of 195 patients with RA or asthma, undergoing GC therapy with less than 20 mg/day of prednisone for longer than a year, did not show any correlation between dose or duration of GC treatment and rise in blood pressure.[54]

Toxicity data from the four trials on low-dose GCs in RA are very reassuring in respect to blood pressure: there were no significant effects of prednisone upon blood pressure in any of the trials. Note that patients with severe hypertension were excluded from most of these trials.

Dyslipidemia and Atherosclerosis

Long-term steroid use is significantly associated with hyperlipemia and coronary artery disease.[55–58] However, the influence of the underlying disease is frequently difficult to discriminate, as increased levels of C-reactive protein are a potent atherosclerotic factor.[59]

Recent data from cohort studies show that RA disease activity unfavorably alters the blood lipid profile, and treatment (including GC treatment) can reverse these changes.[60] A record linkage database study on 68,781 GC-users and 82,202 nonusers was published.[61] The incidence of all cardiovascular diseases, including myocardial infarction, heart failure, and cerebrovascular disease was not increased in patients using $<$7.5 mg prednisolone on a chronic basis. However, it was increased in patients using dosages $\geq$7.5 mg daily: relative risk adjusted for all known risk factors 2.6, 95% CI: 2.2–3. In the four extensively reviewed trials on low-dose GC treatment in RA, no excess cardiovascular events were reported, but the trial duration of 2 years was relatively short for development of these complications.

In summary, evidence does not support a significant role of low-dose GC treatment in the development of cardiovascular disease in RA, in contrast to higher dosages. In patients on low-dose GCs, the disease itself seems to be a greater risk factor.

Edema, Electrolytes, and Renal and Heart Functions

Hypernatremia, hypokalemia, and sodium and water retention leading to edema, and contributing to hypertension and heart failure, are seen in patients with Cushing's disease. However, these are mineralocorticoid effects produced by endogenous GCs at supraphysiological concentrations. Synthetic GCs (prednisone, prednisolone, methylprednisolone, dexamethasone) have little mineralocorticoid effects, and their administration increases glomerular filtration rate and induces kaliuresis and natriuresis without any change in plasma volume.[62–64] A small number of trials have evaluated chronic GC administration in moderate to high doses in patients with heart failure, and no significantly detrimental effect on heart function emerged from these studies.[65,66] In the four reviewed trials of low-dose GCs treatment in RA, no cardiac insufficiency attributable to GCs occurred.

Osteonecrosis

One study reported osteonecrosis in 2.4% of patients receiving GC replacement therapy,[67] but data on low-dose GC treatment is scarce and mostly anecdotal. No case of avascular necrosis was observed in the four extensively reviewed trials of low-dose GCs in RA.

This event seems strongly associated with high-dose therapy, and even then it is sometimes difficult to differentiate whether the treatment or the underlying disease is the cause, as some conditions, such as systemic lupus erythematosus (SLE), are associated with an increased risk of osteonecrosis.[68] Although the occurrence of GC-related osteonecrosis seems to be dose-dependent, this might be confounded by the fact that higher dosages are related to more severe underlying disease (bias by indication), and thus an increased risk of osteonecrosis. This supports the contention that there is limited evidence that GCs are actually responsible for osteonecrosis.[69]

Steroid Myopathy

Chronic steroid myopathy is quite often suspected, but infrequently found and/or documented. The most remarkable finding when searching the literature regarding this topic is the lack of data and proper studies, as illustrated by a recent review.[70] No cases of myopathy were observed in the four trials of low-dose GCs in RA. On the basis of the scarce information available and our own experience, we believe that myopathy is exceedingly rare with GC doses below 7.5 mg prednisolone equivalent daily.

Suppression of Sex Hormone Secretion

High-dose GC therapy has been associated with lower levels of estrogens[71] and testosterone.[72] These suppressing effects can contribute to steroid-induced osteoporosis, but these high GC doses do not seem to have a clinically relevant adverse effect on fertility.[73] Decreased libido has not been reported as a common complaint in patients exposed to low-dose GCs, and it was not spontaneously reported by patients in the four reviewed trials on low-dose GCs in RA.

Infections

The risk of infection increases with dose and duration of GC treatment,[74] and tends to remain low in patients exposed to low doses, even with high cumulative dosages.[75] In a meta-analysis of 71 trials involving over 2,000 patients with different diseases and different dosages of GCs, a relative risk of infection of 1.6 (95% CI: 1.3–1.9) was found.[76] The risk of infection is obviously influenced by the underlying disease. In two studies specifically on RA, the incidence of serious infection was found to be similar to that of placebo or only slightly increased.[5,35] SLE is associated with increased risk of opportunistic infections, exacerbated by therapy with GC.[77] Of the intensively reviewed four studies of low-dose GC therapy in RA, both in the Utrecht and the Woseract trials, prednisone in doses up to 10 mg/day was not associated with increased incidence of any kind of infection over the 2 years of the trials.[5,6] A recent study indicated that GCs are associated with a marked increase in the relative risk of sigmoid diverticular abscess perforation, especially in rheumatic patients, although this seems to be a rare event in terms of absolute risk.[78]

Psychological and Behavioral Disturbances

Steroid psychosis is exceedingly rare with low-dose GCs.[79] No case was observed in any of the four reviewed trials of low-dose GC treatment in RA.

Minor mood disturbances, such as depressed or elated mood (euphoria), irritability or emotional lability, anxiety and insomnia, and memory and cognition impairments are probably more frequent. The exact incidence of such symptoms cannot be drawn from the literature, but doses of less than 20 to 25 mg prednisone equivalent are associated with few or no significant disturbances.[80] These adverse events were not reported in the four index trials on low-dose GC treatment in RA, but they were not systematically assessed either.

Adrenal Crisis on GC Withdrawal

Rapid tapering of GC administration can lead to symptomatic adrenal insufficiency (adrenal crisis), as the atrophic glands cannot meet the rapidly increasing required demand for GC. Major physiologic stress in patients on low-dose GCs may have a similar effect. These patients may experience nausea, vomiting, fatigue, fever, myalgias, hypotension, syncope, and even death.

To avoid the adrenal crisis following chronic GC treatment, GCs should not be tapered too fast. A popular scheme proposed in the 1970s[81] suggests a slow decrease of dose over 3 to 5 months, to taper a dose of 10 mg prednisolone equivalent per day, with several endocrine checks in between. In practice, however, most physicians follow a faster protocol for withdrawal for patients taking chronic low-dose GCs, but the safety of this approach after long-term therapy has not been adequately tested.

A recent study had no cases of adrenal crisis after abrupt suspension of treatment with 7.5 mg of prednisolone daily given for three months in RA.[82] This study also underlines that the fear of rebound of disease activity upon suspension of therapy is not realistic.

CONCLUSIONS AND RESEARCH AGENDA

The overall fear of GC toxicity in RA, as quoted in textbooks and review articles, is probably overestimated based on extrapolation from observations on patients receiving higher-dose therapy. There is surprisingly weak evidence on which to support clear recommendations about toxicity of low-dose GCs, and definitive associations with many adverse effects remain elusive. Obviously, the lack of evidence cannot be taken as a demonstration of safety. Most of the data available come from trials not primarily designed for assessment of adverse effects and from observational studies with possible bias, especially confounding by indication. Subjects participating in randomized clinical trials may not have the same disease characteristics or comorbidities of patients treated in the community, thereby limiting the generalizability of findings of this kind of trial.[83] They certainly do not represent the highest level of evidence, but, they are all that we have at present.

Safety of low-dose GCs needs to undergo serious and systematic reevaluation with properly designed and dedicated studies of adequate size, duration, and state-of-the-art end points. Guidelines for such studies would enhance comprehensiveness and comparability. GC will likely retain an enormous therapeutic value in treatment of a large variety of rheumatic conditions for many years to come, especially since it becomes increasingly clear that these agents have disease-modifying potential in RA. Research on the potential separation of wanted from unwanted GC effects, using newly designed GC-type medicine, provides good reason for hope that an even better safety/efficacy ratio can be achieved in the future.

REFERENCES

1. TOWNSEND, H.B. & K.G. SAAG. 2004. Glucocorticoid use in rheumatoid arthritis: benefits, mechanisms, and risks. Clin. Exp. Rheumatol. **22:** S77–S82.
2. DA SILVA, J.A., J.W. JACOBS, J.R. KIRWAN, *et al.* 2006. Low-dose glucocorticoid therapy in rheumatoid arthritis: a review on safety: published evidence and prospective trial data. Ann. Rheum. Dis. **64:** 285–293.
3. KIRWAN, J.R. 1995. The effect of glucocorticoids on joint destruction in rheumatoid arthritis. The Arthritis and Rheumatism Council Low-Dose Glucocorticoid Study Group. N. Engl. J. Med. **333:** 142–146.
4. RAU, R., S. WASSENBERG & H. ZEIDLER. 2000. Low dose prednisolone therapy (LDPT) retards radiographically detectable destruction in early rheumatoid arthritis—preliminary results of a multicenter, randomized, parallel, double blind study. Z. Rheumatol. **59:** II/90–II/96.
5. VAN EVERDINGEN, A.A., J.W. JACOBS, D.R. SIEWERTSZ VAN REESEMA, *et al.* 2002. Low-dose prednisone therapy for patients with early active rheumatoid arthritis: clinical efficacy, disease-modifying properties, and side effects: a randomized, double-blind, placebo-controlled clinical trial. Ann. Intern. Med. **136:** 1–12.
6. CAPELL, H.A., R. MADHOK, J.A. HUNTER, *et al.* 2004. Lack of radiological and clinical benefit over two years of low dose prednisolone for rheumatoid arthritis: results of a randomised controlled trial. Ann. Rheum. Dis. **63:** 797–803.
7. PISU, M., N. JAMES, S. SAMPSEL, *et al.* 2005. The cost of glucocorticoid-associated adverse events in rheumatoid arthritis. Rheumatology (Oxford) **44:** 781–788.
8. BUTTGEREIT, F., J.A. DA SILVA, M. BOERS, *et al.* 2002. Standardised nomenclature for glucocorticoid dosages and glucocorticoid treatment regimens: current questions and tentative answers in rheumatology. Ann. Rheum. Dis. **61:** 718–722.
9. TON, F.N., S.C. GUNAWARDENE, H. LEE, *et al.* 2005. Effects of low-dose prednisone on bone metabolism. J. Bone Miner. Res. **20:** 464–470.
10. VAN STAA, T.P., P. GEUSENS, H.A. POLS, *et al.* 2005. A simple score for estimating the long-term risk of fracture in patients using oral glucocorticoids. QJM **98:** 191–198.

11. Haugeberg, G., A. Strand, T.K. Kvien, *et al.* 2005. Reduced loss of hand bone density with prednisolone in early rheumatoid arthritis: results from a randomized placebo-controlled trial. Arch. Intern. Med. **165:** 1293–1297.
12. Laan, R.F., P.L. van Riel, L.B. van de Putte, *et al.* 1993. Low-dose prednisone induces rapid reversible axial bone loss in patients with rheumatoid arthritis: a randomized, controlled study. Ann. Intern. Med. **119:** 963–968.
13. de Nijs, R.N., J.W. Jacobs, J.W. Bijlsma, *et al.* 2001. Prevalence of vertebral deformities and symptomatic vertebral fractures in corticosteroid treated patients with rheumatoid arthritis. Rheumatology (Oxford) **40:** 1375–1383.
14. van Staa, T.P., H.G. Leufkens & C. Cooper. 2002. The epidemiology of corticosteroid-induced osteoporosis: a meta-analysis. Osteoporos. Int. **13:** 777–787.
15. Haugeberg, G., B. Griffiths, K.B. Sokoll, *et al.* 2004. Bone loss in patients treated with pulses of methylprednisolone is not negligible: a short term prospective observational study. Ann. Rheum. Dis. **63:** 940–944.
16. Lodder, M.C., W.F. Lems, P.J. Kostense, *et al.* 2003. Bone loss due to glucocorticoids: update of a systematic review of prospective studies in rheumatoid arthritis and other diseases. Ann. Rheum. Dis. **62:** 94.
17. Gluck, O.S., W.A. Murphy, T.J. Hahn, *et al.* 1981. Bone loss in adults receiving alternate day glucocorticoid therapy: a comparison with daily therapy. Arthritis Rheum. **24:** 892–898.
18. Ruegsegger, P., T.C. Medici & M. Anliker. 1983. Corticosteroid-induced bone loss: a longitudinal study of alternate day therapy in patients with bronchial asthma using quantitative computed tomography. Eur. J. Clin Pharmacol. **25:** 615–620.
19. Reid, I.R. & S.W. Heap. 1990. Determinants of vertebral mineral density in patients receiving long-term glucocorticoid therapy. Arch. Intern. Med. **150:** 2545–2548.
20. Lems, W.F., Z.N. Jahangier, J.W. Jacobs, *et al.* 1995. Vertebral fractures in patients with rheumatoid arthritis treated with corticosteroids. Clin. Exp. Rheumatol. **13:** 293–297.
21. van Staa, T.P., H.G. Leufkens, L. Abenhaim, *et al.* 2000. Use of oral corticosteroids and risk of fractures. J. Bone Miner. Res. **15:** 993–1000.
22. Sambrook, P. & N.E. Lane. 2001. Corticosteroid osteoporosis. Best. Pract. Res. Clin. Rheumatol. **15:** 401–413.
23. Kumagai, S., S. Kawano, T. Atsumi, *et al.* 2005. Vertebral fracture and bone mineral density in women receiving high dose glucocorticoids for treatment of autoimmune diseases. J. Rheumatol. **32:** 863–869.
24. Yeap, S.S. & D.J. Hosking. 2002. Management of corticosteroid-induced osteoporosis. Rheumatology (Oxford) **41:** 1088–1094.
25. Sambrook, P.N. 2005. How to prevent steroid induced osteoporosis. Ann. Rheum. Dis. **64:** 176–178.
26. American College of Rheumatology Ad Hoc Committee on Glucocorticoid-Induced Osteoporosis. 2001. Recommendations for the prevention and treatment of glucocorticoid-induced osteoporosis: 2001 update. Arthritis Rheum. **44:** 1496–1503.
27. The Royal College of Physicians, The Bone and Tooth Society of Great Britain & The National Osteoporosis Society. 2002. Glucocorticoid-induced osteoporosis. Guidelines for prevention and treatment. www.rcplondon.ac.uk/pubs/books/glucocorticoid/index.asp.

28. Geusens, P.P., R.N. de Nijs, W.F. Lems, *et al.* 2004. Prevention of glucocorticoid osteoporosis: a consensus document of the Dutch Society for Rheumatology. Ann. Rheum. Dis. **63:** 324–325.
29. Gurwitz, J.H., R.L. Bohn, R.J. Glynn, *et al.* 1994. Glucocorticoids and the risk for initiation of hypoglycemic therapy. Arch. Intern. Med. **154:** 97–101.
30. Black, D.M. & A.T. Filak. 1989. Hyperglycemia with non-insulin-dependent diabetes following intraarticular steroid injection. J. Fam. Pract. **28:** 462–463.
31. Hirsch, I.B. & D.S. Paauw. 1997. Diabetes management in special situations. Endocrinol. Metab. Clin. North Am. **26:** 631–645.
32. Hricik, D.E., M.R. Bartucci, E.J. Moir, *et al.* 1991. Effects of steroid withdrawal on posttransplant diabetes mellitus in cyclosporine-treated renal transplant recipients. Transplantation **51:** 374–377.
33. Hoogwerf, B. & R.D. Danese. 1999. Drug selection and the management of corticosteroid-related diabetes mellitus. Rheum. Dis. Clin. North Am. **25:** 489–505.
34. Greenstone, M.A. & A.B. Shaw. 1987. Alternate day corticosteroid causes alternate day hyperglycaemia. Postgrad. Med. J. **63:** 761–764.
35. Saag, K.G., R. Koehnke, J.R. Caldwell, *et al.* 1994. Low dose long-term corticosteroid therapy in rheumatoid arthritis: an analysis of serious adverse events. Am. J Med. **96:** 115–123.
36. Rooklin, A.R., S.I. Lampert, E.A. Jaeger, *et al.* 1979. Posterior subcapsular cataracts in steroid-requiring asthmatic children. J. Allergy Clin. Immunol. **63:** 383–386.
37. Garbe, E., J. LeLorier, J.F. Boivin, *et al.* 1997. Risk of ocular hypertension or open-angle glaucoma in elderly patients on oral glucocorticoids. Lancet **350:** 979–982.
38. Tripathi, R.C., S.K. Parapuram, B.J. Tripathi, *et al.* 1999. Corticosteroids and glaucoma risk. Drugs Aging **15:** 439–450.
39. Stone, E.M., J.H. Fingert, W.L. Alward, *et al.* 1997. Identification of a gene that causes primary open angle glaucoma. Science **275:** 668–670.
40. Akingbehin, A.O. 1982. Corticosteroid-induced ocular hypertension. I. Prevalence in closed-angle glaucoma. Br. J. Ophthalmol. **66:** 536–540.
41. Brodie, S. 2002. Corticosteroids and the eye. *In* Principles of Corticosteroid Therapy. A.N. Lin & S.A. Paget, Eds.: 131–134. Arnold. London.
42. Allen, D.B. 1996. Growth suppression by glucocorticoid therapy. Endocrinol. Metab. Clin. North Am. **25:** 699–717.
43. Byron, M.A., J. Jackson & B.M. Ansell. 1983. Effect of different corticosteroid regimens on hypothalamic-pituitary-adrenal axis and growth in juvenile chronic arthritis. J. R. Soc. Med. **76:** 452–457.
44. Wang, S.J., Y.H. Yang, Y.T. Lin, *et al.* 2002. Attained adult height in juvenile rheumatoid arthritis with or without corticosteroid treatment. Clin. Rheumatol. **21:** 363–368.
45. Simon, D., N. Lucidarme, A.M. Prieur, *et al.* 2001. Linear growth in children suffering from juvenile idiopathic arthritis requiring steroid therapy: natural history and effects of growth hormone treatment on linear growth. J. Pediatr. Endocrinol. Metab. **14:** 1483–1486.
46. Touati, G., A.M. Prieur, J.C. Ruiz, *et al.* 1998. Beneficial effects of one-year growth hormone administration to children with juvenile chronic arthritis on chronic steroid therapy. I. Effects on growth velocity and body composition. J. Clin. Endocrinol. Metab. **83:** 403–409.
47. Wolverton, S.E. 2002. Corticosteroids and the integument. *In* Principles of Corticosteroid Therapy. A.N. Lin & S.A. Paget, Eds.: 166–172. Arnold. London.

48. COVAR, R.A., D.Y. LEUNG, D. MCCORMICK, *et al.* 2000. Risk factors associated with glucocorticoid-induced adverse effects in children with severe asthma. J. Allergy Clin. Immunol. **106:** 651–659.
49. MARCOCCI, C., L. BARTALENA, M.L. TANDA, *et al.* 2001. Comparison of the effectiveness and tolerability of intravenous or oral glucocorticoids associated with orbital radiotherapy in the management of severe Graves' ophthalmopathy: results of a prospective, single-blind, randomized study. J. Clin. Endocrinol. Metab. **86:** 3562–3567.
50. HATZ, H.J. & K. HELMKE. 1992. [Polymyalgia rheumatica and giant cell arteritis; diagnosis and side effects of low-dose long-term glucocorticoid therapy]. Z. Rheumatol. **51:** 213–221.
51. PIPER, J.M., W.A. RAY, J.R. DAUGHERTY, *et al.* 1991. Corticosteroid use and peptic ulcer disease: role of nonsteroidal anti-inflammatory drugs. Ann. Intern. Med. **114:** 735–740.
52. GARCIA RODRIGUEZ, L.A. & S. HERNANDEZ-DIAZ. 2001. The risk of upper gastrointestinal complications associated with nonsteroidal anti-inflammatory drugs, glucocorticoids, acetaminophen, and combinations of these agents. Arthritis Res. **3:** 98–101.
53. WHITWORTH, J.A. 1987. Mechanisms of glucocorticoid-induced hypertension. Kidney Int. **31:** 1213–1224.
54. JACKSON, S.H., D.G. BEEVERS & K. MYERS. 1981. Does long-term low-dose corticosteroid therapy cause hypertension? Clin. Sci. (Lond.) **61:** 381s–383s.
55. EL-SHABOURY, A.H. & T.M. HAYES. 1973. Hyperlipidaemia in asthmatic patients receiving long-term steroid therapy. Br. Med. J. **2:** 85–86.
56. BECKER, D.M., B. CHAMBERLAIN, R. SWANK, *et al.* 1988. Relationship between corticosteroid exposure and plasma lipid levels in heart transplant recipients. Am. J. Med. **85:** 632–638.
57. MANZI, S., F. SELZER, K. SUTTON-TYRRELL, *et al.* 1999. Prevalence and risk factors of carotid plaque in women with systemic lupus erythematosus. Arthritis Rheum. **42:** 51–60.
58. WALLBERG-JONSSON, S., H. JOHANSSON, M.L. OHMAN, *et al.* 1999. Extent of inflammation predicts cardiovascular disease and overall mortality in seropositive rheumatoid arthritis: a retrospective cohort study from disease onset. J. Rheumatol. **26:** 2562–2571.
59. MUNFORD, R.S. 2001. Statins and the acute-phase response. N. Engl. J Med. **344:** 2016–2018.
60. BOERS, M., M.T. NURMOHAMED, C.J. DOELMAN, *et al.* 2003. Influence of glucocorticoids and disease activity on total and high density lipoprotein cholesterol in patients with rheumatoid arthritis. Ann. Rheum. Dis. **62:** 842–845.
61. WEI, L., T.M. MACDONALD & B.R. WALKER. 2004. Taking glucocorticoids by prescription is associated with subsequent cardiovascular disease. Ann. Intern. Med. **141:** 764–770.
62. BIA, J.M., K. TYLER & R.A. DEFRONZO. 1982. The effect of dexamethasone on renal electrolyte excretion in the adrenalectomized rat. Endocrinology **111:** 882–888.
63. KOHLMANN, O., Jr., A.B. RIBEIRO, O. MARSON, *et al.* 1981. Methylprednisolone-induced hypertension: role for the autonomic and renin angiotensin systems. Hypertension **3:** II-11.
64. WHITWORTH, J.A., D. GORDON, J. ANDREWS, *et al.* 1989. The hypertensive effect of synthetic glucocorticoids in man: role of sodium and volume. J. Hypertens. **7:** 537–549.

65. LATHAM, R.D., J.P. MULROW, R. VIRMANI, *et al.* 1989. Recently diagnosed idiopathic dilated cardiomyopathy: incidence of myocarditis and efficacy of prednisone therapy. Am. Heart J. **117:** 876–882.
66. MASON, J.W., J.B. O'CONNELL, A. HERSKOWITZ, *et al.* 1995. A clinical trial of immunosuppressive therapy for myocarditis. The Myocarditis Treatment Trial Investigators. N. Engl. J. Med. **333:** 269–275.
67. VREDEN, S.G., A.R. HERMUS, P.A. VAN LIESSUM, *et al.* 1991. Aseptic bone necrosis in patients on glucocorticoid replacement therapy. Neth. J. Med. **39:** 153–157.
68. ZIZIC, T.M., C. MARCOUX, D.S. HUNGERFORD, *et al.* 1985. Corticosteroid therapy associated with ischemic necrosis of bone in systemic lupus erythematosus. Am. J. Med. **79:** 596–604.
69. GEBHARD, K.L. & H.I. MAIBACH. 2001. Relationship between systemic corticosteroids and osteonecrosis. Am. J. Clin. Dermatol. **2:** 377–388.
70. KAGEN, L.J. 2002. Steroid myopathy. *In* Principles of Corticosteroid Therapy. N.A. Lin & S.A. Paget, Eds.: 87–90. Arnold. London.
71. NORDIN, B.E., R.G. CRILLY, D.H. MARSHALL, *et al.* 1981. Oestrogens, the menopause and the adrenopause. J. Endocrinol. **89:** 131P–143P.
72. HAMPSON, G., N. BHARGAVA, J. CHEUNG, *et al.* 2002. Low circulating estradiol and adrenal androgens concentrations in men on glucocorticoids: a potential contributory factor in steroid-induced osteoporosis. Metabolism **51:** 1458–1462.
73. JANSSEN, N.M. & M.S. GENTA. 2000. The effects of immunosuppressive and anti-inflammatory medications on fertility, pregnancy, and lactation. Arch. Intern. Med. **160:** 610–619.
74. DALE, D.C. & R.G. PETERSDORF. 1973. Corticosteroids and infectious diseases. Med. Clin. North Am. **57:** 1277–1287.
75. STRACHER, A.R. & R. SOAVE. 2002. Infectious complications of Corticosteroid Therapy. *In* Principles of Corticosteroid Therapy. A.N. Linn & S.A. Paget, Eds.: 419–430. Arnold. London.
76. STUCK, A.E., C.E. MINDER & F.J. FREY. 1989. Risk of infectious complications in patients taking glucocorticosteroids. Rev. Infect. Dis. **11:** 954–963.
77. HELLMANN, D.B., M. PETRI & Q. WHITING-O'KEEFE. 1987. Fatal infections in systemic lupus erythematosus: the role of opportunistic organisms. Medicine (Baltimore) **66:** 341–348.
78. MPOFU, S., C.M. MPOFU, D. HUTCHINSON, *et al.* 2004. Steroids, non-steroidal anti-inflammatory drugs, and sigmoid diverticular abscess perforation in rheumatic conditions. Ann. Rheum. Dis. **63:** 588–590.
79. DEMOPOULOS, A. & B.R. APATOFF. 2002. Corticosteroids and the nervous system. *In* Principles of Corticosteroid Therapy. N.A. Lin & S.A. Paget, Eds.: 150–165. Arnold. London.
80. RECKART, M.D. & S.J. EISENDRATH. 1990. Exogenous corticosteroid effects on mood and cognition: case presentations. Int. J. Psychosom. **37:** 57–61.
81. BYYNY, R.L. 1976. Withdrawal from glucocorticoid therapy. N. Engl. J. Med. **295:** 30–32.
82. KIRWAN, J.R., R. HALLGREN, H. MIELANTS, *et al.* 2004. A randomised placebo controlled 12 week trial of budesonide and prednisolone in rheumatoid arthritis. Ann. Rheum. Dis. **63:** 688–695.
83. JACOBS, J.W. & J.W. BIJLSMA. 2003. Interpretation of trial methodology not always easy: comment on the editorial by Landewé (author reply). Arthritis Rheum. **48:** 2693–2695.

Circadian Rhythms

Glucocorticoids and Arthritis

MAURIZIO CUTOLO,[a] ALBERTO SULLI,[a] CARMEN PIZZORNI,[a] MARIA ELENA SECCHI,[a] STEFANO SOLDANO,[a] BRUNO SERIOLO,[a] RAINER H. STRAUB,[b] KATI OTSA,[c] AND GEORGES J. MAESTRONI[d]

[a]*Research Laboratory and Division of Rheumatology, Department of Internal Medicine, University of Genova, 16132 Genova, Italy*

[b]*Laboratory NeuroEndocrinoImmunology, Department of Internal Medicine I, University Hospital, Regensburg, 93042 Germany*

[c]*Department of Rheumatology, Central Hospital, Tallinn, Estonia*

[d]*Cantonal Institute of Pathology, Locarno, 6601 Switzerland*

ABSTRACT: Circadian rhythms are driven by biological clocks and are endogenous in origin. Therefore, circadian changes in the metabolism or secretion of endogenous glucocorticoids are certainly responsible in part for the time-dependent changes observed in the inflammatory response and arthritis. More recently, melatonin (MLT), another circadian hormone that is the secretory product of the pineal gland, has been found implicated in the time-dependent inflammatory reaction with effects opposite those of cortisol. Interestingly, cortisol and MLT show an opposite response to the light. The light conditions in the early morning have a strong impact on the morning cortisol peak, whereas MLT is synthesized in a strictly nocturnal pattern. Recently, a diurnal rhythmicity in healthy humans between cellular (Th1 type) or humoral (Th2 type) immune responses has been found and related to immunomodulatory actions of cortisol and MLT. The interferon (IFN)-γ/interleukin (IL)-10 ratio peaked during the early morning and correlated negatively with plasma cortisol and positively with plasma MLT. Accordingly, the intensity of the arthritic pain varies consistently as a function of the hour of the day: pain is greater after waking up in the morning than in the afternoon or evening. The reduced cortisol and adrenal androgen secretion, observed during testing in rheumatoid arthritis (RA) patients not treated with glucocoticoids, should be clearly considered as a "relative adrenal insufficiency" in the presence of a sustained inflammatory process, and allows Th1 type cytokines to be produced in higher amounts during the late night. In conclusion, the right timing (early morning) for the glucocorticoid therapy in arthritis is fundamental and well justified by the circadian rhythms of the inflammatory mechanisms.

Address for correspondence: Maurizio Cutolo, Research Laboratory and Division of Rheumatology, Department of Internal Medicine, University of Genova, Viale Benedetto XV6, 16132 Genova, Italy. Voice: +39-010-353-7994; fax: +39-010-353-8885.
e-mail: mcutolo@unige.it

Ann. N.Y. Acad. Sci. 1069: 289–299 (2006).
doi: 10.1196/annals.1351.027

KEYWORDS: **rheumatoid arthritis; circadian rhythms; glucocorticoids; melatonin; tumor necrosis factor (TNF)-α; Th1 cytokines; Th2 cytokines; hypothalamus-pituitary-adrenal (HPA)**

INTRODUCTION

Some clinical signs and symptoms of arthritis, and particularly rheumatoid arthritis (RA), vary within a day and between days, and the morning stiffness observed in RA patients has become one of the diagnostic criteria of the disease.[1]

Among the signs of joint inflammation in RA patients, the intensity of pain varies consistently as a function of the hour of the day: pain is greater after waking up in the morning than in the afternoon or evening (FIG. 1).[2]

Circadian changes are also observed in joint swelling and finger size. The circadian pattern of joint stiffness of an RA patient is in phase with the circadian rhythm of pain. These rhythms differ in phase by approxymately 12 h from the circadian changes of left- and right-hand grip strength: greater grip strength was demonstrated when joint circumferences and the subjective ratings of stiffness and pain were least and *vice versa*.[3]

These rhythms are driven by biological clocks and are endogenous in origin; therefore, clinical signs and symptoms in RA follows a biological clock.

MODULATION OF GLUCOCORTICOID PRODUCTION

The mechanisms of the time-dependent variations of the inflammatory reaction are complex and include several systems of mediators (i.e., histamine, bradykinin, prostaglandins, and mainly, pro- and anti-inflammatory cytokine production).

However, the circadian changes in the metabolism or secretion of endogenous glucocorticoids is certainly responsible in part for the time-dependent changes observed in the inflammatory response.

Diurnal control of the hypothalamus-pituitary-adrenal (HPA) axis is regulated strictly to provide increased glucocorticoid production during the daytime hours in humans and other non-nocturnal animals and increased adrenal androgen–sex hormone precursors at night. In normal subjects, serum levels of proinflammatory cytokines also show diurnal rhythms that peak in the early morning and tend to be related inversely to the rhythms of plasma cortisol.[4] The interaction and relations of serum cortisol and inflammatory cytokine levels are complex. Their relation is believed to be counterregulatory, but the complete controlling factors are not well defined in health or disease.[4,5] Several studies in humans indicate that increase of plasma cortisol within the physiologic range—achieved by administration of cortisone acetate 25 mg at

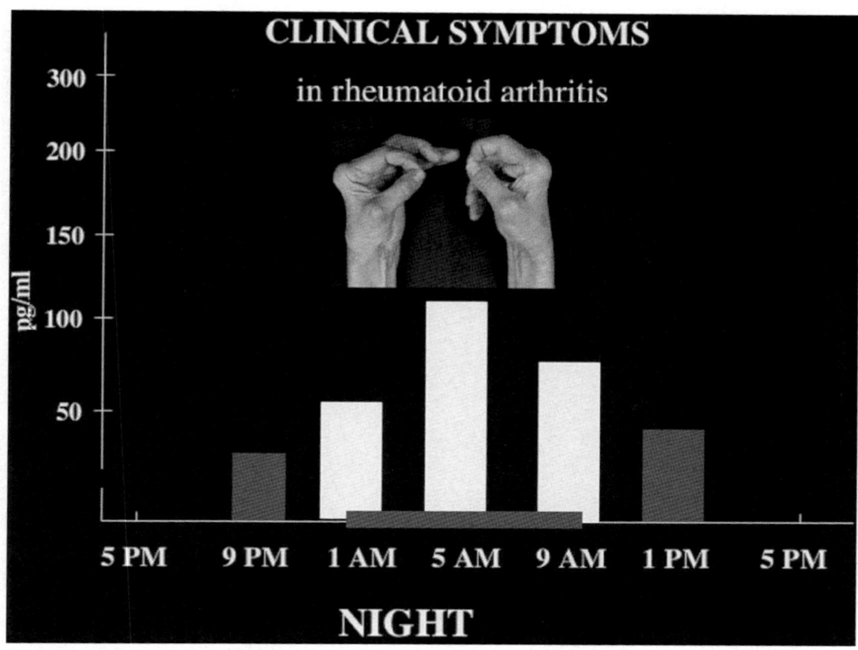

FIGURE 1. Among the signs of joint inflammation in RA patients, the intensity of pain varies consistently as a function of the hour of the day: pain is greater after waking up in the morning than in the afternoon or evening

9 PM—markedly suppressed interferon (IFN)-γ and inflammatory cytokines.[4] The relative efficacy of cortisol to inhibit production of interleukin (IL)-1b, IL-6, and tumor necrosis factor (TNF)-α is not established fully. One study of exercise-induced elevation of cortisol suppressed whole blood production of only TNF-α, without effect on IL-1b or IL-6 production.[6] In addition, the relative effects of individual and combined inflammatory cytokines on central stimulation of the HPA axis are not defined fully.[7]

Normal response to chronic stressors requires appropriate stimulation of the adrenal cortex and maintenance of its appropriate organ size, including its components (i.e., the zona glomerulosa [aldosterone synthesis], zona fasciculata [cortisol synthesis], and zona reticularis [AA synthesis]). Hypocortisolism has been reported in various stress-related bodily disorders, with the deficiency attributed mainly to adrenal cortical insufficiency.[8] Some results imply that hypocortisolism may arise from stressors in humans and in animal models.[8] The mechanisms that permit normal activation of steroidogenesis and preserve the proper size and growth factor stimuli of the adrenal to maintain its structural integrity are really complex and incompletely understood.[9,10] Normal

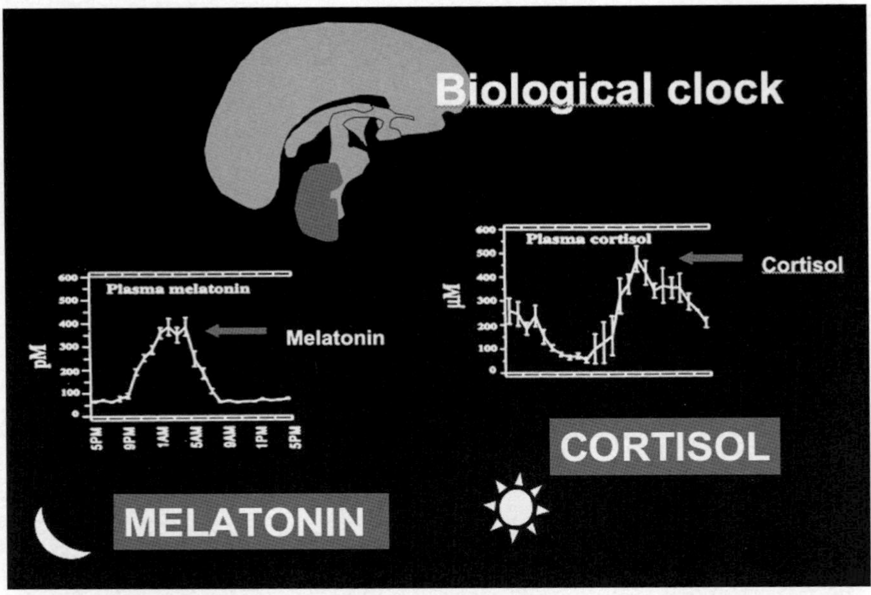

FIGURE 2. The light conditions in the early morning have a strong impact on the morning cortisol peak; MLT is synthesized in a strictly nocturnal pattern.

adrenocortical responses to stress or inflammatory disease require sufficient corticotropin stimulation of steroidogenesis. In addition, maintenance of its structure requires growth hormones and accessory factors that are less well understood.[9,10] Experimental studies of adrenocortical cell growth show that a brief pulse of corticotropin (up to 2 h) stimulated adrenal cell proliferation, whereas continuous treatment with corticotropin (14 h) inhibited cell cycle progress at the midpoint of G1 (mouse model).[11] The possible relevance of such dual effects of corticotropin on cell cycle progress may apply to patients who have RA and their altered diurnal pattern of HPA function (FIG. 2). Potentially, excessive corticotropin pulsing at night in patients who have RA may tend to inhibit the normal adrenal cell proliferation that is required for the maintenance of organ competency, especially under stresses of inflammatory disease. Given the altered status of HPA function in RA, therapy with required glucocorticoids should be provided in optimal dosages and timing to normalize the functional and structural HPA axis dysregulations. Under normal circumstances, corticotropin maintains the size and function of the adrenal cortex. Too little corticotropin—as would result from chronic pharmacologic administration of glucocorticoids—results in adrenal atrophy; increased corticotropin—as occurs in Cushing's disease—results in adrenal hypertrophy. Several studies of patients who had RA and Cushing's disease or syndrome demonstrated remission of RA in the setting of hypercortisolism or flare after surgical treatment.[12–14] These data suggest the important role of cortisol in suppressing inflammation.

CORTISOL AND MELATONIN EFFECTS ON CIRCADIAN CYTOKINE PRODUCTION

More recently, melatonin (MLT), another circadian hormone that is the secretory product of the pineal gland, has been found implicated in the time-dependent inflammatory reaction with effects opposite those of cortisol.[15]

In adult primates, only visible light (400–700 nm) is received by the retina. This photic energy is then transduced and delivered to the visual cortex and, by an alternative pathway, to the suprachiasmatic nucleus (SCN), the hypothalamic region that directs circadian rhythm. Visible light exposure also modulates the pituitary and pineal glands, leading to neuroendocrine changes. MLT, norepinephrine, and acetylcholine decrease with light activation, whereas cortisol, serotonin, γ-aminobutyric acid (GABA), and dopamine levels increase.[16]

Thus, ocular light appears to be the predominant time cue and major determinant of circadian rhythm for many neurohormones.

Therefore, cortisol and MLT show an opposite response to light. The light conditions in the early morning have a strong impact on the morning cortisol peak, whereas MLT is synthesized in a strictly nocturnal pattern. Direct inhibitory effects of light on pineal activity may contribute to phasing of the onset and termination of MLT production.[17,18]

Recently, diurnal rhythmicity in healthy humans between cellular (Th1 type) or humoral (Th2 type) immune responses has been found and related to immunomodulatory actions of cortisol and MLT (FIG. 3).[4]

In particular, LPS- or tetanus-stimulated human whole blood IFN-γ (type 1) and IL-10 (type 2) production, and the IFN-γ/IL-10 ratio exhibited significant diurnal rhythmicity. The IFN-γ/IL-10 ratio peaked during the early morning and correlated negatively with plasma cortisol and positively with plasma MLT. IFN-γ and, to a lesser extent, IL-10 production was sensitive to the inhibition by exogenous cortisone; the IFN-γ/IL-10 ratio decreased by $>70\%$ after the administration of oral cortisone acetate. These findings support the concept that plasma cortisol and possibly MLT regulate diurnal variation in the IFN-γ/IL-10 ratio. As IFN-γ and IL-10 have opposing effects on cellular (type 1) immunity, changes in their balance would be anticipated to impose diurnal rhythmicity on cellular immunity.

As a matter of fact, in normal subjects, MLT peaks at approximately 3 AM, whereas cortisol peaks at approximately 9 AM.[19] Interestingly, IL-1, IL-6 and soluble IL-2 receptors peak between 1 AM and 4 AM and are low throughout the day.[19]

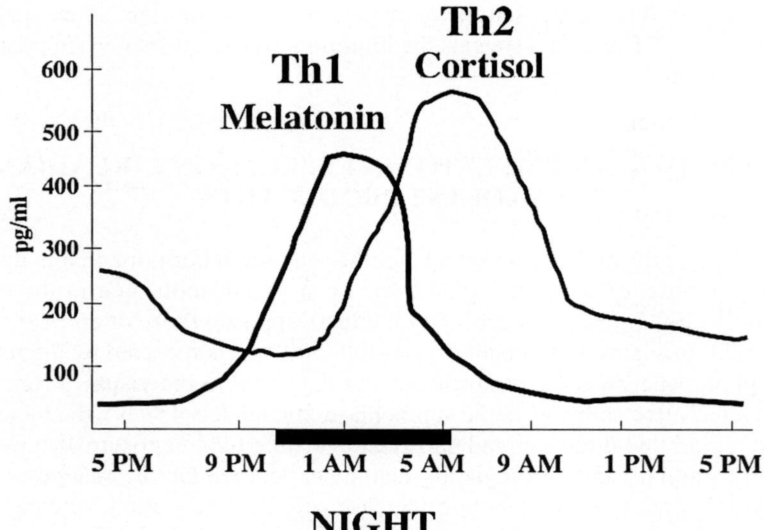

FIGURE 3. A diurnal rhythmicity in healthy humans between cellular (Th1 type cytokines proinflammatory) or humoral (Th2 type cytokines anti-inflammatory) immune responses has been found and related to immunomodulatory action of MLT (Th1) and cortisol (Th2) .

MLT stimulates IL-1 and IFN-γ production by human monocytes and serum IL-2 increases during the night concomitantly to MLT rise, as well MLT seems to enhance IL-2 immunomodulating effects.[20–22]

MLT increases the production of IL-12 and NO by human synovial macrophages, enhances IL-2, IL-6, and IFN-γ production by human circulating $CD4^+$ lymphocytes and upregulate the level of gene expression of TNF-α and macrophage colony-stimulating factor (M-CSF).[23–25]

On the contrary, cortisol was found negatively correlated with the IFN-γ/IL-10 ratio and cortisone administration markedly reduced the ratio with a clear casual relationship.[4] As a matter of fact, there is a positive correlation between whole blood IFN-γ production and plasma MLT, and a negative correlation between IFN-γ and plasma cortisol.

In addition to IFN-γ and IL-1, TNF-α and IL-12 also exhibit distinct diurnal rhythms that peak in the early morning, and are inversely related to the rhythm of plasma cortisol.[26]

Therefore, IFN-γ and IL-10 might be considered markers of cellular (type 1) and humoral (type 2) immunity, respectively. These studies suggest that there is a bias toward cellular immunity during the night and early morning (peak of MLT) when IFN-γ/IL-10 ratio is high and converserly a relative bias toward humoral (type 2) immunity during the day.[27]

CORTISOL AND MLT EFFECTS ON CIRCADIAN RHYTHMS OF RA

The production of corticotropin-releasing hormone (CRH) in the hypothalamus is stimulated by inflammatory cytokines (i.e., IL-6, IL-1, TNF-α) as soluble products of the activated immune system. CRH release leads to pituitary production of adrenocorticotropic hormone (ACTH), followed by glucocorticoid secretion by adrenal cortex (HPA axis).[7,28]

Recently, preserved ACTH secretion, but impaired cortisol response in patients with active RA has been described and this condition was consistent with a relative adrenal glucocorticoid insufficiency, the latter already suggested 40 years earlier.[28,29]

Increased HPA axis function is a normal response to the stress of inflammation and might be mediated by central and peripheral actions of circulating cytokines.

Besides, IL-1 and TNF-α, IL-6 appears as a major factor mediating interactions between the activated immune system and both the anterior pituitary cells and the adrenal steroidogenesis. However, recent studies in RA patients have shown that the overall activity of HPA axis remains inappropriately normal (or low) and is apparently insufficient to inhibit the inflammatory reaction at least in early untreated arthritic patients.[30,31]

In particular, in early morning hours, an earlier surge of plasma ACTH and cortisol was observed in RA patients and significantly increased IL-6 levels and a pronounced circadian variation of plasma levels were detected when compared to healthy subjects.[33]

In addition, in the RA patients, a positive temporal correlation between plasma IL-6 levels and ACTH/cortisol with elevated levels of IL-6 before the elevations of ACTH and cortisol by 1 and 2 h, respectively, was reported.[32]

A negative effect of cortisol upon IL-6 was found exerted with a delay of 5 h in the same patients, confirming that HPA in RA is apparently insufficient to inhibit the inflammatory status.

Another study showed a significantly altered secretion of adrenal androgens in non-glucocorticoid-treated premenopausal RA patients.[33] Low plasma levels of the adrenal androgens dehydroepiandrosterone (DHEA) and its sulfate metabolite DHEAS were found in the same study to be significantly correlated in RA patients with early morning low cortisol concentrations and high basal levels of IL-6.[33]

Early morning IL-6 peak values were recently found to be higher in RA patients than in controls, and significantly correlated to morning C-reactive protein (CRP) levels and Ritchie's index.[34]

The observation of reduced DHEA production, combined with normal cortisol production during CRH and ACTH testing, seems to support the concept of the presence of an adrenal hypofunction in active RA patients.[35]

IL-6 had a strong effect on steroid release and may be one of the factors controlling the long-term adrenal response to stress. In fact, this cytokine is able to act synergistically with ACTH on the adrenal cells to stimulate the release of corticosterone.[36,37]

Therefore, the reduced cortisol and adrenal androgen secretion, observed during testing in RA patients not treated with glucocorticoids, should be clearly considered as a "relative adrenal insufficiency" in the presence of a sustained inflammatory process, as shown by high IL-6 levels.[38]

In a recent investigation on salivary cortisol levels in patients with recent-onset RA, the afternoon concentrations of salivary cortisol levels in patients with high disease activity did not drop, as it did in healthy controls and RA patients with low disease activity.[39] These observations, further indicate that activation of the HPA axis in RA is evident but insufficient. Therefore, the lower-than-required production of cortisol supports the efficacy of low-dose corticosteroid "replacement therapy" in RA patients.[40]

Very recent studies have evaluated MLT levels in RA patients, together with the analysis of circadian variations.[41]

Interestingly, MLT serum levels at 8 PM and 8 AM were found to be significantly higher in RA patients than in controls ($P < 0.05$). The differences that patients resulted were more evident in the older RA patients (age > 60 years) when compared to the younger.

In both RA patients and healthy subjects, MLT levels progressively increased from 8 PM to the early hours of the morning, but in RA patients the peak level was recorded at 12 PM, at least 2 h before than in controls.

Therefore, MLT concentrations showed a plateau in RA patients lasting for 2–3 h not evident in controls. After 2 AM, MLT levels decreased similarly in both RA patients and healthy subjects.

The results of the study confirm the existence of a nocturnal rhythm of MLT also in RA patients, but the peak level was recorded earlier and was of longer duration in the early morning.[41] Interestinlgy, IFN-γ and IL-2, as well as IL-1, IL-6, IL-12, and TNF-α production (Th1 cytokines) reaches the peak during the night and early morning, at the same time when MLT serum levels are highest and plasma cortisol is lower. In conclusion, MLT could be involved in the induction of a more active inflammatory response during the night, at least in RA which is considered to be a Th1-cytokine-driven immune disease.[41] A recent study showed that both MLT and TNF-α serum levels were found to be significantly higher in Estonian RA patients when compared with their controls.[42] Significantly higher serum MLT, IL-6, and TNF-α concentrations were observed again at 10 PM and at midnight in Estonian RA patients when compared with Italian RA patients.

This study showed, for the first time, that in a north European country (Estonia), the circadian serum concentrations of MLT (and TNF-α) are significantly higher than in matched RA patients from a south European country (Italy).

Finally, MLT has been found at a rather high concentration in synovial fluids from RA patients and binding sites for MLT have been detected in synovial macrophages.[43,44]

CONCLUSIONS

The production of the proinflammatory and anti-inflammatory cytokines seems regulated by the two night hormones, namely cortisol and MLT. Both hormones exert opposite effects and their serum (and synovial) levels are altered at least in RA.

Circadian changes in the metabolism or secretion of endogenous glucocorticoids and MLT are certainly responsible, in part, for the time-dependent changes observed in the inflammatory response and arthritis.

The right time (early morning) for the glucocorticoid anti-inflammtory therapy in arthritis is fundamental and well justified by the circadian rhythms of the proinflammatory mediators.

REFERENCES

1. Kowanko, I.C., M.S. Knapp, R. Pownall, *et al.* 1982. Domiciliary self-measurement in rheumatoid arthritis and in the demonstration of circadian rythmicity. Ann. Rheum. Dis. **41:** 453–455.
2. Labrecque, G., J.P. Bureau & A.E. Reinberg. 1995. Biological rhythms in the inflammatory response and in the effects of non-steroidal anti-inflammatory drugs. Pharmac. Ther. **66:** 285–300.
3. Harkness, J.A.P., M.B. Richter, G.S. Panayi, *et al.* 1982. Circadian variations in disease activity in rheumatoid arthritis. Br. Med. J. **284:** 551–554.
4. Petrovsky, N., P. McNair & L. Harrison. 1998. Diurnal rhythms of pro-inflammatory cytokines: regulation by plasma cortisol and therapeutic implications. Cytokine **10:** 307–312.
5. Crofford, L.J., K.T. Kalogeras, G. Mastorakos, *et al.* 1997. Circadian relationships between interleukin (IL)-6 and hypothalamic-pituitary-adrenal axis hormones: failure of IL-6 to cause sustained hypercortisolism in patients with early untreated rheumatoid arthritis. J. Clin. Endocrinol. Metab. **82:** 1279–1283.
6. Cutolo, M., L. Foppiani & F. Minuto. 2002. Hypothalamic-pituitary-adrenal axis impairment in the pathogenesis of rheumatoid arthritis and polymyalgia rheumatica. J. Endocrinol. Invest. **25:** 19–23.
7. Chrousos, G.P. 1995. The hypothalamic-pituitary-adrenal axis and immune-mediated inflammation. N. Engl. J. Med. **332:** 1351–1362.
8. Heim, C., U. Ehlert & D.H. Hellhammer. 2000. The potential role of hypocortisolism in the pathophysiology of stress-related bodily disorders. Psychoneuroendocrinology **25:** 1–35.
9. Bland, M.L., C.A. Jamieson, S.F. Akana, *et al.* 2000. Haploinsufficiency of steroidogenic factor-1 in mice disrupts adrenal development leading to an impaired stress response. Proc. Natl. Acad. Sci. USA **97:** 1448–1493.

10. Bland, M.L., M. Desclozeaux & H.A. Ingraham. 2003. Tissue growth and remodeling of the embryonic and adult adrenal gland. Ann. N. Y. Acad. Sci. **995:** 59–72.
11. Lotfi, C.F., Z. Todorovic, H.A. Armelin, *et al.* 1997. Unmasking a growth-promoting effect of the adrenocorticotropic hormone in Y1 mouse adrenocortical tumor cells. J. Biol. Chem. **272:** 29886–29891.
12. Senecal, J.L., I. Uthman & H. Beauregard. 1994. Cushing's disease-induced remission of severe rheumatoid arthritis. Arthritis Rheum. **37:** 182.
13. Senecal, J.L. 1995. Onset of rheumatoid arthritis after surgical treatment of Cushing's disease. J. Rheumatol. **22:** 1964–1966.
14. Yakushiji, F., M. Kita, N. Hiroi, *et al.* 1995. Exacerbation of rheumatoid arthritis after removal of adrenaladenoma in Cushing's syndrome. Endocr. J. **42:** 219–223.
15. Cutolo, M. & G.J. Maestroni. 2005. The melatonin-cytokine connection in rheumatoid arthritis. Ann. Rheum. Dis. **64:** 1109.
16. Roberts, J.E. 2000. Light and immunomodulation. Ann. N. Y. Acad. Sci. **917:** 435–445.
17. Scheer, F.A. & R.M. Buijs. 1999. Light affects morning salivary cortisol in humans. J. Clin. Endocrinol. Metab. **84:** 3395–3398.
18. Reiter, R.J. 1991. Pineal melatonin: cell biology of its synthesis and of its physiological interactions. Endocr. Rev. **12:** 151–180.
19. Miyatake, A., Y. Morimoto & T. Uishi. 1980. Circadian rhythm of serum testosterone and its relation to sleep: comparison with the variation in serum luteinizing hormone, prolactin, and cortisol in normal men. J. Clin. Endocrinol. Metab. **51:** 1365–1371.
20. Morrey, K.M., J.A. McLachlan & C.D. Serkin. 1994. Activation of human monocytes by pineal hormone melatonin. J. Immunol. **153:** 2671–2680.
21. Lissoni, P., F. Rovelli, F. Brivio, *et al.* 1998. Circadian secretions of IL-2, IL-12, IL-6 and IL-10 in relation to light/dark rhythm of the pineal hormone melatonin in healthy subjects. Nat. Immun. **16:** 1–5.
22. Lissoni, P. 2000. Modulation of anticancer cytokines IL-2 and IL-12 by melatonin and the other pineal indoles 5-methoxytryptamine and 5-methoxytryptolol in the treatment of human neoplasms. Ann. N. Y. Acad. Sci. **917:** 560–567.
23. Garcia-Mauriño, S., M.G. Gonzalez-Haba, J.R. Calvo, *et al.* 1997. Melatonin enhances IL-2, IL-6 and IFN- production by human circulating CD4+ cells. J. Immunol. **159:** 574–581.
24. Cutolo, M., B. Villaggio, F. Candido, *et al.* 1999. Melatonin influences IL-12 and nitric oxide production by primary cultures of rheumatoid synovial macrophages and THP-1 cells. Ann. N. Y. Acad. Sci. **876:** 246–255.
25. Liu, F., T.B. Ng & M.C. Fung. 2001. Pineal indoles stimulates the gene expression of immunomodulating cytokines. J. Neural. Transm. **108:** 397–405.
26. Masi, A.T., S.L. Feigenbaum, R.T. Chatteron, *et al.* 1995. Integrated Hormonal-Immunological-Vascular ("H-I-V" Triad) system interactions in rheumatic diseases. Clin. Exp. Rheumatol. **13:** 203–216.
27. Petrovsky, N. 2001. Towards a unified model of neuroendocrine-immune interaction. Immunol. Cell Biol. **78:** 350–357.
28. Gudbjörnsson, B., B. Skogseid, B. Öberg, *et al.* 1996. Intact adrenocorticotropic hormone secretion but impaired cortisol response in patients with active rheumatoid arthritis. Effect of glucocorticoids. J. Rheumatol. **23:** 596–602.
29. West, H.F. 1993. Corticosteroid metabolism and rheumatoid arthritis. Ann. Rheum. Dis. **16:** 173–181.

30. MASI, A.T. & G.P. CHROUSOS. 1996. Hypothalamic-pituitary-adrenal-glucocorticoid axis function in rheumatoid arthritis. J. Rheumatol. **23:** 577–581.
31. STRAUB, R.H. & M. CUTOLO. 2001. Involvement of the hypothalamic—pituitary—adrenal/gonadal axis and the peripheral nervous system in rheumatoid arthritis: viewpoint based on a systemic pathogenetic role. Arthritis Rheum. **44:** 493–507.
32. CROFFORD, L.J., K.T. KALOGERAS, G. MASTORAKOS, *et al.* 1997. Circadian relationships between interleukin (IL)-6 and hypothalamic-pituitary-adrenal axis hormones: failure of IL-6 to cause sustained hypercortisolism in patients with early untreated rheumatoid arthritis. J. Clin. Endocrinol. Metab. **82:** 1279–1283.
33. CUTOLO, M., L. FOPPIANI, C. PRETE, *et al.* 1999. Hypothalamic-pituitary-adrenocortical axis in premenopausal rheumatoid arthritis patients: not treated with glucocorticoids. J. Rheumatol. **26:** 282–288.
34. ARVIDSON, G.N., G. GUDBJØRSSON, L. ELFMAN, *et al.* 1994. Circadian rhythm of serum interleukin-6 in rheumatoid arthritis. Ann. Rheum. Dis. **53:** 521–524.
35. TEMPL, E., M. KOELLER, M. RIEDL, *et al.* 1996. Anterior pituitary function in patients with newly diagnosed rheumatoid arthritis. Br. J. Rheumatol. **35:** 350–356.
36. MASTORAKOS, G., G.P. CHROUSOS & J.S. WEBER. 1993. Recombinant interleukin-6 activates the hypothalamic-pituitary-adrenal axis in human. J. Clin. Endocr. Metab. **77:** 1690–1694.
37. EHRHART-BORNSTEIN, M., J.P. HINSON, S.R. BORNSTEIN, *et al.* 1998. Intraadrenal interactions in the regulation of adrenocortical steroidogenesis. Endocr. Rev. **19:** 101–103.
38. DEKKERS, J.K., R. GREENEN, G.L.R. GODAERT, *et al.* 2000. Diurnal rhythm of salivary cortisol levels in patients with recent-onset rheumatoid arthritis. Arthritis Rheum. **43:** 465–467.
39. STRAUB, R.H., L. PAIMELA, R. PELTOMAA, *et al.* 2002. Inadequately low serum levels of steroid hormones in relation to IL-6 and TNF in untreated patients with early rheumatoid arthritis and reactive arthritis. Arthritis Rheum. **46:** 654–662.
40. VAN EVERDINGEN, A.A., J.W. JACOBS, D.R. SIEWERTSZ VAN REESEMA, *et al.* 2002. Low-dose prednisone therapy for patients with early active rheumatoid arthritis: clinical efficacy, disease-modifying properties, and side effects: a randomized, double-blind, placebo-controlled clinical trial. Ann. Intern. Med. **136:** 1–12.
41. SULLI, A., G.J.M. MAESTRONI, B. VILLAGGIO, *et al.* 2002. Melatonin serum levels in rheumatoid arthritis. Ann. N. Y. Acad. Sci. **966:** 276–283.
42. CUTOLO, M., G.J. MAESTRONI, K. OTSA, *et al.* 2005. Circadian melatonin and cortisol levels in rheumatoid arthritis patients in winter time: a north and south Europe comparison. Ann. Rheum. Dis. **64:** 212–216.
43. MAESTRONI, G.J.M., A. SULLI, C. PIZZORNI, *et al.* 2002. Melatonin in rheumatoid arthitis: synovial macrophages show melatonin receptors. Ann. N. Y. Acad. Sci. **966:** 271–275.
44. MAESTRONI, G.J.M., A. SULLI, C. PIZZORNI, *et al.* 2002. Melatonin in rheumatoid arthritis: a disease promoting and modulating hormone? Clin. Exp. Rheumatol. **20:** 872–873.

Oral Pulsed Dexamethasone Therapy in Early Rheumatoid Arthritis

A Pilot Study

ERIC-JAN A. KROOT, A. MARGRIET HUISMAN, JENDÉ VAN ZEBEN, JACQUES M.G.W. WOUTERS, AND HENK C. VAN PAASSEN

Department of Rheumatology, St. Franciscus Hospital, Rotterdam, the Netherlands

ABSTRACT: Pulse therapy with high-dose glucocorticoids (GCs) is widely used as "bridging therapy" for the treatment of patients with active rheumatoid arthritis (RA). Oral pulsed dexamethasone therapy has never been used for this purpose. We determined the clinical efficacy of oral pulsed dexamethasone treatment in patients with early active RA, concomitantly starting with disease-modifying anti-rheumatic drugs (DMARDs). Fourteen early RA patients, glucocorticoid-naive and with active disease for less than 1 year were included. Ten patients were treated with oral pulsed dexamethasone therapy for 4 days in a row. Of this group, four patients received 10 mg dexamethasone/day, three patients 20 mg/day, and three patients 40 mg/day. As controls, four patients were treated with intramuscular methylprednisolone injections. Disease activity (ascertained by disease activity score [DAS]) and biochemical variables were measured at base line, and biweekly thereafter for up to 4 weeks, and monthly thereafter for up to 3 months. A decrease in disease activity, similar in all subgroups, was observed. Nine of 10 patients responded favorably (decrease in DAS of >1.2) 4 weeks after the start of the study. This response was sustained in the months thereafter. One patient did not respond at all, and disease progression during treatment was observed in one patient. No side effects were reported. Only once was a decrease in cortisol level observed; this was at 2 weeks after the start of the study (0.03 μmol/L, reference value 0.18–0.70 μmol/L). Oral pulsed dexamethasone therapy seems to be effective and safe as bridging therapy in early rheumatoid arthritis. The results of the present study justify a long-term controlled trial to compare oral pulsed dexamethasone treatment (10 mg dexamethasone, once weekly for 4 weeks) with the standard GC regimes in the near future.

KEYWORDS: rheumatoid arthritis; therapy; oral pulsed dexamethasone

Address for correspondence: Eric-Jan A. Kroot, M.D., Ph.D., Sint Franciscus Gasthuis, Department of Rheumatology, Kleiweg 500, 3045 PM Rotterdam, the Netherlands. Voice: +31-10-461-6167; fax: +31-10-461-2692.
e-mail: ejankroot@yahoo.com

**Ann. N.Y. Acad. Sci. 1069: 300–306 (2006). © 2006 New York Academy of Sciences.
doi: 10.1196/annals.1351.028**

INTRODUCTION

High-dose glucocorticoids (GCs) have already been shown to be beneficial for rheumatoid arthritis (RA).[1,2] Its beneficial effects are generally sustained for 4–12 weeks. Therefore, GCs are widely used as "bridging therapy" for the treatment of patients with RA, with active disease, concomitantly starting with disease-modifying antirheumatic drugs (DMARDs).[1,2] Recently, GCs have also been shown to reduce the progression of joint damage in both mono- and combination therapies with DMARDs.[1,3] Several dosing schemes of high-dose pulsed GC therapy are known: high-dose prednisone according to the COBRA scheme,[4] three intramuscular (i.m.) injections of 120 mg methylprednisolone at 3- or 4-week intervals, and intravenous (i.v.) dexamethasone or methylprednisolone (three infusions of 200 mg dexamethasone or 500 mg methylprednisolone at 3-day intervals). A major advantage of oral pulsed dexamethasone therapy in comparison with the use of i.v. GCs involves the fact that dexamethasone has less mineral corticoid activity in comparison with prednisone, and that patients do not have to stay in the hospital. GC pulse therapy might induce fewer side effects than the more prolonged low dose of oral GC therapy.[1,5] In particular, the possible decreased suppression of the hypothalamic-pituitary-adrenal (HPA) axis of high-dose GC pulse therapy is of importance, especially early in the disease course.[1,2]

Whether oral pulsed dexamethasone therapy is beneficial in patients with RA has never been determined. Oral pulsed dexamethasone therapy has been shown to be effective in other autoimmune diseases, including resistant idiopathic thrombocytopenic purpura, polymyositis, and chronic inflammatory demyelinating polyneuropathy.[6–8] With this in mind, we speculated whether this strategy might be a new therapeutic "pulse" option in RA, with probably fewer side effects than the standard GC strategies.

MATERIALS AND METHODS

Fourteen consecutive eligible patients with newly diagnosed RA (disease duration less than 1 year) and active disease (DAS > 3.2) were included. All patients fulfilled the American College of Rheumatology criteria for RA and were DMARD- and glucocorticoid-naive. Patients with severe comorbidity, including hypertension, diabetes, eye diseases, malignancy, cardiovascular disease, infections, and pulmonary disorders were not included. The patients were assigned into two treatment groups: 10 patients were treated with oral pulsed dexamethasone therapy; four patients were treated with i.m. methylprednisolone. The oral pulsed dexamethasone-treated patients were assigned into three subgroups: four patients received 10 mg/day, three patients 20 mg/day, and three patients 40 mg/day, during four alternate days. These doses of dexamethasone match with cumulative doses of prednisone of successively

TABLE 1. Baseline characteristics of the 14 patients with early RA

Age (years)	62 (30–70)
Male/Female (*n*)	7/7
IgM rheumatoid factor–positive (*n*)	11
Anti-citrulline-containing peptide–positive (*n*)	11
Early morning stiffness (minutes)	70 (30–180)
28 Joint scores for swelling	14 (4–22)
28 Joint scores for tenderness	16 (5–25)
C-reactive protein level (mg/L)	29 (6–74)
Disease activity score (DAS-28)	5.6 (4.01–6.98)

NOTE: Mean values (range) and numbers are given.

265 mg, 530 mg, and 1,060 mg. Patients receiving oral pulsed dexamethasone therapy simultaneously received prophylactic antacid. As mentioned, four patients were treated with i.m. methylprednisolone 120 mg, matching with a cumulative dose of prednisone 150 mg. This procedure was performed at 4-week intervals. Clinical and biochemical variables, including DAS, tension, weight, BSE, CRP, routine blood tests, glucose, and cortisol levels before breakfast were determined at base line and biweekly up to 1 month, and monthly thereafter up to 3 months. The decision to add a particular DMARD was based on clinical grounds (RA disease activity).

RESULTS

Clinical and demographic characteristics of the patients are shown in TABLE 1. Age varied between 30 and 78 years with a mean (±SD) age of 62.2 years. The study group consisted of 7 males and 7 females. Age and sex were equally distributed over the treatment groups, as well as IgM rheumatoid factor (IgM-RF) and anticitrulline-containing peptide antibody (anti-CCP). Ten patients were both IgM-RF- and anti-CCP-positive, one patient only IgM-RF-positive, and one patient only anti-CCP-positive. Treatment with a DMARD was started in all patients. Ten patients were treated with methotrexate, three patients with sulfasalazine, and one patient with leflunomide. Twelve patients completed the study, and two patients were followed up for just 2 months: one patient had moved out of the area and one patient refused further participation. Two patients missed the 2-week follow-up control and one patient missed the 8-week follow-up control because of business abroad and an already planned vacation, respectively (these missing visits have been extrapolated in FIG. 1).

The disease activity of each patient before, during, and after treatment is shown in FIGURE 1. No great differences between the four dosing groups were observed. A decrease in DAS of >1.2 was observed in eight out of 10 patients treated with dexamethasone 2 weeks after the start of the study. Nine out of 10 patients treated with dexamethasone had responded favorably (decrease

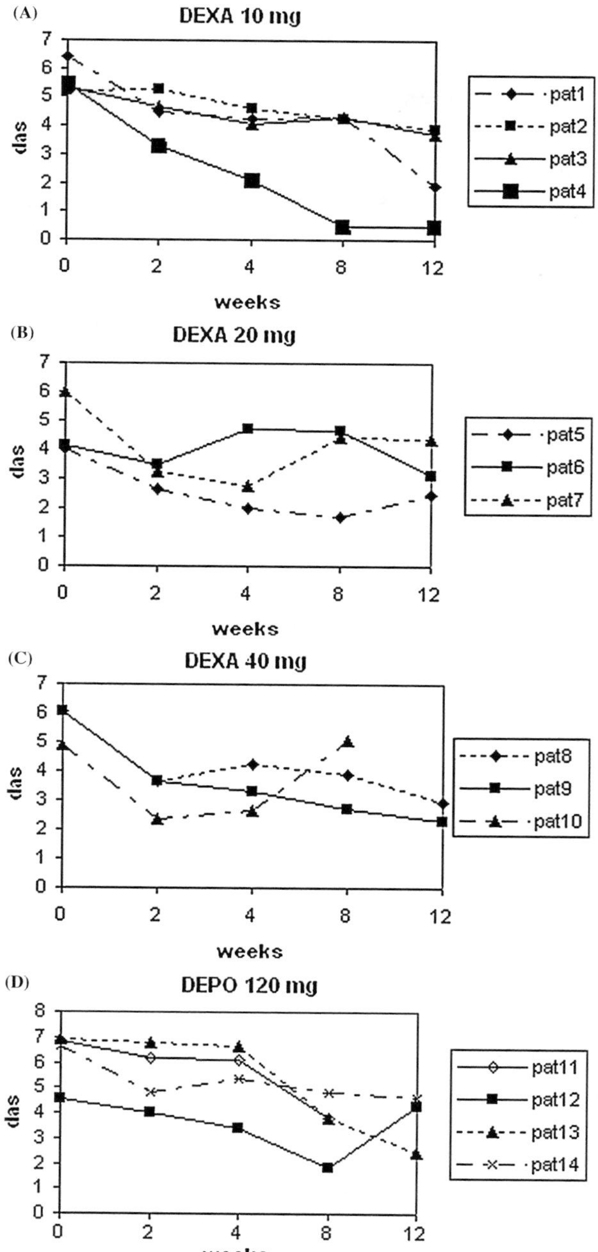

FIGURE 1. Disease activity of each patient for treatment: (**A**) oral dexamethasone 10 mg/day for 4 days, (**B**) oral dexamethasone 20 mg/day for 4 days, (**C**) oral dexamethasone 40 mg/day for 4 days, and (**D**) i.m. methylprednisolone 120 mg given at weeks 0, 4, and 8.

in DAS of >1.2) after 4 weeks of the start of the study. This response was sustained up to 3 months from the start of the study. In most patients, the level of disease activity did not further decrease between weeks 4 and 12. In one patient in the 40-mg group, disease activity severely increased during the second month of study, after which the patient refused to participate further. Only one patient, in the 20-mg dexamethasone group, did not respond at all in the first 4 weeks and received a second dexamethasone pulse of 20 mg/day on four consecutive days at week 4. After this second pulse, the DAS decreased, although less (<1.2) in comparison with the DAS at the start of the study (decrease in DAS from 4.1 to 3.11). In both the 10- and 20-mg dexamethasone groups, higher BSE and CRP levels at the start of the study were observed in patients who responded best. In the 40-mg group, the best responders had higher BSE levels at the start of the study only. Except for one patient in the 10-mg group, a higher number of swollen joints at the start of the study seemed to be associated with better clinical response in all patients. Because of the small number of patients, no statistical analysis was performed to study these correlations.

Patients receiving oral dexamethasone pulse therapy did not report any side effects: no hypertension, weight gain, diabetes, or gastrointestinal complaints were reported, and no abnormal blood-test results were observed. However, some patients experienced flushes after intake of dexamethasone. Only once, was a decrease seen in cortisol level in the oral dexamethasone-treated patients 2 weeks after the start of the study (0.03 μmol/L, reference value 0.18–0.70 μmol/L), which resolved after 4 weeks (0.23 μmol/L).

DISCUSSION

To our knowledge, our study provides the first prospectively investigated results of high-dose oral pulsed treatment with dexamethasone in unselected RA patients with early active disease. We have demonstrated that oral pulsed high-dose dexamethasone is a safe and effective treatment for early RA. Nine out of 10 oral dexamethasone-treated patients responded favorably (decrease in DAS >1.2) after 3 months of follow-up. Decreased disease activity at 4 weeks, usually the time from which DMARDs become effective and therefore considered as the main time point for evaluation of the efficacy of pulse therapy, was observed in nine patients as well. The favorable response was independent of the doses of dexamethasone. That the disease activity did not further decrease between weeks 4 and 12 in most patients might have been due to the fact that only "one pulse" of oral dexamethasone was given. In other autoimmune diseases, patients were treated with high-dose oral dexamethasone during three 28-day cycles.[6–8] Therefore, and due to the results of the present study, in future this strategy should be applied in patients with early RA as well. We chose to test only one dexamethasone pulse cycle, because we considered the dexamethasone doses used, matching with relatively high cumulative doses of prednisolone, sufficient as pulse therapy for early active RA in order to "bridge" until DMARDs become effective.

In the literature, clinical effects of high-dose pulse GCs infusion as a treatment for RA differed considerably between patients.[9–12] The optimal dose of high-dose GC used as bridge therapy for RA, therefore, still has to be established. Some studies suggested that higher doses seem to be more effective than lower doses.[1] With the doses used in the present study, we did not find such a relationship, and therefore suggest that the lowest possible dose of dexamethasone (10 mg orally on four consecutive days or 10 mg orally once weekly for 1 month) should be used in future studies in order to minimize side effects. In contrast to the disagreement in the literature about the most effective dose of GC pulse therapy, higher levels of inflammatory indices correlated with best clinical response in all studies.[5,9–12] The results of the present study, although not statistically analyzed due to the small number of patients, seem to be in line with these studies.

The dexamethasone dosage scheme used in the present study was selected because of good results in several other autoimmune diseases.[6–8] In one of these studies, dexamethasone seemed to be less well tolerated than in the present study, although the side effects were considered acceptable.[6] In this study, dexamethasone pulses were repeated several times and, therefore, much higher cumulative doses of prednisolone in comparison with those in the present study were used.[6] In our study, oral dexamethasone pulses were well tolerated, with no side effects leading to drug discontinuation. Patients could take their pulsed doses at home, without admittance into the hospital.

However, some comments should be made. First, this is an open-label, nonrandomized pilot study with a short period of follow-up encompassing just a small number of patients. Second, we did not compare oral pulsed dexamethasone with a classical dexamethasone pulse therapy scheme and, therefore, the results of our pilot study might be misleading. Third, a very high dose of more than 100 mg prednisolone equivalent per day results in virtually 100% saturation of the cytosolic receptors.[13,14] In addition, with the administration of more than 250 mg prednisolone equivalent per day nongenomic mechanisms come into play as well.[13,14] Therefore, significant differences in therapeutic efficacy between the treatment groups could not be expected.

Nevertheless, the 3-month results of oral pulsed dexamethasone in the present study seem promising. Oral pulsed dexamethasone might be a safe and effective pulse treatment for newly diagnosed RA. A large-scale double-blind, randomized controlled trial might further determine the place of oral pulsed dexamethasone therapy as a "bridging therapy" in patients with active RA in comparison with standard GC strategies.

REFERENCES

1. Laan, R.F., T.L. Jansen & P.L.C.M. van Riel. 1999. Glucocorticosteroids in the management of rheumatoid arthritis. Rheumatology **38:** 6–12.
2. Da Silva, J.A. & J.W. Bijlsma. 2000. Optimizing glucocorticoid therapy in rheumatoid arthritis. Rheum. Dis. Clin. N. Amer. **26:** 859–880.
3. van Everdingen, A.A., J.W. Jacobs, D.R. Siewertsz Van Reesema & J.W. Bijlsma. 2002. Low-dose prednisone therapy for patients with early active rheumatoid arthritis: clinical efficacy, disease-modifying properties, and side effects: a randomized, double-blind, placebo-controlled clinical trial. Ann. Intern. Med. **136:** 1–12.
4. Boers, M., A.C. Verhoeven, H.M. Markusse, *et al.* 1997. Randomised comparison of combined step-down prednisolone, methotrexate and sulphasalazine with sulphasalazine alone in early rheumatoid arthritis. Lancet **350:** 309–318.
5. Frediani, B., P. Falsetti, S. Bisogno, *et al.* 2004. Effects of high dose methylprednisolone pulse therapy on bone mass and biochemical markers of bone metabolism in patients with active rheumatoid arthritis: a 12-month randomized prospective controlled study. J. Rheumatol. **31:** 1083–1087.
6. Andersen, J.C. 1994. Response of resistant idiopathic thrombocytopenic purpura to pulsed high-dose dexamethasone therapy. N. Engl. J. Med. **330:** 1560–1564.
7. Molenaar, D.S., P.A. van Doorn, M. Vermeulen. 1997. Pulsed high dose dexamethasone treatment in chronic inflammatory demyelinating polyneuropathy: a pilot study. J. Neurol. Neurosurg. Psychiatry **62:** 388–390.
8. van der Meulen, M.F., J.E. Hoogendijk, J.H. Wokke & M.DE. Visser. 2000. Oral pulsed high-dose dexamethasone for myositis. J. Neurol. **247:** 102–105.
9. Wenting-Van Wijk, M.J., M.A. Blankenstein, F.P. Lafeber & J.W. Bijlsma. 1999. Relation of plasma dexamethasone to clinical response. Clin. Exp. Rheumatol. **17:** 305–312.
10. Bertouch, J.V., P.J. Roberts-Thomson, M.D. Smith, *et al.* 1986. Methylprednisolone infusion therapy in rheumatoid arthritis patients: the effect on synovial fluid lymphocyte subsets and inflammatory indices. Arthritis Rheum. **29:** 32–38.
11. Nossent, H.C., G. Bakland, H.K. Aslaksen, *et al.* 2001. Efficacy of methylprednisolone pulse therapy versus infliximab in the treatment of severe flares of chronic polyarthritis. Scand. J. Rheumatol. **30:** 335–339.
12. Jacobs, J.W., R. Geenen, A.W. Evers, *et al.* 2001. Short term effects of corticosteroid pulse treatment on disease activity and the wellbeing of patients with active rheumatoid arthritis. Ann. Rheum. Dis. **60:** 61–64.
13. Song, I.H., R. Gold, R.H. Straub, *et al.* 2005. New glucocorticoids on the horizon: repress, don't activate! J. Rheumatol. **32:** 1199–1207.
14. Buttgereit, F., R.H. Straub, M. Wehling & G.R. Burmester. 2004. Glucocorticoids in the treatment of rheumatic diseases: an update on the mechanisms of action. Arthritis Rheum. **50:** 3408–3417.

Glucocorticoid Effects on Adrenal Steroids and Cytokine Responsiveness in Polymyalgia Rheumatica and Elderly Onset Rheumatoid Arthritis

ALBERTO SULLI,[a] CARLO MAURIZIO MONTECUCCO,[b] ROBERTO CAPORALI,[b] LORENZO CAVAGNA,[b] PAOLA MONTAGNA,[a] SILVIA CAPELLINO,[a] LAURA FAZZUOLI,[c] BRUNO SERIOLO,[a] CALVIA ALESSANDRO,[a] MARIA ELENA SECCHI,[a] AND MAURIZIO CUTOLO[a]

[a]*Research Laboratory and Division of Rheumatology, Department of Internal Medicine, San Martino Hospital, University of Genova, 6-16132 Genova, Italy*

[b]*Division of Rheumatology, IRCCS Policlinico San Matteo, University of Pavia, Pavia, Italy*

[c]*Laboratory of Endocrinology, Department of Endocrinology and Metabolism, University of Genova, 16132 Genova, Italy*

Abstract: **Polymyalgia rheumatica (PMR) usually exhibits a good clinical response to glucocorticoid (GC) treatment, but early clinical symptoms may create some difficulties in the differential diagnosis with elderly onset rheumatoid arthritis (EORA), particularly in patients complaining of shoulder and pelvic girdle involvement at onset (PMR-like clinical onset) (EORA/PMR). Since neuroendocrine mechanisms seem to play a pathogenetic role in these clinical conditions, the aim of this study was to evaluate hormone and cytokine responsiveness to GC treatment in these patients. Cortisol (CO), dehydroepiandrosterone sulphate (DHEAS), 17-OH-progesterone (PRG), interleukin-1 receptor antagonist (IL-1Ra), interleukin-6 (IL-6), and tumor necrosis factor-α (TNF-α) were evaluated at base line, and 1 month after GC treatment (prednisone 10 mg/day), in 14 PMR, 11 EORA/PMR, and 13 EORA patients (mean age 73 ± 5 years, ± SD, mean disease duration 3 ± 2 months, ± SD). No patient was taking GCs or immunosuppressive agents at base line. Following GC treatment, CO, DHEAS, and PRG decreased significantly in both PMR and EORA/PMR patients ($P < 0.05$), but not in EORA patients. On the contrary, IL-1Ra was significantly increased in both PMR and EORA/PMR patients ($P < 0.05$). IL-6 and TNF-α serum levels were significantly decreased in all groups of patients**

Address for correspondence: Alberto Sulli, M.D., Research Laboratory and Division of Rheumatology, Department of Internal Medicine, San Martino Hospital, University of Genova, Viale Benedetto XV, 6-16132 Genova, Italy. Voice: +39-010-3538617; fax: +39-010-3537537.
e-mail: albertosulli@unige.it

Ann. N.Y. Acad. Sci. 1069: 307–314 (2006). © 2006 New York Academy of Sciences.
doi: 10.1196/annals.1351.029

($P < 0.05$). In conclusion, PMR and EORA/PMR seem to exhibit similar hormonal variations after GC administration, when compared to EORA patients. These differences suggest a deficient function of the hypothalamic-pituitary-adrenal (HPA) axis in PMR and EORA/PMR patients, with a related higher responsiveness to GC treatment. Interestingly, in PMR and EORA/PMR patients, GC treatment was found to downregulate PRG serum levels.

Keywords: polymyalgia rheumatica; rheumatoid arthritis; elderly onset rheumatoid arthritis; cytokines; hormones

INTRODUCTION

Polymyalgia rheumatica (PMR) is an inflammatory condition characterized by aching and stiffness in the shoulder and in the pelvic girdles, and it has a favorable prognosis after glucocorticoid (GC) treatment.[1,2] However, the occurrence of peripheral arthritis, particularly in both hands, may create some difficulties in the differential diagnosis between PMR and elderly onset rheumatoid arthritis (EORA).[3–5] Furthermore, PMR patients may develop overt rheumatoid arthritis (RA) during the follow-up,[6] while several patients with seronegative EORA show a rapid and complete response to GCs, as well as a nonerosive course.[1] Furthermore, the differential diagnosis might be even more difficult in EORA patients complaining of PMR-like clinical onset (girdle involvement at onset) (EORA/PMR).

Since neuroendocrine mechanisms seem to play a pathogenetic role in these clinical conditions,[7–9] the aim of this article was to evaluate different hormone and cytokine responsiveness to GC treatment in patients with PMR, EORA, and EORA/PMR. GC-naive patients were evaluated at disease onset, and 1 month after prednisone treatment.

PATIENTS AND METHODS

Thirty-eight patients were enrolled in the study, after informed consent was obtained. Fourteen patients complained of PMR (mean age 73 ± 4 years ± SD, mean disease duration 2.8 ± 2 months ± SD), 13 patients EORA (mean age 73 ± 5 years ± SD, mean disease duration 3.5 ± 2.4 months ± SD), and 11 patients EORA/PMR (mean age 73 ± 6 years ± SD, mean disease duration 3.4 ± 2.3 months ± SD). The patients with PMR met the criteria of Chuang.[10] The patients with EORA (disease onset after 60 years of age) met the American College of Rheumatology (ACR) criteria for RA.[11] The EORA/PMR patients complained of aching and stiffness in the shoulder and pelvic girdles (PMR-like clinical onset), along with peripheral arthritis (hands and wrists, knees), and met at least four ACR criteria for RA. No patient was taking GCs or immunosuppressive agents at base line. No patient used immunosuppressive agents during the study period (1 month). No other major diseases were present.

Fasting blood samples for hormone and cytokine evaluation were collected at base line, as well as 1 month after GC treatment (mean prednisone 0.15 mg/kg/day). Blood samples were centrifuged 30 min after collection. Serum tubes were frozen at –70°C, to allow that all samples could be tested at the same time.

The following hormones and cytokines were evaluated: cortisol (CO), dehydroepiandrosterone sulphate (DHEAS), 17-OH-progesterone (PRG), interleukin-1 receptor antagonist (IL-1Ra), interleukin-6 (IL-6), and tumor necrosis factor-α (TNF-α).

Serum levels of CO and DHEAS were assayed by chemiluminescent method (DPC, Los Angeles, CA, and Nichols Institute Diagnostics, San Juan Capistrano, CA, respectively) with a sensitivity of 0.2 μg/dL for CO and 0.1 μg/dL for DHEAS. CVs were 6.5% for CO and 6.7% for DHEAS. The results of CO were expressed in ng/mL, and DHEAS levels were evaluated in μg/dL. Serum levels of PRG were measured by direct immunoenzymatic method (Mascia Brunelli, Milan, Italy) with a sensitivity of 5 pg/mL and CV of 5.4%. The results were reported in μg/mL. Enzyme-linked immunosorbent assay (ELISA) was used to measure serum levels of IL-1Ra (Beckman Coulter, Marseille, France), IL-6, and TNF-α (Cayman, Ann Arbor, MI). Each kit specifically measures both natural and recombinant human TNF-α, IL-6, and IL-1Ra, showing no detectable cross-reaction with other cytokines. Sensitivity was 1.5 pg/mL for TNF-α, 2 pg/mL for IL-6, and 30 pg/mL for IL-1Ra. CV% intra-assay was 1.97% and interassay 3.85% for TNF-α, CV% intra-assay was 2.34% and interassay 3.86% for IL-6, and CV% intra-assay was 4.35% and interassay was 8.6% for IL-1Ra. The results were expressed in pg/mL. All samples were tested three times.

The statistical analysis was performed by nonparametric Wilcoxon signed rank test to compare the continuous variables and Mann–Whitney U test to compare continuous variables with nominal variables. The P value lower than 0.05 was considered statistically significant.

RESULTS

Before GC treatment, no statistically significant difference was observed concerning both CO and PRG serum levels between the three groups of patients, even if CO was found slightly higher in PMR patients when compared to other groups. DHEAS was found significantly higher in EORA patients when compared to both PMR and EORA/PMR patients ($P < 0.05$). IL-1Ra serum levels were found significantly higher in EORA patients when compared with both PMR and EORA/PMR patients ($P < 0.05$). IL-6 serum levels were found significantly higher in both PMR and EORA/PMR patients, when compared with EORA patients ($P < 0.05$), while no statistically significant difference was found for TNF-α serum levels between the three groups of patients.

After 1 month of GC treatment, the following variations were observed. CO, DHEAS, and PRG decreased significantly in both PMR (median 144 → 96 ng/mL, 64 → 41 μg/mL, 83 → 42 μg/mL, before and after GC treatment, for CO, DHEAS, and PRG, respectively) and EORA/PMR patients (median 134 → 70 ng/mL, 25 → 15 μg/mL, 65 → 47 μg/mL, before and after GC treatment, for CO, DHEAS, and PRG, respectively) ($P < 0.05$), but not in EORA patients. IL-1Ra increased significantly in both PMR (median 420 → 677 pg/mL, before and after GC treatment) and EORA/PMR patients (median 458 → 551 pg/mL, before and after GC treatment) ($P < 0.05$), while no statistically significant variation was observed for IL-1Ra in EORA patients. IL-6 and TNF-α serum levels decreased significantly in all groups of patients ($P < 0.05$). See FIGURES 1, 2, and 3 for further details.

No statistically significant difference was found between the groups concerning both age of patients and disease duration.

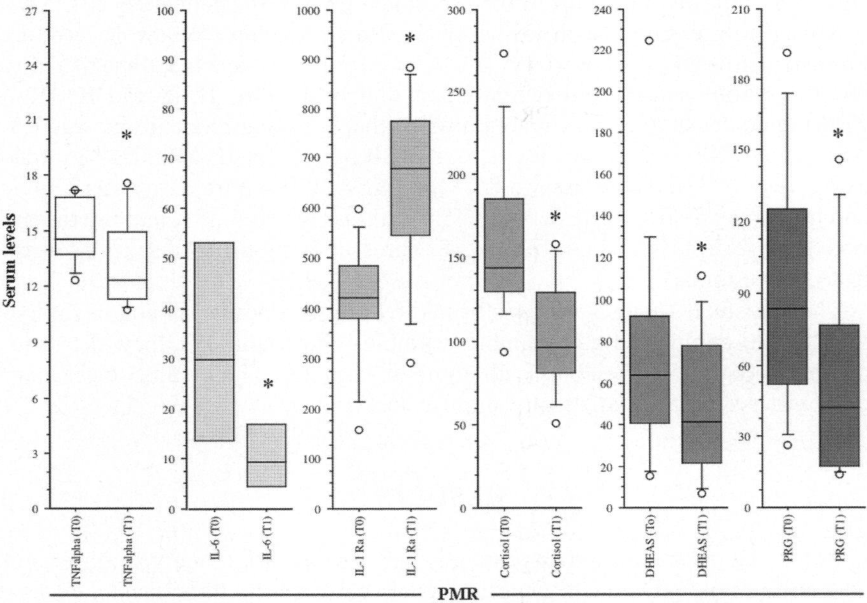

FIGURE 1. Cytokine and hormone serum levels in PMR patients before and after GC treatment. Values are expressed as median, percentiles, maximum, and minimun value in the box plots. Serum levels: TNF-α = pg/mL, IL-6 = pg/mL, IL-1Ra = pg/mL, CO = ng/mL, DHEAS = mcg/mL, PRG = mcg/mL. * = $P< 0.05$ basal (T0) versus post-GC treatment (T1).

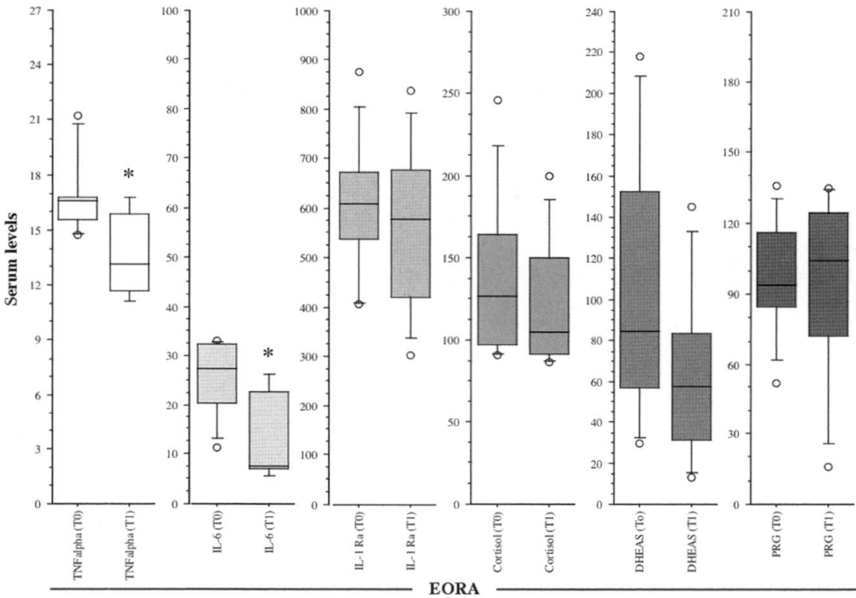

FIGURE 2. Cytokine and hormone serum levels in EORA patients before and after GC treatment. Values are expressed as median, percentiles, maximum, and minimum value in the box plots. Serum levels: TNF-α = pg/mL, IL-6 = pg/mL, IL-1Ra = pg/mL, CO = ng/mL, DHEAS = mcg/mL, and PRG = mcg/mL. ∗ = $P < 0.05$ basal (T0) versus post-GC treatment (T1).

DISCUSSION

Both clinical conditions, PMR and EORA/PMR, seem to exhibit similar hormonal and cytokine variations after GC administration, when compared to EORA patients. These differences suggest a larger impairment of the hypothalamic- pituitary-adrenal (HPA) axis in PMR and EORA/PMR patients, with a related higher responsiveness to GC treatment.

PMR typically affects elderly people. The hypofunction of the HPA axis, as well as a general impairment of the hormone and cytokine production during aging, might contribute to the pathogenesis of PMR. Recently, a reduced synthesis of adrenal hormones, like CO and DHEAS, has been shown in untreated PMR patients with active disease, as well as an increased PRG production following ACTH test.[8,9] In relation to adrenal steroid status, increased production of IL-6 is a characteristic finding in patients with PMR, and GCs rapidly reduce serum levels of IL-6.[7,8,12] Genetic causes, as well as polymorphisms of genes involved in the initiation and regulation of inflammatory reaction have been considered to be possible susceptibility factors for PMR.[13,14] In particular, TNF-α, and IL-1Ra gene polymorphisms are predisposing factors and may be implicated in the pathogenesis of PMR.[15–17]

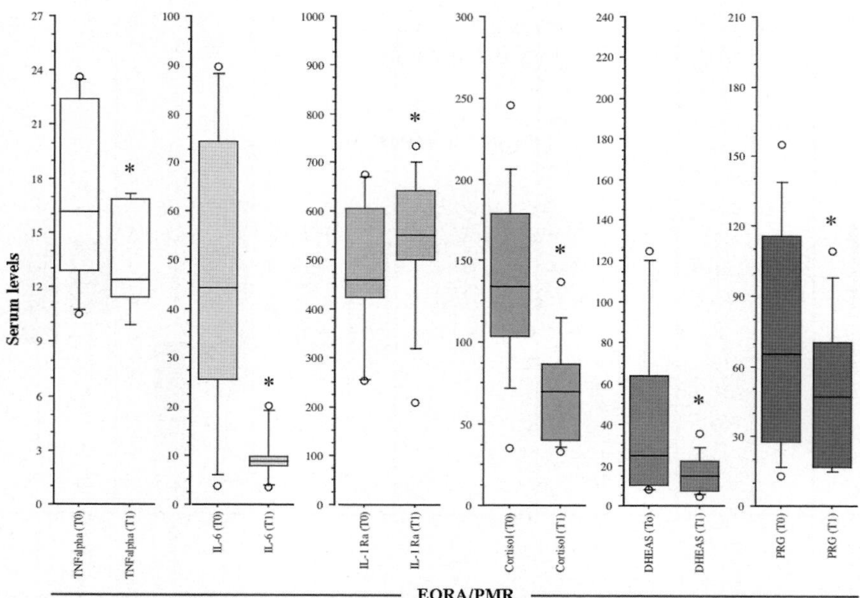

FIGURE 3. Cytokine and hormone serum levels in EORA/PMR patients before and after GC treatment. Values are expressed as median, percentiles, maximum, and minimun value in the box plots. Serum levels: TNF-α = pg/mL, IL-6 = pg/mL, IL-1Ra = pg/mL, CO = ng/mL, DHEAS = mcg/mL, and PRG = mcg/mL. $*$ = $P < 0.05$ basal (T0) versus post-GC treatment (T1).

Interestingly, in PMR and EORA/PMR patients, GC treatment was found to downregulate PRG serum levels. High basal PRG levels in PMR and EORA/PMR might be related to the altered adrenal responsiveness to the ACTH stimulation. PRG represents a precursor of CO biosynthesis at the adrenal level, and a possible partial impairment of the enzyme 21α-hydroxylase might lead to accumulation of PRG. The reasons for a functional 21α-hydroxylase impairment in elderly may include genetic defects, or an age-related increase of serum TNF in healthy women, or elevated serum IL-6 and TNF-α levels during chronic systemic inflammatory stimuli.[8] However, TNF-α was shown to inhibit the 21α-hydroxylase in adrenal cell cultures, and high concentrations of IL-6 and TNF-α have been shown to interfere with enzymes involved in peripheral steroid hormone metabolism.[18,19]

The statistically significant decrease of serum CO levels after 1 month of GC therapy in both PMR and EORA/PMR patients, when compared to EORA patients, suggests an higher HPA axis responsiveness in the former. However, the frequent observation of reduced CO and adrenal androgen secretion during testing in RA patients not treated with GCs, should be regarded as a "relative adrenal insufficiency" in the setting of a sustained inflammatory process, as shown by high serum IL-6 levels.[20,21] The reduction of DHEAS is a general feature of chronic inflammatory diseases, including RA.[20,22,23]

CONCLUSION

GC treatment, acting as a "replacement" on account of the reduced endogenous CO production, seems more effective in both PMR and EORA/PMR patients, than in EORA patients, at least in the short time (significant reduction of IL-6 and TNF-α, and increase of IL-1Ra). As no routine laboratory markers of inflammation allows early differentiation between PMR and EORA,[6] the different clinical and humoral response to GC therapy might differentiate these clinical conditions at onset.

Furthermore, EORA patients with PMR-like clinical onset seem to have better response to GC treatment, than EORA patients. By considering the low erosive potential of EORA, as well as the good response to GC observed in EORA/PMR patients, disease modifying antirheumatic drug employment may be delayed or not necessary in this latter clinical condition.

REFERENCES

1. Salvarani, C., F. Cantini, L. Boiardi, *et al.* 2004. Polymyalgia rheumatica. Best. Pract. Res. Clin. Rheumatol. **18:** 705–722.
2. Cimmino, M.A., G. Moggiana, C. Montecucco, *et al.* 1994. Long term treatment of polymyalgia rheumatica with deflazacort. Ann. Rheum. Dis. **53:** 331–333.
3. Narvaez, J., J.M. Nolla-Sole, J.A. Narvaez, *et al.* 2001. Musculoskeletal manifestations in polymyalgia rheumatica and temporal arteritis. Ann. Rheum. Dis. **60:** 1060–1063.
4. Healey, L.A. 1992. Polymyalgia rheumatica and seronegative rheumatoid arthritis may be the same entity. J. Rheumatol. **19:** 270–272.
5. Bajocchi, G., R. La Corte, A. Locaputo, *et al.* 2000. Elderly onset rheumatoid arthritis: clinical aspects. Clin. Exp. Rheumatol. **18:** S49–S50.
6. Caporali, R., C. Montecucco, O. Epis, *et al.* 2001. Presenting features of polymyalgia rheumatica (PMR) and rheumatoid arthritis with PMR-like onset: a prospective study. Ann. Rheum. Dis. **60:** 1021–1024.
7. Cutolo, M., L. Foppiani & F. Minuto. 2002. Hypothalamic-pituitary-adrenal axis impairment in the pathogenesis of rheumatoid arthritis and polymyalgia rheumatica. J. Endocrinol. Invest. **25:** 19–23.
8. Straub, R.H., T. Gluck, M. Cutolo, *et al.* 2000. The adrenal steroid status in relation to inflammatory cytokines (interleukin-6 and tumour necrosis factor) in polymyalgia rheumatica. Rheumatology **39:** 624–631.
9. Cutolo, M., R.H. Straub, L. Foppiani, *et al.* 2002. Adrenal gland hypofunction in active polymyalgia rheumatica. Effect of glucocorticoid treatment on adrenal hormones and interleukin-6. J. Rheumatol. **29:** 748–756.
10. Chuang, T.Y., G.G. Hunder, D.M. Ilstrup, *et al.* 1982. Polymyalgia rheumatica: a 10-year epidemiologic and clinical study. Ann. Intern. Med. **97:** 672–680.

11. ARNETT, F.C., S.M. EDWORTHY, D.A. BLOCH, *et al.* 1988. The American Rheumatism Association 1987 revised criteria for the classification of rheumatoid arthritis. Arthritis Rheum. **31:** 315–324.
12. WEYAND, C.M., J.W. FULBRIGHT, J.M. EVANS, *et al.* 1999. Corticosteroid requirements in polymyalgia rheumatica. Arch. Intern. Med. **159:** 577–584.
13. LIANG, G.C., P.A. SIMKIN, G.G. HUNDER, *et al.* 1974. Familial aggregation of polymyalgia rheumatica and giant cell arteritis. Arthritis Rheum. **17:** 19–24.
14. SALVARANI, C., P.L. MACCHIONI, F. ZIZZI, *et al.* 1991. Epidemiologic and immunogenetic aspects of polymyalgia rheumatica and giant cell arteritis in Northern Italy. Arthritis Rheum. **34:** 351–356.
15. SALVARANI, C., B. CASALI, L. BOIARDI, *et al.* 2000. Intercellular adhesion molecule 1 gene polymorphisms in polymyalgia rheumatica/giant cell arteritis: association with disease risk and severity. J. Rheumatol. **27:** 1215–1221.
16. MATTEY, D.L., A.H. HAJEER, A. DABABNEH, *et al.* 2000. Association of giant cell arteritis and polymyalgia rheumatica with different tumor necrosis factor microsatellite polymorphisms. Arthritis Rheum. **43:** 1749–1755.
17. BOIARDI, L., C. SALVARANI, J.M. TIMMS, *et al.* 2000. Interleukin-1 cluster and tumor necrosis factor-α gene polymorphisms in polymyalgia rheumatica. Clin. Exp. Rheumatol. **18:** 675–681.
18. JAATTELA, M., V. ILVESMAKI, R. VOUTILAINEN, *et al.* 1991. Tumor necrosis factor as a potent inhibitor of adrenocorticotropin-induced cortisol production and steroidogenic P450 enzyme gene expression in cultured human fetal adrenal cells. Endocrinology **128:** 623–629.
19. HERRMANN, M., J. SCHOLMERICH & R.H. STRAUB. 2002. Influence of cytokines and growth factors on distinct steroidogenic enzymes in vitro: a short tabular data collection. Ann. N. Y. Acad. Sci. **966:** 166–186.
20. CUTOLO, M., A. SULLI, C. PIZZORNI, *et al.* 2003. Hypothalamic-pituitary-adrenocortical and gonadal functions in rheumatoid arthritis. Ann. N. Y. Acad. Sci. **992:** 107–117.
21. CUTOLO, M., B. VILLAGGIO, L. FOPPIANI, *et al.* 2000. The hypothalamic-pituitary-adrenal and gonadal axes in rheumatoid arthritis. Ann. N. Y. Acad. Sci. **917:** 835–843.
22. STRAUB, R.H., M. ZEUNER, E. ANTONIOU, *et al.* 1996. Dehydroepiandrosterone sulfate is positively correlated with soluble interleukin 2 receptor and soluble intercellular adhesion molecule in systemic lupus erythematosus. J. Rheumatol. **23:** 856–861.
23. STRAUB, R.H., D. VOGL, V. GROSS, *et al.* 1998. Association of humoral markers of inflammation and dehydroepiandrosterone sulfate or cortisol serum levels in patients with chronic inflammatory bowel disease. Am. J. Gastroenterol. **93:** 2197–2202.

Is the Course of Steroid-Treated Polymyalgia Rheumatica More Severe in Women?

MARCO A. CIMMINO,[a] MASSIMILIANO PARODI,[a]
ROBERTO CAPORALI,[b] AND CARLOMAURIZIO MONTECUCCO[b]

[a]*Clinica Reumatologica, Dipartimento di Medicina Interna e Specialità Mediche, Università di Genova, 16129 Genova, Italy*

[b]*IRCCS Policlinico S. Matteo, Università di Pavia, 27100 Pavia, Italy*

ABSTRACT: Polymyalgia rheumatica (PMR) has a marked preponderance in women. The female sex has been claimed to be a risk factor for longer-course corticosteroid therapy and to be associated with more severe systemic symptoms and lower hemoglobin levels. Eighty consecutive patients affected by PMR, seen at two tertiary referral centers, were followed-up for a mean period of 14.9 months after initiating corticosteroid treatment. At presentation, women had longer disease duration and lower hemoglobin levels (both $P = 0.05$) than men. In contrast, their systemic signs of PMR were less common ($P = 0.01$). Women were treated with a slightly higher mean daily dose of prednisone ($P = 0.055$), and assumed a significantly higher cumulative dosage of the drug ($P = 0.01$). Accordingly, the mean number of steroid-related side effects was higher among women ($P = 0.003$). The number of relapses during steroid treatment ($P = 0.02$), but not that of recurrences, was increased in women. ESR, which was raised at presentation, significantly declined during follow-up to normal values in both subgroups ($P < 0.00001$ by analysis of variance [ANOVA]). Its decrease was significantly more pronounced in men than in women. Hemoglobin at follow-up was significantly higher in men than in women at any given time point. In conclusion, sex is probably modulating the response to corticosteroids. This finding emphasizes the need to consider differences between males and females in the clinical and therapeutic approach to PMR patients.

KEYWORDS: polymyalgia rheumatica; sex; gender; corticosteroid; treatment

Address for correspondence: Marco A. Cimmino, M.D., Clinica Reumatologica, DI.M.I., Università di Genova, Viale Benedetto XV, 6, 16129 Genova, Italy. Voice: +39010-3538905; fax: +39010-3538638.
e-mail: cimmino@unige.it

**Ann. N.Y. Acad. Sci. 1069: 315–321 (2006). © 2006 New York Academy of Sciences.
doi: 10.1196/annals.1351.030**

INTRODUCTION

Polymyalgia rheumatica (PMR) is a syndrome affecting the elderly, characterized by proximal muscular pain and stiffness. Systemic manifestations and elevated acute phase reactants are often present.[1] The mainstay of therapy is oral steroids, with prednisone at dosages of 10–20 mg usually suppressing inflammation dramatically.[1] However, up to 60% of patients experience disease relapse during steroid tapering, and several studies indicate that only rarely steroid treatment can be discontinued before 1.5 years.[2] PMR has a marked female preponderance, with a female to male ratio of about 2.[1] It is not known why elderly women are preferentially affected, but sex hormones are likely at play. Female sex has been shown to be a risk factor for longer-course corticosteroid therapy in one study.[3] More recently, more severe constitutional symptoms and lower hemoglobin levels have been observed in women with PMR compared with men.[4] However, low hemoglobin concentration in women is not necessarily the consequence of inflammation. In addition, the other signs of PMR as well as erythrocyte sedimentation rate (ESR) were similar between genders. Therefore, it is not clear if women with PMR have more inflammation and a worse prognosis in comparison with men. This article is concerned with an evaluation of a consecutive series of 80 PMR patients to assess if there are gender-related differences in PMR activity at presentation and if women are more resistant to treatment than men.

PATIENTS AND METHODS

Eighty consecutive patients affected by PMR seen at two tertiary referral centers were considered. The centers participating in the study were regional units, where patients are usually referred by general practitioners. The principal investigators responsible for following patients in this study were rheumatologists. PMR was diagnosed according to Chuang *et al.*[5] Accordingly, inclusion criteria were all of the following: (*a*) age >50 years; (*b*) ESR >40 mm/h; (*c*) aching and stiffness at shoulder and/or hip girdle for >1 month; and (*d*) no signs or symptoms of other musculoskeletal or connective tissue conditions, including serum creatine–kinase elevation and polyarthritis.

Demographic data were recorded on a specifically developed protocol, which included disease duration before diagnosis, duration of follow-up, starting dose of corticosteroid, total dosage, mean dose, number of side effects, and mean number of relapses and recurrences. A flare up of signs and symptoms of PMR (i.e., aching and stiffness at shoulder and/or hip girdle) accompanied by an increase of ESR above 30 mm/h and/or C-reactive protein (CRP) levels above 5 mg/L was defined a relapse if observed during steroid tapering or a recurrence if observed after steroid withdrawal. Relapses and recurrences were assessed by the principal investigator at every control visit or whenever an unscheduled visit was requested by the patients.

After the first one, follow-up visits were performed monthly for 6 months, and thereafter every 6 months. Every visit included complete physical examination and a questionnaire designed to assess the patient's symptoms and health status. Adverse events and concomitant therapy were also recorded. At presentation, clinical examination was performed and the following data were recorded: fever, peripheral arthritis, temporal arteritis, weight loss, intensity of pain measured by visual analog scale, and duration of morning stiffness. ESR, CRP, and hemoglobin were evaluated by routine laboratory methods at every visit. Patients were treated with prednisone at a mean starting dose of 15.5 mg/day with range 5–40 mg depending on severity of disease. Prednisone was tapered by about 20% monthly if the patient was asymptomatic and ESR and CRP were reduced to normal.

Statistical analysis included the Student's *t*-test if the variables were continuous and the Wilcoxon's rank sum test in case of non-normal variables. Percentages were compared by the chi-square test. Logistic regression with sex as independent variable was also performed. One-way analysis of variance (ANOVA) was used to test the significance of differences observed in repeated clinical and laboratory examinations. Associations were tested by Spearman's rank correlations test. Statistical significance was defined as $P \leq 0.05$.

RESULTS

The demographic, clinical, and laboratory characteristics at presentation are reported in TABLE 1 where the patients' data are broken down by gender. Sex-related differences of weight loss and hemoglobin shown by univariate analysis remained significant in a logistic regression model weighed for disease duration. At presentation, ESR, CRP, and hemoglobin were not correlated.

Mean duration of follow-up in the 80 patients was 14.9 months (range 4–68 months). Follow-up results are shown in TABLE 2. Women were treated with a slightly higher mean daily dose of prednisone ($P = 0.055$), and assumed a significantly higher cumulative dosage of the drug. Accordingly, the mean number of steroid-related side effects was higher among women. Finally, the number of relapses during steroid treatment, but not that of recurrences, was increased in women.

During the follow-up period, four women were also diagnosed with temporal arteritis. To test if their need for more aggressive treatment could have accounted for the higher total corticosteroid dosage seen in women, we analyzed our data after excluding this small subgroup of patients. Total corticosteroid dosage remained higher in women, although to a lower degree (5.5 ± 4 g versus 3.9 ± 1.9 g; $P = 0.05$), whereas differences in number of relapses and side effects were nearly unchanged.

ESR, which was raised at presentation, significantly declined during follow-up to normal values in both subgroups ($P < 0.00001$ by ANOVA). Its decrease

TABLE 1. Demographic, clinical, and laboratory differences at presentation between women and men with PMR

Feature	Women	Men	*P*
Number	52 (65%)	28 (35%)	
Mean age (years)	67.6 ± 7.8	70.6 ± 9.2	ns
Disease duration (months)	5.3 ± 4.6	3.2 ± 2.3	0.05
Duration of follow-up (months)	14.4 ± 15.4	15.7 ± 17.5	ns
Weight loss	12 (23.1%)	14 (50%)	0.01
Fever	15 (28.8%)	6 (21.4%)	ns
Morning stiffness (minutes)	75.5 ± 48.1	96.2 ± 66.7	ns
Pain (VAS in mm)	69.4 ± 14.5	65.4 ± 15	ns
Arthritis	12 (23.1%)	4 (14.3%)	ns
Arteritis	4 (7.7%)	0	ns
ESR (mm/h)	74.8 ± 24.7	66.9 ± 18.7	ns
CRP (mg/L)	36.9 ± 36.9	30.9 ± 24.3	ns
Hemoglobin (g/L)	12.1 ± 2.1	13.2 ± 2.1	0.05
Corticosteroid starting dose (mg)	17.1 ± 9.9	14.5 ± 6.6	ns

was significantly more pronounced in men than in women (FIG. 1). This was not the case for CRP, which declined significantly after steroid treatment with a course unaffected by gender differences. This behavior at follow-up was shared also by the visual analog scale of pain and by duration of morning stiffness. Hemoglobin at follow-up was significantly higher in men than in women at any given time point (FIG. 2).

DISCUSSION

The amount of inflammation shown by women with PMR at disease presentation was not superior to that of male patients. Conversely, Narváez *et al.*[4] claimed that women with PMR had more severe inflammatory response because they found lower hemoglobin and more constitutional symptoms. However, low hemoglobin levels in women does not point *per se* to chronic inflammation, and in our study no correlation was found between hemoglobin and indexes of inflammation, such as ESR and CRP. On the contrary, weight

TABLE 2. Differences between women and men with PMR at follow-up

Feature	Women	Men	*P*
Duration of treatment (months)	22.6 ± 16.2	17.9 ± 9.3	ns
Corticosteroid mean dosage (mg)	9.6 ± 4.5	7.7 ± 3.2	ns
Corticosteroid total dosage (g)	6.4 ± 4.9	3.9 ± 1.9	0.01
Mean number of relapses	0.7 ± 1	0.3 ± 0.4	0.02
Mean number of recurrences	0.05 ± 0.2	0.09 ± 0.3	ns
Mean number of steroid side effects	2.2 ± 0.8	1.6 ± 0.7	0.003

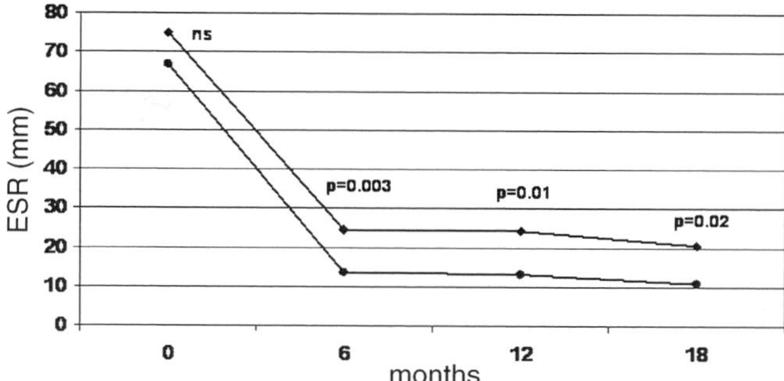

FIGURE 1. Changes in ESR during follow-up according to sex (squares = women, circles = men). ESR significantly declined in women and men ($P < 0.00001$ by ANOVA). The difference between sexes was not seen at presentation but became apparent during follow-up.

loss, which is a systemic symptom frequently seen in PMR, was more frequent in men. In the previously cited study, all clinical findings were considered together and it is impossible to know the sex association of each of them.

Despite the similar degree of inflammation seen in male and female PMR patients at presentation, the amount of steroid needed to control the disease was higher in women with consequent increased incidence of side effects. The number of relapses was also significantly higher in women. The association with temporal arteritis, which was observed only in four women, was not the cause of these differences. In fact, when these four patients were excluded from computation, they persisted. One can postulate that they are related to the protective effect of androgen as well as the enhancing effect of estrogens toward autoimmunity.[6] This last possibility, however, is unlikely because women with PMR are almost exclusively postmenopausal patients who presumably have

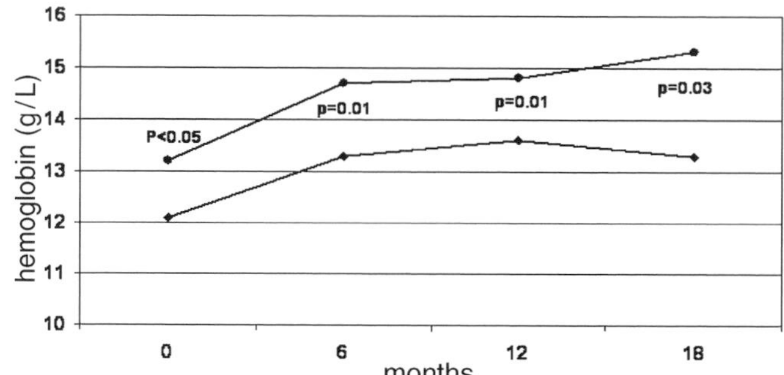

FIGURE 2. Changes in hemoglobin during follow-up according to sex (squares = women, circles = men). Hemoglobin was significantly lower in women at any time point.

low estrogen concentrations. If hormonal factors are implicated in the gender differences, one would expect also a higher severity of the disease before corticosteroid treatment. In addition, a recent epidemiological study has shown that previous pregnancies are protective for temporal arteritis.[7] This finding has been explained by the associated hyperestrogenic effect that could be beneficial by protecting patients from atheromatous arterial wall lesions.

An alternative and speculative hypothesis for the sex-associated differences found in our study is that women with PMR have a low number or low affinity of glucocorticoid receptors, thus explaining the need for higher dosages and the relative lack of efficacy in comparison with men. Glucocorticoid receptors from mononuclear leukocytes isolated from peripheral blood were slightly fewer in normal women and decreased with age.[8] In fact, PMR is usually treated by low-dose corticosteroids acting by classic genomic effects that are mediated by the glucocorticoid receptor.

A surprising finding of this study was the higher delay in diagnosis among women. There is no clear explanation for it, although in a different setting women with HIV infection seeked medical care with more delay than men, primarily for family responsibilities.[9] Another possible explanation is that women more often than men suffer from joint pain and may underestimate PMR symptoms.

A higher incidence of steroid-related side effects in women with PMR has been also shown by Gabriel *et al.*[10] The three variables that increased the risk of side effects were increasing age at diagnosis, a cumulative dosage of prednisone higher than 1.8 g, and female sex. However, these factors were reported to act independently and, in contrast with our findings, no interaction between sex and steroid dosage was found.

In conclusion, gender is probably modulating the response to corticosteroids in PMR patients. This finding emphasizes the need to consider gender differences in the clinical and therapeutic approach to patients.[11] In clinical trials, attention should be paid to the sex ratio of the treated and control groups, because its imbalance could influence results. For the same reason, efficacy and toxicity results should be probably broken down by sex.

REFERENCES

1. Salvarani, C., F. Cantini, L. Boiardi, *et al.* 2002. Polymyalgia rheumatica and giant-cell arteritis. N. Engl. J. Med. **347:** 261–271.
2. Cimmino, M.A., G.L. Moggiana, C. Montecucco, *et al.* 1994. Long term treatment of polymyalgia rheumatica with deflazacort. Ann. Rheum. Dis. **53:** 331–333.
3. Narváez, J., J.M. Nolla-Solé, M.T. Clavaguera, *et al.* 1999. Longterm therapy in polymyalgia rheumatica: effect of coexistent temporal arteritis. J. Rheumatol. **26:** 1945–1952.

4. NARVÁEZ, J., J.M. NOLLA-SOLÉ, J. VALVERDE-GARCÍA, *et al.* 2002. Sex differences in temporal arteritis and polymyalgia rheumatica. J. Rheumatol. **29:** 321–325.
5. CHUANG, T., G.G. HUNDER, D.M. ILSTRUP, *et al.* 1982. Polymyalgia rheumatica. A 10-year epidemiologic and clinical study. Ann. Intern. Med. **97:** 672–680.
6. CUTOLO, M., B. VILLAGGIO, C. CRAVIOTTO, *et al.* 2002. Sex hormones and rheumatoid arthritis. Autoimmun. Rev. **5:** 284–289.
7. DUHAUT, P., L. PINEDE, S. DEMOLOMBE-RAGUE, *et al.* 1999. Giant cell arteritis and polymyalgia rheumatica: are pregnancies a protective factor? A prospective, multicentre case-control study. Rheumatology **38:** 118–123.
8. TANAKA, H., H. AKAMA, Y. ICHIKAWA, *et al.* 1991. Glucocorticoid receptors in normal leukocytes: effects of age, gender, season, and plasma cortisol concentration. Clin. Chem. **37:** 1715–1719.
9. STEIN, M.D., S. CRYSTAL, W.E. CUNNINGHAM, *et al.* 2000. Delays in seeking HIV care due to competing caregiver responsibilities. Am. J. Public Health **90:** 1138–1140.
10. GABRIEL, S.E., J. SUNKU, C. SALVARANI, *et al.* 1997. Adverse outcomes of antiinflammatory therapy among patients with polymyalgia rheumatica. Arthritis Rheum. **40:** 1873–1878.
11. GESENSWAY, D. 2001. Reasons for sex-specific and gender-specific study of health topics. Ann. Intern. Med. **135:** 935–938.

Predicting and Preventing Autoimmunity, Myth or Reality?

MICHAL HAREL[a] AND YEHUDA SHOENFELD[a,b]

[a]*Center for Autoimmune Diseases, Department of Medicine B, Chaim Sheba Medical Center Tel-Hashomer 52621, Tel Aviv, Israel, and the Sackler Faculty of Medicine, Tel-Aviv University, 69978 Tel-Aviv, Israel*

[b]*Incumbent of the Laura Schwarz-Kipp Chair for Research of Autoimmune Diseases, Tel-Aviv University, 69978 Tel-Aviv, Israel*

ABSTRACT: Many autoimmune diseases are chronic conditions that progress over the course of years, and are characterized by the presence of autoantibodies that precede the overt disease by months or years. As examples, the presence of two islet cell antibodies (ICA) are associated with a 50% risk of developing diabetes mellitus in 5 years, anticyclic citrullinated (anti-CCP) antibodies are found in the sera of rheumatoid arthritis (RA) patients a median of 4.5 years before the overt disease, and in systemic lupus erythematosus (SLE), patients accrue antibodies throughout a foreseen course during the 3–4 years prior to the clinical symptoms. This ability to predict autoimmune diseases, or rather their clinical manifestations, leads to the prospect of screening healthy individuals for autoantibodies. The importance of such a notion lies not only in the ability to prevent life-threatening manifestations, such as Addisonian's crisis and thyroid storm, but also in the ability to treat and even prevent overt autoimmune diseases. Among such documented treatment modalities are administration of aspirin in antiphospholipid syndrome, ursodeoxycholic acid in primary biliary cirrhosis (PBC), vitamin D in SLE and autoimmune thyroid diseases (AITD), and more. Although additional studies are still needed to fully assess these notions, as well as the appropriate screening strategies to apply them, one cannot ignore the prospect of predicting and preventing autoimmunity.

KEYWORDS: autoantibodies; diabetes mellitus; rheumatoid arthritis; systemic lupus erythematosus; antiphospholipid syndrome; primary biliary cirrhosis; autoimmune hepatitis; Crohn's; ulcerative colitis; Addison's; thyroid; pemphigus; miscarriages

Address for correspondence: Yehuda Shoenfeld, M.D., F.R.C.P., Department of Medicine 'B' and Center for Autoimmune Diseases, Sheba Medical Center, Tel-Aviv University, Tel-Hashomer 52621, Israel. Voice: 972-3-5302652; fax: 972-3-5352855.
e-mail: Shoenfel@sheba.health.gov.il

Ann. N.Y. Acad. Sci. 1069: 322–345 (2006). © 2006 New York Academy of Sciences.
doi: 10.1196/annals.1351.031

INTRODUCTION

Taken as a group, autoimmune diseases are the third leading cause of morbidity and mortality in the industrialized world, only surpassed by cancer and heart disease.[1] Many autoimmune diseases are chronic diseases that progress over the course of years and are characterized by the presence of autoantibodies that precede the overt disease.[1] Autoantibodies may also predict specific clinical manifestation, disease severity, and rate of progression,[2] as well as specific clinical phenomena, such as autoimmune pregnancy loss.[3] The identification of these markers and the assessment of their predictive value might enable secondary prevention using specific drugs, such as ursodeoxycholic acid in primary biliary cirrhosis (PBC), or by immunological treatment, as is already being studied in type 1 diabetes mellitus. In addition, the ability to predict the severity of disease and its specific clinical manifestation allows tertiary prevention of disease complications. Such prevention may be accomplished by relatively simple adjustments of therapy and lifestyle including administration of aspirin[4] as well as vitamin D,[5] dietary modifications,[6] and avoidance of ultraviolet light exposure[7] or of oral contraceptives.[8]

The following is a brief article of the predictive role of autoantibodies in various autoimmune diseases and of specific pathologic phenomena associated with autoimmune responses.

TYPE 1 DIABETES MELLITUS

Type 1 diabetes is manifested by a destruction of the pancreatic ß cells that lead to insulin deficiency. At the time of clinical symptoms, 60–80% of the ß cells are destroyed. Insulitis, an inflammatory infiltrate containing large numbers of mononuclear cells and CD8 T cells, typically occurs around or within individual islets.[9]

Islet cell antibodies (ICA) in type 1 diabetes were first discovered in the 1970s and later shown to be antibodies directed against an isoform of glutamic acid decarboxylase (GAD65) and a protein tyrosine phosphatase–like molecule (IA-2). Autoantibodies directed against insulin are found in type 1 diabetes patients as well, but are also developed in patients receiving insulin replacement therapy and thus are not useful for classification of diabetes after such treatment has begun. It has been found that these autoantibodies precede the development of diabetes by many months or years, allowing prediction of overt disease and identification of subjects at high risk of developing diabetes.[9] Prospective studies regarding the predictive value of these antibodies have shown that the presence of autoantibodies directed against two or more antigens is far more strongly associated with the risk of disease than is a high titer of autoantibody to any single antigen (up to a 50% risk of developing type 1 diabetes within 5 years in the presence of both anti-GAD65 and IA-2). Moreover, the combination of high-risk human leukocyte antigen (HLA) genes with autoantibodies further increases positive prediction.[9]

In addition, the value of diabetes-associated autoantibodies (anti-GAD and IA-2), as well as HLA type in the prediction of type 1 diabetes after gestational diabetes, has been studied. Twenty-four women out of 43 found positive for at least one diabetes-associated antibody developed type 1 diabetes in a 5-year follow-up. A combination of HLA typing and autoantibody measurements has been found highly predictive of future type 1 diabetes in these cases.[10]

The possibility to predict type 1 diabetes resulted in the development of clinical research protocols for the prevention of type 1 diabetes in high-risk patients. These protocols included randomized treatment with either insulin as in the DPT-1 study,[11] or nicotinamide as in the ENDIT study.[12] None of these treatment modalities were able to change the rate of onset of type 1 diabetes compared to placebo. Nonetheless, these studies have contributed greatly to the assessment of factors that control the progression from islet cell autoimmunity to clinical onset, such as baseline glucose tolerance, age, and the number of ICAs detected.[13]

Another application of antibody testing may be the screening of healthy population or population at risk. In Finland, a population-based birth-to-age-4 screening program[14] has combined HLA typing and autoantibodies testing in 31,526 babies, in order to identify patients prior to overt disease. Genetic susceptibility (2.5–15 times the risk of the general population) was determined in all babies through HLA testing. Only those of HLA–DQB1 genotypes *02/*0302 and *0302/x (x not equal to *02, *0301, and *0602) were invited to autoantibody follow-up. Overall, the program has identified about 75% of the children developing diabetes at an early age. Of the 22 children who developed diabetes, 17 were found to carry the risk genotypes. The importance of such a program lies in both the attempt to prevent the overt disease, but also in the prevention of its life-threatening complications, such as diabetic keto-acidosis and coma.

Screening strategy must take into consideration the sensitivity and specificity of any single serological test as well as their combination. Such evaluation was recently performed in the DPT-1 study.[11] It was found that testing for anti-GAD65 and IA-2 achieved a higher sensitivity compared to the testing of any single antibody. Screening for any three antibodies guaranteed detection of all multiple antibody-positive subjects.

Furthermore, a screening program must also take into consideration the validity, sensitivity, and specificity of different laboratory methods regarding the different antibody testing. In the Diabetes Autoantibody Standardization Program, a proficiency evaluation program has shown that in the majority of participating laboratories, GAD and IA-2 antibody assays perform well. It has been possible to identify GAD antibody, IA-2 antibody, and insulin autoantibody (IAA) assays, which achieved high sensitivity and specificity, and to define the characteristics associated with good levels of discrimination between health and disease. The workshops have shown that good interlaboratory concordance has been achieved if GAD and IA-2 antibody levels are expressed in terms of common WHO units/mL derived from the WHO reference reagent.[15]

In conclusion, the prediction of type 1 diabetes mellitus is now considered feasible by autoantibody testing. In order to achieve significant specificity and sensitivity, multiple-antibody testing, such as anti-GAD and IA-2 would be advised. The combination of such tests with HLA typing may increase sensitivity and specificity. However, its cost and complexity may limit the use of HLA typing as a screening method. As to date, screening of the general population or rather of high-risk population is yet to be justified, mostly on account of the inability to prevent an overt disease. Still, many efforts are being made, and thus further advancement in prevention and treatment of type 1 diabetes mellitus is inevitable.

RHEUMATOID ARTHRITIS

Rheumatoid Arthritis (RA) is a common systemic autoimmune disease with a prevalence of about 1% worldwide. It is marked by a chronic inflammation of the synovial joints that leads to joint swelling, progressive joint erosions, and eventually to disability.[16] The pathogenesis of RA is poorly understood, yet there is evidence of a preclinical or asymptomatic phase of the disease during which there may be already histological evidence of synovitis.[17] Studies have proven that aggressive treatment given early in the course of disease has a great beneficial effect on the outcome. Therefore, early diagnosis prior to joint damage is of great importance.[16]

Several autoantibody systems have been described in association with RA.[16] The autoantibodies most frequently found in patients with RA are antibodies against IgG (IgM rheumatoid factor [IgM-RF]) and antibodies against citrullinated proteins.[17] The latter were originally measured as antibodies against keratin or filaggrin and more recently as anticyclic citrullinated peptide (anti-CCP).[17]

Autoantibodies may be present in RA patients before clinical disease is apparent.[17] It has been shown recently that anti-CCP antibodies are present in the blood of RA patients years before development of overt disease. In a study by Nielen *et al.*,[17] sera of 79 RA patients who had been blood donors, had tested positive for antibodies years before the disease became apparent. About half of the patients were shown to be positive for IgM-RF and/or anti-CCP on at least one occasion before the development of RA symptoms, a median of 4.5 years before symptom onset.

In a similar study by Rantapää-Dahlqvist *et al.*,[18] 83 individuals with RA were identified as having donated blood before presenting with any symptoms of joint disease (median 2.5 years before RA). In samples obtained before the onset of RA, the prevalence of autoantibodies was 33.7% for anti-CCP, 16.9%

for IgG-RF, 19.3% for IgM-RF, and 33.7% for IgA-RF (all highly significant compared with controls). The sensitivities for detecting these autoantibodies >1.5 years and ≤1.5 years before the appearance of any RA symptoms were 25% and 52% for anti-CCP, 15% and 30% for IgM-RF, 12% and 27% for IgG-RF, and 29% and 39% for IgA-RF. In conditional logistic regression models, anti-CCP antibody and IgA-RF were found to be significant predictors of RA.[18]

Several other studies have shown the ability of CCP to predict the erosiveness of the developing RA.[16,19] It has been found that combining the anti-CCP test with the routinely used RF test renders the highest prognostic value for RA. These studies concluded that the presence of anti-CCP antibodies can clearly and specifically predict the development of RA, and may indicate progression to an erosive disease.[16]

In conclusion, anti-CCP antibodies and RF may serve as predictive markers of RA and its severity and thus allow early more appropriate management of the disease. Nevertheless, more large-cohort prospective studies are needed in order to further establish the use of these antibodies in routine serological testing for diagnosed RA patients as well as healthy or high-risk individuals.

SYSTEMIC LUPUS ERYTHEMATOSUS

Systemic lupus erythematosus (SLE) is a prototypic autoimmune disease characterized by multisystem involvement in association with autoantibody production. Clinical manifestations of SLE include inflammation and damage to the skin, joints, serosal surfaces, kidneys, and nervous system, often accompanied by fatigue, malaise, and pain.[20]

Antinuclear antibodies directed against nuclear components of the cell are the most characteristic of SLE, although they have limited specificity. Other autoantibodies in SLE include antibodies directed against other molecules, such as phospholipids, cell surface proteins, and humoral factors.[20]

It has been recently found that some of these antibodies are present in the sera of patients long before the clinical manifestation of SLE. In a study by Arbuckle *et al.*,[21] sera of 130 SLE patients were obtained from the Department of Defense Serum Repository. These samples were originally obtained from U.S. Armed Forces personnel on enlistment and, on average, every other year thereafter, all before the diagnosis of SLE. In 88% of these patients, at least one of the autoantibodies tested was present, a mean of 3.3 years before the diagnosis. Antinuclear, antiphospholipid , anti-Ro, and anti-La antibodies first appeared a mean of 3.4 years prior to the diagnosis of SLE. These antibodies appeared early in the developmental course of disease compared to antidouble-stranded DNA antibodies, which were first detected a mean of 2.2 years before diagnosis. Anti-Sm and antinuclear ribonucleoprotein antibodies appeared a mean of 1.2 years prior to diagnosis, making them the latest predictors of clinical disease. Also described was an accrual of autoantibodies throughout the years, which precedes clinical symptoms and halts upon diagnosis.[21]

Once SLE has been diagnosed, certain autoantibodies can be used as markers for disease activity or organ-specific clinical manifestation.[20] In a study by Ravirajan *et al.*,[22] there was a significant difference in heparan sulphate (HS) reactivity between patients with lupus nephritis compared with patients without renal disease. Also, patients with active disease and lupus nephritis had significantly higher levels of antinucleosome antibodies than patients with inactive disease and nephritis. Global disease activity score was seen to correlate with both antinucleosome and antihistone antibodies. The presence of renal disease correlated with antibodies to dsDNA and HS, but only the latter showed a significant correlation with disease activity in the kidney.[22]

In pregnant women with lupus, the presence of anti-Ro antibodies represents a significant risk factor for neonatal lupus and congenital heart block, prompting more careful monitoring. Monitoring antiphospholipid antibodies is of great importance in pregnancy on account of the greater risk of fetal loss, fetal growth retardation, and premature deliveries associated with the presence of these antibodies. In these cases, anticoagulant therapy may be advised.[20]

Furthermore, positive serology in pregnant women for anti-Ro and anti-La, has been found to be associated with future development of SLE and Sjögren's syndrome. Although most of the mothers with such serological findings are clinically healthy at the time of delivery, different studies have shown that the majority of these women will develop clinical SLE or Sjögren's syndrome in long-term follow-up.[10]

Central nervous system manifestations may be associated with certain antibodies and thus predicted. Among these antibodies are antiphospholipid antibodies associated with strokes, and antiribosomal P protein antibodies associated with cerebritis,[20] psychosis, and depression.[23]

Despite the predictive value of autoantibodies in SLE, and the correlation of specific antibodies with certain disease presentations (TABLE 1), no clinical intervention has been established as management in lack of overt manifestation. Nevertheless, the presence of autoantibodies in asymptomatic individuals as

TABLE 1. Autoantibodies as predictors of specific disease manifestations in SLE

Antibody	SLE manifestation
Anti-HS	lupus nephritis
Antinucleosome	lupus nephritis
Anti-Ro	neonatal lupus,* congenital heart block*
Anti-PL	pregnancy loss,* fetal growth retardation,* premature deliveries,* strokes
Antiribosomal P protein	cerebritis, psychosis, depression

HS = heparan sulphate; PL = phospholipids.

*Disease manifestations when antibody is present during pregnancy.

TABLE 2. Chronological pattern of appearance of autoantibodies predictive of SLE

Antibody	Mean years prior to clinical manifestation
Anti-PL	3.4 years
Anti-Ro	3.4 years
Anti-La	3.4 years
Anti-dsDNA	2.2 years
Anti-Sm	1.2 years
Antinuclear ribonucleoprotein	1.2 years

PL = phospholipids; dsDNA = double-stranded DNA.

well as the typical chronological pattern (TABLE 2) may justify the foundation of screening and follow-up programs for high-risk or general populations.

ANTIPHOSPHOLIPID SYNDROME

Antiphospholipid syndrome (APS) is a disorder of recurrent vascular thrombosis and pregnancy losses associated with persistently positive anticardiolipin or lupus anticoagulant tests.[24] A variety of abnormalities of the skin, the cardiac valves, central nervous system, and other organ systems have been also described.[25]

Many patients with APS have clinical and laboratory features found in other autoimmune disease, particularly SLE. Such patients are defined as having "secondary" APS, as apposed to patients with features of APS alone, thus defined as "primary" APS. Clinical and laboratory features in these two groups are similar.[24]

The similarity of these two entities has led to the notion that some primary APS patients may develop SLE or other autoimmune diseases, thus actually having secondary APS, which has yet to be exposed. A retrospective study[26] following 128 primary APS patients for a mean follow-up period of 9 years has investigated this notion. During the follow-up and after a median disease duration of 8.2 years (range, 1–14 years), 11 (8%) patients developed SLE, 6 (5%) developed lupus-like disease, and 1 (1%) developed myasthenia gravis. The remaining 110 patients (86%) continued to have primary APS. Of the risk factors related to the development of other autoimmune diseases, only the presence of Coomb's positivity had statistical significance (odds ratio, 66.4; 95% confidence interval [CI], 1.6–2714; $P = 0.027$) and was associated with the development of SLE. Hence, this study confirms that progression from primary APS to SLE or lupus-like disease is unusual, even after years of follow-up.[26]

Positive antiphospholipid tests have been known to be found in a variety of patients with drug-induced disorders and miscellaneous infectious disorders, such as syphilis, acquired immunodeficiency syndrome (AIDS), and others.[24] These patients, as opposed to APS patients, do not exhibit the clinical phenomena of APS.[24] This special subgroup, along with healthy individuals positive for antiphospholipid antibodies, confounds the value of antiphospholipid antibodies in asymptomatic individuals as predictors of APS.

Antiphospholipid antibodies have been found to be associated with an increased risk of thrombotic phenomena, such as deep vein thrombosis, myocardial infarction, and stroke.[24] In a prospective nested case–control study by Ginsburg *et al.*,[27] the presence of anticardiolipin was found as a risk factor for deep vein thrombosis or pulmonary embolism in healthy adult men, regardless of age and smoking status. The risk for such a thrombotic event was directly correlated with antibody level, but a significantly increased risk was limited to values above the 95th percentile. In another 4-year-long prospective study,[28] the presence of elevated anticardiolipin antibody levels, 6 months following a venous thrombotic event, was found to be associated with an increased risk of recurrence and of death. The predictive values of the anticardiolipin antibody test increased with antibody levels.

In a large prospective study of SLE patients,[29] the presence of both lupus anticoagulant and anticardiolipin antibodies was found to be associated with an increased risk of venous thrombosis. However, of the two autoantibodies, lupus anticoagulant was found as a better predictor for venous thrombotic events.

In a prospective study performed by Brey *et al.*,[30] an association was demonstrated between the presence of IgG β2 glycoprotein-1-dependent anticardiolipin antibodies and the incidence of myocardial infarction (MI) and stroke. The risk factor for stroke after 15 years of follow-up in positive versus negative subjects for these antibodies was 2.2 (95% CI 1.5–3.4), and for MI was 1.8 (95% CI 1.2–2.6). The association between the presence of anticardiolipin antibodies and MI and stroke was shown to be attenuated in the last 5 years of follow-up.

In conclusion, although the presence of antiphospholipid antibodies may not be specific indicators of "primary" APS, their presence indicate greater risk of both venous and arterial thrombotic events. Therefore, testing for these autoantibodies may allow better risk stratification of healthy individuals in prevention programs, as well as better management of patients following thrombotic events in an attempt to prevent recurrence.

HEPATIC AUTOIMMUNE DISEASES

PBC is a chronic, progressive, cholestatic liver disease characterized histologically by fatal damage to the biliary epithelial cells lining the small intrahepatic bile ducts.[31] This damage is accompanied by a rich T cell mononuclear cell infiltrate with granuloma formation. Patients with late-stage disease can present with end-stage liver failure disease (portal hypertension and hepatocellular failure), although synthetic function is usually reserved till very late end-stages. Other characteristic symptoms are cholestatic itch and profound fatigue, which bare no correlation to biochemical or histological disease severity.[31]

The principal autoantibody responses seen in PBC are directed against a specific mitochondrial (antimitochondrial antibodies [AMA]) and nuclear autoantigens (antinuclear antibodies [ANA]).[31] The main autoantigenic substrate for AMA is the E2 component of a mitochondrial enzyme complex—the pyruvate dehydrogenase complex (anti-PDC),[32] while ANA are directed against the nuclear pore membrane protein gp210. These autoantibodies, along with cholestatic blood biochemistry and appropriate histological findings comprise the diagnostic criteria for PBC.[31]

Numerous studies have attempted to prove the prognostic value of ANA and AMA, rather than their diagnostic value, yet so far most results are questionable. A possible exception is the association found between anti-gp210 antibodies and histologically advanced disease. Still, clinical significance is unclear.[31]

The predictive value of AMA was sought in a prospective study performed by Kisand *et al.*[32] A 9-year follow-up of asymptomatic, anti-PDC positive subjects was carried out. Three out of 8 subjects available for follow-up developed abnormal liver biochemical test results by the ninth follow-up year. Nevertheless, it is not clear whether anti-PDC antibodies mark the initiation of PBC, or rather reflect a predisposition to the disease.[32] Despite the ongoing prospective trials regarding the significance of different autoantibodies to disease development and prognosis, no clinical decisions are currently based upon serological findings.[31]

The sensitivity and specificity of AMA detected by indirect immunofluorescence and anti-PDC detected by ELISA for the diagnosis of PBC are both 95%. In comparison, the reported prevalence of ANA in PBC varies from 10–40%.[31] The predictive value of presence of AMA for PBC disease spectrum is demonstrated by the observation that 24 out of 29 patients who had AMA in the context of normal serum liver biochemistry were found to have histological features diagnostic of PBC on liver biopsy.[31] The vast majority of these patients went on over time to develop cholestatic liver biochemistry and classical symptoms of PBC.[31] The importance of such a finding lies in the ability to treat asymptomatic patients with drugs, such as ursodeoxycholic acid, and thus prevent or postpone the need for liver transplantation, and improve survival.[33]

The ability to identify asymptomatic individuals, the presence of a single specific test, and the ability to effectively treat asymptomatic patients leads to the notion of population screening. Since screening the general population is not cost-effective, specific screening of populations at-risk may be in order. For one, the 10:1 female to male ratio[34] suggests the screening of the female population alone. Furthermore, PBC shows strong heritability according to familial occurrence and monozygotic twin-concordance,[34] suggesting screening family members of diagnosed patients. Interestingly, and in contrast to other autoimmune diseases, PBC shows only weak associations with the usual genetic risk elements for autoimmunity, such as the HLA alleles.[34] Hence, AMA screening of female individuals, especially family members of PBC patients may be greatly beneficial.

Autoimmune hepatitis (AIH) is an inflammatory liver disease characterized histologically by a dense mononuclear cell infiltrate in the portal tract and serologically by the presence of nonspecific autoantibodies and increased levels of transaminases and immunoglobulin G.[35] AIH is divided into two subgroups, AIH type 1 and AIH type 2, on the basis of the presence of ANA or antismooth muscle antibodies versus antibodies to liver/kidney microsome type 1 (LKM 1), respectively.

Primary sclerosing cholangitis (PSC) is a disease characterized by advanced fibroinflammatory damage of intra- and extrahepatic bile ducts, at times accompanied by autoimmune serology. Autoimmune sclerosing cholangitis (ASC) is a variant of PSC, typical of children and young adults, which is clinically characterized by less advanced bile duct lesions and laboratory findings similar to those of AIH type 1.[35]

Positivity to autoantibodies is critical for the diagnosis of AIH and ASC. Furthermore, the levels of these antibodies have been shown to mirror the extent of inflammatory activity in both diseases. The predictive role of autoantibodies in AIH and ASC is yet unknown, although antibody profiles suggestive of AIH type 1 have been found in asymptomatic family members of AIH type 1 patients. Furthermore, autoantibodies typical of AIH type 1 are often detected in formerly seronegative liver transplant patients, a proportion of whom will develop AIH. Still, more prospective studies are needed in order to fully establish the predictive role of autoantibodies in AIH of both types and ASC.[35]

INFLAMMATORY BOWEL DISEASES

Crohn's disease (CD) and ulcerative colitis (UC) are common clinical subtypes of idiopathic inflammatory bowel disease (IBD). These diseases are characterized by excessive, and tissue damaging inflammatory responses of the gastrointestinal tract.[36] Although the etiology is unknown, it is increasingly clear that these diseases represent the outcome of three essential interactive cofactors: environmental factors (e.g., enteric microflora), multigenic host susceptibility, and immune-mediated tissue injury.[36]

Several autoantibodies differentially associated with CD and UC have been investigated of which the most frequently studied in clinical trials are anti-*Saccharomyces cerevisiae* antibodies (ASCA) and perinuclear antineutrophil cytoplasmic antibodies (pANCA). These autoantibodies are considered as disease markers for IBD, although the clinical significance of their presence in healthy individuals up until recently has remained controversial.[36]

In a recent study by Israeli *et al.*,[36] sera of asymptomatic military personnel later diagnosed with CD or UC were obtained from a sera repository. The sera were examined for ASCA and pANCA in an attempt to evaluate the predictive value of these autoantibodies for IBD. ASCA were found in the sera of CD patients up to 60 months prior to diagnosis, but were not found in any of the control sera. The estimated odds ratio calculated for CD in ASCA positive versus negative subjects was 30 (95% CI 4.27–1301.93). Also demonstrated was a significant rise in ASCA titer with time, and until clinical symptoms appear, suggesting that contrary to current beliefs ASCA are a marker of an autoimmune process occurring in IBD rather than a genetic marker alone.

Also demonstrated in this study was a significant association between pANCA and UC[36]; of 8 UC patients, 2 were pANCA positive prior to diagnosis, as opposed to none of the controls ($P = 0.014$).

In conclusion, the presence of autoantibodies, such as ASCA and pANCA in asymptomatic individuals may predict or rather precede clinical IBD. Such serological testing may allow early management or attentive follow-up programs, in an attempt to decrease morbidity associated with the disease as well as with surgical treatment.

AUTOIMMUNE ADDISON'S DISEASE

Primary adrenal insufficiency (PAI) is a clinical condition characterized by the inadequate secretion of corticosteroid hormones resulting from bilateral destruction or impaired function of the adrenal cortex. Among the many etiological agents recognized for this condition, a T cell-mediated autoimmune process (autoimmune Addison's disease [AAD]) is by far the most common cause in Western countries.[37]

AAD is associated with susceptible HLA haplotypes and is characterized by the appearance of autoantibodies to adrenal cortex cells (ACA).[38] ACA recognize an autoantigen located in the microsomal subcellular fraction of the adrenocortical cells, which has been identified as the steroid-synthesizing enzyme 21-hydroxylase (21OH). It has been shown that 21OH autoantibodies (21OHAb) have a high diagnostic sensitivity and specificity for autoimmune adrenal insufficiency. Most likely, the pathogenic role of adrenocortical autoantibodies is irrelevant, but their presence is a useful marker for disease classification at clinical onset.[38]

The determination of adrenal autoantibodies is critical to distinguish between subjects with ADD and subjects with nonautoimmune disease. The importance of a correct etiological classification is largely on account of the frequent association of ADD with other autoimmune endocrine diseases, in the so-called autoimmune polyglandular syndromes.[37]

Adrenal autoantibodies can be used to identify subjects with preclinical AAD, at high risk of progression toward clinical Addison's disease. It has been shown[38] that levels of adrenal autoantibodies correlate with the severity of adrenal dysfunction in the preclinical period. Also, early biochemical signs of adrenal dysfunction have been shown to spontaneously remit, in parallel to the disappearance of both ACA and 21OHAb.

Because of the low prevalence of AAD in the general population and the low frequency of ACA or 21OHAb among healthy subjects, the predictive value of these markers has so far been studied only in patients with organ-specific autoimmune disorders.[37] It has been found that in children with hypoparathyroidism or type 1 diabetes mellitus, the predictive value of ACA for future clinical AAD is as high as 90% at 4 years, becoming 100% at 10 years. In adults, the predictive value of adrenal autoantibodies is lower than that observed in children and is around 20%.[37]

In a recent study of type 1 diabetes patients,[39] it was proposed that 21OHAb can be used as a marker for the large-scale screening of patients with endocrine autoimmune diseases for adrenal insufficiency. However, as also demonstrated by previous studies, the presence of adrenal autoantibodies does not lead necessarily to clinical Addison's disease.[39]

Recently reported[40] was the occurrence of long-term remission of subclinical adrenal failure with disappearance of 21OHAb and ACA in a patient with Graves' ophthalmopathy treated with corticosteroids. This effect of short-term glucocorticoid therapy can be attributed to the well-known immunosuppressive activity of steroids. Alternatively, corticosteroid therapy could act as an iso-hormonal therapy preventing progressive adrenal destruction with restoration to the normal state of adrenal function in subclinical autoimmune Addison's disease.[40] Such findings suggest the possibility of preventing clinical adrenal insufficiency. Nevertheless, such notions need to be independently confirmed.

Hence, adrenal autoantibody testing may serve as a useful tool to distinguish between subjects with ADD as apposed to a nonautoimmune disease, to identify subjects with preclinical AAD, and to predict future AAD in individuals with organ-specific autoimmune disorders, such as hypoparathyroidism or type 1 diabetes mellitus.

AUTOIMMUNE THYROID DISEASES

The term autoimmune thyroid diseases (AITD), encompasses a diverse range of clinical entities including among others Hashimoto's thyroiditis, juvenile thyroiditis, and Graves' disease. All AITD share a variable degree of lymphocytic infiltration of the thyroid gland along with thyroid antibody production. The presence of different AITD in members of the same family suggests a common etiological factor. The overlap extends to the occurrence of thyroid autoantibodies that are directed against three major autoantigens: thyroglobulin (TG), thyroid peroxidase (TPO), and the TSH-receptor (TSH-R).[41]

Several large studies have confirmed the value of anti-TG and anti-TPO antibodies in prediction of autoimmune hypothyroidism.[41] In a 20-year follow-up study in Whickman, UK, it has been shown that the odds ratio of developing hypothyroidism in individuals with positive thyroid antibodies and normal TSH were 8 for women and 25 for men. These values rose up to 38 and 173, respectively, in the presence of elevated TSH levels and normal free T4 (subclinical hypothyroidism). These findings suggest the value of TSH surveillance in subjects with positive thyroid autoantibody serology.[41]

Anti-TPO antibodies found in pregnant women have been found to be correlated with postpartum AITD. It has been shown that 50% of pregnant women found positive for anti-TPO antibodies will develop postpartum thyroiditis.[41] The value of anti-TPO antibodies as predictors of thyroiditis depends upon their titer; a titer of 1:1600 or higher at delivery was found to have a 97% sensitivity and 91% specificity for postpartum AITD.[10] This close relationship between thyroid antibodies and postpartum thyroiditis has led to suggestions that all pregnant women should be offered antenatal screening for TPO autoantibodies, but as yet there is no consensus on its benefits.[41]

In conclusion, the presence of thyroid antibodies may be considered a risk factor for the development of future AITD, and thus renders a careful TSH follow-up. However, the benefits of screening for such antibodies in the general population or pregnant women have not been established.

PEMPHIGUS

Pemphigus comprises a group of chronic cutaneous bullous diseases that are characterized by autoantibody-induced epidermal cell to cell detachment (acantholysis). Pemphigus manifests itself clinically with flaccid blisters and erosions of the skin, histologically with acantholysis, and immunologically with bound and circulating IgG autoantibodies against various keratinocyte desmosomal antigens.[42]

The four major forms of pemphigus are pemphigus vulgaris (PV), pemphigus foliaceus (PF), and its endemic form fogoselvagem (FS), drug-induced pemphigus, and paraneoplastic pemphigus. The diagnosis of any of the clinical forms of pemphigus relies on clinical, histological, and immunological findings. Two desmosomal autoantigens have been characterized as the major targets of PV and PF autoantibodies: desmoglein 3 and desmoglein 1, respectively.[42]

The role of these antibodies as predictive markers has been explored in a study of a special population of Amerindians in Brazil in which the prevalence of FS is especially high. It has been found that antidesmoglein1 can be detected in patients months or years before onset of clinical disease. Also, clinical disease has been shown to be associated with a dramatic increase in these antibodies. In the same study, autoantibodies directed against desmoglein 1 were demonstrated in normal individuals, especially relatives of patients. These findings, along with the findings of a consecutive epitopal study have demonstrated two different types of antidesmoglein 1 antibodies, only one of which is pathogenic. Thus, it has been suggested that individuals developing diseases are those with the appropriate genetic background. These individuals are exposed to environmental factors that allow the formation of pathogenic antibodies by means of epitope spreading.[42]

Hence, the presence of specific autoantibodies may predict pemphigus in asymptomatic individuals. Furthermore, the research of such antibodies in first-degree relatives of pemphigus patients may shed light on the pathogenesis of the disease and the role of genetic versus environmental factors in its development.

RECURRENT MISCARRIAGES

Many autoantibodies have been associated with impaired fertility. Among these are antiphospholipid antibodies, such as anticardiolipin,[43–45] antiphosphatidyl-serine,[46] antiprothrombin,[47,48] antilaminin-1,[49] and anti-β-2-glycoprotein 1, antibodies to thyroid antigens, such as anti-TG and anti-TPO, antibodies to extractable nuclear antigens (anti-ENA),[3,50] autoantibodies associated with SLE, such as anti-DNA,[51] and many more.[52]

Recurrent pregnancy losses are one of the most consistent complications of APS.[24] Losses can occur at any stage of pregnancy, although miscarriages associated with APS are strikingly frequent during the second and third trimester. However, the significance of positive serology for antiphospholipid antibodies on the outcome of the pregnancy depends greatly on previous obstetric outcome. It has been estimated that findings of a positive lupus anticoagulant test, or a moderate level of IgG anticardiolipin in a lupus patient are associated with a 30% risk of miscarriage during the first pregnancy. A history of two previous miscarriages in such a patient raises the risk of miscarriage during the following pregnancy to 70%. Although the risk of fetal loss is directly related to antibody titer, particularly the IgG anticardiolipin, many women with recurrent miscarriages have IgM anticardiolipin while others with persistently elevated antiphospholipid antibodies have no fetal complications at all. In conclusion, the best predictor of pregnancy outcome remains the previous obstetric history.

Several studies have found an association between spontaneous abortions and autoantibodies to the thyroid gland, such as anti-TPO or anti-TG, although the direct role of thyroid autoantibodies in fetal loss is debatable.[50] In a study by Tartakover-Matalon *et al.*,[50] it has been shown that active immunization of mice with human TG results in the production of anti-TG autoantibodies and pregnancy failure manifested by an increased fetal resorption rate (equivalent to human missed abortions) and reduced placental and embryo weights. The mice presented normal thyroid function and normal thyroid histology. This suggests that the higher rate of pregnancy loss observed in this model, as well as that described in women with thyroid antibodies, reflects primarily an autoimmune phenomenon, rather than, or in addition to, a consequence of overt thyroid hormone abnormalities.[50]

Antilaminin antibodies, which may be detected in SLE and APS patients, have been previously shown to be associated with reproductive failures in animal models.[49] In a more recent study, a possible association has been made between anti-DNA antibodies in SLE and recurrent pregnancy loss.[51] It had been shown that exposure of human placentas to anti-DNA, an autoantibody previously shown to cross-react with laminin-1, resulted in abolishment of trophoblast attachment and migration. Laminins are basement membrane glycoproteins believed to play an important role in the remodeling of endometrial stroma, an important aspect of the implantation of the fertilized ovum into the uterus wall. Thus, anti-DNA antibodies which cross-react with laminin-1 may cause pregnancy loss in SLE patients by inhibiting this process.[51] Such knowledge may allow the prediction of possible pregnancy loss in women with high titers of anti-DNA or antilaminin antibodies, as well as contribute to future research regarding its prevention.

In a study testing different panel-kits in women suffering from impaired fertility, a significant association has been shown between recurrent miscarriages and autoantibodies to a combinational panel of anti-TPO, anti-TG, and anti-ENA.[3] In the same study antiphospholipid antibodies have been found to be associated with infertility.

The use of precise kits to anti-TG, anti-TPO, and anti-ENA autoantibodies as screening may diagnose immunologically mediated miscarriages,[3] and thus allow more appropriate and earlier management of such cases. Still, it is not clear which antibodies should be assessed in the evaluation and management of infertility and recurrent miscarriages.[3]

SUMMARY AND CONCLUSIONS

The Profile of an Individual Prone to Develop Autoimmune Diseases

It is now clear that autoimmune diseases, as does the end-organ pathologies they cause, do not begin at the time of clinical appearance, but rather many years before that. The implication of this concept lies in the possibility of predicting autoimmunity. Throughout the years, many risk factors have been found to be associated with autoimmune diseases. Of these, well documented were a female gender, a family history of autoimmune diseases and specific major histocompatibility complex (HLA) alleles.[7] Among these alleles are A1 and DQW1 associated with SLE,[7,53] DQ3-DR4, DQ3-DR9, DQ5-DR1, and DQ5-DR10 associated with RA,[54] DR3 and B8 associated with RA, SLE, autoimmune thyroiditis, celiac, multiple sclerosis, and myasthenia gravis, etc.[7] Other genetic risk factors researched are polymorphisms in specific genes encoding molecules involved in antigen presentation, such as Tap-1 and proteosomes, as well as many other candidate genes.[55–61]

Also documented were specific immune deficiencies associated with autoimmune diseases.[62] These immune deficiencies are genetically determined and in most cases precede or possibly lead to autoimmune phenomena. Complement system abnormalities, for example, have been linked to the development of SLE.[63] Among the different abnormalities, the most prevalent and most severe disease has been found to be associated with deficiency of the proteins of the C1 complex and with total C4 deficiency.[63] Antibodies directed against complement proteins have also been found in SLE patients.[63] Of these antibodies, the most important autoantibody to a complement protein is anti-C1q, which is found in approximately a third of patients with SLE.[63]

Other immune deficiencies associated with autoimmunity are common variable immune deficiencies associated with thrombocytopenia and hemolytic anemia, and selective IgA deficiency associated with SLE and RA.[62] Furthermore, individuals with selective IgA deficiency have been found to be positive for many autoantibodies despite lack of clinical diseases.[64,65] These findings may suggest a common immune disturbance, and/or a tendency to develop future overt autoimmune diseases. Furthermore, immune deficiency creates susceptibility to infections by various agents, thus increasing the risk of a secondary antiself immune response.[66]

All of these risk factors and many others therefore create a profile of an "autoimmune-prone individual" (FIG. 1), which may be prone to develop an autoimmune disease upon exposure to a trigger antigen *via* infection,[66] vaccination,[67] or exposure to chemical substances.[67] While the specific autoimmune disease such an individual may develop depends upon the specific trigger antigen, as well as on the individual's genetics, the date of the disease's future clinical appearance and its specific manifestations may be predicted by specific serological tests (FIG. 1).

Indeed, it is now evident that many autoimmune diseases are preceded by a preclinical phase, which may be manifested by the presence of different autoantibodies (see TABLE 3). Nevertheless, these findings give rise to many questions regarding the management of individuals with positive autoantibody serology, as well as questions regarding future screening policies.

Screening for Autoantibodies as Predictors of Autoimmune Diseases—Practical and Ethical Issues

There is the real prospect that by screening the general population, identification of high-risk individuals for some diseases may be allowed. The goal of such identification would be either prevention of disease, or limitation of clinical impact.[2] However, while having answered the question "why," a number of other questions must be answered for appropriate strategies to be devised:

Who should be screened? Should screening include the general population, or rather first-degree relatives of patients, genetically prone HLA groups, etc? These special groups may benefit more from antibody screening compared to

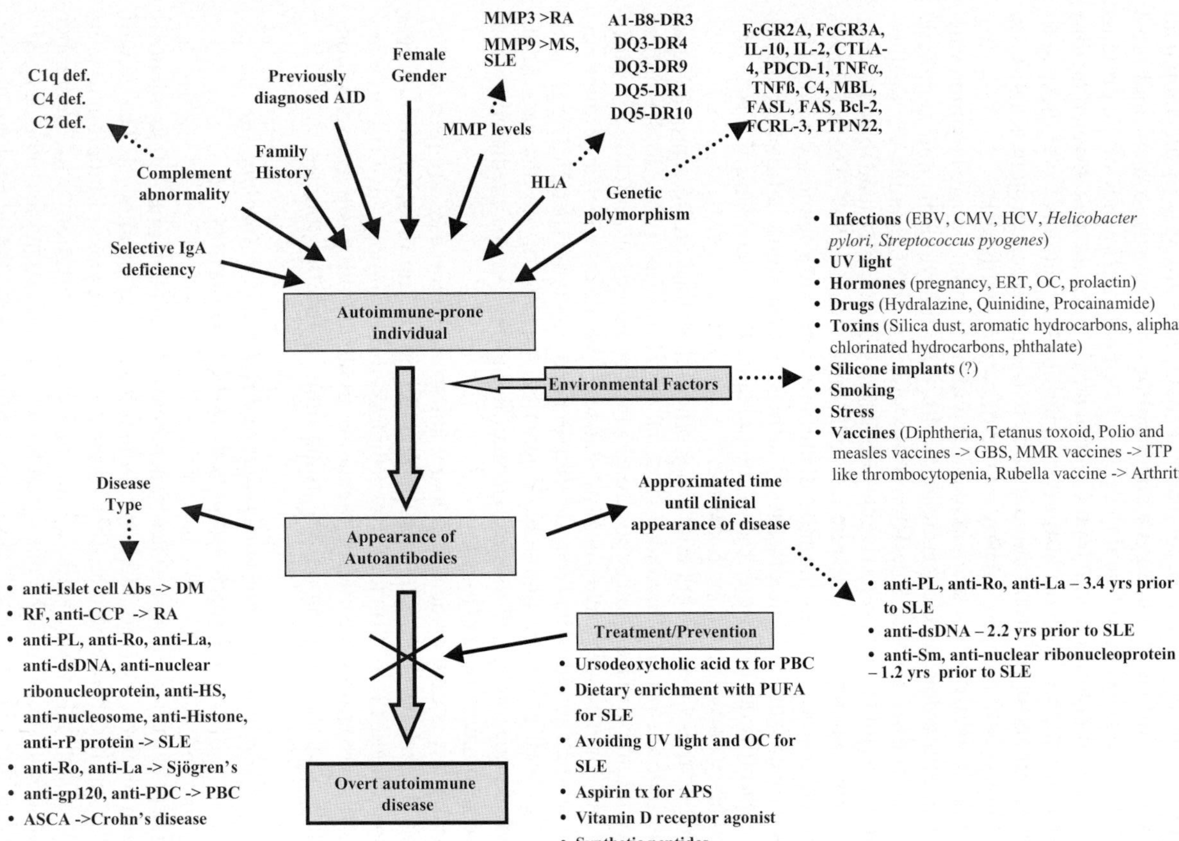
C1q def.
C4 def.
C2 def.
Previously diagnosed AID
Female Gender
MMP3 >RA
MMP9 >MS, SLE
MMP levels
A1-B8-DR3
DQ3-DR4
DQ3-DR9
DQ5-DR1
DQ5-DR10
FcGR2A, FcGR3A, IL-10, IL-2, CTLA-4, PDCD-1, TNFα, TNFß, C4, MBL, FASL, FAS, Bcl-2, FCRL-3, PTPN22,
Family History
Complement abnormality
HLA
Genetic polymorphism
Selective IgA deficiency
Autoimmune-prone individual
Environmental Factors
• Infections (EBV, CMV, HCV, Helicobacter pylori, Streptococcus pyogenes)
• UV light
• Hormones (pregnancy, ERT, OC, prolactin)
• Drugs (Hydralazine, Quinidine, Procainamide)
• Toxins (Silica dust, aromatic hydrocarbons, aliphatic chlorinated hydrocarbons, phthalate)
• Silicone implants (?)
• Smoking
• Stress
• Vaccines (Diphtheria, Tetanus toxoid, Polio and measles vaccines -> GBS, MMR vaccines -> ITP like thrombocytopenia, Rubella vaccine -> Arthritis)
Disease Type
Appearance of Autoantibodies
Approximated time until clinical appearance of disease
• anti-Islet cell Abs -> DM
• RF, anti-CCP -> RA
• anti-PL, anti-Ro, anti-La, anti-dsDNA, anti-nuclear ribonucleoprotein, anti-HS, anti-nucleosome, anti-Histone, anti-rP protein -> SLE
• anti-Ro, anti-La -> Sjögren's
• anti-gp120, anti-PDC -> PBC
• ASCA ->Crohn's disease
• anti-PL, anti-Ro, anti-La – 3.4 yrs prior to SLE
• anti-dsDNA – 2.2 yrs prior to SLE
• anti-Sm, anti-nuclear ribonucleoprotein – 1.2 yrs prior to SLE
Treatment/Prevention
• Ursodeoxycholic acid tx for PBC
• Dietary enrichment with PUFA for SLE
• Avoiding UV light and OC for SLE
• Aspirin tx for APS
• Vitamin D receptor agonist
• Synthetic peptides
Overt autoimmune disease

the general population. Accordingly, testing high-risk groups may change the positive predictive value of autoantibody serological tests.

When should individuals be screened? The best age for screening varies in different diseases; for example, while diabetes-associated antibodies appear by 5 years of age, thyroid antibodies uncommonly appear before 20 years of age.[2]

Which antibodies should be screened for? Different autoantibodies appearing in the same diseases have different predictive values as individual screening test, as well as in combination.

How should the screening be performed? Specificity and sensitivity of different laboratory assays must be considered.

Who should be informed? Once autoantibodies have been found, a risk of future disease is established. This information may have great implication regarding one's future, and thus its distribution should be handled with great care. Should family members be informed, especially taking into account their associated risk? Should employment authorities be notified? Should such information be available to all caring physicians? Should military authorities be informed? Should one be obligated to inform insurance companies?

These seminal practical and ethical questions have to be resolved before any wide screening policy will be implemented.

The Prevention of Overt an Autoimmune Disease in a Prone Individual

As complex as it may be, the identification of positive autoantibody serology in an asymptomatic individual might allow immunological treatment whereby

←

FIGURE 1. Predicting and preventing autoimmunity. Risk factors, such as a female gender, certain HLA haplotypes, such as A1 B8 DR 3,[70] matrix metalloproteases (MMPs) activity,[71–73] specific immune deficiencies, and the presence of already one autoimmune disease, all create a profile of an "autoimmune-prone" individual. Upon exposure to an environmental factor, such as infection, vaccination, or a chemical substance,[67] such an individual may produce autoantibodies detectable by serological tests. These autoantibodies may serve as predicting markers of a specific autoimmune disease, as well as mean of approximation of its date of clinical appearance. Identification of these autoantibodies may allow the treatment and possibly prevention of the overt autoimmune disease. AID, autoimmune disease; MMP, matrix metalloprotease; RA, rheumatoid arthritis; MS, multiple sclerosis; SLE, systemic lupus erythematosus; EBV, Epstein Barr virus; CMV, cytomegalovirus; UV, ultraviolet; ERT, estrogen replacement therapy; OC, oral contraceptives; GBS, Guillian-Barré syndrome; MMR, measles/mumps/rubella; ITP, immune thrombocytopenic purpura; DM, diabetes mellitus; RF, rheumatoid factor; CCP, cyclic citrullinated peptide; PL, phospholipids; dsDNA, double-stranded DNA; HS, heparan sulphate; rP, ribosomal P protein; PDC, pyruvate dehydrogenase complex; PBC, primary biliary cirrhosis; ASCA, anti-*Saccharomyces cerevisiae* antibodies; PUFA, polyunsaturated fatty acids; APS, antiphospholipid syndrome.

TABLE 3. Predictive autoantibodies in autoimmune diseases

Disease	Autoantibodies
Type 1 diabetes mellitus	Anti-GAD
	IA-2
	IAA
RA	RF (anti-IgG)
	Anti-CCP
SLE	Anti-PL
	Anti-Ro
	Anti-La
	Anti-dsDNA
	Anti-Sm
	Antinuclear ribonucleoprotein
	Anti-HS
	Antinucleosome
	Antihistone
	Antiribosomal P protein
Sjögren's disease	Anti-Ro
	Anti-La
APS	Anticardiolipin
	Lupus anticoagulant
PBC	Anti-gp120
	Anti-PDC
AIH	ANA
Crohn's disease	ASCA
UC	pANCA
Autoimmune Addison's disease	ACA (anti-21-hydroxylase)
AITD	Anti-TG
	Anti-TPO
Pemphigus	Antidesmoglein 1

GAD = glutamic acid decarboxylase; IA-2 = protein tyrosine phosphatase-like molecule; IAA = insulin autoantibodies; RF = rheumatoid factor; CCP = cyclic citrullinated peptide; PL = phospholipids; HS = heparan sulphate; PDC = pyruvate dehydrogenase complex; ANA = antinuclear antibodies; ASCA = anti-*Saccharomyces cerevisiae* antibodies; pANCA = perinuclear antineutrophil cytoplasmic antibodies; ACA = adrenal cortex cells antibodies; TG = thyroglobulin; TPO = thyroid peroxidase.

disease is prevented, as is already being studied in diabetes.[10] Additionally, lifestyle modification may be recommended in order to prevent clinical disease or disease flare-ups. Such modifications include ursodeoxycholic acid treatment for PBC,[33] dietary enrichment with polyunsaturated fatty acids,[6] avoiding ultraviolet light exposure[7] and avoiding oral contraceptive agents for SLE,[8] and aspirin treatment in APS.[4] Still in question is the benefit of avoiding vaccination,[67] mainly on account of the relative risk of developing an autoimmune disease versus the risk of serious infection.

Another treatment or rather preventive modality currently being studied is the use of vitamin D receptor (VDR) agonists.[68] Different experimental models have shown the ability of VDR agonists to prevent different autoimmune diseases, such as SLE in MRL$^{lpr/lpr}$ mice, experimental allergic encephalomyelitis (EAE), collagen-induced arthritis, Lyme arthritis, IBD, and autoimmune diabetes in non-obese diabetic (NOD) mice.[68] Furthermore, 1,25$(OH)_2D_3$ analogs are able not only to prevent but also to treat ongoing autoimmune diseases, as demonstrated by their ability to inhibit type 1 diabetes development in adult NOD mice, and to inhibit the recurrence of autoimmune disease after islet transplantation in the NOD mouse. These analogs have also been shown to ameliorate significantly the chronic-relapsing EAE induced in Biozzi mice by spinal cord homogenate.[68]

Recently investigated is the benefit of synthetic peptides in the treatment of autoimmune diseases, and specifically APS.[69] Further research of this modality and its therapeutic and safety profile may enable its use earlier in the clinical course—prior to overt disease.

All of these treatment and preventive modalities underline the great importance that lies in autoantibody testing of asymptomatic individuals. Alternatively, even if disease cannot be prevented, by identification of individuals at risk, perhaps life-threatening conditions, such as thyroid storm and Addisonian's crisis could be avoided.[10]

In conclusion, although many issues remain unresolved, identification of autoimmune diseases in their preclinical stage has become feasible by autoantibody testing. The implementation of this ability is the treatment and possibly the prevention of autoimmune diseases. Nevertheless, many prospective studies are needed in order to assess the predictive value of antibody testing, as well as the means to apply them to clinical management of healthy population and high-risk individuals.

ACKNOWLEDGMENT

This work was partly supported by The Foundation Federico, S.A., for research in Autoimmunity Diseases.

REFERENCES

1. NOTKINS, A.L., A. LERNMARK & D. LESLIE. 2004. Preface. Autoimmunity **37:** 251–252.
2. HAWA, M., H. BEYAN & R.D.G. LESLIE. 2004. Principles of autoantibodies as disease-specific markers. Autoimmunity **37:** 253–256.
3. MARAI, I. *et al.* 2004. Autoantibody panel screening in recurrent miscarriages. Am. J. Reprod. Immunol. **51:** 235–240.
4. TINCANI, A. *et al.* 2003. Treatment of pregnant patients with antiphospholipid syndrome. Lupus **12:** 524–529.
5. MERLINO, L.A. *et al.* 2004. Vitamin D intake is inversely associated with rheumatoid arthritis: results from the Iowa Women's Health Study. Arthritis Rheum. **50:** 72–77.

6. REIFEN, R. *et al.* 1998. Dietary polyunsaturated fatty acids decrease anti-dsDNA and anti-cardiolipin antibodies production in idiotype induced mouse model of systemic lupus erythematosus. Lupus **7:** 192–197.
7. LORBER, M., M.E. GERSHWIN & Y. SHOENFELD. 1994. The coexistence of systemic lupus erythematosus with other autoimmune diseases: the kaleidoscope of autoimmunity. Semin. Arthritis Rheum. **24:** 105–113.
8. PETRI, M. & C. ROBINSON. 1997. Oral contraceptives and systemic lupus erythematosus. Arthritis Rheum. **40:** 797–803.
9. NOTKINS, A.L. & A. LERNMARK. 2001. Autoimmune type 1 diabetes: resolved and unresolved issues. J. Clin. Invest. **108:** 1247–1252.
10. SCOFIELD, R.H. 2004. Autoantibodies as predictors of disease. Lancet **363:** 1544–1546.
11. DIABETES MELLITUS PREVENTION TRIAL – TYPE 1 DIABETES STUDY GROUP. 2002. Effects of insulin in relatives of patients with type 1 diabetes mellitus. N. Engl. J. Med. **346:** 1685–1691.
12. GALE, E.A. *et al.* 2004. European Nicotinamide Diabetes Intervention Trial (ENDIT): a randomized controlled trial of intervention before the onset of type 1 diabetes. Lancet **363:** 925–931.
13. LERNMARK, A. 2004. Type 1 diabetes as a model for prediction and diagnosis. Autoimmunity **37:** 341–345.
14. KUPILA, A. *et al.* 2001. Feasibility of genetic and immunological prediction of type I diabetes in a population-based birth cohort. Diabetologia **44:** 290–297.
15. BINGLEY, P.J. & A.J.K. WILLIAMS. 2004. Validation of autoantibody assays in type 1 diabetes: workshop programme. Autoimmunity **37:** 257–260.
16. ZENDMAN, A.J.W., E.R. VOSSENAAR & W.J. VAN VENROOIJ. 2004. Autoantibodies to citrullinated (poly) peptides: a key diagnostic and prognostic marker for rheumatoid arthritis. Autoimmunity **37:** 295–299.
17. NIELEN, M.M.J. *et al.* 2004. Specific autoantibodies precede the symptoms of rheumatoid arthritis, a study of serial measurements in blood donors. Arthritis Rheum. **50:** 380–386.
18. RANTAPÄÄ-DAHLQVIST, S. *et al.* 2003. Antibodies against cyclic citrullinated peptide and IgA rheumatoid factor predict the development of rheumatoid arthritis. Arthritis Rheum. **48:** 2741–2749.
19. ORBACH, H. *et al.* 2002. Gilburd B, Brickman CM, Gerli R, Shoenfeld Y, anti-Cyclic citrullinated peptide antibodies as a diagnostic test for rheumatoid arthritis and predictor of an erosive disease. Isr. Med. Assoc. J. **4:** 892–893.
20. TRAN, T.T. & D.S. PISETSKY. 2004. Systemic lupus erythematosus and related diseases. Autoimmunity **37:** 301–304.
21. ARBUCKLE, M.R. *et al.* 2003. Development of autoantibodies before the clinical onset of systemic lupus erythematosus. N. Engl. J. Med. **349:** 1526–1533.
22. RAVIRAJAN, C.T. *et al.* 2001. An analysis of clinical disease activity and nephritis-associated serum autoantibody profiles in patients with systemic lupus erythematosus: a cross-sectional study. Rheumatology **40:** 1405–1412.
23. EBERT, T., J. CHAPMAN & Y. SHOENFELD. 2005. Anti-ribosomal P protein and its role in psychiatric manifestations of systemic lupus erythematosus: myth or reality. Lupus **14:** 571–575.
24. KHAMASHTA, M.A., M.L. BERTOLACCINI & G.R.V. HUGHES. 2004. Antiphospholipid (Hughes) syndrome. Autoimmunity **37:** 309–312.
25. SHOENFELD, Y. 2003. Systemic antiphospholipid syndrome. Lupus **12:** 497–498.

26. GOMEZ-PUERTA, J.A. *et al.* 2005. Long-term follow-up in 128 patients with primary antiphospholipid syndrome: do they develop lupus? Medicine (Baltimore) **84:** 225–230.
27. GINSBURG, K.S. *et al.* 1992. Anticardiolipin antibodies and the risk for ischemic stroke and venous thrombosis. Ann. Intern. Med. **117:** 997–1002.
28. SCHULMAN, S., E. SVENUNGSSON & S. GRANQVIST. 1996. Anticardiolipin antibodies predict early recurrence of thromboembolism and death among patients with venous thromboembolism following anticoagulant therapy. Duration of Anticoagulation Study Group. Am. J. Med. **104:** 332–338.
29. SOMERS, E., L.S. MAGDER & M. PETRI. 2002. Antiphospholipid antibodies and incidence of venous thrombosis in a cohort of patients with systemic lupus erythematosus. J. Rheumatol. **29:** 2531–2536.
30. BREY, R.L. *et al.* 2001. β2-Glycoprotein 1-dependent cardiolipin antibodies and risk of ischemic stroke and myocardial infarction, The Honolulu Heart Program. Stroke **32:** 1701–1706.
31. JONES, D.E.J. 2004. Primary biliary cirrhosis. Autoimmunity **37:** 325–328.
32. KISAND, K.E. *et al.* 2001. The follow-up of asymptomatic persons with antibodies to pyryvate dehydeogenase in adult population samples. J. Gastroenterol. **36:** 248–254.
33. NISHIO, A. *et al.* 2001. Primary biliary cirrhosis: from induction to destruction. Semin. Gastrointest. Dis. **12:** 89–102.
34. INVERNIZZI, P. *et al.* 2005. From bases to basis: linking genetics to causation in primary biliary cirrhosis. Clin. Gastroenterol. Hepatol. **3:** 401–410.
35. VERGANI, D. & MIELI-VERGANI. 2004. Autoimmune hepatitis and sclerosing cholangitis. Autoimmunity **37:** 329–332.
36. ISRAELI, E. *et al.* 2005. Anti-*Saccharomyces cerevisiae* and antineutrophil cytoplasmic antibodies as predictors of inflammatory bowel disease. Gut **54:** 1232–1236.
37. MARZOTTI, S. & A. FALORNI. 2004. Addison's disease. Autoimmunity **37:** 333–336.
38. LAURETI, S. *et al.* 1998. Levels of adrenocortical autoantibodies correlate with the degree of adrenal dysfunction in subjects with preclinical Addison's disease. J. Clin. Endocrinol. Metab. **83:** 3507–3511.
39. BREWER, K.W., V.S. PARZIALE & G.S. EISENBARTH. 1997. Screening patients with insulin-dependent diabetes mellitus for adrenal insufficiency. N. Engl. J. Med. **337:** 202.
40. DE BELLIS, A.A. *et al.* 2001. Time course of 21-hydroxylase antibodies and long-term remission of subclinical autoimmune adrenalitis after corticosteroid therapy: case report. J. Clin. Endocrinol. Metab. **86:** 675–678.
41. WEETMAN, A.P. 2004. Autoimmune thyroid disease. Autoimmunity **37:** 337–340.
42. PIAS, E.K. *et al.* 2004. Humoral autoimmunity in pemphigus. Autoimmunity **37:** 283–286.
43. BLANK, M. *et al.* 1991. Induction of anti-phospholipid syndrome in naive mice with mouse lupus monoclonal and human polyclonal anti cardiolipin antibodies. Proc. Natl. Acad. Sci. USA **88:** 3069–3073.
44. BAKIMER, R. *et al.* 1992. Induction of primary antiphospholipid syndrome in mice by immunization with a human monoclonal anti-cardiolipin antibody (H-3). J. Clin. Invest. **89:** 1558–1663.
45. SHURTZ-SWIRSKY, R. *et al.* 1993. In vitro effect of anticardiolipin autoantibodies upon total and pulsatile placental hCG secretion during early pregnancy. Am. J. Reprod. Immunol. **29:** 206–210.

46. TARTAKOVER-MATALON, S. *et al.* 2004. Antiphosphatidylserine antibodies affect rat yolk sacs in culture: a mechanism for fetal loss in antiphopholipid syndrome. Am. J. Reprod. Immunol. **51:** 144–151.
47. VON-LANDENBERG, P. *et al.* 2003. Antiprothrombin antibodies are associated with pregnancy loss in patients with the antiphospholipid syndrome. Am. J. Reprod. Immunol. **49:** 51–56.
48. HAJ-YAHJA, S. *et al.* 2003. Anti-prothrombin antibodies cause thrombosis in a novel qualitative *ex-vivo* animal model. Lupus **12:** 364–369.
49. TARTAKOVER-MATALON, S. *et al.* 2003. Immunization of naïve mice with mouse laminin-1 affected pregnancy outcome in a mouse model. Am. J. Reprod. Immunol. **50:** 159–165.
50. TARTAKOVER-MATALON, S. *et al.* 2003. The pathogenic role of anti-thyroglobulin antibody on pregnancy: evidence from an active immunization model in mice. Hum. Reprod. **18:** 1094–1099.
51. QURESHI, F. *et al.* 2000. Anti-DNA antibodies cross-reacting with laminin inhibit trophoblast attachment and migration: implications for recurrent pregnancy loss in SLE patients. Am. J. Reprod. Immunol. **44:** 136–142.
52. SHOENFELD, Y. & M. BLANK. 2004. Autoantibodies associated with reproductive failure. Lupus **13:** 643–648.
53. WORRALL, J.G. *et al.* 1990. SLE: a rheumatological view. Analysis of the clinical features, serology and immunogenetics of 100 SLE patients during long-term follow-up. Q. J. Med. **74:** 319–330.
54. ZANELLI, E., F.C. BREEDVELD & R.R.P. DE VRIES. 2000. HLA association with autoimmune disease: a failure to protect? Rheumatology **39:** 1060–1066.
55. POWIS, S. J. *et al.*1992. Effect of polymorphism of an MHC-linked transporter on the peptides assembled in a class I molecule. Nature **357:** 211–215.
56. PEARCE, R.B. *et al.* 1993. Polymorphism in the mouse Tap-1 gene. Association with abnormal CD8+ T cell development in the nonobese nondiabetic mouse. J. Immunol. **15:** 5338–5347.
57. MAKSYMOWYCH, W.P. *et al.* 1994. Polymorphism in an HLA linked proteasome gene influences phenotypic expression of disease in HLA-B27 positive individuals. J. Rheumatol. **21:** 665–669.
58. NATH, S.K., J. KILPATRICK & J.B. HARELY. 2004. Genetics of human systemic lupus erythematosus: the emerging picture. Curr. Opin. Immunol. **16:** 794–800.
59. GREGERSEN, P.K. 2005. Pathways to gene identification in rheumatoid arthritis: PTPN22 and beyond. Immunol. Rev. **204:** 74–86.
60. KOCHI, Y. *et al.* 2005. Functional variant in FCRL3, encoding Fc receptor-like 3, is associated with rheumatoid arthritis and several autoimmunities. Nat. Genet. **37:** 478–485.
61. WANDSTRAT, A. & E. WAKELAND. 2003. The genetics of complex autoimmune diseases: non-MHC susceptibility genes. Nat. Immunol. **2:** 802–809.
62. ETZIONI, A. 2003. Immune deficiency and autoimmunity. Autoimmun. Rev. **2:** 364–369.
63. WALPORT, M.J. 2002. Complement and systemic lupus erythematosus. Arthritis Res. **4:** S279–S293.
64. GOSHEN, E. *et al.* 1989. Antinuclear and related autoantibodies in sera of healthy subjects with IgA deficiency. J. Autoimmun. **2:** 51–60.
65. BARKA, N. *et al.* 1995. Multireactive pattern of serum autoantibodies in asymptomatic individuals with immunoglobulin A deficiency. Clin. Diagn. Lab. Immunol. **2:** 469–472.

66. Shoenfeld, Y. & N.R. Rose. 2004. Infection and Autoimmunity. Elsevier Publication. Amsterdam, The Netherlands.
67. Molina, V. & Y. Shoenfeld. 2005. Infection, vaccines and other environmental triggers of autoimmunity. Autoimmunity **38:** 235–245.
68. Adorini, L. 2005. Intervention in autoimmunity: the potential of vitamin D receptor agonists. Cell Immunol. **233:** 115–124.
69. Pierangeli, S.S. *et al.* 2004. A peptide that shares similarity with bacterial antigens reverses thrombogenic properties of antiphospholipid antibodies *in vivo*. J. Autoimmun. **22:** 217–225.
70. Candore, G. *et al.* 2002. Pathogenesis of autoimmune diseases associated with 8.1 ancestral haplotype: effect of multiple gene interactions. Autoimmun. Rev. **1:** 29–35.
71. Goetzl, E.J., M.J. Banda & D. Leppert. 1996. Matrix metalloproteinases in immunity. J. Immunol. **156:** 1–4.
72. Matache, C. *et al.* 2003. Matrix metalloproteinase-9 and its natural inhibitor TIMP-1 expressed or secreted by peripheral blood mononuclear cells from patients with systemic lupus erythematosus. J. Autoimmun. **20:** 323–331.
73. Dubois, B., G. Opdenakker & H. Carton. 1999. Gelatinase B in multiple sclerosis and experimental autoimmune encephalomyelitis. Acta. Neurol. Belg. **99:** 53–56.

Autoimmunity and Pregnancy

Autoantibodies and Pregnancy in Rheumatic Diseases

ANGELA TINCANI,[a] MONICA NUZZO,[a] MARIO MOTTA,[b] SONIA ZATTI,[c] ANDREA LOJACONO,[c] AND DAVID FADEN[c]

[a]*Rheumatology and Clinical Immunology, Brescia Hospital and University, Brescia, Italy*

[b]*Neonatal Intensive Care Unit, Brescia Hospital, Brescia, Italy*

[c]*Obstetrics and Gynecology Department, Brescia Hospital and University, Brescia, Italy*

ABSTRACT: In women who suffer from rheumatic diseases (RDs) the risk of repeated fetal loss, intrauterine growth restriction, and preterm birth remains higher than in the general population. Antiphospholipid antibodies are frequently observed in patients with systemic lupus erythematosus (SLE). They are associated with recurrent pregnancy losses that may occur at any age of gestation. The cause of fetal death is believed to be intraplacental thrombosis, although other pathologic mechanisms have been described. A recent study has described the increased frequency of learning disabilities in the offspring of SLE patients; case reports of neonatal thrombosis are very rare. Transplacental passage of IgG anti-Ro/SS-A antibodies is linked to neonatal lupus (2%). The main manifestation is congenital heart block (CHB) due to the binding of anti-Ro/SS-A antibodies to cardiac conduction tissue and to the consequent inflammatory/fibroid reaction. Neonatal lupus also includes cutaneous, hematologic, and hepatobiliary manifestations, which are typically transient. Incomplete CHB can be treated with fluorinated corticosteroids to prevent the progression and decrease inflammation. Intravenous immunoglobulin, decreasing the tranplacental passage of anti-Ro/SS-A, has been proposed as prophylactic therapy in patients who had one or more child with CHB. Transplacental passage of antiplatelet antibodies, in about 10% of mothers with SLE, can induce thrombocytopenia in the fetus or the neonate. Patients with RD have a higher incidence of anxiety and depression compared to the general population, interfering with parenthood and the upbringing of children.

Address for correspondence: Dr. A. Tincani, Rheumatology and Clinical Immunology, Ospedale Civile, Piazzale Spedali Civili no. 1, 25123 Brescia, Italy. Voice: 030-399-5488; fax: 030-399-5085. e-mail: tincani@bresciareumatologia.it

Ann. N.Y. Acad. Sci. 1069: 346–352 (2006).
doi: 10.1196/annals.1351.032

Keywords: rheumatic disease; pregnancy; antiphospholipid antibodies; anti-Ro/SS-A antibodies; neonatal lupus; corticosteroids; intravenous immunoglobulin; antiplatelet antibodies

INTRODUCTION

Rheumatic autoimmune diseases (RDs) have a higher prevalence in women, particularly in their child-bearing age. Therefore, interest is growing in the possible consequences of maternal disease and the treatment of the fetus and the newborn infant. If maternal disease is characterized by the presence of IgG isotype autoantibodies, these autoantibodies can cross the placenta possibly causing antibody-mediated damage to the fetus.[1] In patients with RD the risk of spontaneous abortion, fetal loss, and preterm births remains higher than in the general population; however, the general improvement in the diagnosis and management of these diseases results in a better quality of life, allowing the planning of a normal family life that includes one or more pregnancies.[2]

ANTIPHOSPHOLIPID ANTIBODIES

Antiphospholipid antibodies (aPLs) are a heterogeneous family of autoantibodies that exhibit a broad range of target specifities and affinities, recognizing various combinations of phospholipids such as cardiolipin, phosphatidylserine, phosphatidylethanolamine, and phospholipid-binding proteins [mainly beta-2-glycoprotein-I (anti-β2GPI), prothrombin, or annexin-V, etc.]. In clinical practice the aPLs are detected by lupus anticoagulant, anticardiolipin (aCL) antibody assays, or anti-β2GPI antibody assays.[3] They are found in 30–80% of patients with systemic lupus erythematosus (SLE) and to a lesser extent in persons with several other RDs or in otherwise healthy subjects (5%).[4] Independent of their clinical setting, these aPLs are related to repeated spontaneous pregnancy losses within the fetal period (10 or more weeks of gestation). The pathogenic role of aPLs was clearly shown in experimental animals that, when infused during pregnancy, developed placental insufficiency and miscarriages.[5] Intraplacental thrombosis does not seem to be the only putative cause, but other pathologic mechanisms have been described (a direct effect on trophoblast cells and induction of complement-mediated placental injury). It has been recently suggested that abnormalities of early trophoblast invasion, by impairing its differentiation, maturation, and decreased human chorionic gonadotropin production, may be the primary pathologic mechanism in the first-trimester pregnancy losses.[6] In addition, the demonstration of the presence of β2GPI on the trophoblast cell membranes explains the aPL placental trophism, β2GPI being one of the most important antigenic targets for aPL.[7] Other pregnancy-related complications among women who have antiphospholipid syndrome (APS) include intrauterine growth restriction (IUGR), placental insufficiency, pre-eclampsia, and maternal thrombosis.[3]

These days, if appropriately managed, APS is "one of the few tractable causes of pregnancy losses" and the rates of successful pregnancy in our and others' experience can be 70% or more.[4] The management of pregnant patients with APS is mainly based on the use of antiaggregant/anticoagulant agents to prevent thrombosis in the uteroplacental circulation, improving maternal and fetal outcome, and to reduce or eliminate the maternal thrombotic risk during pregnancy. In addition, some data indicate that heparin prevents aPL-induced fetal loss by inhibiting complement-activation.[8] Heparin is usually initiated in the early first trimester in association with daily low-dose aspirin. Despite treatment with heparin, recurrent pregnancy losses occur in 20–30% of cases and the best approach to such cases in subsequent pregnancies is unknown. Some trials recommend addition of anticoagulation treatment with low-dose aspirin and an immunomodulatory agent such as glucocorticoids, immunoglobulin, or hydroxychloroquine.[4]

Some studies seem to suggest that the transplacental passage of IgG aPL is low and that aCL can be detected in the blood of neonates; then antibody levels progressively decrease and disappear after about 6 months. In addition, it is observed that at 12 months of age aCL in an infant can be completely negative, while, anti-β2GPI antibody titers can be significantly increased on account of the physiological occurrence of an immune answer to infections or foods antigens.[9] This finding is also observed in children of a similar age with antiphospholipid-negative mothers.[10]

A recent case–control study on babies with APS mothers and healthy mothers did not show any statistically significant difference in the occurrence of neonatal complications, which, therefore, seem to be mainly related to prematurity.[3] However, some case reports described infants who suffered from aPL-associated thrombosis (cerebral ischemia and peripheral thrombosis).

The children of mothers with lupus have a normal intelligence level for their age; what is emerging, however, is an increased occurrence of learning disabilities, and particularly if the child is male, he will have attention deficit, dyslexia, or be left handed, compared to the general population. The influence of the mother's antibody profile was investigated, suggesting that the mothers of children with low scores in specific tests were positive for antiphospholipid antibodies.[11]

ANTI-RO/SS-A ANTIBODIES

Anti-Ro/SS-A and/or anti-La/SS-B antibodies are known to have a high prevalence in patients with Sjögren syndrome (SS), SLE, or rheumatoid arthritis (RA).[12] Contrasting data are reported about the possible association with maternal anti-RO/SS-A and unexplained pregnancy loss and adverse pregnancy outcome; at least in prospective studies, these antibodies are linked to the occurrence of the so-called "neonatal lupus syndrome" and do not affect other pregnancy outcomes. It was reported that the mean gestational age at delivery, the prevalence of pregnancy loss, the preterm birth, the cesarean sections, the premature rupture of membranes, IUGR, newborn small for gestational age, and pre-eclampsia were observed with the same frequency in anti-RO/SS-A-positive and -negative mothers with autoimmune diseases.[13]

These antibodies, if of the IgG isotype, cross the placenta and can be responsible for a complex syndrome that includes complete congenital heart block (CHB), although other less understood pathogenetic factors also seem to be involved in this process. CHB typically is diagnosed *in utero* during the second or third trimester, as first- or second-degree block, eventually evolving to a third-degree block. Complete CHB, once established, appears to be irreversible.[14] It has also been reported that incomplete blocks can progress postnatally, despite the clearance of the maternal antibodies from the neonatal circulation.[15] The frequency of a third-degree block in the offspring of a mother who has anti-Ro/SS-A antibodies is estimated at 1–2%; the rate of recurrence of CHB if the first child had CHB is about 20%.[16] Other cardiac features include congenital malformations, conduction abnormalities, and late-onset cardiomyopathy (some of which display endocardial fibroelastosis). The neonatal lupus syndrome carries a significant mortality (15–30%) and morbidity in the fetus or the newborn because of cardiac manifestations. The early diagnosis of the complete CHB and its potential complications (pericardial/pleural effusion, myocarditis, etc.) usually can prevent the deterioration of the fetal cardiac function. The majority of surviving affected children (67%) require permanent pacing before adulthood.[12] The spectrum of the neonatal lupus syndrome includes some other aspects, typically transient, resolving at about 6 months of life coincident with the disappearance of maternal autoantibodies from the neonatal circulation. Cutaneous manifestations usually appear as erythematous and often annular lesions with a predilection for the eyes, face, and scalp, which are frequently photosensitive. The risk of cutaneous lesions is unknown. In most cases, the rash follows ultraviolet light exposure, the mean age of detection is 6 weeks, and the duration is up to 22 weeks.[17] Cholestatic hepatitis occurs in about 10% of cases. Three types of hepatobiliary disease have been observed: liver failure at birth or *in utero*, transient conjugated hyperbilirubinemia or transient transaminase elevations during infancy.[18] Hematologic abnormalities consisting of thrombocytopenia, neutropenia, or anemia occur in about 27% of cases. It is uncommon for children with neonatal lupus to show the full expression of disease; rather, only one or two organ systems are involved. The long-term prognosis for children who had neonatal lupus is still under investigation, although it is suggested that some of these children have an increased risk of the development of some form of autoimmune disease (systemic or organ-specific) later in childhood.[19]

These days there is no indication to treat a pregnant patient with anti-Ro/SS-A to prevent CHB. Rather, it is important to closely monitor the patients with serial fetal echocardiography weekly starting 16–17 weeks of gestation, through 26 weeks; and then every other week until about 34 weeks in order to allow an early diagnosis. The treatment of identified CHB and the prevention of potential CHB are intended to reduce or eliminate the passage of maternal antibodies, to diminish a generalized inflammatory insult, and to forestall fibrosis. If incomplete heart block is diagnosed, fluorinated corticosteroids are indicated to prevent its progression.[20] Preliminary studies seem to show that prenatal exposure to fluorinated corticosteroids does not have a profound effect on the developing immune system. The main adverse effects observed are neurodevelopmental impairment, preterm delivery, low birth weight, and IUGR.[21] More data and a longer follow-up are needed to confirm these observations.

Prophylactic treatment for anti-Ro/SS-A-positive mothers may be indicated only if the patient already had a child with CHB, and this implies a higher risk in subsequent pregnancies. In these cases a treatment based on intravenous immunoglobulin (IVIG) infusions has been suggested. IVIG is used to treat a number of immune deficiencies and autoimmune diseases. It has been shown that IVIG contains anti-idiotypic antibodies, which explains its immunomodulatory action.[22] It was shown in animal models that the fetal/maternal ratios of anti-Ro/SS-A antibodies were lower in the IVIG-treated group.[23] The mechanism of potential efficacy in the CHB is debated, including a modulation of inhibitory signaling, involving idiotype/anti-idiotype regulation, a decrease in placental transport or perhaps induction of surface expression of the inhibitory Fc receptor on macrophages.[24] The suggested dose of IVIG is 0.4 g/kg given at 12, 15, 18, 21, and 24 weeks of pregnancy.[25] In considering the rarity of CHB in a fetus from a mother with anti-Ro/SS-A antibodies and the low frequency of a subsequent pregnancy in women who have had one or more children with CHB, properly designed multicenter trials would need to be conducted in order to evaluate the efficacy of treatment and to achieve more advances in the treatment of this disease.

ANTIPLATELET ANTIBODIES

Transplacental passage of anti-maternal platelet antibodies can complicate about 10% of pregnancies in patients with SLE, inducing moderate or severe autoimmune thrombocytopenia in the fetus or the newborn. Intracranial neonatal hemorrhages or other major bleeding complications are rare events, occurring in about 1% of the children from antiplatelet-positive mothers; interestingly, among the antiplatelet antibodies described in these children anti-HLA class I antigens were also reported. Neonatal thrombocytopenia usually resolves within 4 to 6 weeks after clearing of the passively acquired maternal autoantibodies.[26]

QUALITY OF LIFE AND PSYCHOLOGICAL IMPLICATIONS FOR MOTHERS WITH RHEUMATIC DISEASE

The presence of the above-cited autoantibody requires appropriate counseling and treatment in patients with RD. In addition, it is important to consider the impact that a chronic illness such as SLE or RA can have on the psychological aspects of the affected mothers' lives. Several articles have found a higher incidence of anxiety (from 15% to 45%) and depression (from 25% to 47%) compared to the general population.[2] Because of this emotional distress, RD can interfere with physiological phenomena as parenthood and the upbringing of children.[11] In addition, the state of anxiety and the worry about pregnancy and family planning are probably enhanced by several questions that are still unanswered. In fact, the persistence of antibodies after birth, the possible pathogenicity of some antibodies, and the long-term outcome of babies born to mothers with RD are questions that are still open. Therefore, psychological support might be an important help in the counseling of patients with RD.[2]

REFERENCES

1. BUYON, J.P., D. NUGENT, E. MELLINS, *et al.* 2002. Maternal immunologic disease and neonatal disorders. NeoReviews **3:** 3–6.
2. NERI, F., L. CHIMINI, E. FILIPPINI, *et al.* 2004. Pregnancy in patients with rheumatic diseases: psychological implication of a chronic disease and neuropsychological evaluation of the children. Lupus **13:** 666–668.
3. TINCANI, A., G. BALESTRIERI, E. DANIELI, *et al.* 2003. Pregnancy complications of the antiphospholipid syndrome. Autoimmunity **36:** 27–32.
4. BRANCH, D.W. & M.A. KHAMASHTA. 2000. Antiphospholipid syndrome: obstetric diagnosis, management and controversies. Am. J. Obstet. Gynecol. **183:** 1008–1012.
5. TINCANI, A., L. SPATOLA, M. CINQUINI, *et al.* 1998. Animal models of antiphospholipid syndrome. Rev. Rheum. **56:** 614–618.
6. DI SIMONE, N., P.L. MERONI & N. DEL PAPA. 2000. Antiphospholipid antibodies affect trophoblast gonadotropin secretion and invasiveness by binding directly and through adhered beta-2 glycoprotein I. Arthritis Rheum. **43:** 140–150.
7. ZURGIL, N., R. BAKIMER, A. TINCANI, *et al.* 1993. Detection of antiphospholipid and anti-DNA antibodies and their idiotypes in newborns of mothers with antiphospholipid sindrome and SLE. Lupus **2:** 233–237.
8. GIRARDI, G., P. REDECHA & J.E. SALMON. 2004. Heparin prevents antiphospholipid antibody-induced fetal loss by inhibiting complement activation. Nat. Med. **10:** 1222–1226.

9. MOTTA, M., C. BIASINI-REBAIOLI, M. FRASSI, *et al*. 2004. Anticardiolipin and anti-beta 2 glycoprotein I in infants born to mothers with and without antiphospholipid antibodies (abstract). Arthritis Rheum. **50:** s69.
10. AVCIN, T., A. AMBROZIC & M. KUHAR. 2001. Anticardiolipin and anti-beta 2 glycoprotein I antibodies in sera of 61 apparently healthy children at regular preventive visits. Rheumatology **40:** 565–573.
11. NERI, F., L. CHIMINI, F. BONOMI, *et al*. 2004. Neuropsychological development of children born to patients with systemic lupus erythematous. Lupus **10:** 805–811.
12. LEE, L.A. 1993. Neonatal lupus erythematosus. J. Invest. Derm. **100:** 9s–13s.
13. BRUCATO, A., A. DORIA, M. FRASSI, *et al*. 2002. Pregnancy outcome in 100 women with autoimmune diseases and anti-Ro/SS-A antibodies: a prospective controlled study. Lupus **11:** 716–721.
14. BRUCATO, A., M. FRASSI, F. FRANCESCHINI, *et al*. 2001. Congenital heart block risk to newborns of mothers with anti-Ro/SSA antibodies detected by counterimmunoelectrophoresis: a prospective study of 100 women. Arthritis Rheum. **44:** 1832–1835.
15. ASKANASE, A.D., D.M. FRIEDMAN, J. COPEL, *et al*. 2002. Spectrum and progression of conduction abnormalities in infants born to mothers with anti-Ro/La antibodies. Lupus **11:** 145–151.
16. BUYON, J.P., A. RUPEL & R.M. CLANCY. 2004. Neonatal lupus syndrome. Lupus **13:** 705–712.
17. NEIMAN, A.R., L.A. LEE, W.L. WESTON, *et al*. 2000. Cutaneous manifestations of neonatal lupus without heart block: characteristics of mothers and children enrolled in a national registry. J. Pediatr. **137:** 674–680.
18. LEE, L.A., R.J. SOKOL & J.P. BUYON. 2002. Hepatobiliary disease in neonatal lupus: prevalence and clinical characteristics in cases enrolled in a national registry. Pediatrics **109:** 11–15.
19. MARTIN, V., L.A. LEE, A.D. ASKANASE, *et al*. 2002. Long-term follow-up of children with neonatal lupus and their unaffected siblings. Arthritis Rheum. **46:** 2377–2383.
20. SALEEB, S., J. COPEL, D. FRIEDMAN, *et al*. 1999. Comparison of treatment with fluorinated glucocorticoids to the natural history of autoantibody-associated congenital heart block: retrospective review of the Research Registry for Neonatal Lupus. Arthritis Rheum. **42:** 2335–2345.
21. PREVOT, A., S. MARTINI & J.P. GUIGNARD. 2002. In utero exposure to immunosuppressive drugs. Biol. Neonate **81:** 73–81.
22. ABU-SHAKRA, M., D. BUSKILA & Y. SHOENFELD. 1997. Introduction idiotypes and anti-idiotypes. *In* Idiotypes in Medicine: Autoimmunity, Infection and Cancer. Y. Shoenfeld, R.C. Kennedy & S. Ferrone, Eds.: 53–74. Elsevier Science B.V. Amsterdam.
23. TRAN, H.B., D. CAVILL, J.P. BUYON, *et al*. 2004. Intravenous immunoglobulin and placental transport of anti-Ro/La antibodies: comment on the letter by Kaaja and Julkunen. Arthritis Rheum. **50:** 337–338.
24. SAMUELSSON, A., T.L. TOWERS & J.V. RAVETCH. 2001. Anti-inflammatory activity of IVIG mediated through the inhibitory Fc receptor. Science **291:** 445–446.
25. HUGHES, G. 2004. The eradication of congenital heart block. Lupus **13:** 489.
26. BUSSEL, J.B. 1997. Immune thrombocytopenia in pregnancy: autoimmune and alloimmune. J. Reprod. Immunol. **37:** 35–61.

Cytokines and Pregnancy in Rheumatic Disease

MONIKA ØSTENSEN, FRAUKE FÖRGER, AND PETER M. VILLIGER

Department of Rheumatology and Clinical Immunology and Allergology, University Hospital, CH-3010 Bern, Switzerland

ABSTRACT: Cytokines are important mediators involved in the successful outcome of pregnancy. The concept of pregnancy as biased toward a Th2 immune response states that Th1 type cytokines are associated with pregnancy failure and that Th2 cytokines are protective and counteract pregnancy-related disorders. Studies at the level of the maternal–fetal interface, in the maternal circulation and in cells of peripheral blood have shown that the Th2 concept of pregnancy is an oversimplification. Both Th1 and Th2 type cytokines play a role at different stages of pregnancy and are adapted to the localization and function of cells and tissues. The changes of local and systemic cytokine patterns during pregnancy correspond to neuroendocrine changes with hormones as powerful modulators of cytokine expression. Several autoimmune disorders show a modulation of disease activity during and after pregnancy. In rheumatic diseases with a predominance of a Th1 immune response, a shift to a Th2 type immune response during pregnancy has been regarded as beneficial. Studies of pregnant patients with rheumatoid arthritis (RA) and systemic lupus erythematosus (SLE) have shown a cytokine expression similar to that found in healthy pregnant women. Significant differences were present only for a few cytokines and seemed related to the activity of the underlying disease. Interestingly, a gestational increase of cytokine inhibitors interleukin 1 receptor antagonist (IL-1ra) and soluble tumor necrosis factor receptor (sTNFR) in the circulation corresponded to low disease activity in RA. The influence of hormones and cytokines on autoimmune disease is an issue for further study.

KEYWORDS: cytokines; pregnancy; Th2 immune response; hormones; rheumatic disease

INTRODUCTION

Successful pregnancy requires a coordinated sequence of events involving a large number of factors acting in concert. Among these factors, cytokines are

Address for correspondence: Professor Monika Østensen, Department of Rheumatology and Clinical Immunology and Allergy, University Hospital, CH-3010 Bern, Switzerland. Voice: 41-31-632-4179; fax: 41-31-632-2600.

e-mail: monika.oestensen@insel.ch

Ann. N.Y. Acad. Sci. 1069: 353–363 (2006).
doi: 10.1196/annals.1351.033

important mediators at different stages of pregnancy. In 1993, Tom Wegmann proposed the concept of successful pregnancy as a Th2 phenomenon.[1] $CD4^+$ T cells can be divided in two subsets: one is the T helper 1 type characterized by the production of interferon-gamma (IFN-γ), interleukin 12 (IL-12), tumor necrosis factor-β (TNF-β), and interleukin-2 (IL-2) and involved in cell-mediated immunity. The other T cell subset consists of Th2 committed cells that mainly produce interleukin 4 (IL-4), interleukin 10 (IL-10), and interleukin 13 (IL-13), thereby enhancing humoral immunity. IFN-γ is a major contributor to a Th1 immune response upregulating Th1 cell differentiation and inhibiting Th2 cell development. IL-10 downregulates production of proinflammatory cytokines by Th1 cells and macrophages. The Th1/Th2 paradigm states that Th1 type cytokines are associated with pregnancy failure like miscarriage and that Th2 cytokines, in particular IL-10 is protective and counteracts pregnancy-related disorders, such as fetal growth restriction as well as fetal death and pre-eclampsia.[2] However, extensive research of the physiology of pregnancy revealed that the concept of a Th2 response is an oversimplification.[3] For example, Th1 type cytokines, such as IFN-γ and tumor necrosis factor-α (TNF-α) are necessary during the early stages of pregnancy to support successful implantation and placenta development.[4,5] However, preferential production of Th1 type cytokines at later stages of pregnancy may be detrimental and may result in pregnancy loss.

CYTOKINES IN THE MATERNAL CIRCULATION

Plasma concentrations of cytokines have been shown to change with the stage of pregnancy.

Conflicting results exist in regard to circulating levels for IFN-γ and IL-1β, which have been found either absent or in low levels during pregnancy.[6,7] In a cross-sectional study of healthy pregnant women, a decrease of IFN-γ was found in maternal plasma.[8] By contrast, another study found no change in maternal plasma levels of IFN-γ or IL-6.[9] In a longitudinal study, IL-10 was not detected in plasma of healthy pregnant women studied at each trimester.[10] By contrast, low levels of IL-10 were found in a cross-sectional study of second and third trimester women.[11]

The immune modulating activities of cytokines are also regulated by soluble cytokine receptors like TNF receptors (TNFR) that can buffer the biological effects of TNF-α. Another natural inhibitory mechanism involves the blocking of receptor binding by cytokine receptor antagonists like IL-1Ra. Regulatory molecules that modify cytokine actions have been found increased in normal pregnancy. The production of soluble IL-6R and IL-1RA in pregnancy was studied by assessing the IL-6R and IL-1RA concentrations in serum samples from healthy pregnant women at different gestational ages.[12] Serum levels of both IL-6R and IL-1RA were increased in pregnant women, as were levels of IL-6 and IL-1. IL-1RA and IL-6 increased with gestational age and with labor activity. Similarly, soluble TNF-α receptor has been found to increase significantly in the second and third trimester of pregnancy compared to nonpregnant values.[13]

A number of studies have investigated whether circulating levels of Th1 type cytokines could predict adverse outcomes like ectopic pregnancy, miscarriage, pre-eclampsia, intrauterine growth retardation (IUGR), preterm labor, or fetal infection. Results have been variable, but with a tendency of higher circulating levels of TNF-α associated with miscarriage, pre-eclampsia,[11,14] IUGR, and pathologic labor.[15] At variance with these studies, another report found an association of pregnancy failure with increased maternal serum levels of IFN-γ and soluble IL-2 receptor, but not with TNF-α.[16]

CYTOKINES IN PERIPHERAL BLOOD CELLS AND REPRODUCTIVE TISSUES

Circulating levels of cytokines reflect only partly what is going on in cell subsets or at the feto–maternal interface. The cytokine profile of cell subsets or in tissues may vary significantly from plasma levels. This has been shown in studies investigating cytokine profiles in cells and reproductive tissues of pregnant women either by staining for intracellular cytokines, by reverse transcriptase polymerase reaction (RT-PCR), or by measuring cytokine secretion in supernatants of cells after stimulation. In the murine placenta, the continuous presence of IL-4, IL-5, and IL-10 has been shown throughout pregnancy, with early and transient expression of IFN-γ.[17] Human placenta at term expresses high mRNA levels of IL-10.[18] Chorionic villous tissue expresses not only Th2 type cytokines, but also IL-1β and TNF-α in the first trimester.[19] Thus, cytokine expression locally is regulated to create optimal conditions for fetal development.

The systemic effects of pregnancy are reflected by a change of the cytokine pattern in peripheral blood lymphocytes and monocytes. Cytokine secretion in whole blood cultures of healthy pregnant women showed a decrease of IL-2 and an increase of TNFR p55 and p75 during pregnancy. Levels of TNF-α and IL-1β were unchanged.[20] An increase of IL-4 secreting peripheral blood mononuclear cells (PBMC), but not of IFN-γ positive cells was found in the second and third trimester of pregnancy in healthy women after stimulation with paternal antigens.[21] The same group found significantly higher numbers of IFN-γ- and IL-4-secreting PBMC in all three trimesters of pregnancy and also post partum, compared with nonpregnant controls indicating a systemic upregulation of both Th1- and Th2-like immune responses during normal pregnancy.[22] Another study investigated *ex vivo* PBMC cytokine patterns of healthy pregnant women throughout pregnancy by RT-PCR. A decrease in mRNA levels was found for IL-6, slightly increased levels for IL-1β and low, mostly unchanged levels for TNF-α and low to undetectable levels for IL-10 during pregnancy. On the day of parturition, all four cytokines were highly upregulated.[23] The study failed to show a distinct Th2 response in PBMC of healthy pregnant women.

THE EFFECT OF HORMONES ON CYTOKINE PRODUCTION

The neuroendocrine system interacts in various ways with the immune system and has a profound effect on cytokine secretion in cells. Pregnancy induces substantial changes in hormone levels. The influence of these hormonal changes on cytokine production has been investigated in several studies.[24]

The effect of androgens on cytokine secretion was investigated in a cross-sectional study of healthy women during and after pregnancy. Serum levels of androstenediol (ADIOL), dehydroepiandrosterone (DHEA), and dehydroepiandrosterone sulfate (DHEAS) were measured as well as secretion of IFN-γ, IL-4, and IL-10 in whole blood cultures.[25,26] ADIOL levels significantly decreased compared to nonpregnant levels in the first trimester and were reversed in the third trimester. After pregnancy, ADIOL levels gradually declined. The serum DHEA levels increased in the first and in the second trimesters and decreased after delivery until 11 months post partum. DHEAS levels were decreased in the second and in the third trimesters and returned to nonpregnant levels after pregnancy. All measured cytokines (IFN-γ, IL-2, IL-4, and IL-10) were decreased during pregnancy and subsequently increased post partum. A significant negative correlation between ADIOL, DHEA, and cytokine levels was found. Androgens were considered to be involved in modifying the maternal immune responses during and after pregnancy.

The effect of pregnancy and of hormones was studied in 18 women with normal pregnancies in their third trimester and during the early postpartum period.[27] During the third trimester of pregnancy, *ex vivo* monocytic IL-12 production was about threefold and TNF-α production was approximately 40% lower than postpartum values. At the same time, urinary cortisol and norepinephrine excretion and serum levels of 1,25-dihydroxyvitamin were two- to threefold higher than postpartum values.

The same group investigated the stress hormones dexamethasone (a synthetic glucocorticoid), and the catecholamines, norepinephrine and epinephrine, to alter the production of IL-12 (p70) and IL-10 induced by bacterial lipopolysaccharide (LPS) in human whole blood.[28] Dexamethasone, norepinephrine, and epinephrine inhibited LPS-induced bioactive IL-12 production in a dose-dependent fashion and at physiologically relevant concentrations. Dexamethasone had no effect on IL-10 secretion whereas both catecholamines dose dependently increased the production of IL-10.

A study of peripheral blood lymphocytes of pregnant women showed that progesterone induced the expression of progesterone-induced immunomodulatory protein (PIBF). PIBF expression was accompanied by an increase of IL-10 production.[29] The same group found low expression of PIBF in peripheral blood lymphocytes of women with preterm labor or recurrent abortions. Compared to women with successful pregnancies, these lymphocytes showed significantly higher expression of IL-12 and low expression of IL-10.[30] Stimulation of antigen-specific T cell clones with progesterone increased the production of IL-4, IL-5, but not of IL-10 in these cells. Interestingly, progesterone also induced the expression of the Th2 marker, CD30.[31] T cell clones exposed to pregnancy levels of estrone and estradiol showed enhancement of IFN-γ and IL-10 secretion, but had an inhibitory effect on the secretion of TNF-α and -β.[32]

Taken together, the studies show the connection between the neuroendocrine system and the cytokine network. Pregnancy influences this interaction both locally and systemically with a fine tuning that creates optimal but not uniform conditions locally and in the circulation. The sometimes seemingly contradicting observations regarding cytokine production locally at the feto–maternal interface and those observed in the maternal circulation may relate to the necessity of inducing tolerance to the fetus without weakening the maternal immune system.

CIRCULATING CYTOKINES IN PREGNANT PATIENTS WITH RHEUMATIC DISEASE

Several autoimmune diseases like multiple sclerosis, autoimmune thyroditis, and rheumatoid arthritis (RA) show a modulation of disease activity during and after pregnancy. RA improves in the majority of patients, whereas ankylosing spondylitis (AS) remains active and is mitigated only in late pregnancy.[33,34] An aggravation of disease symptoms after delivery is commonly seen in both diseases and occurs in general within the first 6 months post partum. In RA, a Th1 type immune response is predominant whereas a Th0 or Th2 type prevails in AS.[35] IL-1β and TNF-α are proinflammatory cytokines that contribute to synovitis and joint destruction in both RA and AS.

In a study of pregnant patients with RA and AS and healthy women, circulating cytokines and regulatory molecules with a focus on the Th1/Th2 balance during and after pregnancy were investigated.[36] In agreement with other studies comparing healthy pregnant women to nonpregnant controls, we found elevated levels of IL-1Ra and soluble TNFR (sTNFR) in pregnant patients and controls whereas IL-1β, IFN-γ, and IL-10 were undetectable (see FIGS. 1 and 2). A negative correlation between IL-1Ra and disease activity was demonstrated. Elevated sTNFR levels in pregnant RA and AS patients were associated with low disease activity in late pregnancy.

Inflammatory rheumatic diseases are associated with a proinflammatory cytokine profile systemically and locally not only at times of active symptoms, but also during quiescent disease.[37] Treatment with the recombinant TNFR:Fc fusion protein and with recombinant IL-1Ra have shown good efficacy in RA and AS. Thus, increased levels of IL-1Ra and TNFR in the third trimester may lead to improvement of the disease in pregnant RA and AS patients.

A rise of sCD30 during pregnancy was observed exclusively in pregnant RA patients who had markedly higher gestational levels of sCD30 compared to the other groups of pregnant women and to nonpregnant patient cohorts.[36] A counterregulatory role of $CD30^+$ T cells providing an attempt to control inflammation in a Th1-driven disease like RA has been discussed and higher circulating levels of sCD30 have been found in nonpregnant RA patients compared to healthy controls.[38] Upregulation of IL-1Ra and sTNFR as well as sCD30 in RA patients during pregnancy may be indirect signs of a Th2 immune response since Th2 cytokines have been shown to induce the production of both sTNFR and IL-1Ra.[39,40]

Circulating cytokines were studied in pregnant patients with SLE and in healthy pregnant women.[41] In SLE patients, IL-6 serum levels did not increase in the third trimester of pregnancy, as was observed in controls. No significant differences between SLE patients and controls were found in either sTNFR I or II levels or profiles before and during pregnancy. IL-10 and sTNFR I levels were significantly higher during pregnancy and post partum in SLE patients with active disease compared to healthy controls.

In a prospective longitudinal study of 4 RA and 10 SLE pregnant women, including healthy pregnant women as a control group the cytokine profile of PBMC was investigated.[42] TNF-α was the most abundant cytokine mRNA expressed in PBMC in all groups studied. However, a general TH2 response reflected by high secretion IL-10 levels was found in RA, as well as SLE, patients. A significant increase in IFN-γ was observed in RA patients but only during the first trimester of pregnancy. This compared with a major TH1 response in healthy pregnant women.

To summarize, pregnancy promotes the secretion of anti-inflammatory cytokines and regulatory molecules. However, the cytokine pattern shows no uniform deviation toward a Th2 response, but is adapted to the localization of cells and tissues, and the stage of pregnancy. How the complex interaction of hormones and cytokines influences autoimmune disease is an intriguing question.[43]

FIGURE 1. Levels of sTNFR before, during (first, second, and third trimester), and after pregnancy (6, 12, and 24 weeks post partum) in patients with RA (A), ankylosing spondylitis (B), and healthy controls (C). Horizontal bar within the box marks the median, the boxes represent the range of $\pm$ 25% around the median (interquartile range). Vertical bars indicate 95% confidence interval. Significant changes are indicated by *P* values (Wilcoxon test for paired data).[36]

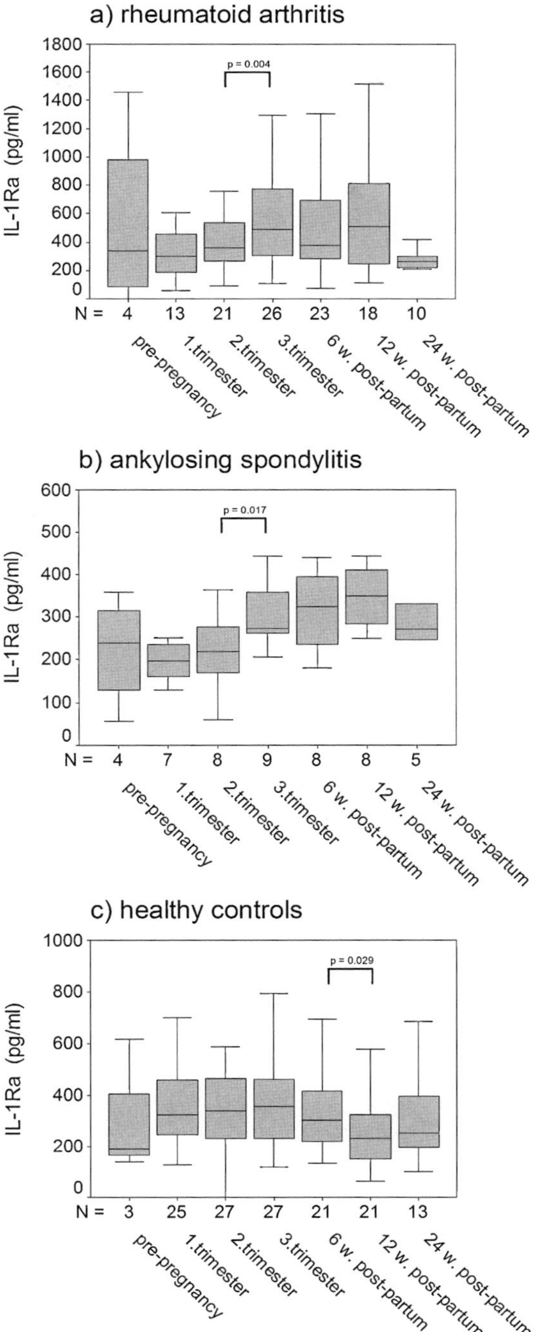

a) rheumatoid arthritis
IL-1Ra (pg/ml)
p = 0.004
N = 4 13 21 26 23 18 10
pre-pregnancy
1.trimester
2.trimester
3.trimester
6 w. post-partum
12 w. post-partum
24 w. post-partum
b) ankylosing spondylitis
IL-1Ra (pg/ml)
p = 0.017
N = 4 7 8 9 8 8 5
pre-pregnancy
1.trimester
2.trimester
3.trimester
6 w. post-partum
12 w. post-partum
24 w. post-partum
c) healthy controls
IL-1Ra (pg/ml)
p = 0.029
N = 3 25 27 27 21 21 13
pre-pregnancy
1.trimester
2.trimester
3.trimester
6 w. post-partum
12 w. post-partum
24 w. post-partum

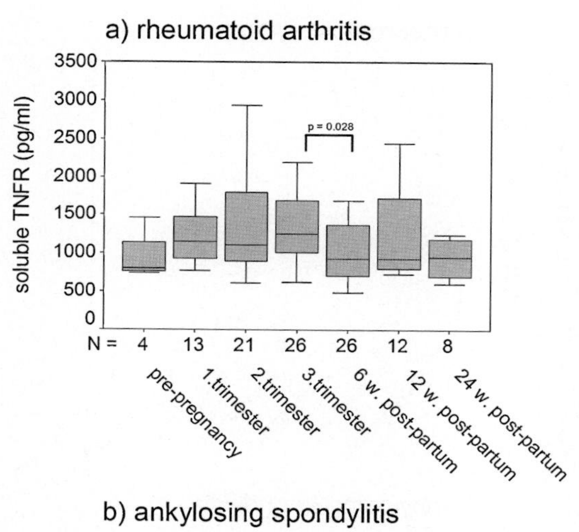
a) rheumatoid arthritis
soluble TNFR (pg/ml)
3500
3000
2500
2000
1500
1000
500
0
p = 0.028
N = 4 13 21 26 26 12 8
pre-pregnancy
1.trimester
2.trimester
3.trimester
6 w. post-partum
12 w. post-partum
24 w. post-partum

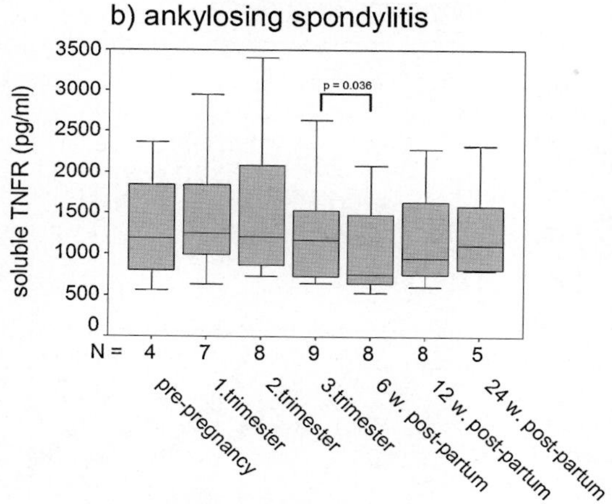
b) ankylosing spondylitis
soluble TNFR (pg/ml)
3500
3000
2500
2000
1500
1000
500
0
p = 0.036
N = 4 7 8 9 8 8 5
pre-pregnancy
1.trimester
2.trimester
3.trimester
6 w. post-partum
12 w. post-partum
24 w. post-partum

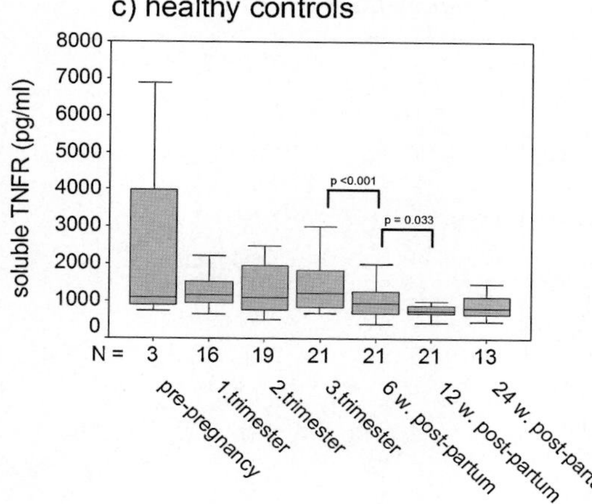
c) healthy controls
soluble TNFR (pg/ml)
8000
7000
6000
5000
4000
3000
2000
1000
0
p <0.001
p = 0.033
N = 3 16 19 21 21 21 13
pre-pregnancy
1.trimester
2.trimester
3.trimester
6 w. post-partum
12 w. post-partum
24 w. post-partum

FIGURE 2. Levels of IL-1Ra before, during (first, second, and third trimester), and after pregnancy (6, 12, and 24 weeks post partum) in patients with RA (A), ankylosing spondylitis (B), and healthy controls (C). Horizontal bar within the box marks the median, the boxes represent the range of $\pm$ 25% around the median (interquartile range). Vertical bars indicate 95% confidence interval. Significant changes are indicated by *P* values (Wilcoxon test for paired data).[36]

REFERENCES

1. WEGMANN, T.G., H. LIN, L. GUILBERT & T.R. MOSMANN. 1993. Bidirectional cytokine interactions in the maternal-fetal relationship: is successful pregnancy a Th2 phenomenon? Immunol. Today **14:** 353–356.
2. CHAOUAT, G., E. MENU, D.A. CLARK, *et al.* 1990. Control of fetal survival in CBA x DBA/2 mice by lymphokine therapy. J. Reprod. Fertil. **89:** 447–458.
3. CHAOUAT, G., N. LEDÉE-BATAILLE, S. DUBANCHET, *et al.* 2004. Th1/Th2 paradigm in pregnancy: paradigm lost? Int. Arch. Allergy Immunol. **139:** 93–119.
4. ASHKAR, A.A., J.P. DI SANTO & B.A. CROY. 2000. Interferon gamma contributes to initiation of uterine vascular modification, decidual integrity, and uterine natural killer cell maturation during normal murine pregnancy. J. Exp. Med. **192:** 259–270.
5. FUKUSHIMA, K., S. MIYAMOTO, K. TSUKIMORI, *et al.* 2005. Tumor necrosis factor and vascular endothelial growth factor induce endothelial integrin repertories, regulating endovascular differentiation and apoptosis in a human extravillous trophoblast cell line. Biol. Reprod. **73:** 172–179.
6. OPSJON, S.L., N.C. WATHEN, S. TINGULSTAD, *et al.* 1993. Tumor necrosis factor, interleukin 1, and interleukin-6 in normal human pregnancy. Am. J. Obstet. Gynecol. **69:** 397–404.
7. HEBISCH, G., P.M. NEUMAIER-WAGNER, R. HUCH & U. VON MANDACH. 2004. Maternal serum interleukin−1 beta, −6 & −8 levels and potential determinants in pregnancy and peripartum. J. Perinat. Med. **32:** 475–480.
8. VEITH, G.L. & G.E. RICE. 1999. Interferon gamma expression during human pregnancy and in association of labour. Gynecol. Obstet. Invest. **48:** 163–167.
9. RUSSWURM, G.P., A.M. MACKLER, O.R. FAGOAGA, *et al.* 1997. Soluble human leukocyte antigens, interleukin-6, and interferon-gamma during pregnancy. Am. J. Reprod. Immunol. **38:** 256–262.
10. MAKHSEED, M., R. RAGHUPATHY, F. Azizieh, *et al.* 2000. Circulating cytokines and CD30 in normal human pregnancy and recurrent spontaneous abortions. Hum. Reprod. **15:** 2011–2017.
11. ELLIS, J., U.B. WENNERHOLM, A. BENGTSSON, *et al.* 2001. Levels of dimethylarginines and cytokines in mild and severe preeclampsia. Acta. Obstet. Gynecol. Scand. **80:** 602–608.
12. AUSTGULEN, R., E. LIEN, N.B. LIABAKK, *et al.* 1994. Increased levels of cytokines and cytokine activity modifiers in normal pregnancy. Eur. J. Obstet. Gynecol. Reprod. Biol. **57:** 149–155.
13. KUPFERMINC, M.J., A.M. PEACEMAN, D. ADERKA, *et al.* 1995. Soluble tumor necrosis factor receptors in maternal plasma and second-trimester amniotic fluid. Am. J. Obstet. Gynecol. **173:** 900–905.

14. Kupferminc, M.J., A.M. Peaceman, D. Aderka, *et al.* 1996. Soluble tumor necrosis factor receptors and interleukin-6 levels in patients with severe preeclampsia. Obstet. Gynecol. **88:** 420–427.
15. Bahar, A.M., H.W. Ghalib, R.A. Moosa, *et al.* 2003. Maternal serum interleukin-6, interleukin-8, tumor necrosis factor-α and interferon-γ in preterm labor. Acta. Obstet. Gynecol. Scand. **82:** 543–549.
16. Fasouliotis, S.J., S.D. Spandorfer, S.S. Wittkin, *et al.* 2004. Maternal serum levels of interferon-gamma and interleukin-2 soluble receptor-alpha predict the outcome of early IVF pregnancies. Hum. Reprod. **19:** 1357–1363.
17. Lin, H., T.R. Mosmann, L. Guilbert, *et al.* 1993. Synthesis of T helper 2-type cytokines at the maternal-fetal interface. J. Immunol. **151:** 4562–4572.
18. Cadet, P., P.L. Rady, S.K. Trying, *et al.* 1995. Interleukin messenger ribonucleic acid in human placenta: implications of a role for interleukin-10 in fetal allograft protection. Am. J. Obstet. Gynecol. **173:** 25–29.
19. Bennett, W.A., S. Lagoo-Deenadaylan, N.S. Whitworth, *et al.* 1999. First trimester human chorionic villi express both immunoregulatory and inflammatory cytokines: a role for interleukin 10 in regulating the cytokine network of pregnancy. Am. J. Reprod. Immunol. **41:** 70–78.
20. Russell, A.S., C. Johnston, C. Chew & W.P. Maksymowych. 1997. Evidence for reduced Th1 function in normal pregnancy: a hypothesis for the remission of rheumatroid arthritis. J. Rheumatol. **24:** 1045–1050.
21. Ekerfelt, C., L. Matthiesen, G. Berg & J. Ernerudh 1997. Paternal leukocytes selectively increase secretion of IL-4 in peripheral blood during normal pregnancies: demonstrated by a novel one-way MLC measuring cytokine secretion. Am. J. Reprod. Immunol. **38:** 320–326.
22. Ekerfelt, C., L. Matthiesen, G. Berg & J. Ernerudh. 1998. Increased numbers of circulating interferon-gamma- and interleukin-4-secreting cells during normal pregnancy. Am. J. Reprod. Immunol. **39:** 362–367.
23. Tranchot-Diallo, J., G. Gras, F. Parnet-Mathieu, *et al.* 1997. Modulations of cytokine expression in pregnant women. Am. J. Reprod. Immunol. **37:** 215–226.
24. Piccini, M.P., C. Scaletti, E. Maggi & S. Romagnani. 2000. Role of hormone-controlled Th1- and Th2-type cytokines in successful pregnancy. J. Neuroimmunol. **109:** 30–33.
25. Tagawa, N., Y. Hidaka, T. Takano, *et al.* 2004. Serum concentrations of androstenediol and androstenediol sulfate, and their relation to cytokine production during and after normal pregnancy. Steroids **69:** 675–680.
26. Tagawa, N., Y. Hidaka, T. Takano, *et al.* 2004. Serum concentrations of dehydroepiandrosterone and dehydroepiandrosterone sulfate and their relation to cytokine production during and after normal pregnancy. Clin. Chim. Acta. **340:** 187–193.
27. Elenkov, I.J., R.L. Wilder, V.K. Bakalov, *et al.* 2001. IL-12, TNF-alpha, and hormonal changes during late pregnancy and early postpartum: implications for autoimmune disease activity during these times. J. Clin. Endocrinol. Metab. **86:** 4933–4938.
28. Elenkov, I.J., D.A. Papanicolaou, R.L. Wilder & G.P. Chrousos. 1996. Modulatory effects of glucocorticoids and catecholamines on human interleukin-12 and interleukin-10 production: clinical implications. Proc. Assoc. Am. Physicians **108:** 374–381.

29. SZEKERES-BARTHO, J., Z. FAUST & P. VARGA. 1995. The expression of a progesterone-induced immunomodulatory protein in pregnancy lymphocytes. Am. J. Reprod. Immunol. **34:** 342–348.
30. SZEREDAY, L., P. VARGA & J. SZEKERES-BARTHO. 1997. Cytokine production by lymphocytes in pregnancy. Am. J. Reprod. Immunol. **38:** 418–422.
31. PICCINI, M.P., M.G. GIUDIZI, R. BIAGIOTTI, *et al.* 1995. Progesterone favors the development of human T helper cells producing Th2-type cytokines and promotes both IL-4 production and membrane CD30 expression in established Th1 cell clones. J. Immunol. **155:** 128–133.
32. CORREALE, J., M. ARIAS & W. GILMORE. 1998. Steroid hormone regulation of cytokine secretion by proteolipid protein-specific CD4+ T cell clones isolated from multiple sclerosis patients and normal control subjects. J. Immunol. **161:** 3365–3374.
33. ØSTENSEN, M., L. FUHRER, R. MATHIEU, *et al.* 2004. A prospective study of pregnant patients with rheumatoid arthritis and ankylosing spondylitis using validated clinical instruments. Ann. Rheum. Dis. **63:** 1212–1217.
34. GRAN, J.T. & M. ØSTENSEN. 1998. Spondylarthritides in females. Ballieres Clin. Rheumatol. **12:** 695–715.
35. VAN ROON, J.A.G. & J.W.J. BIJLSMA. 2002. Th2 mediated regulation in RA and the spondylarthropathies. Ann. Rheum. Dis. **61:** 951–954.
36. ØSTENSEN, M., F. FÖRGER, J. LEE NELSON, *et al.* 2005. Pregnancy in patients with rheumatic disease: anti-inflammatory cytokines increase in pregnancy and decrease post partum. Ann. Rheum. Dis. **64:** 839–844.
37. WAIS, T., W. FIERZ, T. STOLL & P.M. VILLIGER. 2003. Subclinical disease activity in systemic lupus erythematosus: immunoinflammatory markers do not normalize in clinical remission. J. Rheumatol. **30:** 2133–2139.
38. GERLI, R., C. LUNARDI, F. VINANTE, *et al.* 2001. Role of CD30+ T cells in rheumatoid arthritis: a counter-regulatory paradigm for Th1-driven diseases. Trends Immunol. **2:** 72–77.
39. VANNIER, E., L.C. MILLER & C.A. DINARELLO. 1992. Coordinated antiinflammatory effects of interleukin-4: interleukin 4 suppresses interleukin 1 production but up-regulates gene expression and synthesis of interleukin 1 receptor antagonist. Proc. Natl. Acad. Sci. USA **89:** 4076–4080.
40. JOYCE, D.A. & J.H. STEER. 1996. IL-4, IL-10 and IFN-γ have distinct, but interacting, effects of differentiation-induced changes in TNF-a and receptor release by cultured human monocytes. Cytokine **8:** 49–57.
41. DORIA, A., A. GHIRADELLO, L. IACCARINO, *et al.* 2004. Pregnancy, cytokines, and disease activity in systemic lupus erythematosus. Arthritis Rheum. **51:** 989–995.
42. MUNOZ-VALLE, J.F., M.M. VAZQUEZ-DEL, T. GARCIA-IGLESIAS, *et al.* 2003. T(H)1/T(H)2 cytokine profile, metalloprotease-9 activity and hormonal status in pregnant rheumatoid arthritis and systemic lupus erythematosus patients. Clin. Exp. Immunol. **131:** 377–384.
43. ELENKOV, I.J. 1997. Does differential neuroendocrine control of cytokine production govern the expression of autoimmune diseases in pregnancy and the postpartum period? Mol. Med. Today **3:** 379–383.

Anti-Beta-2 Glycoprotein I Antibodies Affect Bcl-2 and Bax Trophoblast Expression without Evidence of Apoptosis

NICOLETTA DI SIMONE,[a] ROBERTA CASTELLANI,[a] ELENA RASCHI,[b] M. ORIETTA BORGHI,[b,c] PIER LUIGI MERONI,[b,c] AND ALESSANDRO CARUSO[a]

[a]*Department of Obstetrics and Gynecology, Università Cattolica del Sacro Cuore, Rome, Italy*

[b]*Allergy, Clinical Immunology & Rheumatology Unit, IRCCS Istituto Auxologico Italiano, University of Milan, Milan, Italy*

[c]*Department of Internal Medicine, University of Milan, Milan, Italy*

ABSTRACT: Antiphospholipid antibodies (aPLs) reacting with beta-2 glycoprotein I (β2GPI) have been associated with recurrent fetal loss and pregnancy complications. The aim of the study was to investigate whether aPLs with anti-β2GPI specificity induce apoptosis of human trophoblasts *in vitro*. To this end, human anti-β2GPI monoclonal IgM derived from a patient with antiphospholipid syndrome and a human irrelevant monoclonal IgM were incubated with human trophoblast cell cultures for 24, 48, and 72 h. In all the cultures we evaluated: (i) Bcl-2 and Bax mRNA and protein expression by Western blot and reverse transcription polymerase chain reaction (RT-PCR), respectively; (ii) DNA fragmentation by a commercial ELISA kit and by agarose gel electrophoresis; and (iii) the percentage of cells reactive with the monoclonal antibody (MAb) M30 by indirect immunofluorescence. The results were: Bcl-2/Bax ratio increased in untreated trophoblast cells during the time of culture, showing the highest values detectable after 72 h (2.68 and 2.28 at protein and mRNA levels, respectively). Cell incubation with anti-β2GPI MAbs induced a significant Bcl-2/Bax ratio reduction in comparison with untreated cells (1.22 and 1.28 at protein and mRNA levels, respectively, after 72 h incubation). No significant difference was detected after cell exposure to irrelevant MAbs. However, neither DNA fragmentation nor increase in cells positive for the caspase-cleaved epitope of cytokeratin 18 cytoskeletal protein (M30) was found. In Conclusion, anti-β2GPI an-

Address for correspondence: Pier Luigi Meroni, M.D., Allergy, Clinical Immunology & Rheumatology Unit, IRCCS Istituto Auxologico Italiano, Via G. Spagnoletto, 3, 20149 Milan, Italy. Voice: +39-02-61911-2553; fax: +39-02-61911-2559.

e-mail: pierluigi.meroni@unimi.it

Ann. N.Y. Acad. Sci. 1069: 364–376 (2006). © 2006 New York Academy of Sciences.
doi: 10.1196/annals.1351.034

tibodies react with trophoblast cells and reduce the Bcl-2/Bax ratio, but without any clear apoptotic effect.

KEYWORDS: beta-2 glycoprotein I; antiphospholipid antibodies; trophoblast; fetal loss; apoptosis

INTRODUCTION

Antiphospholipid antibodies (aPLs) make up a heterogeneous group of pathogenic autoantibodies diagnosed as lupus anticoagulant (LA) or anticardiolipin antibodies.[1] The association between the persistent presence of aPLs and the occurrence of arterial and/or venous thrombosis and recurrent pregnancy loss formally defines the antiphospholipid syndrome (APS).

Rather than being directed against PLs only, these antibodies are specific for PL-binding proteins.[1–3] Among them, beta-2 glycoprotein I (β2GPI) does represent the most important protein.[3]

The mechanisms underlying the recurrent abortions and pregnancy complications in the APS are not completely elucidated, but many hypotheses have been suggested.[4] Although experimental models have emphasized the role of thrombotic phenomena in placental tissue,[5,6] studies in humans have shown that thrombotic events cannot account for all the histopathological findings in placentas from women with APS.[7,8] Evidence from *in vitro* studies with both murine and human monoclonal as well as polyclonal IgG antibodies from APS patients clearly demonstrated that aPLs bind to trophoblast.[9,10] Such a reactivity is mostly due to the expression of β2GPI on the trophoblast cell membranes.[11,12] It has been suggested that β2GPI might bind to anionic PLs exposed on the external cell membranes of trophoblasts undergoing syncytium formation, and, once bound, might behave as a suitable antigenic target for aPLs with anti-β2GPI specificity.[9–13] These findings explain why aPLs passively infused in naïve pregnant mice rapidly disappear from the circulation and are entrapped in the placental tissues.[6,14]

We have previously reported that the anti-β2GPI binding to trophoblasts might directly affect cell functions, such as inhibition of syncytium formation, decreased chorionic gonadotropin production, and defective invasiveness *in vitro*.[9] In line with our findings are the data showing that an anti-β2GPI monoclonal antibody (MAb) affected human choriocarcinoma cell line proliferation *in vitro*.[15] As a whole, these findings do suggest that aPLs with anti-β2GPI specificity might directly affect the critical steps in the development and maturation of the villous trophoblast.

Moreover, it has recently been reported that sera from APS women increased apoptosis in human placental explants, and that IgG purified from systemic lupus erythematosus (SLE)/APS patients displayed a direct damaging effect on embryonic and yolk sac growth.[16–18]

The purpose of the present study was to investigate the *in vitro* ability of human anti-β2GPI MAbs to induce trophoblast apoptosis. From our results, it appears that aPLs reacting with β2GPI affect trophoblast expression of Bcl-2 and Bax, two genes (and proteins) involved in the regulation of programmed cell death. However, no evidence of DNA fragmentation has been observed.

MATERIALS AND METHODS

Human Monoclonal Anti-β2GPI Antibodies

Two human MAbs of the IgM isotype obtained from hybridized Epstein–Barr virus–induced B cell lines from APS patients were used. TM1G2 has been shown to recognize β2GPI, both complexed with anionic PL (in CL-coated plates) and alone in γ-irradiated β2GPI-coated plates. TM1B9 did not display any anti-β2GPI reactivity and was used as a negative control. The characterization of the MAbs had been previously reported in detail.[19]

All the human MAbs were used at a final protein concentration of 50 μg/mL, which has been previously shown to display optimal binding.[9]

Cell Cultures

Placentas were obtained from healthy women immediately after uncomplicated vaginal delivery at 36 weeks of gestation. Cytotrophoblast cells were isolated as detailed elsewhere.[9] The enriched (95%) cytotrophoblast cells (5×10^5 cells/mL) were cultured in DMEM-10% FCS at 37°C in 5% CO_2/95% air. Cell cultures were performed for 24, 48, or 72 h in standard medium.

Each experiment was carried out with primary human trophoblasts in the presence of: (1) medium alone, (2) human anti-β2GPI MAbs (TM1G2; 50 μg/mL), or (3) control MAbs (TM1B9; 50 μg/mL).

Western Blot Analysis

At each time of culture, Bcl-2 and Bax were investigated by Western blot analysis, as previously described.[20] Eighty micrograms of each sample were separated on a 15%-SDS-polyacrylamide gel and, after electroblotting onto polyvinylidene fluoride membrane (Millipore, Bedford, MA), incubated with the primary antibodies (DakoCytomation, Glostrup, Denmark) in 3% nonfat dry milk in 1× TBST (0.1 M Trizma base, 0.15 M NaCl, and 0.05% Tween 20).

Following incubation with an alkaline phosphatase–conjugated goat anti-rabbit antibody, visualization of the bound antibody was performed with the BCIP/NBT Phosphatase Substrate System (Kirkegaard & Perry Laboratories,

Gaithersburg, MD). The levels of the Bcl-2 and Bax were estimated versus the constant level of the 42-kDa β-actin.

Semiquantitative Reverse Transcription Polymerase Chain Reaction Analysis

Confluent cells were collected, centrifuged, and washed, and total RNA was isolated by lysing cells with Trizol™ reagent (Gibco BRL, Grand Island, NY) according to manufacturer's instructions. RNA integrity was confirmed by agarose gel electrophoresis and ethidium bromide staining, as well as by monitoring absorbance at 260/280 nm. The RNA concentration was determined from spectrophotometric analysis and before each reverse transcription polymerase chain reaction (RT-PCR) experiment. The Perkin-Elmer Gene Amp Gold RNA PCR kit was used for all the RT-PCRs, which were performed in the Gene Amp PCR system 9600 (Perkin-Elmer/Cetus, San Diego, CA). After removal of contaminating chromosomal DNA with DNAse I treatment, 1 μg of RNA was reverse-transcribed with 25 units of Moloney murine leukemia virus at 42°C for 20 min. Three microliters of cDNA products were used in each PCR cycle. Primer sequence as well as expected product size are listed in TABLE 1.

Bcl-2 cDNA was coamplified with aldolase-A as internal control,[21] with 1 unit of AmpliTaq Gold DNA polymerase in 1 mM $MgCl_2$, and 35 cycles of 20 sec at 94°C, 60 sec at 62°C, and 7 min at 72°C. Bax was coamplified with aldolase-A, using 1 unit of AmpliTaq DNA polymerase in 5 mM $MgCl_2$, and 32 cycles of 20 sec at 94°C, 60 sec at 62°C, and 7 min at 72°C. The PCR products were loaded onto 2% agarose gels and stained with ethidium bromide. The relative concentration of each Bcl-2 or Bax mRNA was determined by densitometric scanning and normalization to the aldolase-A signal for each sample using the following pair of primers: 5′-CGCAGAAGGGGTCCTGGTGA-3′ and 5′-CAGCTCCTTCTTCTGCTCCGGGGT-3′.[22]

M30 Detection

The percentage of apoptotic cells was determined by M30 CytoDEATH antibody.[20,23] This is a monoclonal mouse immunoglobulin (Ig) G_2b antibody

TABLE 1. Sequences of specific primers for Bcl-2 and Bax

Bcl-2 (385 bp)	
Forward	5′-ACTTGTGGCCCAGATAGGCACCCAG-3′
Reverse	5′-CGACTTCGCCGAGATGTCCAGCCAG-3′
Bax (538 bp)	
Forward	5′-CAGCTCTGAGCAGATCATGAAGACA-3′
Reverse	5′-GCCCATCTTCTTCCAGATGGTGAGC-3′

(clone M30; Roche, Mannheim, Germany) that binds to a caspase-cleaved, formalin-resistant epitope of cytokeratin 18 cytoskeletal protein. The immunoreactivity of the M30 antibody is confined to the cytoplasm of apoptotic cells. Trophoblast cells, treated with human anti-β2GPI MAbs (TM1G2; 50 μg/mL) or control MAbs (TM1B9; 50 μg/mL), for 24 and 48 h, were fixed in 10% neutral-buffered formalin for 15 min, treated with 0.3% hydrogen peroxide in methanol for 10 min to block the endogenous peroxidase activity, washed in phosphate-buffered saline (PBS) solution, and then incubated with M30 antibody at room temperature for 1 h. In negative controls, preimmune mouse serum instead of primary antibody was used. Immunoreactions were revealed by the avidin–biotin complex technique using diaminobenzidine as substrate. We counted the number of M30-positive cells in all fields found at 400× final magnification. For each slide, three randomly selected microscopic fields were observed, and at least 100 cells/field were evaluated.

Measurement of Fragmented DNA by Enzyme-Linked Immunosorbent Assay

Cytotrophoblast cells were detached by EDTA-trypsin (Gibco BRL) treatment and collected by centrifugation at 250 *g* for 10 min at 4°C, then suspended in a fresh culture medium to make 1 × 10^5 cells/mL. A volume of 100 μL of the cell suspension was transferred to each well of a microculture plate and incubated with the test samples (human anti-β2GPI MAbs [TM1G2; 50 μg/mL] or control MAbs [TM1B9; 50 μg/mL]). At 24 and 48 h, the plates were centrifuged at 250 *g* for 10 min at 4°C, the supernatant carefully removed, and 200 μL of lysis buffer were added to each well; the amounts of fragmented DNA were measured with a Cell Death Detection ELISA Plus Kit (Roche Laboratories, Milan, Italy).

The experiments were performed three times on different placentas, in duplicate within each experiment.

DNA Fragmentation Analysis

Cytotrophoblast cells (10^6 cells/mL) were cultured in complete medium. After 48 h culture, the cells were treated for 48 h with the test samples: (1) human anti-β2GPI MAbs (TM1G2; 50 μg/mL) or (2) control MAbs (TM1B9; 50 μg/mL). At the end of the incubation period, cells were washed twice in PBS. Cell pellets were resuspended and incubated with lysis buffer (50 mM Tris–HCl, 100 mM EDTA, and 0.5% SDS), supplemented with proteinase K (0.7 mg/mL; Sigma-Aldrich S.r.l., Milan, Italy), and then incubated for 1 h at 55°C. The DNA was extracted with phenol/chloroform/isoamyl alcohol (25:24:1 v/v), followed by absolute ethanol and addition of 70% ethanol. The

DNA was dissolved in 10 mM Tris (pH 7.5) and 1 mM EDTA (pH 8) after evaporation of ethanol. The DNA was loaded into wells of a 1.5% agarose gel and electrophoresed at 75 mV using 100 mM Tris, 100 mM boric acid, and 0.2 mM EDTA as running buffer. The DNA was visualized by ethidium bromide staining. The experiments were repeated three times on different placentas.

Statistical Analysis

Statistical analysis was performed using two-way analysis of variance for multiple comparisons.

RESULTS

Protein Levels of Bcl-2 and Bax Induced by Anti-β2GPI MAbs

Bcl-2 protein is known to be involved in the inhibition of apoptosis, while other members of the Bcl-2 family, such as Bax, accelerate cell death under various conditions and counteract the protection from apoptosis provided by Bcl-2 protein.[24]

Protein expression analysis by Western blot showed a band of the expected size of 26 kDa for Bcl-2 and of 21 kDa for Bax in all the samples. As previously reported, cytotrophoblasts were single mononuclear cells with two or three aggregates at 24 h of culture; increasing numbers of syncytia were detectable after 48 h (data not shown).[9] As seen in FIGURE 1, analysis of Bcl-2 and Bax protein expression during *in vitro* cytotrophoblast differentiation showed that syncytium formation is associated with a significant change in protein expression: increased expression of Bcl-2 and decreased expression of Bax at 72 h of culture, when syncytia become the dominant form. Trophoblast cells incubated in the presence of anti-β2GPI MAbs (TM1G2) did not display any significant change in Bcl-2 and Bax protein expression from 24 to 72 h of culture (FIG. 1). In contrast, incubation with the irrelevant control MAbs (TM1B9) showed Bcl-2 and Bax protein expression comparable to that found in untreated cells (data not shown).

Bcl-2 and Bax mRNA Expression Correlate with Protein Levels

We also investigated whether the incubation of trophoblast cells with anti-β2GPI MAbs was able to modulate Bcl-2 and Bax expression at mRNA level. The cells' ability to synthesize Bcl-2 and Bax was examined using RT-PCR analysis, and the identity of the PCR products was demonstrated by Southern blot (data not shown).

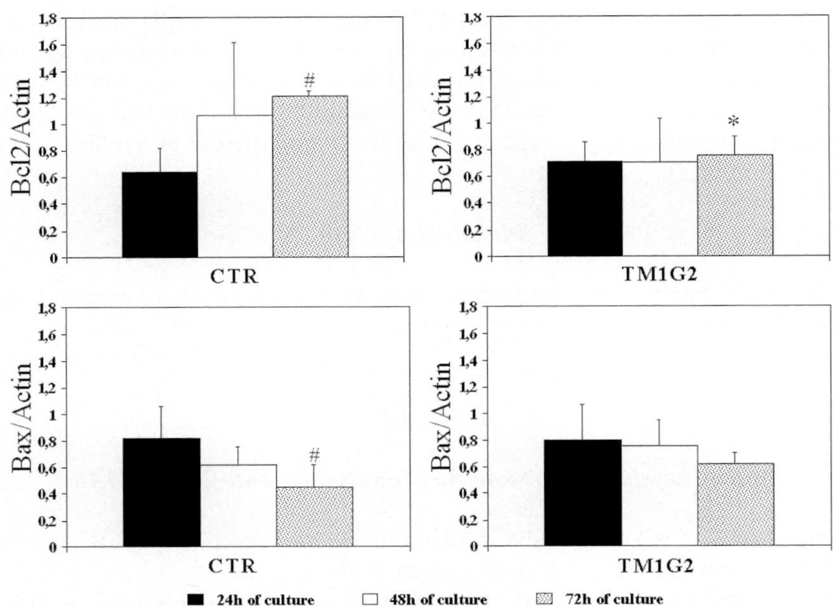

FIGURE 1. Western blot of Bcl-2 and Bax in untreated trophoblast cells (control, CTR) and in the presence of anti-β2GPI MAbs (TM1G2) at different times of culture (24, 48, 72 h). The levels of Bcl-2 and Bax were estimated in comparison with the constant level of β-actin. The values represent the mean ± SD of six independent experiments. Significant increase of Bcl-2 and decrease of Bax expression at 72 h of culture are shown in untreated trophoblast cells (# $P < 0.01$, 72 h vs. 24 h of culture). Bcl-2 expression at 72 h is significantly reduced in TM1G2-treated versus-untreated cells (* $P < 0.01$).

Both Bcl-2 and Bax mRNAs were identified by RT-PCR in untreated trophoblast cells at 24 h of culture and their levels inversely changed during the course of the experiment. As shown in FIGURE 2, Bcl-2 mRNA levels were significantly higher at 72 h than at 24 h of culture; Bax mRNA levels displayed an opposite trend. The presence of anti-β2GPI MAbs inhibited the increase of Bcl-2 and the reduction of Bax levels observed from 24 to 72 h of culture (FIG. 2). Incubation with the irrelevant control MAbs did not modify Bcl-2 and Bax mRNA expression in comparison to untreated cells (data not shown).

Apoptosis Detection

The antibody M30 CytoDEATH recognizes a specific caspase cleavage site and thus is a reliable tool for identifying early apoptosis.[23] The percentages of M30-positive trophoblast cells were comparable both in the cultures carried

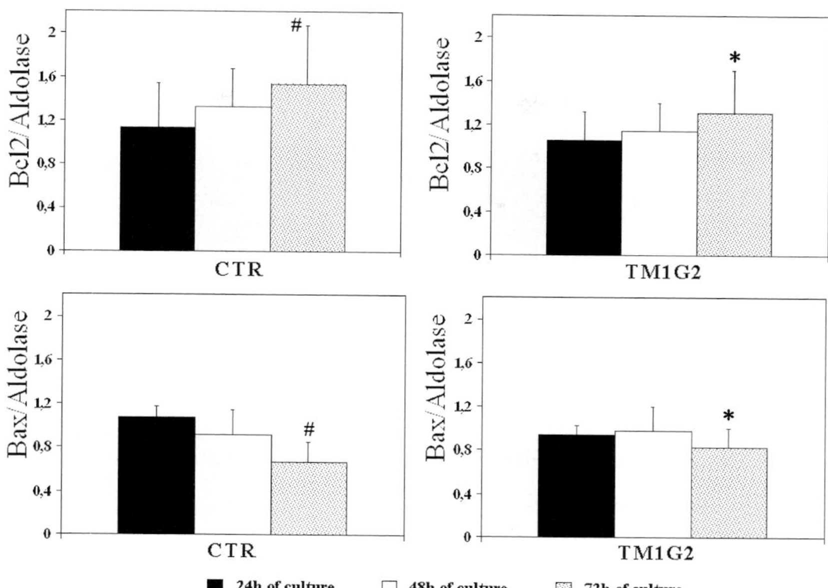

FIGURE 2. Semiquantitative RT-PCR analysis of Bcl-2 and Bax in untreated trophoblast cells (control, CTR) and in the presence of anti-β2GPI MAbs (TM1G2) at different times of culture (24, 48, 72 h). The levels of Bcl-2 and Bax were estimated in comparison with the constant level of aldolase. The values represent the mean ± SD of six independent experiments. Significant increase of Bcl-2 and decrease of Bax expression at 72 h of culture are shown in untreated trophoblast cells (# $P < 0.01$, 72 h vs. 24 h of culture). Bcl-2 expression at 72 h is significantly reduced in TM1G2-treated vs. untreated cells, while Bax is significantly higher in cells treated with anti-β2GPI MAbs (*$P < 0.01$).

out in the presence of the human anti-β2GPI MAbs (TM1G2) and in those with irrelevant control (TM1B9) (0% and 0.5% at 24 h, and 1% and 1.5% at 48 h of culture, respectively).

The time course of apoptosis was also investigated by the appearance of fragmented DNA derived from trophoblast cells. Incubation with TM1G2 MAbs did not induce DNA fragmentation evaluated by enzyme-linked immunosorbent assay (ELISA) (191 ± 56 and 210 ± 26 at 24 and 48 h of culture, respectively; mean optical density [OD] values ± SD). The values for the negative control (TM1B9) were similar to those displayed by untreated cells (142 ± 39 TM1B9 vs. 153 ± 22 untreated cells at 24 h; 269 ± 76 TM1B9 vs. 239 ± 37 untreated cells at 48 h; mean OD values ± SD). As a positive control, trophoblast cells were cultured with tumor necrosis factor-α (100 ng/mL; 820 ± 115 and 1,020 ± 230 at 24 and 48 h, respectively; mean OD values ± SD). Comparable results were obtained when DNA was analyzed by agarose gel electrophoresis (FIG. 3).

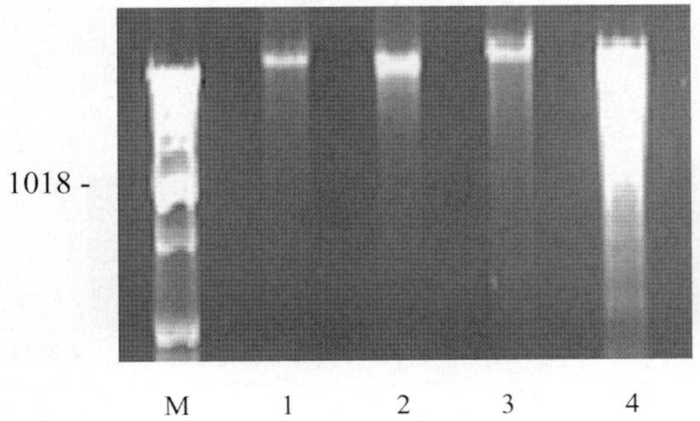

FIGURE 3. Gel electrophoresis of fragmented DNA. In *lane* 1 are shown untreated primary trophoblast cells. *Lanes* 2 and 3 show cells incubated for 48 h with the control MAbs (TM1B9, 50 μg/mL) or with human anti-β2GPI MAbs (TM1G2, 50 μg/mL). TNF-α (100 ng/mL) was used as positive control (*lane* 4). M indicates DNA size markers in base pairs. No differences are observed between untreated and MAb-treated cells.

DISCUSSION

Several studies have shown that β2GPI is expressed on syncytiotrophoblasts and extravillous cytotrophoblasts of normal placentas.[11,12,25,26] Such a finding raises the hypothesis that aPLs with anti-β2GPI specificity might recognize their own antigenic target on trophoblasts and directly affect trophoblast cell functions.

The nature of the binding of β2GPI to trophoblast as well as the ultimate mechanisms responsible for the trophoblast damage are still a matter of investigation.

It has been suggested that exposure of anionic PLs on the external surface during intertrophoblastic fusion might offer a useful substrate for the cationic PL-binding site of β2GPI (reviewed in Ref. 4). In addition, β2GPI was shown to bind to annexin 2, the formal receptor for plasminogen/tissue-plasminogen activator on EC (reviewed in Ref. 4). Furthermore, ApoER2′, a member of the low-density lipoprotein receptor family that is present on placental tissues, has been shown to behave as a receptor for β2GPI, at least on platelets.[27] This finding suggests the possibility for alternative β2GPI-binding modalities to trophoblast cell membrane. Whatever the fine nature of the binding, once bound, the molecule offers suitable epitopes that can be recognized by aPLs with anti-β2GPI specificity. As shown with EC and platelets, antibody binding could trigger a signaling affecting cell functions; thus, comparable events could be also suggested for trophoblasts.[28,29] Accordingly, our recent *in vitro* results are consistent with the possibility that antibody binding inhibits trophoblast differentiation by downregulating gonadotropin release and Matrigel invasiveness. These two mechanisms were suggested to play a pathogenic role for the defective placentation reported in the APS.[9,13]

In addition, the authors suggested that aPL might also display a direct pro-apoptotic effect on trophoblast.[16–18,30] To confirm and extend this finding, we investigated the ability of anti-β2GPI MAbs to regulate the *in vitro* expression of the apoptosis-related genes—Bcl-2 and Bax—by human trophoblast cells. Moreover, the production of the DNA strand breaks (DNA laddering) and the expression of the cytokeratin 18 neoepitope recognized by the M30 MAbs were also evaluated.

Bcl-2 was the first gene that was clearly involved in apoptosis inhibition and promoting cell survival.[31] It belongs to a still-growing family,[32,33] whose members are able to form homo- and/or heterodimers among themselves; their association and the relative ratio between anti- and proapoptotic proteins are responsible for directing the cells toward survival or death.[34,35]

The higher expression of Bcl-2 in syncytiotrophoblast compared to cytotrophoblast has been already observed in previous studies, and it suggests a differentiation-dependent regulation of Bcl-2 expression.[36,37] Furthermore, the increased Bcl-2 expression in syncytiotrophoblast would protect the layer of placental villi from apoptosis.[38] In our experiments, we confirmed the increase in Bcl-2 expression and we showed a decrease of Bax both associated with syncytial fusion and in line with the antiapoptotic phenotype of untreated trophoblast cell cultures. Cell incubation with anti-β2GPI MAbs, but not with the irrelevant control, inhibited such modifications. Thus, a significant reduction ($P < 0.01$) in the Bcl-2/Bax ratio at 72 h of culture was observed in cells treated with the anti-β2GPI MAbs in comparison to untreated cells.

As members of the Bcl-2 family are final common mediators of survival or death in a wide variety of cell types, we speculated that an imbalance between Bax and Bcl-2 expression also could influence the eventual apoptosis for trophoblast cells.

However, we were not able to observe any significant trophoblast M30 staining or DNA fragmentation measured by ELISA or by agarose gel electrophoresis in the presence of anti-β2GPI MAbs. This finding is apparently against the possibility that aPLs with anti-β2GPI specificity induce trophoblast apoptosis at variance with other studies.[16–18,30] The difference in the results might have several explanations. The use of purified anti-β2GPI MAbs in our study instead of whole LA positive sera[18] rules out any effect mediated by soluble serum factors other than the aPLs themselves. Moreover, the use of whole IgG fractions from patients suffering from SLE and APS does not exclude the possibility that other autoantibody specificities, likely present in SLE sera, might display the apoptotic effect.[16,17] Finally, the apoptosis induced *in vitro* by antiphosphatidylserine MAbs on rat yolk sacs cannot be compared with our model because of the different antigenic specificities of the two antibodies.[30]

An alternative explanation for the lack of Bcl-2 increase and Bax decrease in cultures carried out in the presence of anti-β2GPI MAbs might be the fact that these antibodies are able to inhibit trophoblast fusion process, and thus they could just indirectly affect Bcl-2/Bax expression as a consequence of the inhibition of the fusion process itself.[9]

In conclusion, data from our previous studies combined with the present data do suggest that aPLs with anti-β2GPI specificity might bind their own antigenic target expressed on the trophoblast cell membranes, induce cell perturbation that ends in a defective maturation, but do not display a clear pro-apoptotic effect.

REFERENCES

1. Roubey, R.A. 2004. Antiphospholipid antibodies: immunological aspects. Clin. Immunol. **112**: 127–128.
2. Amengual, O., T. Atsumi & T. Koike. 2004. Antiprothrombin antibodies and the diagnosis of antiphospholipid syndrome. Clin. Immunol. **112**: 144–149.
3. Bad de Laat, H., R.H. Derksen & P.G. de Groot. 2004. Beta2-glycoprotein I, the playmaker of the antiphospholipid syndrome. Clin. Immunol. **112**: 161–168.
4. Meroni, P.L. *et al.* 2004. Antiphospholipid antibodies as cause of pregnancy loss. Lupus **13**: 649–652.
5. Piona, A. *et al.* 1995. Placental thrombosis and fetal loss after passive transfer of mouse lupus monoclonal or human polyclonal anti-cardiolipin antibodies in pregnant naive BALB/c mice. Scand. J. Immunol. **41**: 427–432.
6. Ikematsu, W. *et al.* 1998. Human anticardiolipin monoclonal autoantibodies cause placental necrosis and fetal loss in BALB/c mice. Arthritis Rheum. **41**: 1026–1039.
7. Out, H.J. *et al.* 1991. Histopathological findings in placetae from patients with intra-uterine fetal death and anti-phospholipid antibodies. Eur. J. Obstet. Gynecol. Reprod. Biol. **41**: 179–186.
8. Salafia, C.M. *et al.* 1996. Fetal losses and other obstetrical manifestations in the antiphospholipid syndrome. *In* The Antiphospholipis Syndrome. R.A. Asherson, R. Cervera, J.C. Piette & Y. Shoenfeld, Eds.: 117–131. CRC Press. Boca Raton, FL.
9. Di Simone, N. *et al.* 2000. Antiphospholipid antibodies affect trophoblast gonadotropin secretion and invasiveness by binding directly and through adhered β2-glycoprotein I. Arthritis Rheum. **43**: 140–150.
10. Katsuragawa, H. *et al.* 1997. Monoclonal antibody against phosphatidylserine inhibits in vitro human trophoblastic hormone production and invasion. Biol. Reprod. **56**: 50–58.
11. McIntyre, J.A. 1992. Immune recognition at the maternal-fetal interface: overview. Am. J. Reprod. Immunol. **28**: 127–131.
12. La Rosa, L. *et al.* 1994. β2 glycoprotein I and placental anticoagulant protein I in placentae from patients antiphospholipid syndrome. J. Rheumatol. **21**: 1684–1693.
13. Di Simone, N. *et al.* 2005. Pathogenic role of anti-beta 2-glycoprotein I antibodies in antiphospholipid associated fetal loss: characterisation of beta 2-glycoprotein I binding to trophoblast cells and functional effects of anti-beta 2-glycoprotein I antibodies in vitro. Ann. Rheum. Dis. **64**: 462–467.

14. BLANK, M. *et al.* 1991. Induction of anti-phospholipid syndrome in naive mice with mouse lupus monoclonal and human polyclonal anti-cardiolipin antibodies. Proc. Natl. Acad. Sci. USA **88**: 3069–3073.
15. CHAMLEY, L.M. *et al.* 1998. Action of anticardiolipin and antibodies to beta2-glycoprotein-I on trophoblast proliferation as a mechanism for fetal death. Lancet **352**: 1037–1038.
16. YACOBI, S. *et al.* 2002. Effect of sera from women with systemic lupus erythematosus or antiphospholipid syndrome and recurrent abortions on human placental explants in culture. Teratology **66**: 300–308.
17. ORNOY, A. *et al.* 2003. The effects of antiphospholipid antibodies obtained from women with SLE/APS and associated pregnancy loss on rat embryos and placental explants in culture. Lupus **12**: 573–578.
18. BOSE, P. *et al.* 2004. Adverse effects of lupus anticoagulant positive blood sera on placental viability can be prevented by heparin in vitro. Am. J. Obstet. Gynecol. **191**: 2125–2131.
19. ICHIKAWA, K. *et al.* 1994. β2-glycoprotein I reactivity of monoclonal anticardiolipin antibodies from patients with the antiphospholipid syndrome. Arthritis Rheum. **37**: 1453–1461.
20. DI SIMONE, N. *et al.* 2003. Homocysteine induces trophoblast cell death with apoptotic features. Biol. Reproduct. **69**: 1129–1134.
21. DI SIMONE, N. *et al.* 2002. Antiphospholipid antibodies regulate the expression of trophoblast cell adhesion molecules. Fertil. Steril. **77**: 805–811.
22. MARONE, M. *et al.* 1998. Bcl-2, Bax, Bcl-xl, and bcl-xs expression in normal and neoplastic ovarian tissues. Clin. Cancer Res. **4**: 517–524.
23. BREUCKMANN, F. *et al.* 2002. Apoptosis of human dermal endothelial cells as potential side effect following therapeutic administration of UVA irradiation: preliminary results. Arch. Dermatol. Res. **294**: 303–309.
24. ISHIHARA, N. *et al.* 2000. Changes in proliferative potential, apoptosis and Bcl-2 protein expression in cytotrophoblasts and syncytiotrophoblast in human placenta over the course of pregnancy. Endocr. J. **47**: 317–327.
25. CHAMLEY, L.W., J.L. ALLEN & P.M. JOHNSON. 1997. Synthesis of beta 2 glycoprotein 1 by the human placenta. Placenta **18**: 403–410.
26. DONOHOE, S. *et al.* 2000. Ontogeny of beta 2 glycoprotein 1 and annexin V in villous placenta of normal and antiphospholipid syndrome pregnancies. Thromb. Haemost. **84**: 32–38.
27. DE GROOT, P.G. *et al.* 2004. Beta2-glycoprotein I and LDL-receptor family members. Thromb. Res. **114**: 455–459.
28. MERONI, P.L. *et al.* 2004. Endothelial cell activation by antiphospholipid antibodies. Clin. Immunol. **112**: 169–174.
29. PIERANGELI, S.S., M. VEGA-OSTERTAG & E.N. HARRIS. 2004. Intracellular signaling triggered by antiphospholipid antibodies in platelets and endothelial cells: a pathway to targeted therapies. Thromb. Res. **114**: 467–476.
30. MATALON, S.T. *et al.* 2004. Antiphosphatidylserine antibodies affect rat yolk sacs in culture: a mechanism for fetal loss in antiphospholipid syndrome. Am. J. Reprod. Immunol. **51**: 144–151.
31. HOCKENBERY, D.M. *et al.* 1990. Bcl-2 is an inner mitochondrial membrane protein that blocks programmed cell death. Nature **348**: 334–336.
32. YIN, X., Z.N. OLTVAI & S.J. KORSMEYER. 1993. BH1 and BH2 domains of Bcl-2 are required for inhibition of apoptosis and heterodimerization with Bax. Cell **74**: 607–619.

33. RAO, L. & E. WHITE. 1997. Bcl-2 and the ICE family of apoptotic regulators: making a connection. Curr. Opin. Genet. Dev. **7**: 52–58.
34. SEDLAK, T.W. *et al.* 1995. Multiple Bcl-2 family members demonstrate selective dimerization with Bax. Proc. Natl. Acad. Sci. USA **92**: 7834–7838.
35. SATO, T. *et al.* 1994. Interactions among members of the Bcl-2 protein family analyzed with a yeast two-hybrid system. Proc. Natl. Acad. Sci. USA **91**: 9238–9242.
36. SAKURAGI, N. *et al.* 1994. Differentation-dependent expression of the BCL-2 proto-oncogene in the human trophoblast lineage. J. Soc. Gynecol. Invest. **1**: 164–172.
37. MARZIONI, D., *et al.* 1998. BCL-2 expression in the human placenta and its correlation with fibrin deposits. Hum. Reprod. **13**: 1717–1722.
38. LEVY, R. & D.M. NELSON. 2000. To be, or not to be, that is the question. Apoptosis in human trophoblast. Placenta **21**: 1–13.

Endocrine Regulation of Suppressor Lymphocytes

Role of the Glucocorticoid-Induced TNF-Like Receptor

SIMONE NEGRINI,[a] DANIELA FENOGLIO,[a,b] PIERCESARE BALESTRA,[b] MARCO FRAVEGA,[b] GILBERTO FILACI,[a,b] AND FRANCESCO INDIVERI[a,b]

[a]*Department of Internal Medicine, University of Genoa, Genoa, Italy*

[b]*Centre of Excellence for Biomedical Research (CEBR), University of Genoa, Genoa, Italy*

ABSTRACT: Mechanisms responsible for peripheral immune tolerance are currently under investigation in several laboratories, in order to define the role of immune homeostasis in physiological processes and pathologic conditions, such as autoimmunity and cancer. In this context, recent studies attributed a relevant role to the glucocorticoid-induced TNFR-related gene (GITR). GITR is expressed at high levels on CD4$^+$CD25$^+$. T regulatory (Treg) cells, but only at low levels on resting responder T lymphocytes, and is upregulated after activation. GITR triggering induces both pro- and anti-apoptotic effects through different intracellular pathways, abrogates the suppressive activity of Treg cells, and co-stimulates responder T cells. These data hint that GITR triggering overstimulates the immune system. Indeed, *in vivo* studies demonstrated that GITR stimulation may both induce autoimmune diseases and strengthen anti-virus and anti-tumor immune responses. Therefore, the GITR–GITRL system appears crucial in regulating immunity. Currently, the majority of studies about GITR's role on regulatory cells are focused on CD4$^+$CD25$^+$ Treg cells, while very little is known about the importance of this molecule in other Treg subtypes. We have recently characterized a subpopulation of CD8$^+$ T suppressor lymphocytes able to inhibit both T cell proliferation and cytotoxicity. Preliminary data show that GITR is expressed on such CD8$^+$ T suppressor cells and that its activation by a specific antibody inhibits generation, but not function, of these cells. These early results suggest the importance of GITR in human T suppressor lymphocytes other than CD4$^+$CD25$^+$ Treg cells.

KEYWORDS: GITR; GITRL; T suppressor lymphocytes; T regulatory lymphocytes; glucocorticoid hormones

Address for correspondence: Prof. Francesco Indiveri, Department of Internal Medicine (DIMI), University of Genoa, Genoa, Italy. Voice: +39-010-3538987; fax: +39-010-3538994.
e-mail: frindi@unige.it

**Ann. N.Y. Acad. Sci. 1069: 377–385 (2006). © 2006 New York Academy of Sciences.
doi: 10.1196/annals.1351.035**

MODULATION OF LYMPHOCYTES BY GLUCOCORTICOID HORMONES

A novel scientific discipline that examines the complex interdependence of the neural, endocrine, and the immune systems in health and disease has emerged in recent years.[1,2] These systems both express and respond to a large number of common regulatory molecules including steroids, neuropeptides, cytokines, and neurotransmitters, which provide the molecular basis for coordinated neuroendocrine-immune responses in health and in pathologic conditions, such as inflammation, infection, or tumor.[3–6] Among these complex and largely still unknown interactions, the relations between glucocorticoids and the immune system are certainly the deepest investigated.[7–11]

Glucocorticoid hormones (GCHs) influence a variety of immune functions through specific alteration in gene expression.[12,13] Indeed, GCH activity involves the inhibition of the production of many cytokines, such as IL-2 and interferon-gamma (IFN-γ), as well as the synthesis and surface expression of several membrane-bound proteins, including melanin-concentrating hormone molecules, cytokine receptors, and adhesion molecules. Consequently, GCHs inhibit the antigen presentation process, as well as the migration of immune cells and intercommunication among cells involved in inflammatory response.[14–16]

GCHs regulate the negative selection of immature T cells in the thymus and also the maintenance of immune tolerance, increasing apoptosis in mature activated peripheral blood lymphocytes.[17–19]

Glucocorticoids not only break down the effector arm of the immune response, but also upmodulate the regulatory counterpart. Indeed, GCHs directly promote differentiation to T regulatory (Treg) cells by a FOXP3-dependent mechanism.[20,21] In addition, corticosteroids (CTSs) inhibit dendritic cell (DC) maturation; in this way, GCHs strongly reduce T cell-mediated responses and allow the selective expansion of Treg cells induced by the immature DCs.[22]

These data indicate the existence of an intricate network of immunoregulatory mechanisms in which CTSs play a strong role supporting their documented efficacy in the treatment of inflammatory and immunologic diseases.

Furthermore, it has been recently described that GCHs upregulate the expression of glucocorticoid-induced TNFR-related gene (GITR), a receptor belonging to the TNFR superfamily (TNFRSF) with complex and essential modulatory functions in the immune system, especially in Treg cells.[23]

GLUCOCORTICOID-INDUCED TNF-LIKE RECEPTOR (GITR)

The TNFRSF includes more than 20 proteins; all these molecules have the cysteine-rich domain as a common structural feature.[24,25] The TNFRSF comprises crucial molecules in the immune system and is mainly involved in the control of cell survival and differentiation of different cell lineages.[23–25] The GITR was cloned in 1997 in a hybridoma T cell line treated with dexamethasone, and recently has been classified as the 18th member of TNFRSF, (TNFRSF18).[23] In 1999, its human ligand, GITRL, a type-II transmembrane protein belonging to the TNFRSF, was cloned.[26]

GITR is expressed at basal levels in responder resting T cells, with CD4$^+$ cells having a higher GITR expression than CD8$^+$ cells.[27,28] After T cell activation, GITR is upregulated in both CD4$^+$ and CD8$^+$ cells.[27,29] It is expressed constitutively at high levels in CD4$^+$CD25$^+$ Treg cell, and further upregulated upon activation.[27,30] GITR is expressed at such high levels in murine and human Treg cells as to be considered a Treg marker.[27,31–33] Some studies suggest that GITR is also expressed at a low level in B cells and macrophages.[27,30,34] GITRL is expressed in macrophages, immature and mature DCs, B cells, and endothelium-derived cell lines.[35,36] It is not expressed in resting or activated T cells.[23,35,37] Functionally, GITR acts as co-stimulatory molecules. The capability of GITR to increase T cell proliferation and activation was confirmed in many studies by cell cycle analysis, activation markers, and cytokine production.[29,38]

Although some investigators [23,29] indicate that GITR plays a role in protecting from apoptosis, evidence has also emerged that GITR stimulation induces apoptosis.[37,39–41] These different and apparently opposite results may derive from different experimental settings. Pro-apoptotic versus anti-apoptotic effect of GITR triggering may depend on the biological environment or intrinsic characteristics of the cell, such as phenotype or level of activation.[37,40,41]

GITR triggering abrogates the *in vitro* suppressor function of murine Treg cell.[28,42] Various experimental data suggested that this was due to GITR triggering rather than GITR blocking.[27–29,31,35,37] Triggering of GITR stimulates Treg cell proliferation with loss of anergy and suppressor activity.[43]

Although GITR is also expressed at high levels on human Treg cells, a recent study suggests that triggering the receptor by an anti-hGITR mAb or by an hGITRL recombinant protein does not interfere with suppression.[33] Therefore, it seems that GITR plays a different role in mice and in humans. Nevertheless, further studies are necessary to define better the role of GITR in Treg cells and other Treg subtypes described in humans.

Signaling via GITR both turns off Treg cells and directly co-stimulates conventional T cells. With these notions, one might expect GITR triggering to over-activate immune systems *in vivo*. This indeed occurred in various experimental models in mice. There are several studies which report that GITR exacerbates inflammatory responses in autoimmune diseases such as autoimmune gastritis,[27] autoimmune diabetes,[44] and experimental allergic encephalitis.[45]The stimulatory effects of GITR triggering in inflammatory response have been described using a graft-versus-host disease (GVHD) murine model[41] and ischemic lesions after arterial occlusion.[46] Other *in vivo* studies reported that GITR stimulation may strengthen anti-virus and anti-tumor immune responses.[47,48]

If these data apply also in human disease, blocking or triggering GITR by Ab or fusion proteins could be useful in the treatment of immunology-related diseases, including tumors and autoimmune diseases. The large majority of the studies on GITR are based on animal models and are focused only on a subtype of regulatory cells ($CD4^+CD25^+$ Treg cells). Little is known about GITR activity in human regulatory circuits *in vivo* and, above all, there are no data on the role of this molecule in other subtypes of Treg lymphocytes.

REGULATORY/SUPPRESSOR T LYMPHOCYTES

Several mechanisms control discrimination between self and nonself, preventing the onset of autoimmune diseases. The immune system homeostasis is assured by different mechanisms of central and peripheral immune tolerance including thymic deletion of autoreactive T cells and induction of anergy in the periphery. Among these systems, evidence has accumulated for the active suppression of autoreactivity by regulatory or suppressor T cells (Ts).

The cells that were first assumed to have an immunosuppressive function are the $CD8^+$ T lymphocytes, as proposed by Gershon and Kondo in 1971.[49]

Several subsets of Treg cells with distinct phenotypes and mechanisms of action have now been identified. They constitute a network of heterogeneous $CD4^+$ or $CD8^+$ T cell subsets and other minor T cell populations, such as nonpolymorphic CD1d-responsive natural killer T cells.[50–57]

Among these cells, a subset of $CD8^+CD28^-$ T suppressor lymphocytes has recently been characterized by our group for the capacity to mediate their effects without antigen restriction. These non-antigen-specific $CD8^+$ T suppressor lymphocytes originate from circulating $CD8^+CD28^-$ T lymphocytes after stimulation with interleukin-2 and interleukin-10. $CD8^+$ suppressor cells inhibit both antigen-specific $CD4^+$ T cell proliferation and cellular cytotoxicity. $CD8^+$ suppressor cells operate through secretion of cytokines such as interferon-gamma, interleukin-6, and interleukin-10, and do not need direct cell-to-cell contact to exert their inhibitory functions.[58,59]

Previous work has shown the impairment of *in vitro* generation of $CD8^+$ Ts cells from the peripheral blood of relapsed patients with multiple sclerosis, systemic lupus erythematosus, or systemic sclerosis.[60,61] Similar findings are demonstrated for patients with human immunodeficiency virus or chronic hepatitis C virus infection. Furthermore, the presence of $CD8^+$ Ts cells infiltrating pathologic tissues in patients with autoimmune thyroiditis or cancer has been shown.[58,62] Collectively, these findings suggest that $CD8^+$ Ts cells may be involved in the control of pathologic chronic immune responses, contributing in some cases to the pathogenesis of the disease.

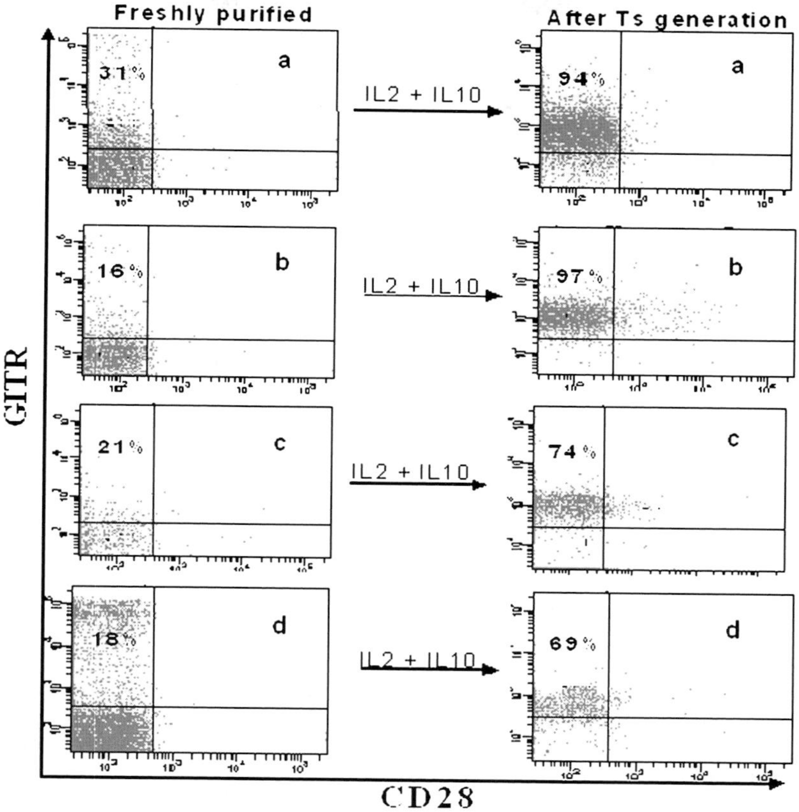

FIGURE 1. CD8^{+} T lymphocytes were purified from peripheral blood of four healthy subjects (a, b, c, and d) as described by Filaci *et al.*[59] Cells were stained with a FITC-conjugated anti-GITR and a PE-conjugated anti-CD28 monoclonal antibody, before analysis by an FACSCalibur cytometer (Beckton–Dickinson). Percentages of CD8^{+}-CD28^{-}-GITR^{+} T cells are indicated in each graph.

GITR IS EXPRESSED IN ANTIGEN NONSPECIFIC CD8^{+} T SUPPRESSOR LYMPHOCYTES

GITR was found expressed in a variable proportion (ranging from 15% to 30%) of circulating CD8^{+}CD28^{-} T lymphocytes isolated *ex vivo* from different healthy donors (FIG. 1). Stimulation with interleukin-2 and interleukin-10 in order to generate T suppressor lymphocytes determines a strong upregulation of GITR on CD8^{+}CD28^{-} cells when compared with basal levels. Indeed, a percentage variable from 70% to 95% of $CD8^+CD28^-$ Ts is $GITR^+$. Experiments are ongoing to analyze the existence of functional diversities between $CD8^+$CD28-$GITR^+$ and $CD8^+$CD28-$GITR^-$ T cells. Concerning the activity of GITR in $CD8^+CD28^-$ Ts lymphocytes, preliminary data suggest that GITR expression is mandatory for the generation of this subset of suppressor cells (personal observation). Further investigations are needed in order to define better the functional implication of GITR in the activation processes of regulatory circuits and in the maintenance of immune homeostasis.

ACKNOWLEDGMENTS

This study has been supported by grants from MIUR National Program "Meccanismi umorali e cellulari di modulazione dell'immunoflogosi" (No. 9706117821-001) and from Compagnia di San Paolo, Torino.

REFERENCES

1. STEINMAN, L. 2004. Elaborate interactions between the immune and nervous systems. Nat. Immunol. **5:** 575–581.
2. BESEDOVSKY, H. *et al.* 1996. Immune-neuro-endocrine interactions: facts and hypothesis. Endocr. Rev. **18:** 206–228.
3. TURNBULL, A.V. *et al.* 1999. Regulation of the hypothalamic-pituitary-adrenal axis by cytokines: actions and mechanisms of action. Physiol. Rev. **79:** 1–71.
4. WILDER, R.L. 1995. Neuroendocrine-immune system interactions and autoimmunity. Annu. Rev. Immunol. **13:** 307–338.
5. CHROUSOS, G. 1998. Stressors, stress and neuroendocrine integration of the adaptive response. Ann. N.Y. Acad Sci. **851:** 311–335.
6. STRAUB, R.H., M. CUTOLO, B. ZIETZ, *et al.* 2001. The process of aging changes the interplay of the immune, endocrine and nervous systems. Mech. Ageing Dev. **122:** 1591–1611.
7. COLE, T.J. *et al.* 2005. Intrathymic glucocorticoid production and thymocyte survival: another piece in the puzzle. Endocrinology **146:** 2499–2500.
8. TUCKERMANN, J.P. *et al.* 2005. Molecular mechanisms of glucocorticoids in the control of inflammation and lymphocyte apoptosis. Crit. Rev. Clin. Lab. Sci. **42:** 71–104.
9. REICHARDT, H.M. 2004. Immunomodulatory activities of glucocorticoids: insights from transgenesis and gene targeting. Curr. Pharm. Des. **10:** 2797–2805.
10. ELENKOV, I.J. 2004. Glucocorticoids and the Th1/Th2 balance. Ann. N.Y. Acad. Sci. **1024:** 138.
11. CUTOLO, M. *et al.* 2003. Hypothalamic-pituitary-adrenocortical and gonadal functions in rheumatoid arthritis. Ann. N.Y. Acad. Sci. **992:** 107–117.
12. KUMAR, R. *et al.* 2005. Gene regulation by the glucocorticoid receptor: structure: function relationship. J. Steroid. Biochem. Mol. Biol. **94:** 383–394.
13. SMOAK, K.A. *et al.* 2004. Mechanisms of glucocorticoid receptor signaling during inflammation. Mech. Ageing Dev. **125:** 697–706.

14. SCUDELETTI, M. *et al.* 1999. Immune regulatory properties of corticosteroids: prednisone induces apoptosis of human T lymphocytes following the CD3 down-regulation. Ann. N.Y. Acad. Sci. **876:** 164–179.
15. SCUDELETTI, M. *et al.* 1990. New glucocorticoids: mechanisms of immunological activity at the cellular level and in the clinical setting. Ann. N. Y. Acad. Sci. **595:** 368–382.
16. INDIVERI, F. *et al.* 1983. Inhibitory effect of a low dose of prednisone on PHA-induced Ia antigen expression by human T cells and on proliferation of T cells stimulated with autologous PHA-T cells. Cell Immunol. **80:** 320–328.
17. SCUDELETTI, M. *et al.* 1999. Immune regulatory properties of corticosteroids: prednisone induces apoptosis of human T lymphocytes following the CD3 down-regulation. Ann. N.Y. Acad. Sci. **876:** 164–179.
18. FRANCHIMONT, D. 2004. Overview of the actions of glucocorticoids on the immune response: a good model to characterize new pathways of immunosuppression for new treatment strategies. Ann. N.Y. Acad. Sci. **1024:** 124–137.
19. LANZA, L. *et al.* 1996. Prednisone increases apoptosis in in vitro activated human peripheral blood T lymphocytes. Clin. Exp. Immunol. **103:** 482–490.
20. BARRAT, F.J. *et al.* 2002. In vitro generation of interleukin 10-producing regulatory CD4($^+$) T cells is induced by immunosuppressive drugs and inhibited by T helper type 1 (Th1)- and Th2-inducing cytokines. J. Exp. Med. **195:** 603–616.
21. KARAGIANNIDIS, C. *et al.* 2004. Glucocorticoids upregulate FOXP3 expression and regulatory T cells in asthma. J. Allergy Clin. Immunol. **114:** 1425–1433.
22. MATYSZAK, M.K. *et al.* 2000. Differential effects of corticosteroids during different stages of dendritic cell maturation. Eur. J. Immunol. **30:** 1233–1242.
23. NOCENTINI, G. *et al.* 1997. A new member of the tumor necrosis factor/nerve growth factor receptor family inhibits T cell receptor-induced apoptosis. Proc. Natl. Acad. Sci. USA **94:** 6216–6221.
24. WAJANT, H. *et al.* 2003. Tumor necrosis factor signaling. Cell Death Differ. **10:** 45–65.
25. MACEWAN, D. 2002. TNF ligands and receptors—a matter of life and death. Br. J. Pharmacol. **135:** 855–875.
26. GURNEY, A.L. *et al.* 1999. Identification of a new member of the tumor necrosis factor family and its receptor, a human ortholog of mouse GITR. Curr. Biol. **9:** 215–218.
27. SHIMIZU, J. *et al.* 2002. Stimulation of CD25(+)CD4(+) regulatory T cells through GITR breaks immunological self-tolerance. Nat. Immunol. **3:** 135–142.
28. JI, H.B. *et al.* 2004. Cutting edge: the natural ligand for glucocorticoid-induced TNF receptor-related protein abrogates regulatory T cell suppression. J. Immunol. **172:** 5823–5827.
29. RONCHETTI, S. *et al.* 2002. Role of GITR in activation response of T lymphocytes. Blood **100:** 350–352.
30. MCHUGH, R.S. *et al.* 2002. CD4(+)CD25(+) immunoregulatory T cells: gene expression analysis reveals a functional role for the glucocorticoid-induced TNF receptor. Immunity **16:** 311–323.
31. LI, Z. *et al.* 2003. Expression of glucocorticoid induced TNF receptor family related protein (GITR) on peripheral T cells from normal human donors and patients with non-infectious uveitis. J. Autoimmun. **21:** 83–92.
32. ZELENIKA, D. *et al.* 2002. Regulatory T cells overexpress a subset of Th2 gene transcripts. J. Immunol. **168:** 1069–1079.

33. LEVINGS, M.K. *et al.* 2002. Human CD25$^+$CD4$^+$ T suppressor cell clones produce transforming growth factor, but not interleukin 10, and are distinct from type 1 T regulatory cells. J. Exp. Med. **196:** 1335–1346.
34. SHIN, H.H. *et al.* 2002. Recombinant glucocorticoid induced tumor necrosis factor receptor (rGITR) induces NOS in murine macrophages. FEBS Lett. **514:** 275–280.
35. KIM, J.D. *et al.* 2003. Cloning and characterization of GITR ligand. Genes Immun. **4:** 564–569.
36. KWON, B. *et al.* 1999. Identification of a novel activation-inducible protein of the tumor necrosis factor receptor superfamily and its ligand. J. Biol. Chem. **274:** 6056–6061.
37. TONE, M. *et al.* 2003. Mouse glucocorticoid-induced tumor necrosis factor receptor ligand is co-stimulatory for T cells. Proc. Natl. Acad. Sci. USA **100:** 15059–15064.
38. KANAMARU, F. *et al.* 2004. Co-stimulation via glucocorticoid-induced TNF receptor in both conventional and CD25$^+$ regulatory CD4$^+$ T cells. J. Immunol. **172:** 7306–7314.
39. SPINICELLI, S. *et al.* 2002. GITR interacts with the pro-apoptotic protein Siva and induces apoptosis. Cell Death Differ. **9:** 1382–1384.
40. PRASAD, K.V. *et al.* 1997. CD27, a member of the tumor necrosis factor receptor family, induces apoptosis and binds to Siva, a proapoptotic protein. Proc. Natl. Acad. Sci. USA **94:** 6346–6351.
41. MURIGLAN, S.J. *et al.* 2004. GITR activation induces an opposite effect on alloreactive CD4(+) and CD8(+) T cells in graft-versus-host disease. J. Exp. Med. **200:** 149–157.
42. LA CAVA, A. *et al.* 2004. Ig-reactive CD4$^+$CD25$^+$ T cells from tolerized (New Zealand Black × New Zealand White) F1 mice suppress in vitro production of antibodies to DNA. J. Immunol. **173:** 3542–3548.
43. NOCENTINI, G. *et al.* 2005. GITR: a multifaceted regulator of immunity belonging to the tumor necrosis factor receptor superfamily. Eur. J. Immunol. **35:** 1016–1022.
44. SURI, A. *et al.* 2004. Regulation of autoimmune diabetes by non-islet-specific T cells—a role for the glucocorticoid-induced TNF receptor. Eur. J. Immunol. **34:** 447–454.
45. KOHM, A.P. *et al.* 2004. Cutting edge: ligation of the glucocorticoid-induced TNF receptor enhances autoreactive CD4$^+$ T cell activation and experimental autoimmune encephalomyelitis. J. Immunol. **172:** 4686–4690.
46. CUZZOCREA, S. *et al.* 2004. Glucocorticoid-induced TNF receptor family gene (GITR) knockout mice exhibit a resistance to splanchnic artery occlusion (SAO) shock. J. Leukoc. Biol. **76:** 933–940.
47. DITTMER, U. *et al.* 2004. Functional impairment of CD8(+) T cells by regulatory T cells during persistent retroviral infection. Immunity **20:** 293–303.
48. CALMELS, B. *et al.* 2005. Bypassing tumor-associated immune suppression with recombinant adenovirus constructs expressing membrane bound or secreted GITR-L. Cancer Gene Ther. **12:** 198–205.
49. GERSHON, R.K. *et al.* 1971. Infectious immunological tolerance. Immunology **21:** 903–913.
50. DIECKMANN, D. *et al.* 2001. Ex vivo isolation and characterization of CD4(+)CD25(+) T cells with regulatory properties from human blood. J. Exp. Med. **193:** 1303–1310.

51. JONULEIT, H. *et al.* 2002. Identification and functional characterization of human CD4(+)CD25(+) T cells with regulatory properties isolated from peripheral blood. J. Exp. Med. **193:** 1285–1294.
52. BANCHEREAU, J. *et al.* 2001. Dendritic cells and the control of immunity. Nature **392:** 245–252.
53. CASSIS, L. S. AIELLO & M. NORIS. 2005. Natural versus adaptive regulatory T cells. Contrib. Nephrol. **146:** 121–131.
54. DAMLE, N.K. *et al.* 1989. Antigen-specific suppressor T lymphocytes in man. Clin. Immunol. Immunopathol. **53:** S17–S24.
55. SERCARZ, E. *et al.* 1991. The distinctive specificity of antigen-specific suppressor T cells. Immunol. Today **12:** 111–118.
56. YUEN, M.H. *et al.* 1995. Immunoregulatory $CD8^+$ cells recognize antigen-activated $CD4^+$ cells in myasthenia gravis patients and in healthy controls. J. Immunol. **154:** 1508–1520.
57. FILACI, G. *et al.* 2002. $CD8^+$ T suppressor cells are back to the game: are they players in autoimmunity? Autoimmun. Rev. **1:** 279–283.
58. FILACI, G. *et al.* 2004. Non-antigen specific $CD8^+$ T suppressor lymphocytes. Clin. Exp. Med. **4:** 86–92.
59. FILACI, G. *et al.* 2004. Non-antigen specific $CD8^+$ T suppressor lymphocytes originate from $CD8^+CD28^-$. T cells and inhibit both T-cell proliferation and CTL function. Hum. Immunol. **65:** 142–156.
60. BALASHOV, K.E. *et al.* 1995. Inhibition of T cell responses by activated human $CD8^+$ T cells is mediated by interferon-γ and is defective in chronic progressive multiple sclerosis. J. Clin. Invest. **95:** 2711–2719.
61. FILACI, G. *et al.* 2001. Impairment of $CD8^+$ T suppressor cell function in patients with active systemic lupus erythematosus. J. Immunol. **166:** 6452–6457.
62. FILACI, G. *et al.* 2005. Non-antigen-specific $CD8^+$ T suppressor lymphocytes in diseases characterized by chronic immune responses and inflammation. Ann. N.Y. Acad. Sci. **1050:** 115–123.

Neuroendocrine Manifestations of Phospholipid Antibody Disease Identified by Long-Term Follow-Up Study of Patients with Phospholipid Antibodies

WILLIAM TRAVERSE, BEATRIZ TENDLER, CHARLES GALEA, SANTHANAN LAKSHMINARAYAN, AND ANN PARKE

Department of Medicine, University of Connecticut Health Center, Farmington Avenue, Farmington, CT, USA

Abstract: Recurrent clinical thrombotic episodes and/or recurrent fetal wastage are the clinical features of phospholipid antibody (aPL) syndrome, which is characterized by a bland thrombosis, but is not inflammatory, as is found in other connective tissue diseases such as systemic lupus erythematosus (SLE). Previous reports have suggested that some patients with primary aPL syndrome may progress to develop other autoimmune diseases, including inflammatory diseases such as SLE. The aim of this study was to determine the long-term outcome of women with aPL antibodies, with regard to progression of their underlying autoimmune disease. To that end, a retrospective study was made of women with aPL and primary aPL syndromes who had been followed at our institution for a minimum of 3 years. Charts were reviewed, patients interviewed, and laboratory tests were performed to determine whether the clinical nature of the disease and/or its autoantibody profile had changed. Thirty patients were enrolled into the study (29 with aPL syndrome, 1 with consistent aPL and no syndrome). Follow-up ranged from 3 to 22 years. Results were as follows: The autoimmune clinical features were unchanged in 27 patients, but 3 patients developed inflammatory disease, presenting with nasal chondritis (2), cutaneous vasculitis (3), and mucosal ulcer (1). In each case, these changes occurred during pregnancy or the immediate postpartum period. One patient fulfilled criteria for SLE as seen by a change in her autoantibody profile. Another incidental finding was that three other patients were diagnosed with papillary thyroid cancer, two being diagnosed during the follow-up period. In conclusion: (1) Inflammatory disease may develop in some patients with aPL and appears to be set off by pregnancy, a known trigger for clinical thrombotic events in aPL patients. (2) Thyroid cancer may be associated with

Address for correspondence: Ann Parke, Department of Medicine, University of Connecticut Health Center, Farmington Avenue, Farmington, CT, USA. Voice: 860-679-2161; fax: 860-679-1287 e-mail: parke@nso.uchc.edu

Ann. N.Y. Acad. Sci. 1069: 386–390 (2006).
doi: 10.1196/annals.1351.036

aPL, and this association warrants further study with larger number of patients.

KEYWORDS: **phospholipid antibodies; pregnancy; systemic lupus erythematosus; thrombosis; HELLP syndrome; papillary carcinoma of the thyroid**

INTRODUCTION

Antiphospholipid antibody syndrome (aPLS) is an autoimmune disease characterized clinically by (1) recurrent arterial and/or venous thrombosis and (2) recurrent early or unexplained late fetal losses. These clinical complaints are found associated with antibodies to phospholipid protein complexes (aPL).[1] Some experimental studies have suggested that these antibodies are directly involved in the pathogenesis of this disease.[2,3] Other clinical features have been described in patients with aPL syndrome, but these are not included in the current criteria. By definition, primary aPLS (PaPLS) occurs in the absence of a well-defined connective tissue disease. Some PaPLS patients produce other autoantibodies in addition to aPL and may be considered to have a lupus-like disease, but it is important to remember that the basic thrombotic pathology occurring in PaPLS is a bland noninflammatory thrombosis[4] and not an inflammatory vasculitis as is found in systemic lupus erythematosus (SLE). Some previous studies have, however, suggested that, in time, some PaPLS patients may progress to develop the clinical features of SLE,[5] or a lupus-like disease (LLD), that is, a disease that does not fulfill 4 of 11 ACR criteria for SLE. Because the basic pathology of SLE is an inflammatory vasculitis, this clinical change would suggest that a change in pathology may occur over time in some PaPLS patients. Not every patient with aPL develops the classical clinical syndrome, but in many of these aPL patients development of a clinical thrombotic event can be triggered by certain pathologic and physiological states, one of which is pregnancy.

Objective

Our goal was to determine whether, over time, patients with aPL or PaPLS present with new clinical complaints suggesting the development of an inflammatory pathology or they go on to develop 4 of 11 American Rheumatism Association criteria for SLE or fulfill criteria for another connective tissue disease.

METHODS

Forty-nine female patients followed for more than 3 years at the University of Connecticut Health Center (UCHC) with consistently positive aPL antibodies (lupus anticoagulant [LAC] or cardiolipin [aCL] antibodies), but not fulfilling criteria for any connective tissue disease, were eligible for inclusion in the study.

Disease progression was assessed by retrospective chart review, a questionnaire, physical examination and repeat tests for autoantibodies, and determination of complement levels, and complete blood count (CBC) and erythrocyte sedimentation rate (ESR). The autoantibody tests ordered included: antinuclear antibodies (ANA), double-stranded DNA antibodies, antibodies to Ro, La, Sm, RNP, aCL antibodies, and LAC.

RESULTS

To date, 30 patients have been enrolled into the study (29 with aPL syndrome and 1 patient with persistently positive aPL, follow-up of 14 years at UCHC, but no clinical complaints attributable to PaPLS).

Twenty-nine subjects were Caucasian and one Hispanic, with an age range of 17–58 years at the time of presentation. Follow-up varied from 3 to 20 years with a mean of approximately 10 years. Our initial studies, presented at an earlier meeting, suggested that despite consistently positive phospholipid antibodies, complement abnormalities, and elevated ESRs, these primary phospholipid antibody patients did not develop new clinical complaints suggestive of inflammatory disease. However, additional study has now identified three PaPLS patients who have developed new clinical complaints suggestive of an inflammatory pathology; and in each case, these changes occurred during pregnancy or in the immediate postpartum period. The first patient with a history of a deep venous thrombosis, pulmonary embolus, and late fetal wastage developed a malar rash, oral mucosal ulcers, chondritis of the nasal cartilage, and an infarct of her ear 8 days post partum after her third pregnancy. This patient had never previously had any clinical complaints consistent with SLE, but she went on to develop anti-ds-DNA antibodies and low levels of complement, which had not been found at initial presentation and so fulfilled criteria for SLE. Two other patients both developed hemolysis, elevated liver enzymes, and low platelet (HELLP)/HELLP-like syndrome at 19- and 21-weeks of gestation, respectively. One HELLP patient also developed severe preeclampsia with hypertension and 14 g of proteinuria. At the time of the HELLP syndrome both of these patients developed inflammatory skin lesions on the palms and soles, not usually a feature of HELLP syndrome. One of these HELLP patients also developed nasal chondritis. These two patients did not develop any change in their autoantibody profiles. All three patients responded to high-dose corticosteroids and have done well.

An incidental finding detected during this study determined that 3 of the 30 PaPLS patients studied have been diagnosed with papillary carcinoma of the thyroid, two after the diagnosis of PaPLS/apl positivity. A variety of malignancies have been described in association with aPL syndrome, but to our knowledge papillary carcinoma of the thyroid is not one of these reported associations.[6]

DISCUSSION

The immunology of pregnancy is extremely complex.[7] The known immune modulation, switching from Th1cytokine production to Th2 cytokines,[8,9] can help to explain the known benefit of pregnancy for patients with rheumatoid arthritis.[10] The effect of pregnancy on the clinical expression of other autoimmune diseases is less predictable, and an abnormal pregnancy may be one of the earliest manifestations of an underlying, subclinical autoimmune diathesis.[11,12] This study suggests that pregnancy is a particularly dangerous time for some patients with phospholipid antibodies, as both clinical thrombotic events and *de novo* clinical inflammatory events may be precipitated by pregnancy and/or the immediate postpartum period.

CONCLUSIONS

1. Most patients with aPL/PaPLS remain clinically stable and do not progress to develop SLE despite persistent laboratory abnormalities.
2. Some patients never develop the clinical features of the syndrome despite persistently high levels of aPL.
3. Pregnancy appears to be a physiological event capable of triggering some PaPLS patients into developing new clinical complaints consistent with an inflammatory pathology and even SLE.
4. Papillary carcinoma of the thyroid may be associated with aPL and aPL syndromes and this association warrants further study with larger number of patients.

REFERENCES

1. Wilson, W., A.E. Gharavi, T. Koike, *et al.* 1999. International consensus statement on preliminary classification criteria for definite antiphospholipid syndrome. Arthritis Rheum. **42:** 1309–1311.
2. Shoenfeld, Y., Y. Sherer, M. Blank. 1998 Antiphospholipid syndrome in pregnancy—animal models and clinical implications. Scand. J. Rheumatol. Suppl. **10:** 33–36.
3. Ornoy, A., S. Yacobi, S.T. Matalon, *et al.* 2003. The effects of antiphospholipid antibodies obtained from women with SLE/APS and associated pregnancy loss on rat embryos and placental explants in culture. Lupus **8:** 573–578.
4. Lie, J.T. 1996. Pathology of antiphospholipid syndrome. *In* The Antiphospholipid Syndrome. 89–104. CRC Press. Boca Raton, FL.

5. CARBONE, J., M. ORERA, M. RODRIGUEZ-MAHOU, *et al.* 1999. Immunological abnormalities in primary APS evolving into SLE: 6 years follow-up in women with repeated pregnancy loss. Lupus **8:** 274–278.
6. GOMEZ-PUERTA, J.A., R. CERVERA, G. ESPINOSA, *et al.* 2006. Antiphospholipid antibodies associated with malignancies: clinical and pathological characteristics of 120 patients. Semin. Arthritis Rheum. **35:** 322–332.
7. VAN NIEUWENHOVEN, A.L., M.J. HEINEMAN, M.M. FAAS. 2003. The immunology of successful pregnancy. Hum. Reprod. Update **9:** 347–357.
8. MARZI, A. VIGANO, D. TRABATTONI, *et al.* 1996. Characterization of type 1 and type 2 cytokine production profile in physiologic and pathologic human pregnancy. Clin. Exp. Immunol. **106:** 127–133.
9. PICCINNI, M.P., C. SCALETTI, M. MAGGI, *et al.* 2000. Role of hormone controlled T cell cytokines in the maintenance of pregnancy. Biochem. Soc. Trans. **28:** 212–215.
10. HENCH, P.S. 1938. The ameliorating effect of pregnancy on chronic atrophic (infectious rheumatoid) arthritis, fibrositis, and intermittent hydrarthrosis. Mayo Clin. Proc. **13:** 161–167.
11. GLEICHER, N., A. EL-ROEIY, E. CONFINO, *et al.* 1989. Reproductive failure because of autoantibodies: unexplained infertility and pregnancy wastage. Am. J. Obstet. Gynecol. **160:** 1376–1385.
12. ROTE, N.S. & B.P. STETZER. 2003. Autoimmune diseases as a cause of reproductive failure. Clin. Lab. Med. **23:** 265–293.

Anti-TNF and Sex Hormones

MAURIZIO CUTOLO,[a] ALBERTO SULLI,[a] SILVIA CAPELLINO,[b] BARBARA VILLAGGIO,[a] PAOLA MONTAGNA,[a] CARMEN PIZZORNI,[a] SABRINA PAOLINO,[a] BRUNO SERIOLO,[a] LAMBERTO FELLI, AND RAINER H. STRAUB[b]

[a]*Research Laboratory and Division of Rheumatology, Department of Internal Medicine–University of Genova, 16132 Genova, Italy*

[b]*Laboratory NeuroEndocrinoImmunology, Department of Internal Medicine I, University Hospital, Regensburg, Germany*

ABSTRACT: Whenever serum estrogen concentrations are normal in rheumatoid arthritis (RA) patients, lower androgen concentrations (i.e., testosterone, androstenedione, and dehydroepiandrosterone sulfate [DHEAS]) are detected in the serum as well as in the synovial fluid of male and female RA patients. The presence in the RA synovial fluid of a significant altered sex hormone balance resulting in lower immunosuppressive androgens and higher immuno-enhancing estrogens, might determine a favorable condition for the development of the immunomediated RA synovitis. The inflammatory cytokines (i.e., TNF-α), particularly increased in RA synovitis, are able to markedly stimulate the aromatase activity in peripheral tissues and, therefore, induce the peripheral metabolism from androgens to estrogens. The effects of TNF blockers (and generally of anticytokine agents) on peripheral sex hormone levels seem exerted in a faster way at the level of the RA synovial tissue (before any influence on serum levels) where they seem to block the conversion from androgens (anti-inflammatory) to estrogens (proinflammatory) induced by aromatase. Therefore, the beneficial effects of restoring synovial androgens might be clinically more evident in male RA patients (as recently observed in ANTARES study) since they suffer more for the lack of androgens (anti-inflammatory) on account of the action of TNF-α on peripheral hormonal conversion. However, therapy (3 months) with anti-TNF did not change serum levels of typical sex hormones in patients with RA, although baseline values were largely different from controls. In patients with at least long-standing RA, this indicates that alterations of serum sex hormones and altered activity of respective converting enzymes are imprinted for a long-lasting period over at least 12 weeks.

Address for correspondence: Maurizio Cutolo, Research Laboratory and Division of Rheumatology, Department of Internal Medicine–University of Genova, Viale Benedetto XV6, 16132, Genova, Italy. Voice: +39-010-353-7994; fax: +39-010-353-8885.

e-mail: mcutolo@unige.it

Ann. N.Y. Acad. Sci. 1069: 391–400 (2006).
doi: 10.1196/annals.1351.037

Keywords: anti-TNF-α therapy; adalimumab; biologic drugs; TNF-α blockers; estrogens; androgens; sex hormones; rheumatoid arthritis; synovial fluid; macrophages

INTRODUCTION

Tumor necrosis factor (TNF) is supposed to have a pivotal role in the pathogenesis of rheumatoid arthritis (RA) synovitis.[1] The direct pathogenic effects of TNF are amplified by its ability to induce other proinflammatory cytokines, such as IL-1, as well as granulocyte macrophage colony stimulating factor, adhesion molecules, prostaglandin E2, and matrix metalloproteinases, involved in the joint degradation exerted by the synovial tissue. TNF also stimulates the production of the soluble TNF receptors (sTNF-R), which may act as its natural inhibitors. Recently, levels of TNF-α, p55, and p75 sTNF-R were higher in the serum of patients with RA with follicular synovitis than in patients with diffuse synovitis ($P < 0.001$, $P < 0.01$, and $P < 0.05$, respectively). Serum concentrations of TNF-α, p55, and p75 sTNF-R correlated with markers of disease activity.[2]

Monocytes/macrophages contribute to autoimmune events in rheumatic diseases, such as RA or systemic lupus erythematosus (SLE), mainly acting

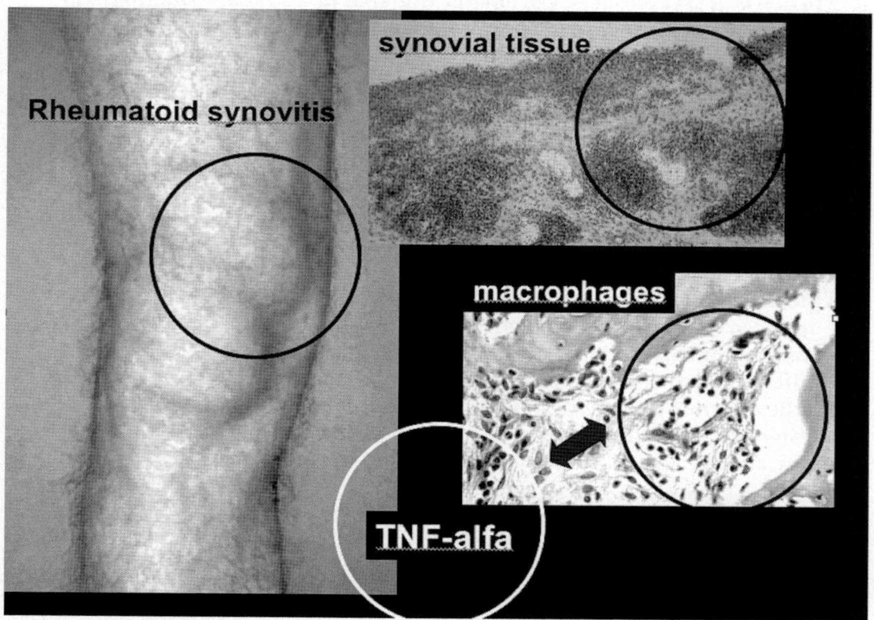

FIGURE 1. Synovial tissue of a patient affected by RA. Synovial macrophages are the more active inflammatory cells and produce large amounts of TNF-α.

as antigen-processing and presenting cells in the presence of an autoimmune rheumatic disease as well as major producers of TNF-α[3] (FIG. 1).

Clinical symptoms, such as morning stiffness and gelling, at least in RA, that peak during the late night and early morning, are consistent with the hypothesis that the immune function of activated cells (i.e., Th1 cells and monocytes/macrophages) and their mediators (cytokines and reactive oxygen intermediates) is increased at these times in relation to neuroendocrine pathway rhythmicity.[4]

In addition, functional gonadal hormones have been detected in synovial macrophages.[5] Therefore, monocytes/macrophages seem to be the "link" between the steroid hormone environment (i.e., gonadal hormones) and the immune response effectors (i.e, TNF-α).

PERIPHERAL ESTROGEN METABOLISM IN RA SYNOVIAL TISSUE: ROLE OF TNF-α

Whenever serum estrogen concentrations are normal in RA patients, lower androgen concentrations (i.e., testosterone, androstenedione, and dehydroepiandrosterone sulfate [DHEAS]) are detected in the serum as well as in the synovial fluid of male and female RA patients.[6,7]

The presence in the RA synovial fluid of an altered sex hormone balance resulting in lower immunosuppressive androgens and higher immuno-enhancing estrogens, might determine a favorable condition for the development of the immuno-mediated RA synovitis.

The appropriate explanation of lower androgen and higher estrogen levels in both female and male RA synovial fluid might be related to the increase of the inflammatory cytokines in RA synovitis (i.e.,TNF-α, IL-6, and IL-1) that are able to markedly stimulate the aromatase activity in peripheral tissues (FIG. 2).[8–10]

As a matter of fact, the aromatase enzyme complex is involved in the peripheral conversion of androgens (testosterone and androstenedione) to

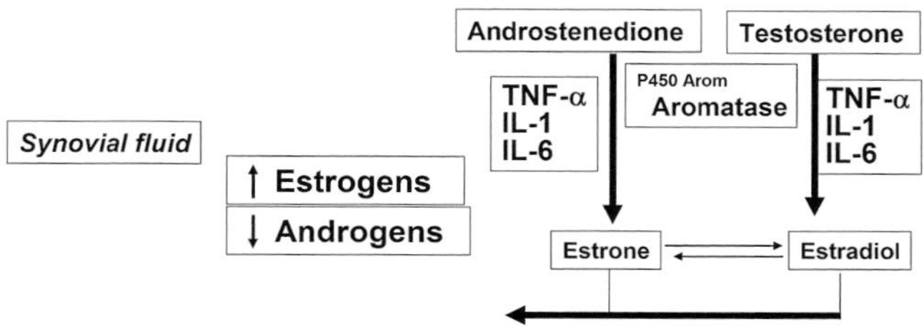

FIGURE 2. The appropriate explanation of lower androgen and higher estrogen levels in both female and male RA synovial fluid might be related to the increase of the inflammatory cytokines in RA synovitis (i.e., TNF-a, IL-6, and IL-1) that are able to markedly stimulate the aromatase activity in peripheral tissues.

estrogens (estrone and estradiol, respectively). In tissues rich of macrophages, a significant correlation was found between the aromatase activity and the IL-6 production, and aromatase has been found also in synoviocytes.[11]

Therefore, the increased aromatase activity induced by locally produced inflammatory cytokines (i.e., TNF-α, IL-1, and IL-6) might explain the altered balance resulting in lower androgens and higher estrogens in the synovial RA fluids, as well as their effects on synovial cells, first described by us.[12] The role of local sex hormone concentrations at the level of inflammatory foci is of great value in order to explain the modulatory effects exerted by these hormones on the immune–inflammatory reaction. Recently, they were tested in 12 patients with RA and 8 patients with traumatic knee injury (noninflammatory controls), synovial fluid steroid concentrations that were measured by HPLC and mass spectrometry.[13]

Overall synovial fluid concentration of free estrogens tended to be higher in RA as compared to controls ($P = 0.06$). Molar ratio of free synovial fluid estrogens/synovial fluid androgens was elevated in RA as compared to controls ($P = 0.017$). Synovial fluid concentration of the precursor androstenedione was higher in RA as compared to controls ($P = 0.011$), and synovial fluid estrone, the aromatase conversion product of androstenedione, was also elevated in RA versus controls ($P = 0.035$). The most biologically active estrogens, 16a-hydroxyestrone and 4-hydroxyestradiol, were higher in RA as compared to controls ($P = 0.085$ and $P = 0.044$, respectively). In mixed synoviocytes, DHEA conversion yielded high local levels of estrogens as compared to androgens. This study clearly demonstrates that local levels of proinflammatory estrogens relative to androgens are significantly elevated in patients with RA as compared to controls, which is most probably on account of increased aromatase activity (TNF-α induced). Thus, available steroid prehormones (mainly androgens) are rapidly converted to proinflammatory estrogens in the synovial tissue.

In addition, *in situ* estrogen synthesis through local aromatase activity in the tumor and adjacent tissue is probably a very important growth-stimulating system in hormone-dependent breast cancer.[14]

This synthesis can be blocked with aromatase inhibitors. There seems to be a complex interaction between malignant cells and adjacent cells in which factors, such as TNF-α, IL-6 and its soluble receptor, and prostaglandin E2 play an important role in stimulating aromatase activity.

PREVALENCE OF HYDROXYLATED ESTROGENS IN RA SYNOVIAL FLUID

The increased estrogen concentrations observed in RA synovial fluid of both sexes are characterized by the hydroxylated forms, in particular 16a-hydroxyestrone and 4-hydroxyestradiol, whereas the 2-hydroxyestrone was found similar to the controls.[12,13] Other studies in breast cancer research delineated that 16a-hydroxyestrone is a mitogenic and proliferative endogenous hormone that covalently binds to the estrogen receptor leading to nuclear translocation.[15,16]

16a-Hydroxyestrone is converted from upstream estrone and E2, and shows persistent biological responses consisting in a mitogenic tumor growth-stimulating role.

Other conversion products of estrone and E2 are the 2-hydroxylated estrogens, such as 2-hydroxyestrone and 2-hydroxyestradiol. In contrast to 16a-hydroxylated estrogens, the 2-hydroxylated forms inhibit growth-promoting effects of E2.[17] In this respect, 2-hydroxyestrone has anticarcinogenic properties and, thus, it is most likely a naturally occurring antiestrogen.[18] In a recent study, urinary levels of 2-hydroxylated estrogens were found 10 times lower in RA patients than in healthy controls, whereas the ratio 16a-hydroxyestrone2-hydroxyestrogens was found 20 times higher in RA patients then in healthy controls.[13]

The relative loss of 2-hydroxylated estrogens in relation to the mitogenic 16a-hydroxyestrone might thus be an important switch to support the proliferative state of the synovial cells in RA. Therefore, dose-related conversion to pro- or anti-inflammatory downstream metabolites of estrogens might also support the dual role of estrogens (pro- or anti-inflammatory) for example during estrogen replacement therapy, depending on local concentration (i.e., synovial fluid in RA) of 16a-hydroxyestrone or 2-hydroxyestrogens.

ESTROGENS REGULATE TNFR EXPRESSION BY BREAST FIBROBLASTS

Recently, it was demonstrated that malignant epithelial cells produce large amounts of TNF-α that inhibit the differentiation of breast fibroblasts. TNF action is mediated by its two receptors (TNFRs), TNFR1, which mediates inhibition of adipocyte differentiation, and TNFR2, which was linked to the proliferation of thymocytes.[19] There is evidence that estrogen modulates the synthesis of receptors for TNF in human adipose fibroblasts (HAFs) from breast tissue in a paracrine fashion, which may serve as a mechanism for the inhibition of adipocyte differentiation in breast cancer. Estradiol treatment increased TNFR1 mRNA and protein levels in primary HAFs in a dose- and time-dependent manner, which could be reversed by the estrogen antagonist ICI182,780. Interestingly, higher concentration of estradiol inhibited whereas lower concentrations stimulated TNFR2 mRNA levels in HAFs.

EFFECTS OF ANTI-TNF-α THERAPY ON SERUM SEX HORMONES IN RA PATIENTS

Androgens, such as DHEAS and testosterone are markedly lower in postmenopausal women with RA than in controls. In contrast, compared to controls, serum levels of estrogens are normal or elevated in women with RA. Since TNF alters production of these hormones, it is interesting to investigate changes of these hormones during 12 weeks of anti-TNF antibody (anti-TNF) therapy with adalimumab in long-standing RA.

In a recent longitudinal anti-TNF therapy study, 13 patients with long-standing RA without prior prednisolone (7 infusions of anti-TNF: Week 0, 2, 4, 6, 8, 10, and 12 serum concentrations of IL-6, androstenedione, DHEA, DHEAS, free testosterone, estrone, and 17ß-estradiol[20]) were measured. Levels of these hormones in patients were compared to serum levels of 31 age- and sex-matched healthy controls.

Upon treatment with anti-TNF, there was an impressive decrease of clinical markers of inflammation, erythrocyte sedimentation rate, and serum levels of IL-6. Serum levels of DHEAS and free testosterone were markedly lower at baseline in patients compared to controls, but this did not change during anti-TNF therapy. Serum levels of DHEA and 17ß-estradiol were significantly elevated in patients compared to controls, but similarly, anti-TNF therapy did not change initially increased levels. Molar ratios of hormones, which reflect hormone shifts via converting enzymes, showed typical alterations at base line, but did not change markedly during anti-TNF therapy.

In conclusion, therapy (3 months) with anti-TNF did not change altered serum levels of typical sex hormones in patients with RA, although baseline values were largely different. In patients with at least long-standing RA, this indicates that alterations of sex hormones and altered activity of respective converting enzymes are imprinted for a long-lasting period over at least 12 weeks.

EFFECTS OF ANTI-TNF-α THERAPY ON CLINICAL RESPONSIVENESS IN RA PATIENTS OF BOTH SEXES

Interesting results have been recently observed in a very recent Italian post-marketing study on anti-TNF-α agents in RA therapy (ANTARES study). Over a total number of 1707 RA patients treated with biologic agents (60% infliximab, 38% embrel, and 3.7% anakinra) significant results gender linked were apparently obtained concerning the responsiveness after 14 weeks of treatment (Momtecucco CM, personal communication).

As a matter of fact, the American College of Rheumatology (ACR) criteria responsiveness was found significantly higher ($P < 0.05$) in male RA patients when compared to female ones (ratio 1.36:1.00) (FIG. 3).

There are several possible explanations. The effects of TNF blockers (and generally of anticytokine agents) on peripheral sex hormone levels seem exerted in a faster way at the level of the RA synovial tissue (before any influence on serum levels) where they seem to block the conversion

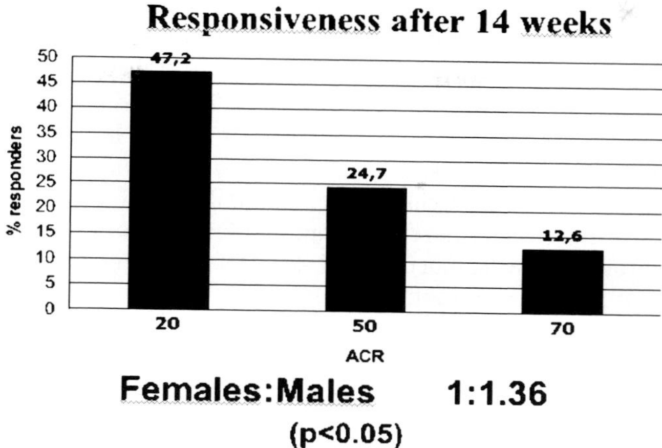

FIGURE 3. In the ANTARES study the ACR criteria responsiveness was found significantly higher ($P < 0.05$) in male RA patients when compared to female ones (ratio 1.36:1.00) (Montecucco CM personal communication).

from androgens (anti-inflammatory) to estrogens (proinflammatory) through aromatase.

Therefore, the beneficial effects of restoring synovial androgens might be clinically more evident in male RA patients since they suffer more from the lack of androgens (anti-inflammatory) on account of the action of TNF-α on peripheral hormonal conversion.

Androgens exert anti-inflammatory activities when compared to estrogens.[21] In particular, testosterone has immune modulating properties, and current *in vitro* evidence suggests that testosterone may suppress the expression of the proinflammatory cytokines TNF-α, IL-1β, and IL-6 and potentiate the expression of the anti-inflammatory cytokine IL-10.

A recent randomized, single-blind, placebo-controlled, crossover study of testosterone replacement (Sustanon 100) versus placebo in 27 men (age, 62 ± 9 years) with symptomatic androgen deficiency (total testosterone, 4.4 ± 1.2 nmol/L; bioavailable testosterone, 2.4 ± 1.1 nmol/L) was realized for 1 month.[22]

Compared with placebo, testosterone induced reductions in TNF-α (−3.1 ± 8.3 versus 1.3 ± 5.2 pg/mL; $P = 0.01$) and IL-1β (−0.14 ± 0.32 versus 0.18 ± 0.55 pg/mL; $P = 0.08$) and an increase in IL-10 (0.33 ± 1.8 versus −1.1 ± 3.0 pg/mL; $P = 0.01$); the reductions of TNF-α and IL-1β were positively correlated [$r(S) = 0.588$; $P = 0.003$].

The study seems to confirm that testosterone replacement shifts the cytokine balance to a state of reduced inflammation.

OTHER ACTIONS OF GONADAL HORMONES MIGHT BE MODULATED BY TNF-α BLOCKING

Recently, the effects of 17β-estradiol and of testosterone were tested on the cultured human monocytic/ macrophage cell line (THP-1) activated with IFN-γ in order to investigate their role in cell proliferation and apoptosis.[23]

Activated human THP-1 cells were cultured in the presence of 17β-estradiol and testosterone (final concentration, 10 nM). The evaluation of markers of cell proliferation included the NF-kB DNA-binding assay, the NF-kB inhibition complex, the proliferating cell nuclear antigen expression and the methyltetrazolium salt test. Apoptosis was detected by the annexin Vpropidium assay and by the cleaved poly-ADP ribose polymerase expression. Increased poly-ADP ribose polymerase-cleaved expression and decreased proliferating cell nuclear antigen expression, as well as an increase of IkB-α and a decrease of the IkB-α phosphorylated form (ser 32), were found in testosterone-treated THP-1 cells. However, the NF-kB DNA binding was found increased in 17β-estradiol-treated THP-1 cells, confirming that estrogens enhance the proliferative/inflammatory cell activity. Therefore, treatment of THP-1 by sex hormones was found to influence cell proliferation and apoptosis. Androgens were found to increase the apoptosis, and estrogens showed a protective trend on cell death both acting as modulators of the NF-kB complex.

Therefore, the reduction of aromatase-induced synovial estrogen formation by blocking TNF-α, might further exert antiproliferative/anti-inflammatory effects on RA synovitis.

CONCLUSIONS

TNF-α increases the peripheral (i.e., synovial tissue) conversion of androgens to estrogens through increase of the aromatase activity. Estrogens mainly exert cell proliferative and proinflammatory activities and are involved in RA synovitis in both sexes.

The TNF-α blockers seem to induce more significant clinical effects in male RA patients since they suffer more for the lack of androgens (anti-inflammatory) on account of the action of TNF-α on peripheral hormonal conversion.

Androgens exert potent anti-inflammatory activities.

Further studies on synovial sex hormone metabolism in RA patients during anti-TNF therapy are in progress.

REFERENCES

1. Firestein, G.S. 2005. Pathogenesis of rheumatoid arthritis: how early is early? Arthritis Res. Ther. **7:** 157–159.

2. KLIMIUK, P.A., S. SIERAKOWSKI, R. LATOSIEWICZ, *et al.* 2003. Circulating tumour necrosis factor alpha and soluble tumour necrosis factor receptors in patients with different patterns of rheumatoid synovitis. Ann. Rheum. Dis. **62:** 472–475.
3. CUTOLO, M. 1999. Macrophages as effectors of the immunoendocrinologic interactions in autoimmune rheumatic diseases. Ann. N. Y. Acad. Sci. **876:** 32–41.
4. CUTOLO, M. & A.T. MASI. 2005. Circadian rhythms and arthritis. Rheum. Dis. Clin. North Am. **31:** 115–129.
5. CUTOLO, M., S. ACCARDO, B. VILLAGGIO, *et al.* 1996. Androgen and estrogen receptors are present in primary cultures of human synovial macrophages. J. Clin. Endocrinol. Metab. **81:** 820–827.
6. CUTOLO, M., E. BALLEARI, M. GIUSTI, *et al.* 1986. Sex hormone status in women suffering from rheumatoid arthritis. J. Rheumatol. **13:** 1019–1023.
7. DE LATORRE, B., M. HEDMAN, E. OLESEN, *et al.* 1997. Relationship between blood and joint tissue DHEAS levels in rheumatoid arthritis and osteoarthritis. Clin. Exp. Rheumatol. **56:** 281–284.
8. NESTLER, J.E. 1993. Interleukin-1 stimulates aromatase activity of human placental cytotrophoblasts. Endocrinology **132:** 566–570.
9. MACDIARMID, F., D. WANG & L.G. DUNCAN. 1994. Stimulation of aromatase activity in breast fibroblasts by tumor necrosis factor alpha. Mol. Cell. Endocrinol. **106:** 17–21.
10. PUROHIT, A., M.W. GHILCHIC & L. DUNCAN. 1995. Aromatase activity and interleukin-6 production by normal and malignant breast tissues. J. Clin. Endocrinol. Metab. **80:** 3052–3058.
11. LE BAIL, J., B. LIAGRE, P. VERGNE, *et al.* 2001. Aromatase in synovial cells from postmenopausal women. Steroids **66:** 749–757.
12. CASTAGNETTA, L., M. CUTOLO, O. GRANATA, *et al.* 1996. Endocrine end-points in rheumatoid arthritis. Ann. N. Y. Acad. Sci. **876:** 180–192.
13. CASTAGNETTA, L., G. CARRUBA, O. GRANATA, *et al.* 2003. Increased estrogen to androgen ratio in the synovial fluid of patients with rheumatoid arthritis. J. Rheumatol. **30:** 2597–2605.
14. DE JONG, P.C., M.A. BLANKENSTEIN, J. VAN DE VEN, *et al.* 2001. Importance of local aromatase activity in hormone-dependent breast cancer: a review. Breast **10:** 91–99.
15. SWANECK, G.E. & J. FISHMAN. 1988. Covalent binding of the endogenous estrogen 16 alpha-hydroxyestrone to estradiol receptor in human breast cancer cells: characterization and intranuclear localization. Proc. Natl. Acad. Sci. USA **85:** 7831–7835.
16. TELANG, N.T., A. SUTO, G.Y. WON, *et al.* 1992. Induction by estrogen metabolite 16 alpha-hydroxyestrone of genotoxic damage and aberrant proliferation in mouse mammary epithelial cells. J. Natl. Cancer. Inst. **15:** 634–638.
17. SCHNEIDE, J., M.M. HUH, H.L. BRADLOW, *et al.* 1984. Antiestrogen action of 2-hydroxyestrone on MCF-7 human breast cancer cells. J. Biol. Chem. **259**(Suppl): 4840–4845.
18. BRADLOW, H.L., N.T. TELANG, D.W. SEPKOVIC, *et al.* 1992. 2-hydroxyestrone: the 'good' estrogen. J. Endocrinol. **150:** S259–S265.
19. DEB, S., S. AMIN, A.G. IMIR, *et al.* 2004. Estrogen regulates expression of tumor necrosis factor receptors in breast adipose fibroblasts. J. Clin. Endocrinol. Metab. **89:** 4018–4024.

20. STRAUB, R.H., P. HARLE, F. ATZENI, *et al.* 2005. Sex hormone concentrations in patients with rheumatoid arthritis are not normalized during 12 weeks of anti-tumor necrosis factor therapy. J. Rheumatol. **32:** 1253–1258.
21. CUTOLO, M. & R.G. LAHITA. 2005. Estrogens and arthritis. Rheum. Dis. Clin. North. Am. **31:** 19–27.
22. MALKIN, C.J., P.J. PUGH, R.D. JONES, *et al.* 2004. The effect of testosterone replacement on endogenous inflammatory cytokines and lipid profiles in hypogonadal men. J. Clin. Endocrinol. Metab. **8:** 3313–3318.
23. CUTOLO, M., P. MONTAGNA, S. CAPELLINO, *et al.* 2005. Sex hormone modulation of cell growth and apoptosis of human monocytic/macrophage cells. Arthritis. Res. Ther. **7:** R1124–R1132.

DHEA Metabolism in Arthritis

A Role for the p450 Enzyme Cyp7b at the Immune–Endocrine Crossroad

JOHN DULOS AND ANNEMIEKE H. BOOTS

Department of Pharmacology, N.V. Organon, 5340 BH Oss, The Netherlands

ABSTRACT: For dehydroepiandrosterone (DHEA) both immunosuppressive and immuno-stimulating properties have been described. The immunosuppressive effects may be explained by the conversion of DHEA into androgens and/or estrogens. The described immuno-stimulating effects of DHEA may be due to the conversion of DHEA into 7α-hydroxy-DHEA (7α-OH-DHEA) by the activity of the p450 enzyme, Cyp7b. 7α-OH-DHEA is thought to have anti-glucocoticoid activity preventing the anti-inflammatory action of endogenous glucocorticoids. To investigate a putative role of Cyp7b in the arthritic process, tissues from both the murine collagen-induce arthritis (CIA) model and from patients with rheumatoid arthritis (RA) were studied. We determined the Cyp7b expression levels in synovial tissue and the level of 7α-OH-DHEA in both serum and arthritic joints of mice with CIA. Our studies showed that the severity of arthritis correlates with increased Cyp7b activity. Next, we investigated Cyp7b expression and activity in RA patients where the proinflammatory cytokines tumor necrosis factor-α (TNF-α) and interleukin-1β (IL-1β) are known to control the disease process. Fibroblast-like synoviocytes (FLS), isolated from RA synovial biopsies were found to express Cyp7b mRNA. In addition, Cyp7b enzymatic activity was detected in these cells. We also investigated whether Cyp7b activity is regulated by cytokines. Proinflammatory (e.g., TNF-α and IL-1β) cytokines were found to stimulate Cyp7b activity and the anti-inflammatory cytokine transforming growth factor-β (TGF-β) was found to suppress Cyp7b activity in FLS. Next, we studied which signal transduction pathway is involved in the TNF-α-mediated induction of Cyp7b activity in human FLS. The results show a role for nuclear factor κ B (NFκB) and activator protein-1 (AP-1) in the regulation of Cyp7b expression. Finally, we established that the effects of DHEA or 7α-OH-DHEA on the immune system can not be explained by glucocorticoid receptor (GR) engagement. The role of the p450 enzyme Cyp7b in DHEA metabolism and its relevance in the arthritic process will be discussed.

Address for correspondence: John Dulos, Department of Pharmacology, Section Autoimmunity, Room RE3211, N.V. Organon, PO Box 20, 5340 BH Oss, The Netherlands. Voice: +31-0-412- 663748; fax: +31-0-412-663532.
e-mail: John.Dulos@Organon.com

Ann. N.Y. Acad. Sci. 1069: 401–413 (2006).
doi: 10.1196/annals.1351.038

Keywords: rheumatoid arthritis; DHEA 7-hydroxylase; Cyp7b; TNF-α; IL-1β; cytokines

INTRODUCTION

Rheumatoid arthritis (RA) is characterized by a chronic inflammation of the joints ultimately resulting in the destruction of cartilage and bone. The pathogenesis of RA is still unknown. Mediators of the endocrine system like dehydroepiandrosterone (DHEA), androgen, estrogen, and glucocorticoids are all known to influence the disease process in RA.[1,2] Among these endocrine mediators, DHEA and its sulfate form DHEAS, are the most abundant prohormones formed *in vivo*[3] and can be found in blood and synovial fluid.[4]

For DHEA both immunosuppressive[5–7] and immuno-stimulating[8–10] properties have been described. The immunosuppressive effects may be explained by the conversion of DHEA into androgens and/or estrogens.[1,11] The described immuno-stimulating effects of DHEA may be due to the conversion of DHEA into 7α-hydroxy-DHEA (7α-OH-DHEA).[9] Previous studies suggested that 7α-OH-DHEA acts as an anti-glucocorticoid that can block the glucocorticoid-induced immuno-suppression.[12,13] If so, the local balance between DHEA metabolites and endogenous glucocorticoids might be disturbed in inflammatory diseases.[13]

To date, three p450 7α-hydroxylase isoenzymes are known, Cyp7A, Cyp39A, and Cyp7b. Cyp7A[14] is expressed in liver and Cyp39A1[15] is expressed in brain; both are involved in the elimination of cholesterol. Cyp7b is not restricted to the liver or the brain and is expressed in various tissues and cells including thymus and lymphocytes.[16] The DHEA metabolite 7α-OH-DHEA and to a lesser extent 7β-OH-DHEA are formed by the activity of the cytochrome P450 enzyme, Cyp7b.[17–21] We propose that enhanced Cyp7b activity, resulting in enhanced levels of 7α-OH-DHEA, might play a proinflammatory role in the disease process.[20,21] Increased Cyp7b activity is thought to result in increased 7α-OH-DHEA levels but may also result in a decline in DHEA levels as observed in inflammatory diseases like RA.[11]

To investigate the possible involvement of Cyp7b in the arthritic process, tissue samples from the murine collagen-induced arthritis (CIA) model and from patients with RA were studied. First, we determined the level of 7α-OH-DHEA in both serum and arthritic joints of mice with CIA. Second, the effect of cytokines (proinflammatory and anti-inflammatory) on Cyp7b mRNA expression and Cyp7b activity in fibroblast-like synoviocytes (FLS) from RA patients was studied. After establishing that tumor necrosis factor-α (TNF-α), known to play a crucial role in the pathogenesis of RA,[22] mediates an increase in Cyp7b activity, we investigated which signal transduction pathway is involved in the TNF-α-mediated increase in Cyp7b activity in human FLS. Finally, we investigated whether the mechanism of action of DHEA (or its catabolized metabolites) can be explained by the engagement (agonistic or antagonistic activity) of the glucocorticoid receptor (GR).

RESULTS AND DISCUSSION

Increased 7α-OH-DHEA Levels in Arthritic Joints

We studied 7α-OH-DHEA levels in knee synovial biopsies of arthritic versus nonarthritic collagen-II-immunized mice. A fivefold increase in 7α-OH-DHEA levels was observed in knee joint synovial biopsies of arthritic mice versus non-arthritic mice (FIG. 1A). The increase in 7α-OH-DHEA proved to be a local phenomenon because enhanced levels of 7α-OH-DHEA were not found in the serum of these mice (FIG. 1A). Interestingly, the 7α-OH-DHEA levels in the knee synovial biopsies were higher than the levels in the total hind paws suggesting enhanced Cyp7b activity at the site of inflammation.

Our data show a disease-dependent increase in the amount of 7α-OH-DHEA in the affected joints of arthritic mice.

Correlation of Arthritis Scores with Increases in Synovial Cyp7b and IL-1β mRNA Expression

In order to investigate whether there is a relation between the joint score and the level of Cyp7b mRNA, cDNA of synovial biopsies from knees with different knee joint scores were used. Interleukin-1β (IL-1β) mRNA levels were measured, besides Cyp7b, as a reference cytokine for inflammation in murine CIA.[23] Glyceraldehyde-3-phosphate dehydrogenase (GAPDH) was used as an internal control to check for possible differences in the amount of RNA per sample. The mRNA level of GAPDH was compared with those of Cyp7b and IL-1β, using the same amount of cDNA. No or only a weak signal for Cyp7b and IL-1β mRNA was observed in nonarthritic mice (FIG. 1B: score 0). When arthritis develops, an increase in the arthritic score of the knee joints is associated with a gradual increase in both Cyp7b- and IL-1β-mRNA levels in the synovium (FIG. 1B: score 1, 1.5, 2).

We were the first to report in the field of endocrine immunology that Cyp7b, responsible for the conversion of the adrenal prohormone DHEA into its metabolite 7α-OH-DHEA, is present locally in the arthritic joint.[21] Our hypothesis is that increases in Cyp7b may contribute to the severity of inflammation. To elucidate the mechanism by which Cyp7b interferes with the inflammatory process, studies with overexpression of the Cyp7b gene are needed. In addition, it would be of interest to assess whether inflammation and arthritis development are reduced in Cyp7b knockout mice.

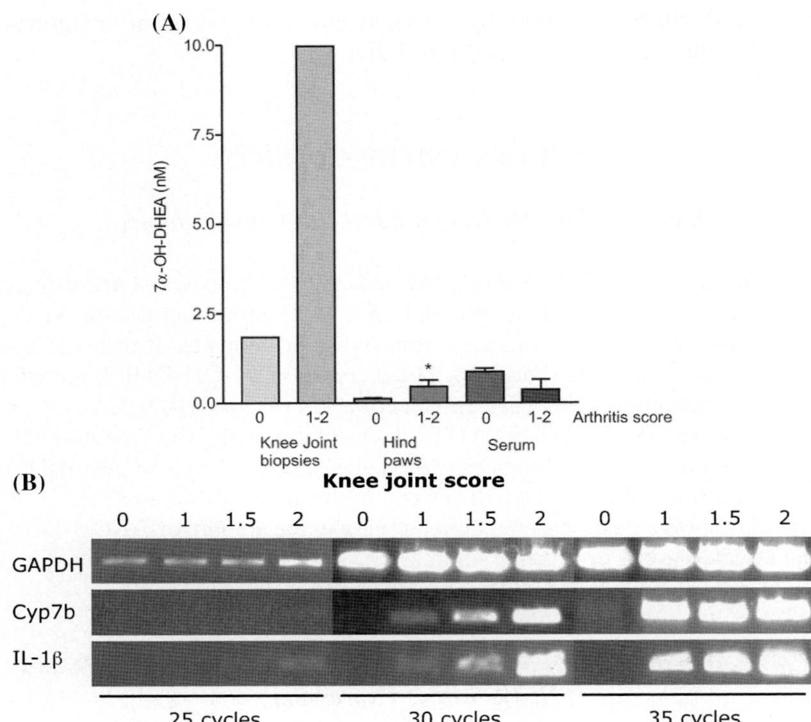

FIGURE 1. Correlation between knee joint score and Cyp7b and IL-1 mRNA levels in collagen-II-induced arthritis. (**A**) Levels of 7α-OH-DHEA and 7β-OH-DHEA in serum, hind paws, and knee joint synovial biopsies of arthritic and nonarthritic collagen-II-immunized mice. All mice were immunized at day 0 and boosted at day 21 with collagen type II. Levels of 7α-OH-DHEA were measured in extracts of hind paws ($n = 3$), pooled knee joint synovial biopsies and serum extracts ($n = 3$) using radioimmunoassay analysis as described.[28] Thirty biopsies with a knee score of 0 were pooled (103 mg total weight) and 30 biopsies with a knee score of 1–2 were pooled (116 mg total weight). Hind paws and knee joints of arthritic mice with a knee score of 1–2 were compared with non-arthritic mice (knee score 0). The level of 7α-OH-DHEA in joint synovial biopsies and hind paws is displayed as nM, normalized to 7α-OH-DHEA concentration per 100 mg tissue. The concentration 7α-OH-DHEA in sera is displayed as nM. (**B**) Reverse transcription polymerase chain reaction (RT-PCR) analysis of knee synovial biopsies. Synovial biopsies of five mice were pooled for each knee joint score. RNA was isolated, cDNA was made, and RT-PCR was performed with GAPDH, Cyp7b and IL-1β specific primers as described.[21] Results shown are representative of three experiments with three mice (two synovial biopsy samples per mouse).

Regulation of Cyp7b Activity in a Human FLS Cell Line

The findings in murine arthritis prompted us to study a putative role for Cyp7b in RA, where the proinflammatory cytokines TNF-α and IL-1β are known to govern the disease process.

The SCRO.14.SF FLS cell line, isolated from snovial biopsy tissue of a patient with RA, was used to study regulation of Cyp7b activity, by cytokines. As a measure of Cyp7b activity, we determined the amount of radiolabeled 7α-OH-DHEA measured in supernatant from FLS cultured in the presence of radiolabeled DHEA. In untreated SCRO.14.SF FLS, Cyp7b activity was already detectable (FIG. 2A). Our data show that the proinflammatory cytokines TNF-α, IL-1α, and IL-1β, stimulated Cyp7b activity significantly (FIG. 2A). In addition, the T-cell-derived cytokine IL-17 increased 7α-OH-DHEA formation, although to a lesser extent than TNF-α, IL-1α, and IL-1β (FIG. 2A). In contrast, the anti-inflammatory cytokine transforming growth factor-β (TGF-β) downregulates Cyp7b activity in FLS isolated from RA patients (FIG. 2A). Interestingly, IL-10, another anti-inflammatory cytokine, did not affect the (TNF-α-induced increase in) Cyp7b activity, which may be explained by the fact that IL-10 and TGF-β use different signaling pathways. Other cytokines (IL-2, IL-4, IL-6, IL-10, IL12, IL-15, interferon-γ [IFN-γ]) and chemokines (IL-8, granulocyte-macrophage colony-stimulating factor [GM-CSF]) did not have an effect on Cyp7b activity (FIG. 2A).

Thus, our data show that the stimulation of FLS with the proinflammatory cytokines TNF-α, IL-1α, IL-1β, or IL-17 increases Cyp7b activity (schematically depicted in FIG. 2B) which is probably due to the increase of Cyp7b mRNA levels.[20]

Considerable evidence over the last years indicates an important role for TNF-α and IL-1β in arthritis,[22,24,25] to which we can now add the increased expression of Cyp7b. Importantly, the increased generation of the Cyp7b metabolite 7α-OH-DHEA by TNF-α/IL-1β is restricted to this isoform, because other p450 enzymes such as Cyp7a, Cyp2C11, and Cyp3A2 are downregulated by TNF-α.

TNF-α Stmulates DHEA Metabolism in Human FLS: A Role for NFκB and AP-1 in the Regulation of Cyp7b Expression

Cyp7b is constitutively expressed in RA FLS and can be activated in response to TNF-α (FIG. 2). The findings described prompted us to study which signal transduction pathway is involved in the TNF-α-mediated induction of Cyp7b activity in human FLS. TNF-α signaling includes mitogen-activated protein kinases (MAPKs) and nuclear factor κ B (NFκB). Our investigations suggest a role for NFκB and activator protein-1 (AP-1) in the regulation of the expression of Cyp7b (schematically depicted in FIG. 3), which is in line with the presence of AP-1 and NFκB binding sites in the Cyp7b promotor.[26] It is known that NFκB activation increases expression of adhesion molecules and proinflammatory cytokines, whereas NFκB inhibition reduces leukocyte adhesion and transmigration. NFκB is also involved in inhibition of apoptosis together with AP-1. Moreover, NFκB, and AP-1 are important in the expression of matrix metalloproteinases, involved in the destruction of cartilage and bone in RA.

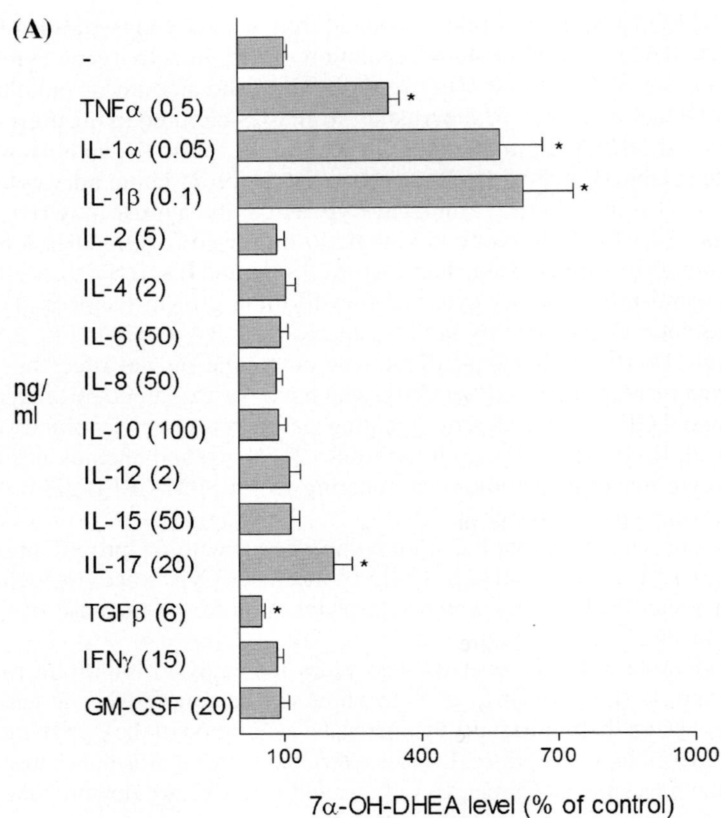
(A)
-
TNFα (0.5)
IL-1α (0.05)
IL-1β (0.1)
IL-2 (5)
IL-4 (2)
IL-6 (50)
IL-8 (50)
IL-10 (100)
IL-12 (2)
IL-15 (50)
IL-17 (20)
TGFβ (6)
IFNγ (15)
GM-CSF (20)
ng/ml
100
400
700
1000
7α-OH-DHEA level (% of control)

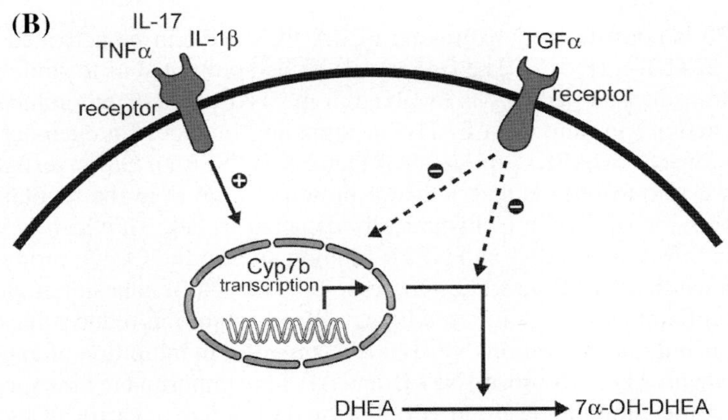
(B)
IL-17
IL-1β
TNFα
receptor
TGFα
receptor
Cyp7b
transcription
DHEA
7α-OH-DHEA

However, other approaches are needed, such as deletion mutants for NFκB and/or AP-1 in Cyp7b transfected cell lines or the use of synoviocytes from AP-1 and NFκB knockout mice, to further substantiate the role of NFκB and AP-1 in the TNF-α-induced increase in Cyp7b activity.

ANTI-GLUCOCORTICOID ACTIVITY OF 7α-OH-DHEA

The reported immuno-stimulating effects of DHEA may be due to the conversion of DHEA into 7α-OH-DHEA. The DHEA metabolite 7α-OH-DHEA is formed by the activity of the cytochrome P450 enzyme, Cyp7b. It has been suggested that 7α-OH-DHEA acts as an anti-glucocorticoid that can block the endogenous glucocorticoid-induced immuno-suppression.[12,13,16,27,28] Moreover, Morfin *et al.* hypothesized that in inflammatory diseases the local balance between DHEA metabolites and endogenous glucocorticoids might be disturbed.[29] Thus, the mechanism of action of DHEA or its Cyp7b catalyzed metabolites 7α-OH-DHEA and 7β-OH-DHEA may occur via binding to the GR, thereby explaining the putative antagonistic effect. In this context, we studied the ability of DHEA, 7α-OH-DHEA, and 7β-OH-DHEA to bind the GR using Chinese hamster ovary (CHO) cells stably transfected with the human GR. For this purpose two different assays were employed in which we studied whether the metabolites displayed agonistic activity (measured by GR transactivation) or antagonistic activity (measured by inhibition of transactivation with a reference glucocorticoid). The data show that DHEA and its metabolites do not bind to the GR (neither in an agonistic nor antagonistic mode: FIG. 4A and B).

←

FIGURE 2. Regulation of Cyp7b activity in a human FLS cell line. (**A**) Human FLS (SCRO.14.SF) were plated at 1×10^5 cells/well in a 24-well plate and incubated for 24 h in medium in the presence or absence of different cytokines. Thereafter the cells were washed and incubated for another 24 h with 1.5×10^{-8} M ^{3}H-DHEA in a steroid-deprived medium. Steroids were extracted by solid phase extraction (SPE) and analyzed by high-performance liquid chromatography (HPLC). Results shown for the amount of 7α-OH-DHEA are the average of two independent experiments, with triplicates for each condition in the experiments. The percentage [^{3}H]-7α-OH-DHEA formed in the incubations without cytokines was 5.4 ± 0.6 and 8.7 ± 0.3 for the two independent experiments. 7α-OH-DHEA was measured in human FLS (SCRO.14.SF) for 24 h. Results shown for the amount of 7α-OH-DHEA are the average of two independent experiments, with triplicates for each condition in the experiments. The percentage [^{3}H]-7α-OH-DHEA formed in the incubations without cytokines was 3.7 ± 0.1 and 4.2 ± 0.2 for the two independent experiments. $^*P < 0.0005$ versus medium control (−) using Student's *t*-test. (**B**) Illustration of the role of cytokines in Cyp7b mRNA expression and Cyp7b activity in FLS from patients with RA. Shown are stimulation (+) and inhibition (−) of Cyp7b mRNA expression and Cyp7b activity. Cyp7b activity is measured by the conversion of DHEA to 7α-OH-DHEA. Cyp7b mRNA expression is measured by RT-PCR. It is not known whether TGF-β exerts its effect via direct or indirect mechanisms (broken lines).

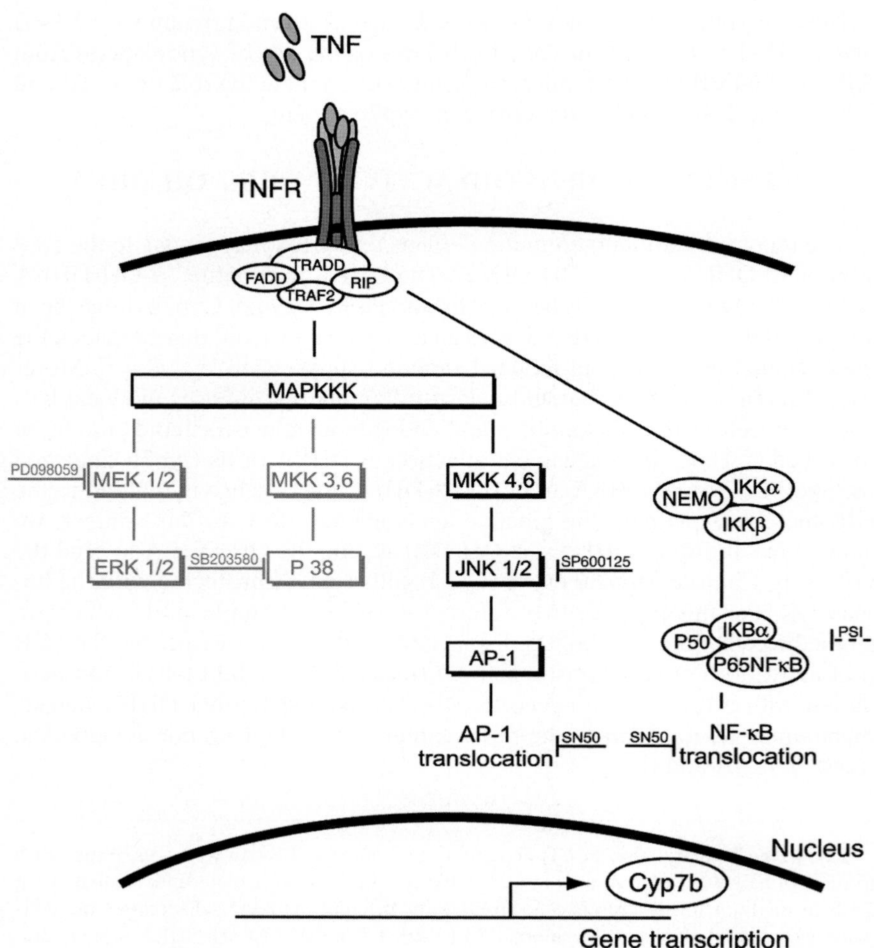

FIGURE 3. Simplified diagram of the proposed signaling events leading to Cyp7b gene transcription in synovial fibroblasts. Using inhibitors of the MEK1/ERK1/2 pathway PD98059, the p38 MAP kinase pathway SB203580, the JNK pathway SP600125, the IκB/NFκB pathway PSI (dashed line), and the NFκB/AP-1 pathway SN50, it was established that the NFkB and AP-1 pathway is relevant to Cyp7b activity. All experiments were performed using synovial fibroblasts derived from RA patients. TNFR = TNF-α receptor; TRADD = TNF receptor associated death domain; TRAF2 = TNF receptor associated factor 2; RIP = receptor interacting protein; IKBα = inhibitor of nuclear factor κB; the IkappaB kinase (IKK) complex is composed of three subunits, IKKα, IKKβ, and IKKγ (NEMO), RelA (p65), and NFκB1 (p50/p105) are subunits of NFκB. ERK1/2 = extracellular signal-(mitogenic) regulated kinases 1/2; JNK = c-Jun-NH_2-terminal kinases; p38 = p38 mitogen-activated protein kinases (MAPKs). MAPKKinase = MEK.

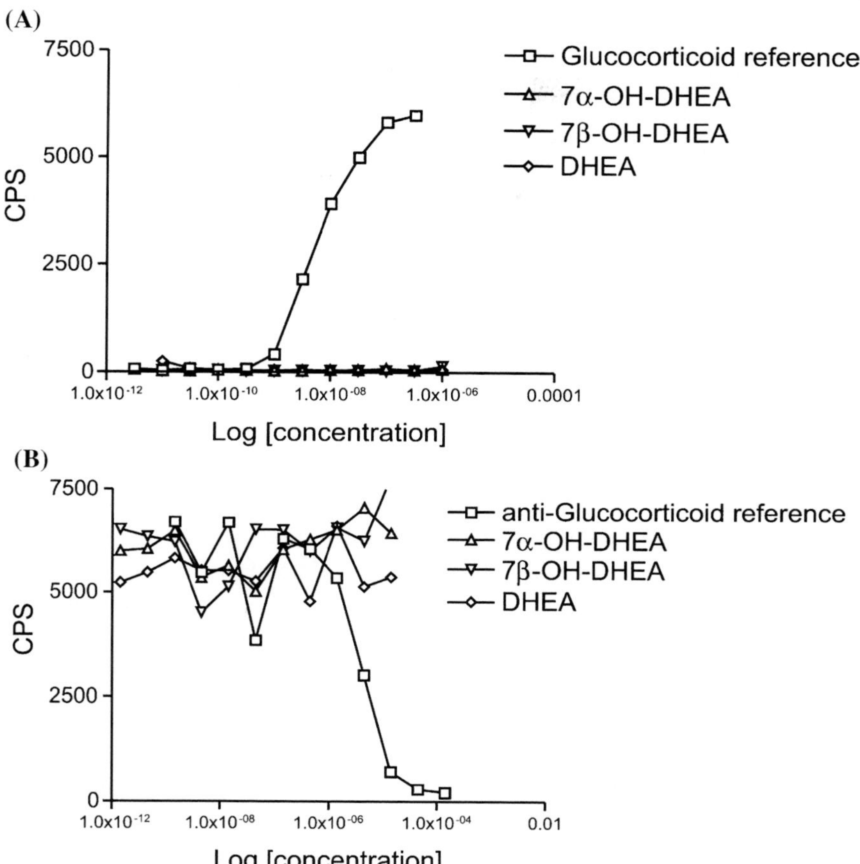

FIGURE 4. Dose-dependent effect of 7α-OH-DHEA, 7β-OH-DHEA, DHEA, and (anti-) glucocorticoid reference on glucocorticoid and anti-GR transactivation. Glucocorticoid (**A**) and anti-glucocorticoid (**B**) activity in GR transfected (mouse mammary tumor virus) CHO cells, measured by luciferase activity. Cps = counts per second.

In conclusion, the reported immuno-stimulating activities of DHEA, 7α-OH-DHEA, and 7β-OH-DHEA can not be explained by GR blockade (and thus preventing anti-inflammatory activity of endogenous glucocorticoids).

HPA-AXIS

A defect in the hypothalamus-pituitary-adrenal (HPA)-axis response after stimulation with corticotropin-releasing hormone (CRH) or after stress has been reported in a variety of autoimmune diseases including RA.[30] One aspect of the defect in the HPA-axis response could be due to 7α-OH-DHEA which may be caused by: (*a*) the adrenocorticotropic hormone (ACTH)-increased secretion of glucocorticoids by the adrenals, (*b*) the increased activity of the Cyp7b enzyme in the brain and locally in the joint, (*c*) the increased production of proinflammatory cytokines like TNF-α, IL-1, and IL-6, and (*d*) the increased amount of cells like macrophages, lymphocytes, and FLS.

We suggest that a disbalance in the amount of 7α-OH-DHEA may influence the immune-endocrine crossroad by an as yet unknown mechanism.

ROLE OF CYP7B IN DHEA METABOLISM

In the liver, Cyp7b promotes 7α-hydroxylation of 25- and 27-hydroxycholesterol and therefore could contribute to the elimination of cholesterol from the circulation.[17] A role for Cyp7b in cholesterol elimination has also been described in a newborn child with severe cholestasis with a mutation in the Cyp7b gene.[31] This is in contrast to the findings in mice by Schwarz *et al.*[19] showing that Cyp7b is not present in liver of newborn mice but may be upregulated later in life. In Cyp7b knockout mice, no accumulation of cholesterol or bile acids was found,[32] which makes a role for Cyp7b in the elimination of cholesterol of less importance in rodents. The latter data were substantiated by the observation that elimination of cholesterol is more efficiently performed by the liver-specific Cyp7a than Cyp7b, in parallel with 24-hydroxycholesterol 7α-hydroxylase Cyp39A1 enzyme.[32] Despite the similarities in elimination of cholesterol between Cyp7a, Cyp39A1, and Cyp7b, the enzymes display different substrate preferences. As reported by Wu *et al.*, cloned human Cyp7b 7-hydroxylates DHEA a hundred times more efficiently than it hydroxylates 27-hydroxycholesterol.[33] It should be noted that Cyp7a, in contrast to Cyp7b, is not capable of hydroxylating DHEA at the 7α position,[34] which already suggests a different function for these genes. Cyp7b predominantly catalyzes DHEA into 7α-OH-DHEA. Importantly, the production of 7α-OH-DHEA out of DHEA, by the activity of the Cyp7b enzyme, is irreversible.[35]

In conclusion, we were the first to report in the field of endocrine immunology that Cyp7b, responsible for the conversion of the adrenal prohormone DHEA into its metabolite 7α-OH-DHEA, is present locally in the arthritic joint. Our hypothesis is that increases in Cyp7b may contribute to the severity of inflammation.

THERAPEUTIC POSSIBILITIES OF CYP7B INHIBITION

To definitely solve this issue the development of selective Cyp7b inhibitors that can be used orally should be developed. The inhibitors, selected for inhibition of conversion of DHEA into the immune stimulatory 7α-OH-DHEA, could be tested first *in vitro* for their capacity to suppress the development and maintenance of arthritic processes in animal models of arthritis. Moreover, studies in the Cyp7b knockout mouse should add to our understanding of the role of Cyp7b activity in arthritic processes. Intra-articular delivery of Cyp7b inhibitors could be a valid and specific approach as well. All together, it is anticipated that these types of experiments will help to solve the question whether Cyp7b inhibition would present a novel treatment option in arthritis.

ACKNOWLEDGMENTS

We thank Dr. C. Heijnen, Dr. A. Kavelaars, and Dr. A. Kaptein for their help to conceive the studies. We thank Mrs. N. Bisseling for photographic reproductions.

REFERENCES

1. Straub, R.H. & M. Cutolo. 2001. Involvement of the hypothalamic-pituitary-adrenal/gonadal axis and the peripheral nervous system in rheumatoid arthritis: viewpoint based on a systemic pathogenetic role. Arthritis Rheum. **44:** 493–507.
2. Dulos, G.J. & W.M. Bagchus. 2001. Androgens indirectly accelerate thymocyte apoptosis. Int. Immunopharmacol. **1:** 321–328.
3. Bradlow, H.L., J. Murphy & J.J. Byrne. 1999. Immunological properties of dehydroepiandrosterone, its conjugates, and metabolites. Ann. N. Y. Acad. Sci. **876:** 91–101.
4. Cutolo, M., B. Seriolo, B. Villaggio, *et al.* 2002. Androgens and estrogens modulate the immune and inflammatory responses in rheumatoid arthritis. Ann. N. Y. Acad. Sci. **966:** 131–142.
5. Giltay, E.J., D. van Schaardenburg, L.J. Gooren, *et al.* 1998. Effects of dehydroepiandrosterone administration on disease activity in patients with rheumatoid arthritis. Br. J. Rheumatol. **37:** 705–706.
6. Williams, P.J., R.H. Jones & T.W. Rademacher. 1997. Reduction in the incidence and severity of collagen-induced arthritis in DBA/1 mice, using exogenous dehydroepiandrosterone. Arthritis Rheum. **40:** 907–911.
7. Du, C., M.W. Khalil & S. Sriram. 2001. Administration of dehydroepiandrosterone suppresses experimental allergic encephalomyelitis in SJL/J mice. J. Immunol. **167:** 7094–7101.
8. Daynes, R.A., D.J. Dudley & B.A. Araneo. 1990. Regulation of murine lymphokine production in vivo. II. Dehydroepiandrosterone is a natural enhancer of interleukin 2 synthesis by helper T cells. Eur. J. Immunol. **20:** 793–802.
9. Morfin, R. & G. Courchay. 1994. Pregnenolone and dehydroepiandrosterone as precursors of native 7-hydroxylated metabolites which increase the immune response in mice. J. Steroid Biochem. Mol. Biol. **50:** 91–100.
10. Wolvers, D.A., J.M. Bakker, W.M. Bagchus & G. Kraal. 1998. The steroid hormone dehydroepiandrosterone (DHEA) breaks intranasally induced tolerance, when administered at time of systemic immunization. J. Neuroimmunol. **89:** 19–25.

11. WILDER, R.L. 1996. Adrenal and gonadal steroid hormone deficiency in the pathogenesis of rheumatoid arthritis. J. Rheumatol. **44**(Suppl): 10–12.
12. CHMIELEWSKI, V., F. DRUPT & R. MORFIN. 2000. Dexamethasone-induced apoptosis of mouse thymocytes: prevention by native 7alpha-hydroxysteroids. Immunol. Cell Biol. **78:** 238–246.
13. MORFIN, R. 2002. Involvement of steroids and cytochromes P(450) species in the triggering of immune defenses. J. Steroid Biochem. Mol. Biol. **80:** 273–290.
14. CHIANG, J.Y.L. 1998. Regulation of bile acid synthesis. Front. Biosci. **3:** D176–D193.
15. BJORKHEM, I. & G. EGGERTSEN. 2001. Genes involved in initial steps of bile acid synthesis. Curr. Opin. Lipidol. **12:** 97–103.
16. LATHE, R. 2002. Steroid and sterol 7-hydroxylation: ancient pathways. Steroids **67:** 967–977.
17. STAPLETON, G., M. STEEL, M. RICHARDSON, *et al.* 1995. A novel cytochrome P450 expressed primarily in brain. J. Biol. Chem. **270:** 29739–29745.
18. ROSE, K., A. ALLAN, S. GAULDIE, *et al.* 2001. Neurosteroid hydroxylase CYP7B: vivid reporter activity in dentate gyrus of gene-targeted mice and abolition of a widespread pathway of steroid and oxysterol hydroxylation. J. Biol. Chem. **276:** 23937–23944.
19. SCHWARZ, M., E.G. LUND, R. LATHE, *et al.* 1997. Identification and characterization of a mouse oxysterol 7alpha-hydroxylase cDNA. J. Biol. Chem. **272:** 23995–24001.
20. DULOS, J., M.A. VAN DER VLEUTEN, A. KAVELAARS, *et al.* 2005. CYP7B expression and activity in fibroblast-like synoviocytes from patients with rheumatoid arthritis: regulation by proinflammatory cytokines. Arthritis Rheum. **52:** 770–778.
21. DULOS, J., E. VERBRAAK, W.M. BAGCHUS, *et al.* 2004. Severity of murine collagen-induced arthritis correlates with increased CYP7B activity: enhancement of dehydroepiandrosterone metabolism by interleukin-1beta. Arthritis Rheum. **50:** 3346–3353.
22. ELLIOTT, M.J., R.N. MAINI, M. FELDMANN, *et al.* 1993. Treatment of rheumatoid arthritis with chimeric monoclonal antibodies to tumor necrosis factor alpha. Arthritis Rheum. **36:** 1681–1690.
23. JOOSTEN, L.A., M.M. HELSEN, T. SAXNE, *et al.* 1999. IL-1 alpha beta blockade prevents cartilage and bone destruction in murine type II collagen-induced arthritis, whereas TNF-alpha blockade only ameliorates joint inflammation. J. Immunol. **163:** 5049–5055.
24. AREND, W.P. & J.M. DAYER. 1995. Inhibition of the production and effects of interleukin-1 and tumor necrosis factor alpha in rheumatoid arthritis. Arthritis Rheum. **38:** 151–160.
25. MORELAND, L.W., M.H. SCHIFF, S.W. BAUMGARTNER, *et al.* 1999. Etanercept therapy in rheumatoid arthritis. A randomized, controlled trial. Ann. Intern. Med. **130:** 478–486.
26. DULOS, J., A. KAPTEIN, A. KAVELAARS, *et al.* 2005. TNFα stimulates DHEA metabolism in human fibroblast-like synoviocytes: a role for NFκB and AP-1 in the regulation of Cyp7b expression. Arthritis Research & Therapy **7:** In press.
27. HAMPL, R., O. LAPCIK, M. HILL, *et al.* 2000. 7-Hydroxydehydroepiandrosterone—a natural antiglucocorticoid and a candidate for steroid replacement therapy? Physiol. Res. **49**(Suppl 1): S107–S112.

28. HAMPL, R., M. HILL & L. STARKA. 2001. 7-Hydroxydehydroepiandrosterone epimers in the life span. J. Steroid Biochem. Mol. Biol. **78:** 367–372.
29. MORFIN, R., P. LAFAYE, A.C. COTILLON, *et al.* 2000. 7 alpha-hydroxy-dehydroepiandrosterone and immune response. Ann. N. Y. Acad. Sci. **917:** 971–982.
30. WEBSTER, E.L., R.M. BARRIENTOS, C. CONTOREGGI, *et al.* 2002. Corticotropin releasing hormone (CRH) antagonist attenuates adjuvant induced arthritis: role of CRH in peripheral inflammation. J. Rheumatol. **29:** 1252–1261.
31. SETCHELL, K.D., M. SCHWARZ, N.C. O'CONNELL, *et al.* 1998. Identification of a new inborn error in bile acid synthesis: mutation of the oxysterol 7alpha-hydroxylase gene causes severe neonatal liver disease. J. Clin. Invest. **102:** 1690–1703.
32. LI-HAWKINS J., E.G. LUND, A.D. BRONSON, *et al.* 2000. Expression cloning of an oxysterol 7 alpha-hydroxylase selective for 24-hydroxycholesterol. J. Biol. Chem. **275:** 16543–16549.
33. WU, Z., K.O. MARTIN, N.B. JAVITT & J.Y. CHIANG. 1999. Structure and functions of human oxysterol 7alpha-hydroxylase cDNAs and gene CYP7B1. J. Lipid Res. **40:** 2195–2203.
34. NORLIN, M. & K. WIKVALL. 1998. Biochemical characterization of the 7alpha-hydroxylase activities towards 27-hydroxycholesterol and dehydroepiandrosterone in pig liver microsomes. Biochim. Biophys. Acta **1390:** 269–281.
35. DOOSTZADEH, J. & R. MORFIN. 1996. Studies of the enzyme complex responsible for pregnenolone and dehydroepiandrosterone 7 alpha-hydroxylation in mouse tissues. Steroids **61:** 613–620.

Effects of Anti-TNF-α Treatment on Lipid Profile in Patients with Active Rheumatoid Arthritis

BRUNO SERIOLO, SABRINA PAOLINO, ALBERTO SULLI, DANIELA FASCIOLO, AND MAURIZIO CUTOLO

Division of Rheumatology, Department of Internal Medicine and Medical Specialities, University of Genova, Genova, Italy

ABSTRACT: Cardiovascular morbidity and mortality appear to be increased in rheumatoid arthritis (RA), which might be due to increased prevalence of risk factors for cardiovascular disease, such as an accelerated progression of atherosclerosis. Patients with active RA frequently show an atherogenic lipid profile, which has been linked with the inflammatory reaction. Tumor necrosis factor-α (TNF-α), a pivotal proinflammatory cytokine implicated in the pathogenesis of atherosclerosis in RA, may be involved in the development of the altered lipid profile observed in active RA. Our aim was to investigate the effects of anti-TNF-α treatment in combination with methotrexate (MTX) and corticosteroid therapy on lipid profile in patients with active RA. In this prospective study 34 consecutive RA patients were included (all women, mean age 51.6 ± 7.9 years, range 46–72 years) with active (defined as Disease Activity Index 28 joint score [DAS-28], of at least 3.2) and refractory RA, in stable treatment with MTX (7.5–10 mg/week) and prednisone (7.5–10 mg/day) for 3 months. All patients received TNF-α blockers ($n = 16$, etanercept 25 mg twice weekly; $n = 14$, infliximab 3 mg/kg on 0, 2, 6, and every 8 weeks thereafter; and finally, $n = 4$, adalimumab 40 mg every other week). Total cholesterol, high-density lipoprotein cholesterol (HDL cholesterol), triglycerides (TG) and lipoprotein (a) [Lp(a)] levels and the atherogenic index (ratio cholesterol/HDL cholesterol) were measured at base line, and at 16 and 24 weeks. Results were as follows: The DAS-28 was 6.9 ± 2.1 at base line and decreased to 4.6 ± 1.8 after 16 weeks, and further to 4.1 ± 1.3 after 24 weeks (both, $P < 0.01$). Following anti-TNF-α treatment, the mean levels of total cholesterol were 168 ± 24 mg/dL at base line and increased to 188 ± 28 mg/dL at 16 weeks ($P < 0.01$), and 197 ± 26 mg/dL at 24 weeks ($P < 0.001$). However, also the mean levels of HDL cholesterol were significantly higher than basal values after 16 and 24 weeks of treatment (34 ± 12 mg/dL versus 36 ± 18 mg/dL [$P < 0.05$] and 38 ± 14 mg/dL [$P < 0.01$], respectively). TG and Lp(a) levels, as well as the atherogenic index were

Address for correspondence: Prof. B. Seriolo, Clinica Reumatologica, Dipartimento Medicina Interna e Specialità Mediche, Università di Genova, Viale Benedetto XV, n 6, 16132 Genova, Italy. Voice: +39-010-353-8616/+39-010-353-8609; fax: +39-010-353-8877.
e-mail: seriolob@unige.it

Ann. N.Y. Acad. Sci. 1069: 414–419 (2006).
doi: 10.1196/annals.1351.039

not significantly changed. Interestingly, variations in disease activity were significantly and inversely correlated with HDL cholesterol levels. In conclusion: Short anti-TNF-α treatment was associated with a significant increase of both total cholesterol and HDL cholesterol levels, and correlated with decreased disease activity. The atherogenic index showed no changes during the study. Therefore, anti-TNF-α treatment might affect lipid profile in RA patients.

KEYWORDS: **lipid profile; anti-TNF-α therapy; rheumatrid arthritis**

INTRODUCTION

Epidemiologic studies have shown an increased risk of cardiovascular disease among patients with rheumatoid arthritis (RA) when compared with the general population.[1,2] Several investigators reported an excess of cardiovascular morbidity and mortality in active RA; and the majority of cardiovascular deaths in RA result from accelerated atherosclerosis.[3,4] The potential mechanisms involved in the accelerated atherosclerosis associated with RA may involve various cellular and humoral inflammatory mediators, immune complex–mediated endothelial cell damage, prothrombotic states, and autoantibodies.[2]

Patients with active RA are associated with an unfavorable lipid profile, such as decreased total cholesterol and relatively more depressed high-density lipoprotein cholesterol (HDL cholesterol) in comparison with RA patients in remission.[5]

In addition, tumor necrosis factor-α (TNF-α), a pivotal proinflammatory cytokine implicated in the pathogenesis of RA, may be involved in the development of accelerated atherosclerosis observed in active RA.[6,7]

In the present study, we investigated the pattern of lipid profiles and the relationships of the inflammatory activity of RA with lipid profiles before and after anti-TNF-α treatment.

PATIENTS AND METHODS

Patients

In this prospective study, 34 consecutive female patients with RA in stable treatment with methotrexate (MTX) and prednisone for 3 months were included. Patients fulfilled the American College of Rheumatology 1987 criteria, had an active disease as defined by a Disease Activity Index 28 joint score (DAS-28) >3.2 at base line, and all patients received TNF-α blockers ($n = 16$, etanercept 25 mg twice weekly; $n = 14$, infliximab 3 mg/kg on 0, 2, 6, and every 8 weeks thereafter; and finally, $n = 4$, adalimumab 40 mg every other week). Stable doses of nonsteroidal anti-inflammatory drugs, prednisone (<10 mg/day) and MTX (10 mg/week), were allowed during the study. Measurements of the variables studied were made on blood samples collected before the administration of an anti-TNF-α dose, at base line, and 16 and 24 weeks after the starting treatment.

Methods

Fasting blood samples were collected in Vacutainer tubes (Beckton & Dickinson, Rutherford, NJ, USA) containing K3-EDTA (1 mg/mL), centrifuged at 3,600 rpm for 8 min at 4°C, supplemented with saccharose as a cryoprotectant (final concentration 6 mg/mL), and frozen at −70°C until assay. The concentrations of total cholesterol and triglyceride (TG) were determined by commercially available enzymatic reagents on the Hitachi 747 analyzer (Boehringer Mannheim, Germany), while the levels of HDL cholesterol were determined by the phosphotungstate/Mg^{2+} method.[8] The low-density lipoprotein cholesterol (LDL cholesterol) value was calculated with the Friedewald formula, which provides reliable values up to a TG concentration of 8.0 mmol/L. Lipoprotein (a) [Lp(a)] concentrations were assayed by enzyme-linked immunosorbent assay.[9] At each visit, erythrocyte sedimentation rate (ERS), C-reactive protein (CRP), a visual analogic scale for general health, and the number of swollen and tender joints were assessed to determine disease activity (DAS-28).

Statistical Analysis

The differences of the levels of total cholesterol, HDL cholesterol, TG, Lp(a), and the total cholesterol/HDL cholesterol ratio (the atherogenic index), and DAS-28 at 16 and 24 weeks were compared to base line with paired *t*-test. To investigate the association between the changes in lipid profiles and those in disease activity, Pearson's correlation was performed for the period from base line to 16 weeks and the period from base line to 24 weeks. Significance was set at the 0.05 level. Values are expressed as mean and standard deviation.

RESULTS

The baseline characteristics of the patients with RA are presented in TABLE 1. Total cholesterol and HDL cholesterol levels were 168 ± 24 and 34 ± 12 mg/dL at base line, respectively. Total cholesterol and HDL-cholesterol levels were significantly higher during treatment at 16 and 24 weeks than at base line (188 ± 28 mg/dL [$P < 0.01$] and 197 ± 26 mg/dL [$P < 0.001$] for levels of total cholesterol and 36 ± 18 mg/dL [$P < 0.05$] and 38 ± 14 mg/dL [$P < 0.01$] for levels of HDL cholesterol, respectively, at 16 and 24 weeks).

TABLE 1. Baseline characteristics of patients with active RA

Age, yr	
Median	51.6 ± 7.9
Range	46–72
Rheumatoid factor–positive, *n* (%)	32 (94%)
Mean duration of disease, yr (range)	14 ± 9 (2–34)
HAQ score	1.5 ± 0.5
ERS (mm/h)	46 ± 21
CRP level (mg/dL)	16 ± 5
Cigarette smoking, *n* (%)	
Never smoked	18 (53%)
Past smoked	14 (41%)
Current smoker	2 (6%)
BMI (kg/m^2)	25.7 ± 2.8
Hypertension, *n* (%)	7 (21%)
Systolic blood pressure (mmHg)	140 ± 24
Diastolic blood pressure (mmHg)	77 ± 26

HAQ = Health Assessment Questionnaire; ERS = erythrocyte sedimentation rate; CRP = C-reactive protein; BMI = body mass index.

In contrast, TG and Lp(a) concentrations were not significantly changed following anti-TNF-α treatment at 16 and 24 weeks (TG: 126 ± 15 mg/dL [base line] vs. 123 ± 17 mg/dL [at 16 weeks] and 124 ± 17 mg/dL [at 24 weeks]; Lp(a): 31 ± 4 mg/dL [base line] versus 31 ± 3 mg/dL [at 16 weeks] and 30 ± 4 mg/dL [at 24 weeks], respectively). The atherogenic index, however, remained constant during the 24 weeks of anti-TNF treatment (3.9 ± 0.3 [base line] versus 3.9 ± 0.2 [at 16 weeks] and 3.8 ± 0.4 [at 24 weeks]). The DAS-28 was 6.9 ± 2.1 at base line and decreased to 4.6 ± 1.8 after 16 weeks and further to 4.1 ± 1.3 after 24 weeks (both, $P < 0.01$). The change in HDL cholesterol and total cholesterol levels from base line to 16 weeks showed no significant associations with changes in DAS-28. However, changes in DAS-28 from base line to 24 weeks were significantly inversely associated with changes in both total cholesterol and HDL cholesterol levels ($P < 0.01$, see TABLE 2).

TABLE 2. Correlations between the changes in DAS-28 at base line–16 wk and base line–24 wk and the changes in total cholesterol and HDL cholesterol at base line–16 wk and base line–24 wk

	Changes in DAS-28 at base line–16 wk	Changes in DAS-28 at base line–24 wk
Changes in total cholesterol at base line–16 wk	−0.03	−0.34
Changes in total cholesterol at base line–24 wk	−0.29	−0.48*
Changes in HDL cholesterol at base line–16 wk	−0.12	−0.28
Changes in HDL cholesterol at base line–24 wk	−0.34	−0.52*

*$P < 0.01$.

DISCUSSION

In this study, we found that anti-TNF-α treatment in patients with active RA significantly increased both the total cholesterol and HDL cholesterol concentrations. However, these changes did not modify the atherogenic index, which is an important prognostic marker for future cardiovascular disease. The increases in total cholesterol and HDL cholesterol concentrations were significantly associated with a decrease in disease activity. In contrast, there were no significant changes in the TG and Lp(a) concentrations. Recently, several studies have examined the relationships between carotid atherosclerosis and markers associated with systemic inflammation in patients with RA. Kumeda *et al.* demonstrated that the duration and clinical severity of RA were independently associated with increased intima-media thickness of the common carotid artery.[10] DelRincon *et al.* showed that the presence of carotid plaque was associated with markers of systemic inflammation, such as CRP levels and ERS determinations, both in RA patients and in healthy subjects.[11] These studies have suggested a close relationship between systemic inflammation and the progression of atherosclerosis in patients with RA. In our study, RA disease activity was reduced by anti-TNF treatment together with increase of HDL cholesterol levels. Other small studies have assessed the effect of TNF neutralization with the chimeric monoclonal antibody infliximab on lipoproteins in patients with RA. Hurlimann *et al.* also found a slight increase in total cholesterol in 11 patients treated for 12 weeks, but no data were provided about HDL cholesterol, LDL, and TG.[12] In another study, Cauza *et al.* found an increase in TG and decrease in HDL cholesterol concentrations in seven patients with RA after 3 weeks' treatment.[13] Finally, Popa *et al.* found increased HDL cholesterol concentrations with an improvement in the cardiovascular risk profile after treatment with anti-TNF therapy.[14] In conclusion, our results show that the anti-TNF-α treatment produces benefits, changing the lipid profile and possibly the cardiovascular risk by decreasing inflammation in RA patients. However, long-term studies are needed to confirm this hypothesis and to identify which anti-TNF-α blocker is more protective versus accelerated atherosclerosis in RA.

REFERENCES

1. Watson, D.J. *et al.* 2003. All-cause mortality and vascular events among patients with rheumatoid arthritis, osteoarthritis, or no arthritis in the UK General Practice Research Database. J. Rheumatol. **30:** 1196–2002.
2. Solomon, D.H. *et al.* 2004. Cardiovascular risk factors in women with and without rheumatoid arthritis. Arthritis Rheum. **11:** 3444–3449.
3. Van Doornum, S. *et al.* 2002. Seropositive rheumatoid arthritis in Northern Sweden. Arthritis Rheum. **46:** 862–873.

4. GOODSON, N. 2002. Coronary artery disease and rheumatoid arthritis. Curr. Opin. Rheumatol. **14:** 115–120.
5. SERIOLO, B. *et al.* 1995. Lipid profile and anticardiolipin antibodies in rheumatoid arthritis. Clin. Exp. Rheumatol. **13:** 406–407.
6. RIDKER, P.M. 2003. Clinical application of C-reactive protein for cardiovascular disease detection and prevention. Circulation **107:** 363–369.
7. VIS, M. *et al.* 2005. Short term effects of infliximab on the lipid profile in patients with rheumatoid arthritis. J. Rheumatol. **32:** 252–255.
8. DEMACKER, P.N.M. *et al.* 1997. Precipitation methods for high-density lipoprotein cholesterol measurement compared, and final evaluation under routine operating conditions of a method with a low sample to reagent ratio. Clin. Chem. **43:** 663–668.
9. SERIOLO, B. *et al.* 1995. Lipoprotein (a) and anticardiolipin antibodies as risk factors for vascular disease in rheumatoid arthritis. Thromb. Haemost. **74:** 799–800.
10. KUMEDA, Y. *et al.* 2002. Increased thickness of the arterial intima-media detected by ultrasonography in patients with rheumatoid arthritis. Arthritis Rheum. **46:** 1489–1497.
11. DELRINCON, I. *et al.* 2003. Association between carotid atherosclerosis and markers of inflammation in rheumatoid arthritis patients and healthy subjects. Arthritis Rheum. **48:** 1833–1840.
12. HURLIMANN, D. *et al.* 2002. Antitumor necrosis factor-α treatment improves endothelial function in patients with rheumatoid arthritis. Circulation **106:** 2184–2187.
13. CAUZA, E. *et al.* 2002. Intravenous anti-TNFα antibody therapy leads to elevated triglyceride and reduced HDL-cholesterol levels in patients with rheumatoid arthritis and psoriatic arthritis. Wien. Klin. Wochenschr. **114:** 1004–1007.
14. POPA, C. *et al.* 2005. Influence of anti-tumor necrosis factor therapy on cardiovascular risk factors in patients with active rheumatoid arthritis. Ann. Rheum. Dis. **64:** 303–305.

Bone Metabolism Changes During Anti-TNF-α Therapy in Patients with Active Rheumatoid Arthritis

BRUNO SERIOLO, SABRINA PAOLINO, ALBERTO SULLI, VALENTINO FERRETTI, AND MAURIZIO CUTOLO

Division of Rheumatology, Department of Internal Medicine and Medical Specialities, University of Genova, Italy

ABSTRACT: Osteoporosis (OP) occurs more frequently in patients with rheumatoid arthritis (RA) than in healthy individuals. Specific treatments of RA may increase susceptibility to OP, but at the same time decrease inflammatory activity, which is associated with accelerated bone loss. Treatment with TNF-α blockers might influence bone metabolism and prevent structural bone damage in RA, in particular at the periarticular level. Our aim was to assess the influence of anti-TNF-α therapy on bone metabolism in RA patients. To that end we evaluated a group of 30 RA patients [mean age 50.6 $\pm$ 6.8 years; median disease duration 82 $\pm$ 38 months; median disease activity score (DAS-28) 5.8 $\pm$ 1.2: 70% of whom were positive for the rheumatoid factor IgM (>40 IU/mL)]. Patients were treated with stable therapy of prednisone (7.5 mg/day) and methotrexate (MTX = 10 mg/week). Eleven of these RA patients further received etanercept (25 mg, twice/weekly) and 10 infliximab (3 mg/kg on 0, 2, 6, and every 8 weeks thereafter). A control group included 10 RA patients with stable therapy (prednisone and MTX) and without anti-TNF-α therapy. All the patients fulfilled the ACR criteria for the diagnosis of adult RA and were treated for 6 months. Quantitative ultrasound (QUS) bone densitometry was performed at the metaphyses of the proximal phalanges of both hands with a DBM Sonic 1200 QUS device (IGEA, Carpi, Italy). Amplitude-dependent speed of sound (AD-SoS) was evaluated at base line and at 3 and 6 months. Bone mineral density (BMD) of the hip and lumbar spine (L_1–L_4) was determined by a densitometer (GE Lunar Prodigy, USA) at base line at after 6 months. Soluble bone turnover markers [osteocalcin (BGP) and deoxypyridinoline/creatinine (Dpd/Cr) ratio] were measured in all patients at the same times, using enzyme-linked immunosorbent assay tests. All data were compared using Wilcoxon signed rank test. Results were as follows: AD-SoS values were found increased by 1.3% after 6 months of treatment in the RA patients treated with anti-TNF-α therapy. On the contrary,

Address for correspondence: Prof. B. Seriolo, Clinica Reumatologica, Dipartimento Medicina Interna e Specialità Mediche, Università di Genova, Viale Benedetto XV, n 6, 16132 Genova, Italy. Voice: +39-010-3538616/+39-010-3538609; fax: +39-010-353-8877.
e-mail: seriolob@unige.it

Ann. N.Y. Acad. Sci. 1069: 420–427 (2006). © 2006 New York Academy of Sciences.
doi: 10.1196/annals.1351.040

the Ad-SoS levels decreased by 4.6% during the same period in the untreated RA group. BMD increased by 0.2% at lumbar spine and 0.1% at the hip in TNF-α-blocker-treated patients and decreased by 0.8% and 0.6% (at lumbar spine and at the hip, respectively) in RA patients without anti-TNF-α therapy. However, BMD variations were not significant. In RA patients treated with TNF-α blockers, BGP levels were found significantly increased (14.8 ± 3.8 mg/mL vs. 22.4 ± 4.2 mg/mL; $P < 0.01$) and Dpd/Cr levels were found significantly decreased (8.2 ± 2.1 nM vs. 4.6 ± 1.8 nM; $P < 0.01$) at 6 months when compared to base line values. On the contrary, there were no significant differences in the untreated RA patients concerning these latter parameters (BGP = 12.2 ± 3.1 mg/mL vs. 10.8 ± 2.8 mg/mL and Dpd/Cr = 8.9 ± 2.4 nM vs. 10.2 ± 1.8 nM, respectively). In conclusion, during 6 months of treatment of RA patients with TNF blockers, bone formation seems increased while bone resorption seems decreased. The reduced rate of OP appears to be supported by the same mechanisms involved in the decreased bone joint resorption during anti-TNF-α therapy, that is, the marked decrease of the proinflammatory (i.e., TNF-α) cytokine effects on bone metabolism.

KEYWORDS: bone metabolism; osteoporosis; anti-TNF-α therapy; rheumatoid arthritis

INTRODUCTION

Osteoporosis (OP) is frequently observed in patients with rheumatoid arthritis (RA) in two forms: periarticular OP around inflamed joints, which is a characteristic of early disease, and generalized OP as one of the extra-articular manifestations of RA which results in an increased risk of fractures and associated morbidity, mortality and health care cost.[1,2]

OP in RA is, in addition to a risk factor for primary OP, believed to be a consequence of three major factors: inflammation, the use of corticosteroids, and inactivity as an inevitable consequence of a disabling disease.

Treatment of RA with disease-modifying antirheumatic drugs and corticosteroids may not only increase susceptibility to OP, but also suppress inflammatory activity, which is an important risk factor for OP in RA.

Although the underlying cause of RA is unknown, tumor necrosis factor α (TNF-α)—a proinflammatory cytokine produced by macrophages and T cells—contributes to the pathogenesis of synovitis and joint destruction. A critical role for TNF-α in the pathogenesis of RA has been established in studies demonstrating profound proinflammatory properties of TNF-α *in vitro*, the presence of high levels of cytokines in rheumatoid sera and joints, and the ability of TNF antagonists to reduce significantly joint inflammation in animal models of arthritis. Biological therapy with TNF-blocking agents represents the most effective therapy so far available to patients with RA.[3]

This prospective study considers a homogeneous group of RA patients with active disease to assess the effects of treatment with TNF-α blockers on bone metabolism.

MATERIALS AND METHODS

Thirty postmenopausal women with early, active RA were enrolled; they fulfilled the American College of Rheumatology criteria for adult RA and attended our outpatient rheumatology clinic, to the exclusion of patients who were receiving drugs that could affect bone mass or bone metabolism.[4] The age of the patients in the study group ranged from 45 to 68 years [mean age ± standard deviation (SD), 51 ± 7 years]. None was in perimenopausal status and none was taking estrogen replacement therapy. Patients were treated with stable therapy of methotrexate (MTX) at a dose of 10 mg/weekly and prednisone at a dose of <7.5 mg/day. Eleven of these RA patients further received etanercept (25 mg, twice/weekly) and nine infliximab (3 mg/kg on 0, 2, 6, and every 8 weeks thereafter). None had evidence of concurrent disease known to interfere with bone metabolism, such as liver or renal diseases or extra-articular manifestations of RA. Informed consent was obtained from all subjects. A control group included 10 RA postmenopausal patients with stable therapy (prednisone at dose of <7.5 mg/day and MTX at dose of 10 mg/weekly).

Disease activity was measured by the disease activity score (DAS) composite index, using a 28-joint score (DAS-28). This includes number of swollen joints, number of tender joints, patient's global assessment of disease activity, and erythrocyte sedimentation rate. Levels of C-reactive protein (CRP) and rheumatoid factor were also determined by standard methods. Functional disability was evaluated using the Italian version of the Stanford Health Assessment Questionnaire (HAQ), a self-reporting instrument measuring disability of daily life activities. The score created for the disability index ranges from 0 to 3, where a higher score indicates a higher degree of disability.

Bone Mineral Densitometry

Scans of the proximal phalanges were taken with a DBM Sonic 1200 ultrasound unit (IGEA, Carpi, Italy). This instrument is equipped with two probes mounted on an electronic caliper. The emitter is positioned on the medial surface of the phalange, and the receiver is positioned on the opposite side. The emitter probe generates a ultrasound (US) signal with a frequency of 1.25 MHz. A good coupling between the probes and skin is achieved with interfacing gel. The DBM Sonic 1200 measures a velocity depending on amplitude of trace [amplitude-dependent speed of sound (AD-SoS), expressed in m/s]. The results are expressed as averages of AD-SoS values for the four phalanges. The intraoperator errors are less than 1%.[5] A quantitative analysis of the pattern of the transmitted ultrasound signal was performed and the Ultrasound Bone Profiler Index (UBPI), expressing the probability of the tested subject belonging to the control group to have a fracture at the time of the measurement, was calculated according to the following optimum multivariate logistic model:

$$\text{UBPI} = 1/[1 + \exp(-0.0018\,\text{SD}\mu - 0.056\,\text{FWA} - 1.1467\,\text{TF} + 3.03)]$$

where SDy (dynamic of the US signal, mV/μsec[sup2]) is the mean value of the second derivative of amplitude versus time of the first two peaks of the US signal, FWA (fast-wave amplitude, mV) is the first highest peak in the first part of the US received and digitized signal, and TF (time frame, μsec) is the time interval between the first received signal and the speed value of 1,700 m/sec. Results were expressed as arbitrary units. Spine and hip bone mineral density (BMD) determinations were measured before start of biologic therapy using dual-energy X-ray absorptiometry (DXA) with GE Lunar Prodigy densitometer (GE Lunar, Madison, Wisconsin, software version 5.0). Bone mass measurements were made at the lumbar spine (L_1–L_4) and at the left hip (femoral neck, greater trochanter, and Ward's triangle). BMD value was expressed as gram of bone mineral per square centimeter (g/cm^2), as the number of standard deviations of young healthy people, T score, and the number of standard deviations from the mean of healthy age- and sex-matched people, Z score, values obtained from Lunar's combined European/U.S. reference population.[6] The coefficients of variation for bone measurements made in our bone densitometry laboratory are $<1\%$.

Collection of Blood and Urine Samples for Deoxypyridinoline (Dpd) Assay

Blood samples were collected in the morning after overnight fasting from patients and controls. A spot urine sample was collected from each patient and control subjects during the day, avoiding the first morning urine. Sera were separated by centrifugation, and aliquots of urine samples were kept without additives and frozen at $-70°$C until they could be analyzed.

Serum Osteocalcin Assay

The osteocalcin Immunoradiologic Assay (IRMA) Kit (Incstar Co. Stillwater, MN, USA) was used for the quantification of serum osteocalcin in serum samples. The kit measures intact human osteocalcin (1–49) with no cross reactivity to the (1–43) fragment. This assay uses human osteocalcin (1–49) as a standard for controls and two polyclonal antibodies that have been purified by affinity chromatography. The first antibody, specific for the amino terminus of human osteocalcin, is bound to a solid phase (polystyrene beads). The second antibody, which is specific for the carboxy terminus of human osteocalcin, is labeled with ^{125}I. In brief: samples are incubated at room temperature for 2 h. Following the incubation period, each bead is washed to remove unbound labeled antibody. The radioactivity present in the remaining bound labeled antibody is then measured on a gamma counter. The concentration of osteocalcin in the sample is directly proportional to the radioactivity measured. The sensitivity of the assay is of 0.2 ng/mL, and the concentrations of osteocalcin could be determined in all subjects. The intra-assay variation is below 8% and the interassay variation is below 12%.

Determination of Urinary Dpd Concentration

The Pyrilinks-D Assay (Metra Biosystems, Inc., Mountain View, CA, USA), a competitive immunoassay in a microtiter strip well format using a monoclonal anti-deoxypyridinoline antibody coated on the strip to capture Dpd, was used to determine the urinary concentration of Dpd. Manufacturer's instructions for the assay were followed. Dpd in the urine samples competed with conjugated Dpd-alkaline phosphatase for the antibody and the reaction was detected with a pNPP substrate. Duplicate measurements were performed for each urine sample and the results were expressed as nmol Dpd/mmol creatine measured on a Hitachi 911 autoanalyzer. The intra-assay and interassay coefficients of variation were 4.8% and 4.6%, respectively.[7]

Statistical Analysis

Results are expressed as mean and standard deviation. BMD and bone marker results were compared with baseline values using paired Student's *t*-test.

The significance cut-off was $P < 0.05$.

RESULTS

The base line characteristics of the RA patients are shown in TABLE 1. AD-SoS values were found increased by 1.3% after 6 months of treatment in the RA patients treated with anti-TNF-α therapy. On the contrary, the AD-SoS levels decreased by 4.6% during the same period in the untreated RA group. BMD increased by 0.2% at the lumbar spine and 0.1% at the hip in TNF-α-blocker-treated patients and decreased by 0.8 % and 0.6% (at lumbar spine and at the hip, respectively) in RA patients without anti-TNF-α therapy. (FIG. 1).

However, BMD variations were not significant. In RA patients treated with TNF-α blockers, BGP levels were found significantly increased (14.8 ± 3.8 mg/mL vs. 22.4 ± 4.2 mg/mL; $P < 0.01$) and Dpd/Cr levels were found significantly decreased (8.2 ± 2.1 nM vs. 4.6 ± 1.8 nM; $P < 0.01$) at 6 months when compared to baseline values. On the contrary, there were no significant differences in the untreated RA patients concerning these latter parameters

TABLE 1. Baseline characteristics of patients with active RA

	All patients ($n = 30$)	With anti-TNF-α therapy ($n = 20$)	Without anti-TNF-α therapy ($n = 10$)
Age, yr median	51 ± 8	50 ± 4	51 ± 9
Range	45–68	45–64	51–68
Rheumatoid factor IgM–positive, n (%)	21 (70%)	14 (70%)	7 (70%)
Mean duration of disease, months (range)	82 ± 38 (12–134)	76 ± 24 (36–134)	88 ± 38 (12–98)
HAQ score	1.5 ± 0.5	1.6 ± 0.4	1.4 ± 0.5
DAS-28 joint score	5.8 ± 1.2	6.1 ± 0.9	5.5 ± 1.8
ERS, mm/hr	46 ± 21	48 ± 18	44 ± 20
CRP level, mg/dL	16 ± 5	15 ± 4	16 ± 8
BMI, kg/m^2	25.7 ± 2.8	26.1 ± 1.8	25.2 ± 0.4

HAQ = Health Assessment Questionnaire; DAS-28 joint score = disease activity score; ERS = erythrocyte sedimentation rate; CRP = C-reactive protein; BMI = body mass index.

(BGP = 12.2 ± 3.1 mg/mL vs. 10.8 ± 2.8 mg/mL and Dpd/Cr = 8.9 ± 2.4 nM vs. 10.2 ± 1.8 nM, respectively).

Z scores and T scores did not correlate significantly with the disease variables DAS-28 or CRP or with the HAQ score at base line or after 6 months.

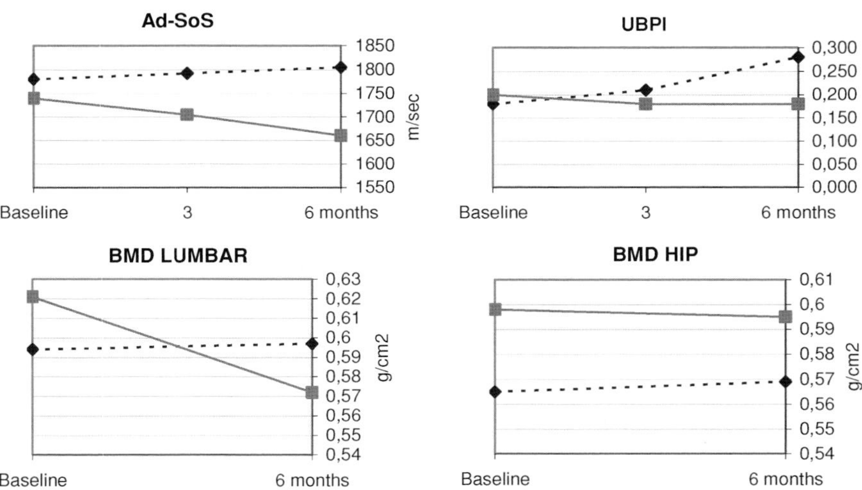

FIGURE 1. Changes of measurements of AD-SoS, UBPI, and BMD of the lumbar spine and hip at base line and after 3 and 6 months in patients with rheumatoid arthritis with anti-TNF-α therapy (*dotted line*) and without anti-TNF-α therapy *(continous line)*. AD-SoS: amplitude-dependent speed of sound; UBPI: ultrasound bone profile index; BMD: bone mineral density.

DISCUSSION

The mechanism by which the inflammatory cytokines from active rheumatoid joints affects bone turnover has recently been studied. Inflamed RA synovial tissue releases inflammatory cytokines, such as TNF-α, which can exert effects on bone locally and throughout the skeleton, possibly by acting via complex signaling pathways, such as the newly identified osteoprotegerin pathways.[8]

It is well known that inflammation is one of the strong risk factor of OP. Cytokines have been postulated to be important mediators of inflammation due to their role in cell–cell interactions. TNF-α cytokine plays an important role in the inflammatory processes of RA and the resulting joint pathology; *in vitro* studies have shown that TNF-α cytokine can induce bone resorption. Anti-TNF-α treatment inhibits the acute-phase response, proliferation of fibroblasts, and recruitment and activation of leukocytes.

In our study, we found that anti-TNF-α treatment significantly decreased disease activity.

Our data indicate that values of both BMD of the spine and hip and AD-SoS have a tendency to increase during 6 months of treatment with anti-TNF-α treatment. This is in contrast with the values of BMD and the levels of AD-SoS in RA patients without anti-TNF-α treatment during the same period. These data suggest that treatment with anti-TNF-α can reduce generalized and periarticular OP in RA patients. This view is supported by the observation that markers of bone formation increased and markers of bone resorption decreased in the first 6 months of treatment with anti-TNF-α treatment.

In conclusion, this study supports the already assessed finding that treatment with anti-TNF-α has a positive effect on bone-joint metabolism in patients with RA. In addition, this treatment might represent an additional advantage, in particular by reducing the general risk of bone loss and subsequently osteoporotic fractures.

REFERENCES

1. Gough, A.K.S. *et al.* 1994. Generalised bone loss in patients with early rheumatoid arthritis. Lancet **344:** 23–27.
2. Kroot, E.J.A. *et al.* 2001. Change in bone mineral density in patients with rheumatoid arthritis during the first decade of the disease. Arthritis Rheum. **44:** 1254–1260.
3. Emery, P. & Y. Seto. 2003. Role of biologics in early arthritis. Clin. Exp. Rheumatol. **21:** S191–S194.
4. Arnett, F.C. *et al.* 1988. The American Rheumatism Association 1987 revised criteria for the classification of rheumatoid arthritis. Arthritis Rheum. **31:** 315–324.

5. CAMOZZI, V. *et al.* 2003. Phalangeal quantitative ultrasound technology and dual energy X-ray densitometry in patients with primary hyperthyroidism: influence of sex and menopausal status. Osteoporos. Int. **14:** 602–608.
6. LUNAR CORPORATION. 1998. Operator's Manual, Expert-XL, Version 1.7. Lunar Corporation. Madison, WI.
7. ROBINS, S.P. *et al.* 1986. Measurement of the cross linking compound pyridinoline in urine as an index of collagen degradation in joint disease. Ann. Rheum. Dis. **45:** 969–973.
8. HOFBAUER, L.C. *et al.* 2000. The roles of osteoprotegerin and osteoprotegerin ligand in the paracrine regulation of bone resorption. J. Bone Miner. Res. **15:** 2–12.

Neuroendocrine Modulation Induced by Selective Blockade of TNF-α in Rheumatoid Arthritis

GABRIELE DI COMITE,[a] ALESSANDRO MARINOSCI,[a] PAOLA DI MATTEO,[b] ANGELO MANFREDI,[a] PATRIZIA ROVERE-QUERINI,[a] ELENA BALDISSERA,[a] PATRIZIA AIELLO,[a] ANGELO CORTI,[b] AND MARIA GRAZIA SABBADINI[a]

[a]*Clinical Immunology and Rheumatology Unit, H. San Raffaele Scientific Institute and Vita-Salute University, 20132 Milan, Italy*

[b]*Department of Biological and Technological Research, H. San Raffaele Scientific Institute, 20132 Milan, Italy*

ABSTRACT: Tumor necrosis factor-α (TNFα) is a main actor in the pathogenesis of rheumatoid arthritis (RA), interacting with other molecules in complex mechanisms. The neuroendocrine system is known to be involved and Chromogranin A (CHGA) serum levels are elevated in patients with RA. We evaluated the effect of the selective blockade of TNF-α, induced by treatment with anti-TNF-α monoclonal antibodies (mAbs), on the serum levels of CHGA and on its correlation with TNF-α and TNF-α receptors (TNFRs) serum levels. Seven patients with RA have been treated with the anti-TNF-α mAb, infliximab. We measured the serum levels of TNF-α, its receptors (tumor necrosis factor receptor-I [TNFR-I] and tumor necrosis factor receptor-II [TNFR-II]), and CHGA before and during the treatment. We also measured, as a control, the serum levels of CHGA, TNF-α, and soluble TNFRs in 14 patients who were being treated with infliximab, adalimumab, or etanercept and in 20 matching negative controls. The serum levels of TNFR-I and TNFR-II, which are a sensitive marker for the TNF-α pathway, correlated with those of CHGA before treatment (Pearson's coefficient, respectively, 0.59 and 0.53). Treatment with anti-TNF-α mAb provided a significant clinical response in all patients and the correlation between CHGA and TNFR-I and TNFR-II was no more evident during treatment (respectively, −0.09 and −0.07). TNF-α blockade allows a clinical effect in patients with RA and modifies the correlation between CHGA and TNFRs, suggesting that TNF-α and CHGA reciprocally interfere in the pathogenesis of RA, through intermediate adaptors, whose identification warrants further studies.

Dr. Gabriele Di Comite and Dr. Alessandro Marinosci equally contributed to this study.

Address for correspondence: Gabriele Di Comite, Clinical Immunology and Rheumatology Unit, CIGTP, H. San Raffaele Scientific Institute—DIBIT, 3A1-Lab 3, via Olgettina 58, 20132 Milan, Italy. Voice: +39-02-2643-4864; fax: +39-02-2643-4786.

e-mail: dicomite.gabriele@hsr.it

Ann. N.Y. Acad. Sci. 1069: 428–437 (2006).
doi: 10.1196/annals.1351.041

KEYWORDS: Chromogranin A; tumor necrosis factor-α; tumor necrosis factor receptor-I; tumor necrosis factor receptor-II; rheumatoid arthritis; anti-TNF-α monoclonal antibodies

INTRODUCTION

Chromogranin A (CHGA) is a 48-kDa acidic polypeptide, stored in the dense-core secretory granules of the chromaffin cells of the exocrine, endocrine, and the nervous systems.[1,2] It plays a central role in the trafficking and storage of the hormones, enzymes, neuropeptides, and neurotransmitters contained in the granules and it is involved in the regulation of granule biogenesis.[2,3] Along with this, CHGA exerts various extracellular actions after secretion, as a precursor of biologically active fragments such as pancreastatin (CHGA 250–301 fragment), chromacin (CHGA 176–197), vasostatin (CHGA 1–76), and catestatin (CHGA 352–372).[2]

Full-length CHGA and its processed products have been shown to play a role in immunity against microbes[4] and to be implicated in neurodegenerative disorders and cardiovascular diseases, such as hypertension.[2,5] Thanks to its ubiquitous presence into the neuroendocrine cells, CHGA is currently used in the follow-up of neuroendocrine malignancies.[2]

Recently, CHGA has been shown to take part in the regulation of the endothelial barrier function. It protects vessels against plasma leakage in inflammatory diseases, inhibiting tumor necrosis factor-α (TNF-α)-induced endothelial cytoskeleton rearrangement.[6,7]

A growing body of evidence suggests that the neuroendocrine system could be implicated in the pathogenesis of rheumatoid arthritis (RA), interfering with complex inflammatory mechanisms, including TNF-α networks and vascular endothelial dysfunctions.[8–10]

Clinical observations demonstrate that, when RA patients, who almost always present symmetric upper limb involvement, develop hemiplegia, arthritis of the paralytic limb improves and it may even reach complete remission with resolution of bone erosions.[11] Sensory neurons release inflammatory peptides which could be involved in a pathway leading to symmetric arthritis and continuous pain stimulation.[12] Sensory, sympathetic, and parasympathetic neurotransmitters and cytokines released in the periphery signal to the central nervous system, causing feedbacks that may be involved in maintaining the pannus.[8]

Anti-TNF-α monoclonal antibodies (mAbs) are a major breakthrough in the management of RA, not only because they provide good responses in patients with arthritis refractory to treatment with conventional therapies,[13–15] but also because they represent a unique opportunity to selectively block a single pathogenetic factor in an *in vivo* system. The serum levels of the TNF-α receptors (TNFRs) represent a more sensitive parameter compared with TNF-α to measure the activity of TNF-α itself, because they finely modulate its action and they are more stable molecules.[16,17] Upon activation by TNF-α, membrane-bound TNFR-I and TNFR-II form homotrimers which in turn activate the transduction of the signal into the cell. TNFR-II has a greater affinity and half-life of ligand binding compared with TNFR-I and thus it binds and holds the cytokine, increasing the TNF-α concentration in vicinity of the TNFR-I, which then accepts it from TNFR-II. Membrane TNFRs are readily cleaved by the metalloprotease TNF-α converting enzyme (TACE) into the soluble forms which are still capable of TNF-α binding.[16] This fine modulation of the biologic form of TNFRs and the different tissue distribution of TNFR-I and TNFR-II, suggest that these molecules are crucial in the regulation of the cell responsiveness to TNF-α.[17]

We recently found that high levels of CHGA identify a subset of patients with RA at increased risk for systemic involvement (submitted for publication). To better understand how CHGA and TNF-α reciprocally interact in RA, we performed this study which evaluates the direct effect of the use of anti-TNF-α mAbs on the serum levels of CHGA in patients with RA and the effect on the correlation between CHGA and TNF-α and TNFR-I and TNFR-II.

MATERIALS AND METHODS

Population

From November 2001 to February 2004 we enrolled into this study 21 patients with RA who were being followed at the Division of Rheumatology and Clinical Immunology of the Scientific Institute Hospital San Raffaele, Milan (TABLE 1). Fourteen of them were being treated with anti-TNF-α mAbs. Seven patients started biologic therapy at the moment of enrollment.

Diagnosis of RA had been made in accordance with the 1987 American Rheumatism Association (ARA/ACR) diagnostic criteria.[18] Patients were eligible to start anti-TNF-α mAbs if they had active disease despite treatment with methotrexate 15 mg per week or more, in association with at least another disease modifying antirheumatic drug (DMARD), including azathioprine, leflunomide, cyclosporine, sulfasalazine, hydroxychloroquine, gold salts, and penicillamine. Active RA was defined by the presence of a ≥ 3.5 DAS28 value. The DAS28 is determined by a complex formula which takes in account three parameters (the number of affected joints, the erythrocyte sedimentation rate level, and the patient VAS for the pain) and can be calculated using computing devices.[19] Patients were not eligible if they had concomitant NYHA stage III or IV cardiac failure, uncontrolled hypertension, neuroendocrine malignancies, sepsis or severe infections, severe renal failure (< 50 mL/min creatinine clearance), and hepatic insufficiency (Child class B or C).

TABLE 1. Characteristics of patients at enrollment and their anti-TNF-α treatment

Pts	Age	VAS	DAS28	Erosions	Treatment
1	72	0	2.71	+	Etanercept
2	73	50	4.96	+	Etanercept
3	42	70	6.48	–	Infliximab
4	51	75	6.40	+	Infliximab
5	23	40	4.68	–	Adalimumab
6	28	20	4.40	–	Infliximab
7	68	10	2.72	+	Etanercept
8	39	35	7.15	+	Infliximab
9	53	20	6.46	–	Infliximab
10	51	20	4.12	–	Etanercept
11	53	0	4.08	+	Infliximab
12	67	50	4.32	+	Etanercept
13	57	10	4.59	+	Infliximab
14	55	50	5.45	+	Infliximab
15	52	30	2.52	+	Etanercept
16	61	55	3.46	–	Adalimumab
17	54	5	3.92	+	Adalimumab
18	30	20	4.21	–	Adalimumab
19	61	0	7.04	+	Infliximab
20	43	80	6.92	+	Adalimumab
21	54	40	4.25	–	Adalimumab

The mean age of the entire population (15 females and 6 males) was 52 years (range 23–78) (TABLE 1). Seven of 21 patients (5 females and 2 males) started anti-TNF-α treatment at the moment of enrollment: their mean age was 51.42 (range) and the mean DAS28 was 5.89 (range 4.08–7.15) (TABLE 2). All patients provided written informed consent to this study. We also selected 20 matching negative controls.

Treatment

Patients received one of the three anti-TNF-α mAbs accepted for the treatment of RA in our country:

(*a*) Nine patients received intravenous 3 mg/kg infliximab (Remicade, ®Centocor, Inc., Horsham, PA), at the initiation of treatment (week 0), at week 2, at week 6, and then every 8 weeks, in association with weekly oral methotrexate 7.5–15 mg;

(*b*) Six patients received subcutaneous 50 mg etanercept (Embrel, ®Immunex Corporation, Thousand Oaks, CA), twice a week;

(*c*) Six patients received subcutaneous 40 mg adalimumab (Humira, ®Abbott Laboratories, Abbott Park, IL) every 2 weeks, in association with weekly oral methotrexate 7.5–15 mg.

Concomitant treatment with daily prednisone, 10 mg or less, and/or nonsteroidal anti-inflammatory drugs (NSAIDs) was permitted.

TABLE 2. Response to therapy, measured using DAS28, in seven patients who started treatment with infliximab

Pts	DAS28 prior treatment	DAS28 after treatment	No. infusions
3	6.48	6.01	4
8	7.15	3.94	3
9	6.46	2.48	3
11	4.08	1.92	4
13	4.59	2.45	3
14	5.45	4.29	4
19	7.04	3.28	3

Disease Activity

We calculated the DAS28 at enrollment in all 21 patient and in the occasion of each drug infusion in the 7 patients who started *de novo* treatment with infliximab.

Assays for Cytokines and Neuroendocrine Factors

Blood samples were taken in all patients and in negative controls at the moment of enrollment from peripheral veins. In the seven patients starting infliximab samples were also collected in the occasion of each drug infusion (total 24 samples) (TABLE 2). The serum was obtained by centrifugation (2200 revolutions per min [RPM]; 5′) and stored at −30°C.

We measured, through sandwich enzyme-linked immunosorbent assay (ELISA), the serum levels of TNF-α, TNFR-I, TNFR-II, and CHGA. The TNF-α, TNFR-I, and TNFR-II serum levels were measured using the DuoSet R & D Systems ELISA kit (Minneapolis, MN), based on a solid phase-bound mouse antibody and a goat biotinylated reporter antibody. Results were converted to ng/mL using the standard curves. CHGA was measured by coating plates with B4E11 (a mouse IgG1 anti-CHGA mAb that recognizes an epitope corresponding to residues 68–79 of human CHGA) and using the rabbit anti-rCHGA-7–439 antiserum to human CHGA. Both B4E11 mAb and 7–439 antiserum were developed at the department of biotechnology, DIBIT, of our institution. The plates were further incubated with goat anti-rabbit IgG-peroxidase conjugated.

Statistical Analysis

We calculated the correlation between the serologic parameters through Pearson's coefficient.

RESULTS

Efficacy of the Functional Blockade of TNF-α in Treated RA Patients

Treatment with anti-TNF-α mAbs achieved a significant response. TABLE 2 reports data of patients who started treatment with infliximab at enrollment. DAS28 significantly decreased during treatment. The mean value varied from 5.89 to 3.48.

Serum Levels of TNF-α, TNFR-I, TNFR-II, and CHGA

To calculate the serum levels of TNF-α, TNFRs, and CHGA we collected a single blood sample from the 14 patients who were already being treated with anti-TNF-α mAbs and from negative controls. In the seven patients who started treatment at enrollment, we collected blood samples at baseline and subsequently in the occasion of the drug infusions (24 samples).

TNF-α was detectable in 32 out of 45 serum samples from RA patients. Its mean concentration was 71.2 pg/mL (range 10.7–556.5). The mean TNFR-I concentration was 2218.7 pg/mL (range 445.3–4048.8). TNFR-II levels were not considered in patients treated with etanercept because this drug is a recombinant molecule corresponding to the soluble form of the receptor II. The mean TNFR-II value was 3064.1 pg/mL (range1881.8–5430.4). The mean serum concentration of CHGA was 280.2 ng/mL (range 29.9–3594.5). Notably, TNF-α was detectable in none of the serum samples from negative controls and TNFR-I, TNFR-II, and CHGA mean levels (respectively, 1281.4, 1859,2, and 82.1) were significantly lower compared with patients.

The serum levels of TNF-α in patients showed no correlation with the serum levels of TNFR-I, TNFR-II, and CHGA. The correlation values, measured through Pearson's coefficient, resulted respectively, −0.03, 0.18, and −0.02.

In a previous study, we observed that patients with RA present higher levels of CHGA and TNFRs, but not of TNF-α, compared with the normal population and that CHGA and TNFR-I significantly correlate (submitted for publication). We thus focused our attention on the effect of the selective blockade of TNF-α on the correlation between CHGA and TNFRs.

TNF-α-Blockade Abrogates the Correlation Between CHGA and TNFRs

We measured the mean values of CHGA, TNFR-I, and TNFR-II in the samples collected before the initiation of treatment (respectively, 191.2, 1952.2, and 3104.7) and observed no difference with those measured during treatment (respectively, 173.6, 1095.6, and 3165.9). We then investigated the correlation between serum TNFRs and CHGA levels measured at baseline: the Pearson's coefficient between TNFR-I and CHGA resulted 0.59 (FIG. 1A) and between

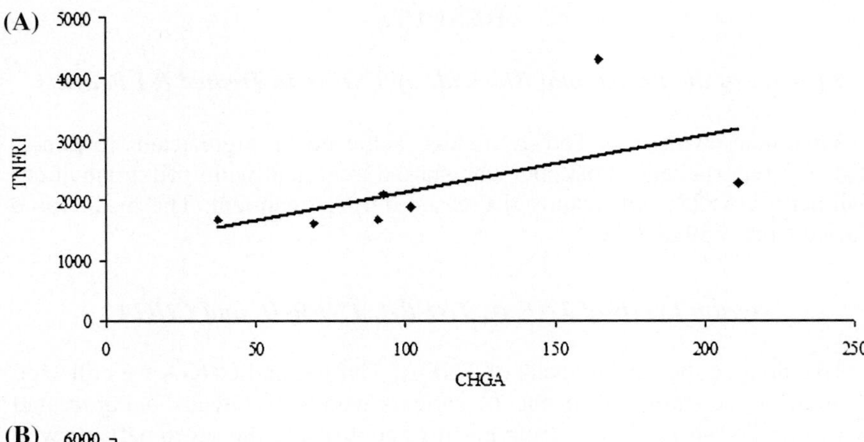

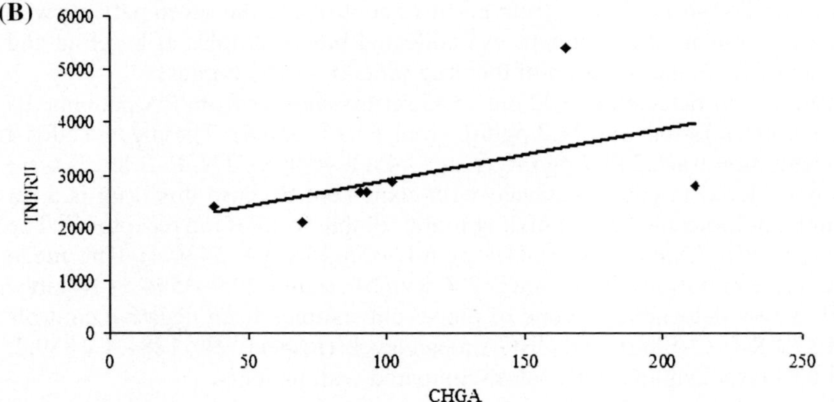

FIGURE 1. Correlation between serum CHGA, ng/mL, and TNFR-I **(A)** and TNFR-II **(B)**, pg/mL, levels before treatment in seven patients.

TNFR-II and CHGA resulted 0.53 (FIG. 1B), indicating that a correlation between CHGA and the receptors for TNF-α exists before treatment.

The correlation, calculated in the same patients during treatment with anti-TNF-α mAbs (24 samples at different times) was no more evident. The Pearson's coefficient between CHGA and TNFR-I and TNFR-II resulted respectively, −0.09 (FIG. 2A) and −0.07 (FIG. 2B), suggesting that TNF-α blockade interferes with the regulation of the CHGA pathway in RA.

DISCUSSION

Recent advances in the understanding of the pathogenetic mechanisms of RA led to identifying different factors reciprocally interacting in different pathways. Many evidences suggest that RA can be considered a systemic disease

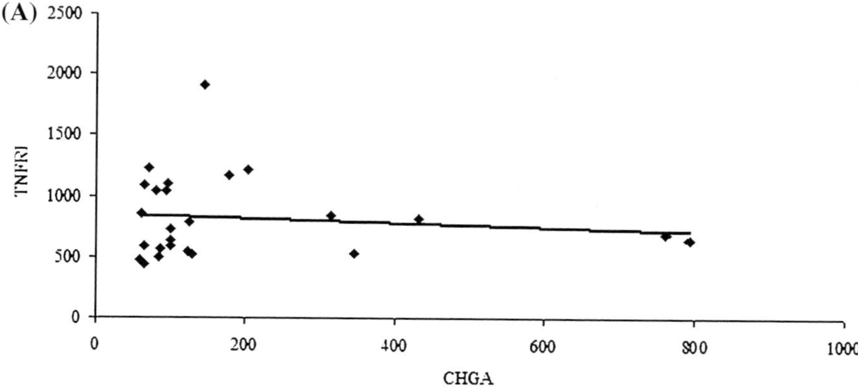

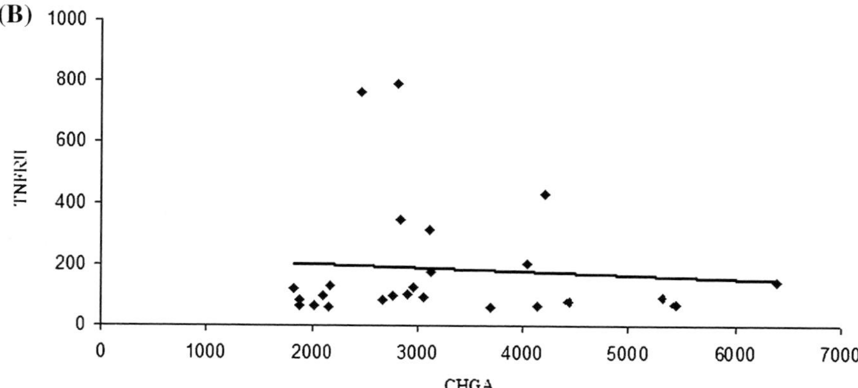

FIGURE 2. Correlation between serum CHGA, ng/mL, and TNFR-I **(A)** and TNFR-II **(B)**, pg/mL, levels during treatment with infliximab.

and that biohumoral factors must contribute to its pathogenesis.[9] Attention has always focused on cytokines, which are considered the main actors in the pathogenesis of RA. Among them TNF-α certainly plays a crucial role.[9] The circulating levels of its soluble receptors,TNFR-I and TNFR-II, are a sensitive parameter to evaluate the activity of the pathway of TNF-α itself, because they are stable molecules and are responsible for the fine regulation of TNF-α. The soluble receptors derive from cleavage of the membrane-bound molecules by the metalloprotease TACE. When circulating TNF-α levels are low, they bind it in order to prolong its bioavailability, representing a biologic reservoir. Instead, when circulating TNF-α is present at high concentrations, they compete for its binding with the membrane receptors, preventing excessive activation.[16,17]

Other humoral factors have proved to be involved in the pathogenesis of RA.[9] Among them many hormones and neuropeptides are contained in the secretory granules of the cells of the neuroendocrine system.[8] CHGA is commonly considered a marker for the activation of these cells and thus is monitored in the follow-up of neuroendocrine malignancies. In fact CHGA is contained in the secretory granules along with the other molecules and plays a main role in the regulation of their trafficking, storage, and secretion.[2,3] Recently CHGA has been shown to take part in the regulation of the endothelial barrier function in inflammatory diseases, interacting with TNF-α.[6]

We recently performed a study on a large cohort of patients with RA aimed at evaluating whether CHGA could be a useful marker in the clinical setting and could provide new insights in the role of the neuroendocrine system in the pathogenesis of RA. We observed that patients with RA have significantly higher serum levels of CHGA and TNFRs compared with controls and that the highest levels of CHGA identify the population of patients with extra-articular manifestations. In patients with RA, CHGA correlated with TNFR-I, suggesting that CHGA might be involved in the pathogenesis of the disease through an interaction with TNF-α (submitted for publication).

We therefore measured the serum levels of TNF-α, TNFR-I, TNFR-II, and CHGA in a population of 21 patients (45 blood samples) treated with one of the three anti-TNF-α mAbs available in the clinical setting: infliximab, etanercept, and adalimumab. Those patients had persistently active disease despite previous treatment with methotrexate in association with at least another DMARD. Anti-TNF-α treatment in these patients achieved a good response, consistent with that reported in the literature.[13–15] We evaluated the correlation between CHGA and TNFR-I and between CHGA and TNFR-II in patients before the initiation of treatment with infliximab and compared it with the value calculated during treatment. We observed a high correlation between CHGA and both the receptors. Moreover, we found that treatment with anti-TNF-α mAbs abrogated both the correlation between CHGA and TNFR-I and the correlation between CHGA and TNFR-II.

In conclusion, treatment with anti-TNF-α mAbs induces a good clinical response in patients with refractory disease, demonstrating its capability of interfering with key pathogenetic factors. These drugs do not vary the mean levels of CHGA and TNFRs but they lead to the abrogation of the correlation between CHGA and TNFRs. Taken together our results seem to suggest that CHGA might be involved in the pathogenesis of RA through a complex interaction with TNF-α, mediated by yet undefined factors. A better understanding could be derived by the analysis of wider cohorts of patients, identifying different subgroups according to the response to treatment with anti-TNF-α mAbs.

REFERENCES

1. Winkler, H. & R. Fischer-Colbrie. 1992. The chromogranins A and B: the first 25 years and future perspectives. Neuroscience **49:** 497–528.

2. TAUPENOT, L., K.L. HARPER & D.T. O'CONNOR. 2003. Mechanisms of disease: the chromogranin-secretogranin family. N. Engl. J. Med. **348:** 1134–1149.
3. KIM, T. *et al.* 2001. Chromogranin A, an "on/off" switch controlling dense-core secretory granule biogenesis. Cell **106:** 499–509.
4. METZ-BOUTIGUE, M.H. *et al.* 2003. Innate immunity: involvement of new neuropeptides. Trends Microbiol. **11:** 585–592.
5. TAKIYYUDDIN, M.A. *et al.* 1990. Chromogranin A. Storage and release in hypertension. Hypertension **15:** 237–246.
6. FERRERO, E. *et al.* 2004. Chromogranin A protects vessels against tumor necrosis factor alpha-induced vascular leakage. FASEB J. **18:** 554–556.
7. FERRERO, E. *et al.* 2002. Regulation of endothelial cell shape and barrier function by chromogranin A. Ann. N. Y. Acad. Sci. **971:** 355–358.
8. HARLE, P. *et al.* 2005. Predictive and potentially predictive factors in early arthritis: a multidisciplinary approach. Rheumatology (Oxford) **44:** 426–433.
9. FIRESTEIN, G.S. *et al.* 2003. Evolving concepts of rheumatoid arthritis. Nature **423:** 356–361.
10. HARRIS, E.D. *et al.* 1990. Rheumatoid arthritis: pathophysiology and implications for therapy. N. Engl. J. Med. **322:** 1277–1289.
11. MILLER, L.E. *et al.* 1999. In vitro superfusion method to study nerve-immune cell interactions in human synovial membrane in long-standing rheumatoid arthritis or osteoarthritis. Ann. N. Y. Acad. Sci. **876:** 266–275.
12. SEGOND VON BANCHET, G.G. *et al.* 2000. Monoarticular antigen-induced arthritis leads to pronounced bilateral upregulation of the expression of neurokinin 1 and bradykinin 2 receptors in dorsal root ganglion neurons of rats. Arthritis Res. **2:** 424–427.
13. LIPSKY, P.E. *et al.* 2000. Infliximab and methotrexate in the treatment of rheumatoid arthritis. Anti-tumor necrosis factor trial in rheumatoid arthritis with concomitant therapy study group. N. Engl. J. Med. **343:** 1594–1602.
14. MORELAND, L.W. *et al.* 1999. Etanercept therapy in rheumatoid arthritis. A randomised controlled trial. Ann. Intern. Med. **130:** 478–486.
15. WEINBLATT, M.E. *et al.* 2003. Adalimumab, a fully human anti-tumor necrosis factor alpha monoclonal antibody, for the treatment of rheumatoid arthritis in patients taking concomitant methotrexate: the ARMADA trial. Arthritis Rheum. **48:** 35–45.
16. TARTAGLIA, L.A. *et al.* 1993. Ligand passing—the 75-kDa tumor-necrosis-factor (TNF) receptor recruits TNF for signaling by the 55-kDa TNF receptor. J. Biol. Chem. **268:** 18542–18548.
17. PENNICA, D. *et al.* 1992. Biochemical-properties of the 75-kDa tumor-necrosis-factor receptor—characterization of ligand-binding, internalization, and receptor phosphorylation. J. Biol. Chem. **267:** 21172–21178.
18. ARNETT, F.C. *et al.* 1988. The American Rheumatism Association 1987 revised criteria for the classification of rheumatoid arthritis. Arthritis Rheum. **31:** 315–324.
19. The home of the DAS. http://www.das-score.nl/www.das-score.nl/. September 2005.

Nerve Growth Factor and Brain-Derived Neurotrophic Factor Levels in Patients with Rheumatoid Arthritis Treated with TNF-α Blockers

FLAVIA DEL PORTO,[a] LUIGI ALOE,[b] BRUNO LAGANÀ,[a] VIVIANA TRIACA,[b] ITALO NOFRONI,[c] AND RAFFAELE D'AMELIO[a,d]

[a]*Cattedra ed U.O.C di Allergologia, Immunologia Clinica e Reumatologia, II Facoltà di Medicina e Chirurgia, Università "La Sapienza," Ospedale Sant'Andrea, 00189 Roma, Italy*

[b]*Istituto di Neurobiologia e Medicina Molecolare, CNR, EBRI, Roma, Italy*

[c]*I Facoltà di Medicina e Chirurgia, Dipartimento di Medicina Sperimentale e Patologia, II Facoltà di Medicina e Chirurgia, Università "La Sapienza," Roma, Italy*

[d]*Ministero della Difesa, Direzione Generale della Sanità Militare, Roma, Italy*

ABSTRACT: Twenty consecutive rheumatoid arthritis (RA) patients (mean age 50.4 ± 10.5 years; 17 females; mean disease duration 5.78 ± 3.75 years) enrolled for tumor necrosis factor-α (TNF-α) blockers therapy (10 infliximab and 10 etanercept) were selected. Before starting therapy, 3 and 6 months thereafter all patients were evaluated for disease activity score (DAS), erythrocyte sedimentation rate (ESR), serum levels of C-reactive protein (CRP), interleukin-6 (IL-6), nerve growth factor (NGF), and brain-derived neurotrophic factor (BDNF). After 3 and 6 months a significant reduction in DAS, ESR, CRP, and IL-6 was observed, whereas no significant differences of NGF and BDNF serum levels were found. These preliminary results confirm that TNF-α blockers significantly improve disease activity and inflammation in RA; nevertheless further studies are needed to explain the mechanisms regulating NGF and BDNF release in RA patients treated with TNF-α blockers.

KEYWORDS: NGF; BDNF; rheumatoid arthritis; TNF-α blockers

Address for correspondence: Flavia Del Porto, M.D., Cattedra e U.O.C di Allergologia, Immunologia Clinica e Reumatologia, II Facoltà di Medicina e. Chirurgia, Università "La Sapienza," Ospedale Sant'Andrea, Via di Grottarossa 1035-1039, 00189 Roma, Italy. Voice: +39-06-33775495 fax: +39-06-33775074

e-mail: flavia.delporto@uniroma1.it

Ann. N.Y. Acad. Sci. 1069: 438–443 (2006). © 2006 New York Academy of Sciences.
doi: 10.1196/annals.1351.042

BACKGROUND

Rheumatoid arthritis (RA) is a systemic autoimmune disease characterized by chronic inflammation and cytokine release. Among cytokines, tumor necrosis factor-α (TNF-α) plays a pivotal role in the induction and maintenance of synovial immune-inflammation[1]; therefore, it is considered an effective target for therapy.[2] Nerve growth factor (NGF) and brain-derived neurotrophic factor (BDNF) are polypeptides that exert trophic, differentiative, and repairing effects on peripheral and central populations of neurons.[3] Moreover, they act on a wide variety of immune cells, being involved in the inflammatory response modulation.[4–6] NGF and BDNF have been detected in the synovial fluid of patients with chronic autoimmune arthritis[7]; furthermore, it has been demonstrated that proinflammatory cytokines such as interleukin-1 (IL-1), IL-6, and TNF-α may promote neurotrophin secretion.[8,9] Monoclonal antibodies against TNF-α have been shown to reduce the expression of receptor for NGF and BDNF, but the effect on NGF and BDNF serum levels, to our knowledge, has not yet been studied.

The aim of this study was therefore to evaluate, in RA patients, the possible effect of TNF-α blockers on NGF and BDNF serum levels.

PATIENTS AND METHODS

Patients

Twenty consecutive RA patients (mean age 50.4 ± 10.5 years; 17 females; mean disease duration 5.78 ± 3.75 years) selected from those attending our outpatient clinic and diagnosed on the basis of American College of Rheumatology (ACR) criteria[10] were selected. All the patients met the requirement for anti-TNF-α therapy. Ten of them were treated with infliximab and 10 with etanercept. The type of biological drug as well as therapeutic strategy adopted was decided independently of the study.

Patients with past or current central or peripheral nervous system diseases were excluded from the study. An informed written consent was obtained from each patient before the inclusion in the study.

Methods

In all the patients the below-listed clinical and laboratory parameters have been evaluated before starting the therapy, 3 and 6 months thereafter.

Clinical Measurement

Disease activity score (DAS) has been measured according to the ACR guidelines[11] by evaluating Ritchie index, number of swollen joints, erythrocyte sedimentation rate (ESR), and general health.

Therapeutic effect has been assessed on the basis of European League Against Rheumatism (EULAR) criteria by evaluating the improvement of DAS.[12]

Laboratory Tests

NGF and BDNF were assessed by ELISA. The levels of NGF were measured using the R&D Duoset ELISA Development System (DY256) and the levels of BDNF were measured using an ELISA kit "BDNF EmaxTm ImmunoAssay System" number G6891 by Promega (Madison, WI, USA), following the instructions suggested by the manufacturer. The sensitivity of the assays was 3 pg/mL; cross-reactivity with other molecules of the NGF family was <3%; and all assays were performed in duplicate. Data were represented as pg/mL NGF and as pg BDNF/mg of total protein.

Before and after 6 months after the beginning of the therapy, IL-6 levels were measured by flow cytometry using commercially available kits (BD CBA Bead Array, BD Biosciences, San Josè, CA, USA) according to the manufacturer's instructions. C-reactive protein (CRP) and rheumatoid factor (RF) were evaluated by nephelometry.

Statistical Analysis

Data were expressed as mean $\pm$ SD. A perspective analysis of results (times 3 and 6 versus time 0) was performed using Wilcoxon signed rank test ($P <$ 0.05 significant).

RESULTS

Since no differences were found between patients treated with infliximab and those treated with etanercept, results have been taken as a whole.

Three and 6 months after the beginning of therapy, a significant improvement of DAS ($P < 0.0001$), ESR ($P < 0.001$), CRP($P <$ 0. 0001), and IL-6 ($P < 0.011$) has been observed whereas no significant difference of NGF and BDNF serum levels ($P < 0.170$ and $P < 0.679$, respectively) has been found (see TABLE 1).

DISCUSSION

These preliminary results confirm that TNF-α blockers significantly improve RA disease activity and inflammation.[1] Nevertheless, we did not find any modification of NGF and BDNF levels after TNF-α blockers administration. The concept that neurotrophins operate only as interneural mediators has been recently revised by the finding that NGF and BDNF act both on immune

TABLE 1. Results from the perspective analysis of mean values (times 3 and 6 versus time 0)

	DAS	ESR (mm/h)	CRP (mg/L)	IL-6 (pg/mL)	NGF (pg/mL)	BDNF (pg/mg)
Time 0	5.54 ± 0.93	33.21 ± 23.74	23.15 ± 31.35	20.02 ± 51.88	190.58 ± 243.55	6469.26 ± 4526.89
3 months	3.59 ± 0.71	19.78 ± 18.70	4.46 ± 5.58	N.D.	235.22 ± 282.92	6506.77 ± 4756.18
6 months	2.97 ± 0.55	13.78 ± 8.81	5.15 ± 5.42	4.61 ± 11.43	220.48 ± 189.97	5696.42 ± 4648.62
P	< 0.0001	< 0.001	< 0.0001	< 0.011	N.S.	N.S.

N.D. not done; N.S. not significant.

cells.[13] Moreover, these neutrotrophins are constitutively secreted by peripheral blood mononuclear cells and synoviocytes.[9–14] It has been demonstrated that neurotrophin levels increase in inflamed tissues, such as brain lesions of multiple sclerosis,[15] airways in asthma,[16] synovial fluid in chronic autoimmune arthritis, and synovium of pharmacologically induced arthritis in animal models.[13] Neurotrophins, in fact, are involved in the modulation of the inflammatory response.[17] The bidirectional relationship occurring between the nervous and the immune system is mediated by cytokines. In particular, it has been demonstrated that proinflammatory cytokines, such as TNF-α and IL-6, specifically promote NGF and BDNF secretion by immune cells.[8,9] Moreover, TNF-α participates in the death of NGF-dependent neurons during the development of the central nervous system.[18] In patients with chronic autoimmune diseases, inflammation and cytokine release may only in part account for the overexpression of NGF and BDNF; several other factors, such as chronic stress and therapies, in fact, may interfere with neurotrophin release. Stress, which is characterized by immune cell activation, has been documented to increase NGF levels,[19] while corticosteroids downregulate neurotrophin synthesis.[15]

Data regarding neurotrophin levels in sera from chronic autoimmune diseases do not seem to be unequivocal; some authors, in fact, found increased levels of NGF in sera from RA and systemic lupus erythematosus (SLE) patients,[20] whereas Rhil *et al*. reported that NGF was not detectable in sera from RA patients.[7] NGF and BDNF were both detectable in sera from our patients, but their levels did not show any significant reduction after TNF-α administration. In the literature it has been reported that BDNF levels were higher in sera from healthy subjects than in those from patients with chronic autoimmune arthritis,[7] suggesting that, although proinflammatory cytokines play a key role in promoting neurotrophin secretion, several other mechanisms are probably involved in regulating NGF and BDNF release during the inflammatory response. Further studies are needed to clarify the elements involved in NGF and BDNF secretion in RA patients treated with TNF-α blockers.

ACKNOWLEDGMENTS

This study was financially supported by the Ateneo Project number C26A049040, University "La Sapienza," Rome, Italy.

REFERENCES

1. Harris, E.D. 1990. Rheumatoid arthritis. Pathophysiology and implications for therapy. N. Engl. J. Med. **322:** 1277–1289.
2. Redlich, K., G. Schett, G. Steiner, *et al.* 2003. Rheumatoid arthritis therapy after tumor necrosis factor and interleukin 1 blockade. Arthritis Rheum. **48:** 3308–3319.

3. LYNCH, M.A. 2004. Long-term potentiation and memory. Physiol. Rev. **84:** 87–136.
4. ALOE, L., L. BRACCI-LAUDIERO, S. BONINI, *et al.* 1997. The expanding role of nerve growth factor: from neurotrophin activity to immunologic diseases. Allergy **52:** 883–894.
5. ALOE, L., M.D. SIMONE & F. PROPERZI. 1999. Nerve growth factor: a neurotrophin with activity on cells of the immune system. Microsc. Res. Tech. **45:** 285–291.
6. STANISZ, AM. & J.A. STANISZ. 2000. Nerve growth factor and neuroimmune interactions in inflammatory diseases. Ann. N. Y. Acad. Sci. **917:** 268–272.
7. RIHL, M., E. KRUITHOF, C. BARTHEL, *et al.* 2005. Involvement of neurotrophins and their receptors in spondyloarthritis synovitis: relation to inflammation and response to therapy. Ann. Rheum. Dis. **64**(11): 1542–1549.
8. CARLSON, N.G., W.A. WIEGGEL, J. CHEN, *et al.* 1999. Inflammatory cytokines IL-1α, IL-1β, IL-6 and TNF-α in part neuroprotection to an exitotoxin through distinct pathways. J. Immunol. **163:** 3936–3968.
9. HERBRUGGEN, O.S., C. NASSENSTEIN, M. LOMMATZSCH, *et al.* 2005. Tumor necrosis factor-α and interleukin-6 regulate secretion of brain derived neurotrophic factor in human monocytes. J. Neuroimmunol. **160:** 204–209.
10. ARNETT, F.C., S. EDWORTHY, D.A. BLOCH, *et al.* 1988. The American Rheumatism Association 1987 revised criteria for the classification of rheumatoid arthritis. Arthritis Rheum. **31:** 315–324.
11. FELSON, D.T., J.J. ANDERSON, M. BOERS, *et al.* 1993. The American College of Rheumatology preliminary core set of disease activity measures for rheumatoid arthritis clinical trials. The Committee on Outcome Measures in Rheumatoid Arthritis Clinical Trials. Arthritis Rheum. **36:** 729–740.
12. VAN GESTEL, A.M., M.L.L. PREVOO, M.A. VAN'T HOF, *et al.* 1996. Development and validation of the European League Against Rheumatism response criteria for rheumatoid arthritis. Arthritis Rheum. **39:** 34–40.
13. ALOE, L. & M.A. TUVERI. 1997. Nerve growth factor and autoimmune rheumatic diseases. Clin. Exp. Rheumatol. **15:** 433–438.
14. MANNI, L., T. LUNDEBERG, S. FIORITO, *et al.* 2003. Nerve growth factor release by human synovial fibroblasts prior to and following exposure to tumor necrosis factor-alpha, interleukin-1 beta and cholecystokinin-8: the possible role of NGF in the inflammatory response. Clin. Exp. Rheumatol. **21:** 617–624.
15. KERSCHENSTEINER, M., E. GALLMEIER, L. BEHRENS, *et al.* 1999. Activated human T cells, B cells and monocytes produce brain derived neurotrophic factor in vitro and in inflammatory brain lesions: a neuroprotective role of inflammation? J. Exp. Med. **185:** 865–870.
16. FROSSARD, N., V. FREUND & C. ADVENIER. 2004. Nerve growth factor and its receptors in asthma and inflammation. Eur. J. Pharmacol. **500:** 453–465.
17. BONINI, S., G. RASI, M.L. BRACCI-LAUDIERO, *et al.* 2003. Nerve growth factor: neurotrophin or cytokine? Intl. Arch. Allergy Immunol. **131:** 80–84.
18. BAKER, V., G. MIDDLETON, F. DAVEY, *et al.* 2001. TNFα contributes to the death of NGF-dependent neurons during development. N. Neurosci. **12:** 1194–1198.
19. ALOE, L., E. ALLEVA & M. FIORE. 2002. Stress and nerve growth factor: findings in animal models and humans. Pharmacol. Biochem. Behav. **73:** 159–166.
20. DICOU, E., C. MASSON, W. JABBOUR, *et al.* 1993. Increased frequency of NGF in sera of rheumatoid arthritis and systemic lupus erythematosus patients. Neuroreport **5:** 321–324.

Adipose Tissue Has Anti-Inflammatory Properties

Focus on IL-1 Receptor Antagonist (IL-1Ra)

JEAN-MICHEL DAYER,[a] RACHEL CHICHEPORTICHE,[a]
CRISTIANA JUGE-AUBRY,[b] AND CHRISTOPH MEIER[b]

[a]*Division of Immunology & Allergy, University Hospital / Faculty of Medicine, 1211 Geneva 14, Switzerland*

[b]*Endocrine Unit, Division of Endocrinology & Diabetology, University Hospital/ Faculty of Medicine, 1211 Geneva 14, Switzerland*

ABSTRACT: The formation of adipose tissue could result from abnormal metabolic processes and, at the local level, from chronic inflammatory processes such as those occurring in the synovial cavity in rheumatoid arthritis or osteoarthritis, or the peritoneal cavity in various inflammatory processes of the digestive system. Adipocytes are said to produce many hormones and proinflammatory mediators. So far, however, little attention has been paid to cytokine inhibitory molecules. Based on our observation of high levels of serum interleukin receptor antagonist (IL-1Ra) in obese patients contrasting with decreased levels after gastric bypass surgery, we found white adipose tissue (WAT) in the human system to be the main source of IL-1Ra. IL-10 was also present in WAT. Furthermore, we found that interferon-β (IFN)-β was the principal cytokine inducing IL-1Ra in various WAT, such as that present in the synovium. We suggest that in addition to other functions adipose tissue may give rise to a host-defense mechanism against local inflammation and that fibrotic tissue in the vicinity may further induce IL-1Ra in adipocytes via the production of IFN-β.

KEYWORDS: adipocytes; arthritis; inflammation; obesity; synovial tissue; IL-1Ra; IFN-β; IL-10; MCP-1

OBESITY AND IL-1Ra

It has been shown that obesity is associated with the increased secretion of metabolic and inflammatory mediators by white adipose tissue (WAT), for

All studies performed by the authors were approved by the Ethical Committee of Geneva University Hospital.

Address for correspondence: Jean-Michel Dayer, M.D., Division of Immunology & Allergy, 24 Rue Micheli-du-Crest, 1211 Geneva 14, Switzerland. Voice: +41-22-372-94 09; fax: +41-22-372-94 18.
e-mail: jean-michel.dayer@hcuge.ch

**Ann. N.Y. Acad. Sci. 1069: 444–453 (2006). © 2006 New York Academy of Sciences.
doi: 10.1196/annals.1351.043**

instance tumor necrosis factor-α (TNF-α) which is implicated in the pathogenesis of cardiovascular complications and insulin resistance, respectively.[1–4] Adipocytes also produce other factors to control obesity.

Hyperleptinemia appears to correlate with obesity, as determined by the percentage of body fat.[5] However, cytokine antagonists have not been studied so far, and interleukin receptor antagonist (IL-1Ra) for instance has never been measured in these conditions. IL-1Ra is a natural antagonist specific to the proinflammatory cytokine IL-1 and is commonly thought to play an important role in the regulation of inflammatory responses *in vitro* and *in vivo*.[6–8] Based on the findings that the mitigating effect of leptin on food intake and body temperature is mediated by IL-1, it was hypothesized that IL-1Ra also plays a regulatory part in the homeostasis of energy[9]; the authors demonstrated that the hypothalamic effects of leptin depend markedly on the action of IL-1 and that the injection of IL-1Ra into the cerebral ventricles inhibited leptin-induced reduction of food intake as well as the simultaneous increase in body temperature by more than 60%. Furthermore, we observed *in vitro* that leptin increased the expression and secretion of IL-1Ra in human monocytes, whereas it had a lesser effect, or none at all, on IL-1 secretion.[10] Leptin activates the promotor of IL-1Ra through p42/44 mitogen-activated protein kinase and a composite nuclear factor κB/PU.1 binding site.[11] It was thus tempting to speculate that the leptin-induced increase in IL-1Ra secretion might antagonize the hypothalamic effects of IL-1 on food intake.

In accordance with this premise, we investigated the putative relationship between IL-1Ra serum concentrations and leptin levels, as well as other metabolic parameters in lean and obese subjects before and after gastric bypass surgery. We demonstrated that IL-1Ra levels are highly elevated in human obesity and that its concentrations decrease after weight loss from bypass surgery. However, lean body mass (LBM) and insulin resistance were better predictors of serum IL-1Ra concentrations than were leptin levels, suggesting that additional metabolic factors control the secretion of this cytokine antagonist.[12] However, we only found IL-6 levels to be slightly, but not significantly, higher in obese patients than in the lean control subjects, neither group presenting inflammatory conditions as demonstrated by C-reactive protein (CRP) levels. Of note, knockout mice lacking the IL-1Ra gene were significantly lighter than their wild-type littermates.[13]

ADIPOSE TISSUE AS A MAJOR SOURCE OF IL-1Ra

The observation that IL-1Ra levels were higher in obese patients and decreased after weight loss induced by intestinal bypass surgery, highlighted the importance of identifying the main tissular origin of IL-1Ra. In mice, IL-1Ra mRNA was expressed in liver, spleen, and in epididymal and inguinal WAT and in very low amounts in brown adipose tissue, kidney, skeletal muscle, and heart. In comparison to lean mice, most tissue from ob/ob animals expressed higher amounts of IL-1Ra, with a 37- and 5-fold increase in WAT epididymal and WAT inguinal tissue, respectively. In contrast, the expression of IL-1β mRNA and TNF mRNA in WAT was lower in obese animals than in lean ones. Consequently, the ratio of proinflammatory to anti-inflammatory cytokines was in favor of the latter. In the human system, IL-1Ra protein and mRNA are clearly present in WAT and markedly increased in obesity, the ratio of IL-1Ra to IL-1β protein in tissue being clearly in favor of IL-1Ra. The production of IL-1Ra as compared to that of IL-6, TNF, and IL-1 is much higher by far. IL-1Ra serum levels are elevated in human obesity to a similar extent as in systemic inflammation.[14]

REGULATION OF IL-1Ra PRODUCTION IN THE ADIPOSE TISSUE

The next question was to determine which factors could favor the production of IL-1Ra. It is well known that IL-1Ra levels increase markedly in response to fever and inflammation as a host-defense mechanism, which seminal observation was made in patients with systemic juvenile rheumatoid arthritis[7] and then confirmed by many investigators (for review see Ref. 15) and that IL-1Ra acts as an acute-phase protein.[16] Cytokines such as IL-1, IL-3, IL-4, IL-10, TNF-α, granulocyte-macrophage colony-stimulating factor (GM-CSF), and interferon-β (IFN-β) have been found to modulate IL-1Ra, IFN-β having proved the most potent of them on human monocytes.[17,18] This was confirmed on human WAT both at the protein level and mRNA expression.[14,19] Peroxisome proliferator-activated receptor-γ (PPAR-γ) ligands, such as rosiglitazone, failed to induce the secretion of IL-1Ra. This contrasts with the observation that PPAR-γ ligands enhance the expression and secretion of IL-1Ra by stimulated monocytes.[20] Because IFN-β is not only derived from fibroblasts but also produced by other types of cells such as macrophages, epithelial, endothelial, and lymphoid cells[21] it is tempting to speculate that stromal cells and preadipocytes might be involved in IL-1Ra secretion via a paracrine mechanism. Taking into account the fact that IL-4 and IL-10 were also known to induce IL-1Ra in human monocytes, we observed that the addition of IL-4 also enhanced the stimulatory effect of IL-1 (∼ twofold), but alone neither IL-4 nor IL-10 induced the production of IL-1Ra, although IL-1 alone slightly induced IL-1Ra as did lipopolysaccharide (LPS).[19]

Furthermore, the human system expresses the receptors and proteins required for IL-1 action, that is, IL-1 receptor type I rather than IL-1 receptor type II (decoy receptor) and IL-1 receptor accessory protein. Besides increasing IL-1RII, IFN-β also increases the IFN-α / -β subunits IFNAR1 and IFNAR2.[19]

PRODUCTION OF CYTOKINES AND CHEMOKINES BY ADIPOSE TISSUE

As discussed, human WAT produced far more IL-1Ra than IL-1, TNF, IL-6, and IL-8.[14] Others have reported the production of the latter four cytokines by adipose tissue.[3,22–26] All these proinflammatory cytokines may amplify the inflammatory process at the local level. However, the ratio of IL-1Ra/IL-1 is in favor of IL-1Ra. We have therefore investigated the production of other cytokines and chemokines that might possibly be involved in the regulation of inflammation. Indeed, adipose tissue also produced IL-10, a molecule also possessing anti-inflammatory properties.[27] In WAT explants, IL-1 was upregulated by LPS and TNF *in vitro*, as well as in obese patients. It has been previously demonstrated that obesity is associated with increasing circulating levels of IL-10,[28] which is consistent with our finding that IL-10 expression is increased in the adipose tissue of obese humans and rodents. Noteworthy, other chemokines—such as IL-8, monocyte chemotactic protein-1 (MCP-1), and Regulated upon Activation Normal T cell Express Sequence (RANTES)—are expressed to a greater extent in obese than in lean subjects[29]; however, IP-1+, but not RANTES, is upregulated by leptin in monocytic cells.[30,31]

PRODUCTION OF CYTOKINES AND OTHER MEDIATORS BY SYNOVIAL ADIPOSE TISSUE IN THE PRESENCE OF IFN-β

On investigating the action of IFN-β in synovial adipose tissue we found that in the presence of IFN-β, the levels of IL-1Ra and MCP-1 were markedly increased, contrary to those of IL-1β, IL-6, IL-8, metalloproteinase 1 (MMP-1), prostaglandin E2 (PGE2), leptin, and adiponectin (TABLE 1). The levels of the latter parameters, with the exception of adiponectin, are even lower in the presence of IFN-β, although not to a significant extent. The results are consistent when adjusting the levels of mediators either to milligram of wet tissue weight or to microgram of DNA. In these experiments, TNF-α levels were at the limit of detection and IL-1α undetectable. These results were similar in three different preparations of synovial adipose tissue (FIG. 1).

When compared in micrograms of protein or DNA, IL-1Ra levels at base line appear to be markedly higher (∼threefold) in adipose tissue originating from inflammatory tissue, that is, synovial tissue, as compared to subcutaneous adipose tissue from obese patients.

DISCUSSION

At the present stage of the study, we can draw the following conclusion: (*a*) IL-1Ra levels in serum and adipose tissue from obese patients are higher

TABLE 1. Production of cytokines and other mediators by adipose tissue of the human synovium (two separate experiments)

	IFN-β (1)		IFN-β (2)	
	–	+	–	+
Mediators	(per mg of wet tissue) Mean ± SD		(per mg of wet tissue) Mean ± SD	
IL-1Ra (pg)	40 ± 22	155 ± 20	996 ± 643	9526 ± 2483
MCP-1 (ng)	196 ± 114	665 ± 92	4810 ± 3340	18795 ± 8014
IL-1β (pg)	0.3 ± 0.1	0.2 ± 0.1	6.6 ± 3.8	4.1 ± 1.7
IL-6 (ng)	10 ± 5	3 ± 1	256 ± 151	85 ± 37
IL-8 (ng)	4 ± 2	2 ± 1	106 ± 55	41 ± 18
MMP-1 (ng)	3 ± 1	1 ± 1	71 ± 39	21 ± 2
PGE2 (ng)	13 ± 8	3 ± 2	318 ± 216	93 ± 67
Adiponectin (ng)	1.1 ± 0.3	1.1 ± 0.2	27 ± 8	29 ± 8

NOTE: Adipose tissue was dissected from synovial tissue and incubated for 48 h in Ultracult medium (BIO WHITTAKER, Walkersville, MD, USA) in the presence or absence of IFN-β (10^4 U/mL). At the end of the culture time, supernatants were assayed for the various mediators by enzyme-linked immunosorbent assay (ELISA). Values represent the mean of triplicate fragments (mean ± SD). Values were adjusted either to milligram of wet tissue weight or microgram of DNA.

than in normal controls, and the ratio of IL-1Ra to IL-1β is in favor of IL-1Ra; (*b*) of the cytokines tested so far, that modulate mediator production by WAT, IFN-β is among those that induce IL-1Ra the most; (*c*) IFN-β elicits a marked selective increase in some chemokines such as MCP-1 but not IL-8, but adiponectin and leptin are not modulated by IFN-β; (*d*) adipose

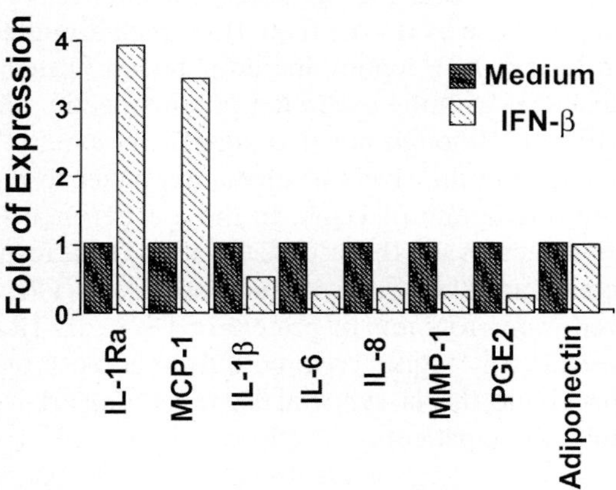

FIGURE 1. Induction by IFN-β (10 U/mL) of IL-1Ra and MCP-1 on synovial adipose tissue. Fragments of synovial tissue were incubated for 48 h. Supernatant was tested for mediators by enzyme-linked immunosorbent assay (ELISA). Values were normalized to the protein tissue content and represent the mean of three separate experiments on different human synovial tissue.

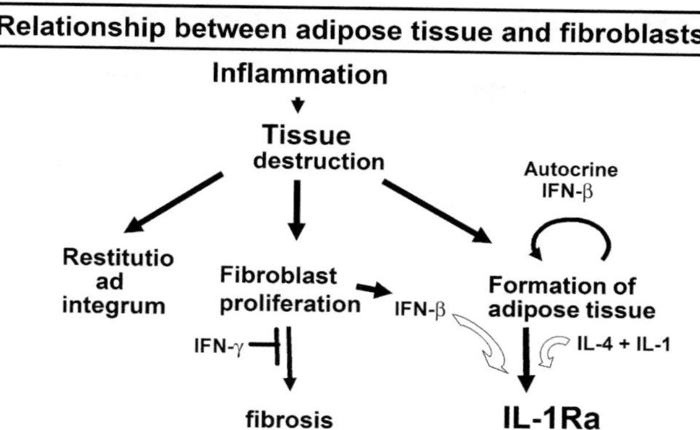

FIGURE 2. Induction of IL-1Ra in adipose tissue by IFN-β and IL-4 in synergism with IL-1.

tissue from the inflammatory site has a higher content in IL-1Ra and releases higher amounts than does adipose tissue from normal or obese patients; and (*e*) in the supernatant tested we did not find significant amounts of IL-1β, IL-6, and IL-8; TNF-α was at the limit of detection whether in the presence or absence of IFN-β and IL-1β was undetectable.

The question arises as to whether adipose tissue produces more inhibitory cytokines like IL-1Ra and IL-10 than proinflammatory cytokines. The situation may differ between "obese" adipose tissue and inflammatory adipose. From our preliminary results it would appear that this is indeed the case, at least as far as synovial adipose tissue is concerned. It is possible that during chronic inflammation, adipocytes are prone to produce anti-inflammatory molecules, whereas within the context of fibrosis, fibroblasts produce significant amounts of IFN-β which further increase IL-1Ra production by adipose tissue. Furthermore, autocrine or paracrine production by adipocytes can further increase the production of IL-1Ra as well simultaneously that of IL-1 and IL-4 (FIG. 2). This could therefore be considered a local mechanism of host defense, but it may also counteract the systemic effect of IL-1. In contrast, at the metabolic level, IL-1Ra produced by adipocytes may favor the decrease of other mediators such as leptin along with its effect on the central nervous system, thus favoring obesity. In this regard, the recent report of a paradoxical effect of body mass index on the survival of patients with rheumatoid arthritis (RA) is intriguing.[32] These investigators report a lower mortality among the heaviest patients in an RA cohort contrasting with a greater risk of dying in underweight RA patients. However, others also observed that a program aimed to reduce body weight was associated with a reduction in markers of vascular inflammation and insulin resistance.[33] Of interest, while the tendency to obesity in the Western population is increasing, the incidence of RA is decreasing.[34] This observation is supported by the fact that after a surgical intervention for cholesteatoma—a

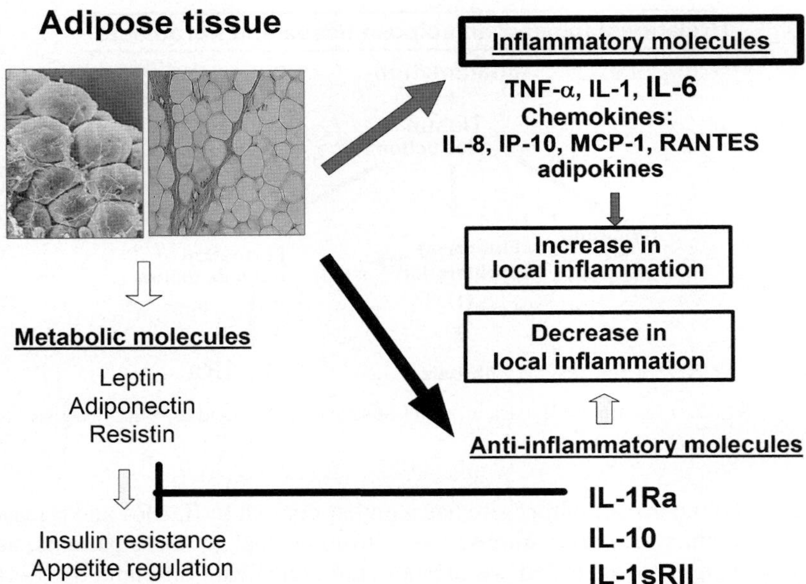

FIGURE 3. Adipocytes can produce both inflammatory and anti-inflammatory molecules at the local level.

highly inflammatory and destructive process—when autologous fat tissue is placed in the cavity, and no further inflammation occurs.[35]

The issue is even more complex because other molecules produced by adipocytes, other cells found in synovial fluid such as adiponectin and resistin could have proinflammatory properties and are linked to obesity.[36–39] Besides, obesity has been shown to induce inflammatory changes in adipose tissue which could be associated with the accumulation of macrophages in adipose tissue.[40,41] Recently, it has been reported that other molecules such as IL-18 were secreted by human adipocytes and might consequently play a part in innate immunity.[42]

In conclusion, depending probably on the stage of the pathological process or of the differentiation-maturation of adipocytes, the balance of production of pro- and anti-inflammatory mediators by adipocytes can tip to either side, and if obesity can induce inflammation, the inflammatory reaction in a reactive phase could then also induce anti-inflammatory molecules like IL-1Ra and IL-10 as part of a host-defense mechanism (FIGS. 3 and 4). It remains to be elucidated which are the triggering events and which are the subsequent events, which may be different depending on whether the primary events are of metabolic or of inflammatory origin. Surprisingly, in our experiments on human adipose tissue derived from human synovium the level of IL-1Ra was much higher than the levels of either IL-1β or IL-1α; besides, those of proinflammatory cytokines such as TNF-α, IL-6, and IL-8 were extremely low.

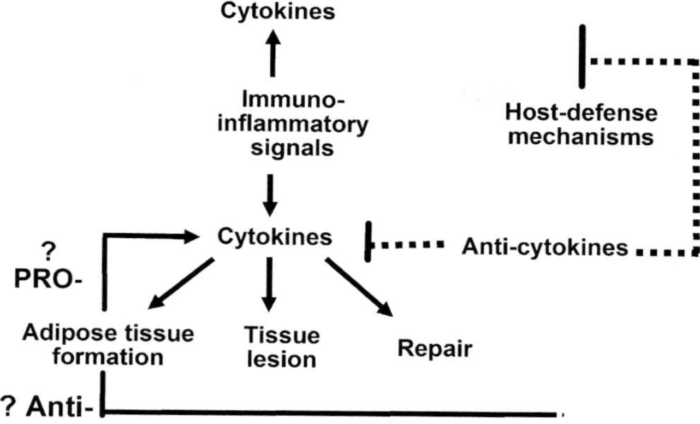

FIGURE 4. Adipose tissue produces both pro- and anti-inflammatory cytokines: consequences.

ACKNOWLEDGMENTS

We thank Professor Pierre Hoffmeyer (Clinic of Orthopedics) for supplying surgical specimens. Part of the study was funded by the Swiss National Science Foundation (grant No 3200-68286.02 to Jean-Michel Dayer).

REFERENCES

1. MOHAMED-ALI, V., J.H. PINKNEY & S.W. COPPACK. 1998. Adipose tissue as an endocrine and paracrine organ. Int. J. Obes. Relat. Metab. Disord. **22:** 1145–1158.
2. KAHN, B.B. & J.S. FLIER. 2000. Obesity and insulin resistance. J. Clin. Invest. **106:** 473–481.
3. YUDKIN, J.S., M. KUMARY, S.E. HUMPHRIES & V. MOHAMED-ALI. 2000. Inflammation, obesity, stress and coronary heart disease: is interleukin-6 the link? Atherosclerosis **148:** 209–214.
4. HOTAMISLIGIL, G.S. & B.M. SPIEGELMAN. 1994. Tumor necrosis factor alpha: a key component of the obesity-diabetes link. Diabetes **43:** 1271–1278.
5. CONSIDINE, R.V., M.K. SINHA, M.L. HEIMAN, *et al.* 1996. Serum immunoreactive-leptin concentrations in normal-weight and obese humans. N. Engl. J. Med. **334:** 292–295.
6. SECKINGER, P., J.W. LOWENTHAL, K. WILLIAMSON, *et al.* 1987. A urine inhibitor of interleukin 1 activity that blocks ligand binding. J. Immunol. **139:** 1546–1549.
7. PRIEUR, A.-M., M.-T. KAUFMANN, C. GRISCELLI, *et al.* 1987. Specific interleukin-1 inhibitor in serum and urine of children with systemic juvenile chronic arthritis. Lancet **28:** 1240–1242.
8. DAYER, J.-M. & B. BRESNIHAN. 2002. Targeting interleukin-1 in the treatment of rheumatoid arthritis. Arthritis Rheum. **46:** 574–578.

9. LUHESHI, G.N., J.D. GARDNER, D.A. RUSHFORTH, *et al.* 1999. Leptin actions on food intake and body temperature are mediated by IL-1. Proc. Natl. Acad. Sci. USA **96:** 7047–7052.
10. GABAY, C., M. DREYER, N. PELLEGRINELLI, *et al.* 2001. Leptin directly induces the secretion of interleukin 1 receptor antagonist in human monocytes. J. Clin. Endocrinol. Metab. **86:** 783–791.
11. DREYER, M., C.E. JUGE-AUBRY, C. GABAY, *et al.* 2003. Leptin activates the promoter of the interleukin-1 receptor antagonist through p42/44 mitogen-activated protein kinase and a composite nuclear factor kappa B/PU.1 binding site. Biochem. J. **370:** 591–598.
12. MEIER, C.A., E. BOBBIONI, C. GABAY, *et al.* 2002. IL-1 receptor antagonist serum levels are increased in human obesity: a possible link to the resistance to leptin? J. Clin. Endocrinol. Metab. **87:** 1184–1188.
13. HIRSCH, E., V.M. IRIKURA, S.M. PAUL, *et al.* 1996. Functions of interleukin 1 receptor antagonist in gene knockout and overproducing mice. Proc. Natl. Acad. Sci. USA **93:** 11008–11013.
14. JUGE-AUBRY, C.E., E. SOMM, V. GIUSTI, *et al.* 2003. Adipose tissue is a major source of interleukin-1 receptor antagonist: upregulation in obesity and inflammation. Diabetes **52:** 1104–1110.
15. BURGER, D. & J.-M. DAYER. 2000. IL-1Ra. *In* Cytokine Reference. J.J. Oppenheim & M. Feldmann, Eds.: 319–336. Academic Press. New York.
16. GABAY, C., M.F. SMITH, D. EIDLEN, *et al.* 1997. Interleukin 1 receptor antagonist (IL-1Ra) is an acute-phase protein. J. Clin. Invest. **15:** 2930–2940.
17. JUNGO, F., J.-M. DAYER, C. MODOUX, *et al.* 2001. IFN-beta inhibits the ability of T lymphocytes to induce TNF-alpha and IL-1beta production in monocytes upon direct cell-cell contact. Cytokine **7:** 272–278.
18. MOLNARFI, N., L. GRUAZ, J.-M. DAYER, *et al.* 2004. Opposite effects of IFN beta on cytokine homeostasis in LPS- and T cell contact-activated human monocytes. J. Neuroimmunol. **146:** 76–83.
19. JUGE-AUBRY, C., E. SOMM, R. CHICHEPORTICHE, *et al.* 2004. Regulatory effects of interleukin (IL)-1, interferon-β, and IL-4 on the production of IL-1 receptor antagonist by human adipose tissue. J. Clin. Endocrinol. Metab. **89:** 2652–2658.
20. MEIER, C.A., R. CHICHEPORTICHE, C.E. JUGE-AUBRY, *et al.* 2002. Regulation of the interleukin-1 receptor antagonist in THP-1 cells by ligands of the peroxisome proliferator-activated receptor gamma. Cytokine **18:** 320–328.
21. KUNZI, M.S. & P.P. ROWE. 2000. IL-Ra *In* Cytokine Reference. J.J. Oppenheim & M. Feldmann, Eds.: 627–638. Academic Press. New York.
22. FRIED, S.K., D.A. BUNKIN & A.A. GREENBERG.1998. Omental and subcutaneous adipose tissues of obese subjects release interleukin-6: depot difference and regulation by glucocorticoid. J. Clin. Endocrinol. Metab. **83:** 847–850.
23. BRUUN, J.M., S.B. PEDERSEN & B. RICHELSEN. 2001. Regulation of interleukin 8 production and gene expression in human adipose tissue in vitro. J. Clin. Endocrinol. Metab. **86:** 1267–1273.
24. HOTAMISLIGIL, G.S., N.S. SHARGILL & B.M. SPIEGELMAN. 1993. Adipose expression of tumor necrosis factor-alpha: direct role in obesity-linked insulin resistance. Science **259:** 87–91.
25. BASTARD, J.P., C. JARDEL, E. BRUCKERT, *et al.* 2000. Elevated levels of interleukin 6 are reduced in serum and subcutaneous adipose tissue of obese women after weight loss. J. Clin. Endocrinol. Metab. **85:** 3338–3342.

26. MATSUKI, T., R. HORAI, K. SUDO, *et al.* 2003. IL-1 plays an important role in lipid metabolism by regulating insulin levels under physiological conditions. J. Exp. Med. **198:** 877–888.
27. JUGE-AUBRY, C., E. SOMM, A. PERNIN, *et al.* 2005. Adipose tissue is a regulated source of interleukin-10. Cytokine **29:** 270–274.
28. ESPOSITO, K., A. PONTILLO, F. GIUGLIANO, *et al.* 2003. Association of low interleukin-10 levels with the metabolic syndrome in obese women. J. Clin. Endocrinol. Metab. **88:** 1055–1058.
29. HENRICHOT, E., C.E. JUGE-AUBRY, A. PERNIN, *et al.* 2005. Production of chemokines by perivascular adipose tissue: a role in the pathogenesis of atherosclerosis? Arterioscler. Thromb. Vasc. Biol. **25:** 2594–2599.
30. MEIER, C.A., R. CHICHEPORTICHE, M. DREYER, *et al.* 2003. IP-10, but not RANTES, is upregulated by leptin in monocytic cells. Cytokine **21:** 43–47.
31. WOLF, A.M., D. WOLF, H. RUMPOLD, *et al.* 2004. Adiponectin induces the anti-inflammatory cytokines IL-10 and IL-1Ra in human leukocytes. Biochem. Biophys. Res. Comm. **323:** 630–635.
32. ESCALANTE, A., R.W. HAAS & I. DEL RINCÓN. 2005. Paradoxical effect of body mass index on survival in rheumatoid arthritis. Role of comorbidity and systemic inflammation. Arch. Intern. Med. **165:** 1624–1629.
33. ESPOSITO, K., A. PONTILLO, C. DI PALO, *et al.* 2003. Effect of weight loss and lifestyle changes on vascular inflammatory markers in obese women: a randomized trial. JAMA **289:** 1799–1804.
34. UHLIG, T. & T.K. KVIEN. 2005. Is rheumatoid arthritis disappearing? Ann. Rheum. Dis. **64:** 7–10.
35. GRAY, R.F., J. RAY & D.J. MCFERRAN. 1999. Further experience with fat graft obliteration of mastoid cavities for cochlear implants. J. Laryngol. **113:** 881–884.
36. GOMEZ-AMBROSI, J. & G. FRUHBECK. 2001. Do resistin and resistin-like molecules also link obesity to inflammatory diseases? Ann. Intern. Med. **135:** 306–307.
37. SCHÄFFLER, A., A. EHLING, E. NEUMANN, *et al.* 2003. Adipocytokines in synovial fluid. JAMA **290:** 1709–1710.
38. STEFAN, N., H.-U. HÄRING & M. STURMVOLL. 2004. Regulation of synovial adipocytokines. JAMA **291:** 694–695.
39. BOKAREWA, M., I. NAGAEV, L. DAHLBERG, *et al.* 2005. Resistin, an adipokine with potent proinflammatory properties. J. Immunol. **174:** 5789–5795.
40. WEISBERG, S.P., D. MCCANN, M. DESAI, *et al.* 2003. Obesity is associated with macrophage accumulation in adipose tissue. J. Clin. Invest. **112:** 1796–1808.
41. WELLEN, K.E. & G.S. HOTAMISLIGIL. 2003. Obesity-induced inflammatory changes in adipose tissue. J. Clin. Invest. **112:** 1785–1788.
42. SKURK, T., H. KOLB, S. MÜLLER-SCHOLZE, *et al.* 2005. The proatherogenic cytokine interleukin-18 is secreted by human adipocytes. Eur. J. Endocrinol. **152:** 863–868.

Leptin Is a Link between Adipose Tissue and Inflammation

PETER HÄRLE AND RAINER H. STRAUB

Laboratory of Experimental Rheumatology and Neuroendocrino-Immunology, Department of Internal Medicine I, University Hospital, Regensburg, Germany

ABSTRACT: Leptin is a hormone of the pluripotent white adipose tissue and confers a multitude of regulatory functions within the organism. It controls the energy storage, lipoprotein metabolism, acute phase reactants, sex hormones and glucocorticoid metabolism, and immune function. In this review, we describe these multiple functions of leptin, the regulation of leptin expression, and how leptin can modulate the immune system via direct and indirect mechanisms. We show how leptin can be a link between the adipose tissue and inflammation.

KEYWORDS: leptin; immune system; neuroendocrine system

INTRODUCTION

Leptin is a nonglycosylated polypeptide and a member of the adipokine family. Adipokines are synthesized mainly by white adipose tissue, the predominant type of adipose tissue in humans.[1] It has a molecular size of 16 kD and is highly conserved among mammals. Structurally, leptin belongs to the type I cytokine superfamily. Levels of leptin decrease during weight loss and correlations were found between the amount of body fat and the circulating levels of leptin.[2] This suggests that leptin might act as part of a feedback mechanism signaling to the brain the size of the available energy resources in the body as function of the body's fat stores.[3,4] It has long been known that leptin-deficient (ob/ob) mice and leptin-receptor-deficient (db/db) mice have an altered immune response, suffering from obesity, displaying hormonal imbalances, abnormalities in thermoregulation, infertility, and evidence of immune and hematopoietic defects.[5,6]

The leptin receptor (Ob-R) is encoded by the diabetes (db) gene that was initially cloned from mouse choroid plexus.[7] The mRNA is alternatively spliced, resulting in six different splice products known as Ob-R, OB-Rb, OB-Rc, Ob-Rd, Ob-Re, and Ob-Rf.[8,9] The Ob-Rb is primarily expressed at high levels

Address for correspondence: Peter Härle, M.D., Laboratory of Experimental Rheumatology and Neuroendocrino-Immunology, Division of Rheumatology, Department of Internal Medicine I, University Hospital, 93042 Regensburg, Germany. Voice: +49 941 944 7116; fax: +49 941 944 7121.
e-mail: peter.haerle@klinik.uni-regensburg.de

**Ann. N.Y. Acad. Sci. 1069: 454–462 (2006). © 2006 New York Academy of Sciences.
doi: 10.1196/annals.1351.044**

in nuclei of the hypothalamus. Other isoforms are expressed in many tissues, such as muscle, liver, kidney, vascular endothelial cells, adrenal glands, and leukocytes.[10–12] The occurrence of leptin receptors in these tissues reveals the morphological correlate to link the body energy status, the nervous system, the endocrine system, and the immune system. Next to the direct, receptor-mediated effects of leptin, there are indirect effects resulting from hypercortisolism, diabetes, altered thyroid, and growth hormone levels in ob/ob and db/db mice, which indirectly influence the immune system.[13]

MULTIPLE FUNCTIONS OF ADIPOSE TISSUE

White adipose tissue not only stores energy, but also serves to produce and metabolize multiple other molecules (FIG. 1). One group of molecules produced are the adipokines leptin, adiponectin, and resistin. Leptin is positively correlated with body mass index (BMI) and reveals a circadian rhythm with peak levels at night and low levels in the morning reciprocal to the diurnal cortisol rhythm.[14,15] Leptin also signals to the hypothalamus, where it decreases the food intake, increases the energy expenditure, inhibits the HPA-axis function,[16] as well as the steroid production in adrenal cells.[17] Leptin and resistin are considered to mainly confer proinflammatory properties, in contrast to adiponectin.[10,18] Adiponectin seems to act in an antagonistic way to leptin, being negatively correlated with the BMI. It is also negatively correlated with the degree of hyperinsulinemia and insulin resistance.[19]

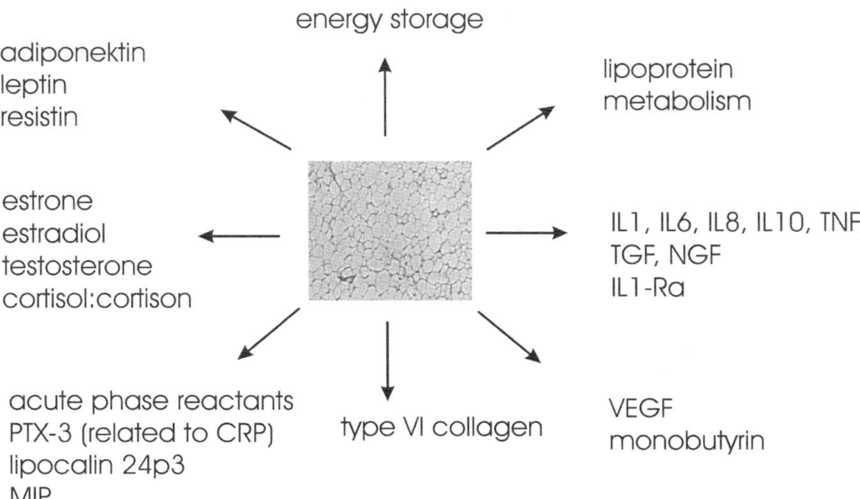

FIGURE 1. The multiple functions of adipose tissue in upregulation of multiple factors. PTX-3 = pentraxin.

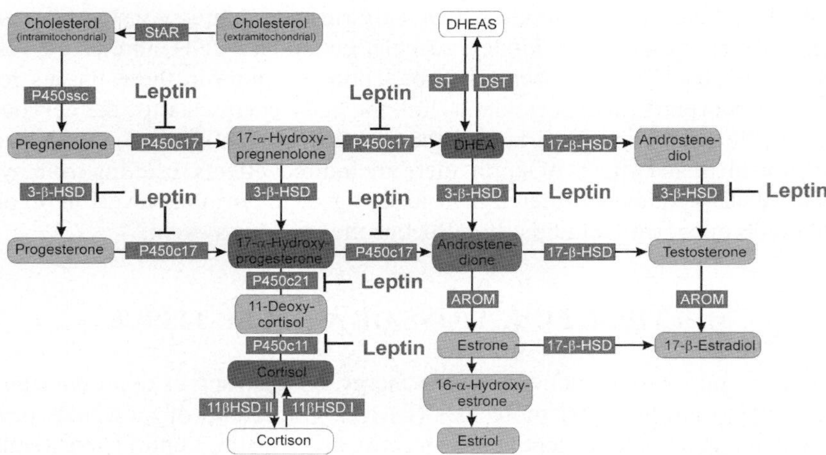

FIGURE 2. Leptin downregulates the steroid-producing system in the adrenal glands.

Adipose tissue is involved in the conversion of sex steroids and glucocorticoids, and leptin is able to influence enzymatic processes (FIG. 2). The biologically active cortisol can be converted into the biologically inactive cortisone via the 11-β-hydroxysteroid dehydrogenase type II and vice versa by the 11-β-hydroxysteroid dehydrogenase type I. In addition, the adipose tissue is capable of converting androgens into estrogens by aromatization. Next to the anti-inflammatory effects of androgens and proinflammatory effects of certain estrogens, adipocyte-conditioned medium was shown to promote tumorigenesis, including increased cell proliferation, invasive potential, survival, and angiogenesis of breast cancer cells.[20] This observation was found to be estrogen-dependent and emphasizes the proinflammatory properties of estrogens. Acute-phase reactants, including the pentraxin family member PTX-3,[21] which is closely related to the C-reactive peptide (CRP) molecule, is expressed in white adipose tissue. In addition, iron-binding proteins, such as the lipocalin 24p3 have recently been found to be secreted.[22] Next to coeruloplasmin, serum amyloid A, and macrophage migration inhibitory factor, the anti-inflammatory factor IL-1-receptor antagonist (IL1-Ra) is also being secreted in major amounts.[23] There is growing evidence that adipose tissue produces cytokines, such as TNF, IL-1β, IL-6, IL-8, IL-10, TGF-β, and NGF.[24] Many more substances are being produced in adipose tissue, which characterizes this tissue as pluripotent with respect to its regulatory function within metabolism, immune and endocrine system, and the central nervous system (CNS).[25]

REGULATION OF LEPTIN EXPRESSION

The regulation of synthesis and release of adipokines from adipose tissue is complex and not completely understood. Constantly cycling vesicles to and

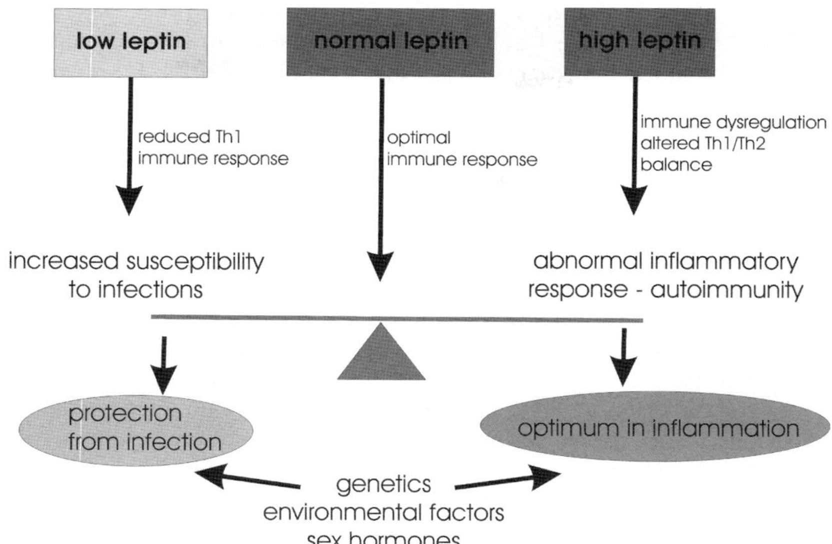

FIGURE 3. A possible model of leptin action on infection and autoimmunity.

from the plasma membrane do not represent an attractive vehicle for triggered release of soluble molecules.[26] Leptin is mainly cleared by the kidneys and the serum levels depend on the energy stored as fat as well as the status of energy balance. Patients with liver cirrhosis reveal elevated leptin levels. Whether this is the result of a reduced clearance of leptin by the liver or caused secondary by a reduced renal clearance in the context of the liver disease is not known. The nutritional regulation of leptin is mediated at least in part by insulin with increasing leptin levels under feeding conditions accompanied by high insulin serum levels (FIG. 3). In addition, leptin levels are higher in weight- and age-matched females compared with males, partly as a result of inhibition by androgens and stimulation by estrogens.[27,28] Various transcription factors have been located in the ob gene promotor region.[29] Leptin is increased by glucocorticoids, sex steroids, cytokines, and toxins as seen in acute infection. Furthermore, the sympathetic nervous system mediates, via the liberation of catecholamines, probably via the β3-receptor, a suppression of leptin serum levels as has been demonstrated in an acute cold-stress model.[30] Leptin signals mainly via a Jak/STAT signaling pathway and induces SOCS-3 to inhibit leptin signaling in a negative feedback loop fashion.

LEPTIN AND THE IMMUNE SYSTEM

As stated above, circulating levels of leptin are proportional to the fat mass, but may be lowered rapidly in fasting conditions or increased in acute inflammatory situations. Leptin- or leptin-receptor-deficient mice suffer from impaired T cell immunity. T cells from leptin-deficient mice were incubated *in vitro* with increasing concentrations of leptin, which positively correlated to increasing levels of T helper cell type 1 (Th1) cytokines over type 2 (TH2) cytokines.[10] This may add an enhanced susceptibility to infections in a leptin-deficient situation, such as starvation. In addition, the allogenic response of T cells was enhanced in the presence of leptin. Furthermore, Gainsford *et al.* showed that phagocytosis of peritoneal macrophages was concentration-dependently enhanced in the presence of leptin.[31] Leptin not only modulates peripheral T cell function, but it also acts on primary lymphoid organs, such as the thymus. Thymic atrophy is a prominent feature of malnutrition. Under conditions of leptin deficiency, the cortical-medullary structure of the thymus is disrupted. This is accompanied by a reduced $CD4^+CD8^+$ thymocyte subpopulation caused by enhanced apoptosis. Preventing the decrease in leptin in starving mice by peripheral administration of leptin prevents these starvation-induced thymic changes. Administration of recombinant leptin to leptin-deficient mice reduced thymocyte apoptosis and increased the thymic cellularity and $CD4^+/CD8^+$ and $CD4^-/CD8^-$ ratio.[32]

In contrast to a reduced capacity for immunologic defense in a situation of reduced leptin serum concentration, high leptin concentration may lead to an abnormally strong immune response predisposing to autoimmune phenomena.[33] To study the influence of leptin on autoimmunity, susceptibility to experimental autoimmune encephalomyelitis induced by immunization with a myelin-derived peptide was examined in leptin-deficient, C57BL/6J-ob/ob mice, with or without leptin replacement, and in wild-type controls. Leptin replacement converted disease resistance to susceptibility in the C57BL/6J-ob/ob mice, which was accompanied by a switch from a Th2 to Th1 pattern of cytokine release and consequently a reversal of immunoglobulin subclass production. These findings suggest that leptin is required for the induction and maintenance of an effective proinflammatory immune response in the CNS.

Another study showed an enhanced proinflammatory effect of leptin in the model of autoimmune diabetes in nonobese diabetic mice. The administration of leptin accelerated autoimmune destruction of pancreatic islets and significantly enhanced IFN-γ production in peripheral T cells.[34] Finally, it was shown that adjuvant-induced arthritis in wild-type C57/Bl6 mice compared to leptin-deficient C57/Bl6 mice showed enhanced arthritis scores. This phenomenon is accompanied by enhanced BSA-specific antibody levels, increased IFN-γ levels, reduced IL-10 levels, and enhanced lymphocyte proliferation in the wild-type mice compared to the leptin-deficient mice.[12]

Next to the direct effects of leptin on lymphocytes, there are other mechanisms by which leptin may cause an immune stimulation. The first indirect mechanism is the inhibition of the HPA-axis in stress, such as in hypoglycemia, which has been shown in explanted and superfused rat hypothalamus. Corticotropin-releasing hormone (CRH) was measured as read-out parameter for the HPA axis function. Leptin clearly suppressed the increase of CRH in hypoglycemic conditions in a concentration-dependent way.[35] Furthermore, the diurnal rhythm of leptin runs anticyclic to the diurnal rhythm of corticosterone in mice with low leptin serum concentrations and high corticosterone concentrations in the afternoon and high leptin concentrations and low corticosterone concentrations at night.[14,15]

The second indirect mechanism is that leptin is able to inhibit the expression of multiple enzymes within the steroid metabolic pathway (FIG. 2).[17] This leads to a reduced production of cortisol and androgens in the adrenal glands. At the local level in fat tissue, leptin stimulates the expression of 11-β-hydroxysteroid dehydrogenase type 1, which converts the biologically inactive cortisone into cortisol. Cortisol is able to upregulate the expression of aromatase in the fat tissue resulting in an enhanced synthesis of estrogens. If we consider certain estrogen metabolites, especially 4- and 16-hydroxylated forms, as being proinflammatory it might well be that via the shift toward more proinflammatory estrogens, leptin confers this indirect proinflammatory effect. Recently, it was shown that androgens conferring anti-inflammatory effects have a negative correlation to serum leptin concentrations underlining the above-described changes in steroid metabolism.[28]

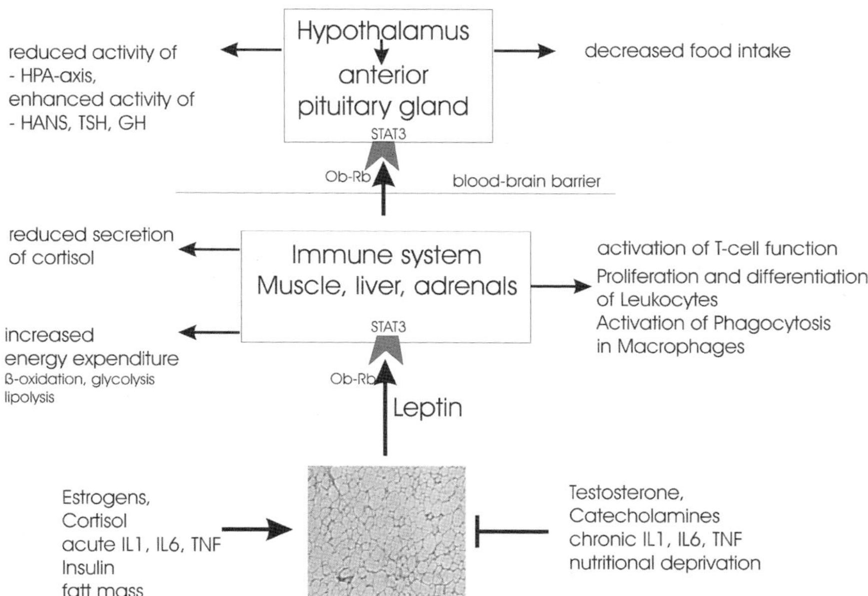

FIGURE 4. Some molecules influencing the secretion of leptin from white adipose tissue and the effect of leptin on different systems in the organism are described. Ob-Rb = long form of the leptin receptor, STAT3 = signal transducer and activator of transcription.

In summary, leptin deficiency might induce enhanced susceptibility to infections, and leptin excess may result in enhanced susceptibility to autoimmune phenomena (FIG. 3). The question appears as to how the secretion of leptin is regulated by inflammatory mediators. The recent data show that acute stimulation with proinflammatory cytokines leads to an increase in serum leptin concentrations.[15] In contrast to the acute proinflammatory stimulus, chronic IL-1, IL-6, or TNF stimulation results in a reduction of leptin levels. This has been shown in adipose tissue cultures[36] and in a clinical study in patients with rheumatoid arthirtis (RA) where the inflammatory index, measured by IL-6 and CRP serum concentrations, negatively correlated with the serum leptin level.[37] However, anti-TNF therapy over a period of 12 weeks did not alter serum leptin concentrations.[38] Finally, FIGURE 4 gives a graphic summary of the regulation of leptin expression and the physiologic effects on systems in the organism involved in the regulation of inflammation.

REFERENCES

1. ZHANG, Y., R. PROENCA, M. MAFFEI, *et al.* 1994. Positional cloning of the mouse obese gene and its human homologue. Nature **372:** 425–432.
2. CONSIDINE, R.V., M.K. SINHA, M.L. HEIMAN, *et al.* 1996. Serum immunoreactive-leptin concentrations in normal-weight and obese humans. N. Engl. J. Med. **334:** 292–295.
3. VAN GAAL, L.F., M.A. WAUTERS, I.L. MERTENS, *et al.* 1999. Clinical endocrinology of human leptin. Int. J. Obes. Relat. Metab. Disord. **23:** 29–36.
4. FLIERS, E., F. KREIER, P.J. VOSHOL, *et al.* 2003. White adipose tissue: getting nervous. J. Neuroendocrinol. **15:** 1005–1010.
5. CHANDRA, R.K. 1980. Cell-mediated immunity in genetically obese C57BL/6J ob/ob) mice. Am. J. Clin. Nutr. **33:** 13–16.
6. FERNANDES, G., B.S. HANDWERGER, E.J. YUNIS, *et al.* 1978. Immune response in the mutant diabetic C57BL/Ks-dt+ mouse: discrepancies between in vitro and in vivo immunological assays. J. Clin. Invest. **61:** 243–250.
7. TARTAGLIA, L.A., M. DEMBSKI, X. WENG, *et al.* 1995. Identification and expression cloning of a leptin receptor, OB-R. Cell **83:** 1263–1271.
8. KISHIMOTO, T., T. TAGA & S. AKIRA. 1994. Cytokine signal transduction. Cell **76:** 253–262.
9. HELDIN, C.H. 1995. Dimerization of cell surface receptors in signal transduction. Cell **80:** 213–223.
10. LORD, G.M., G. MATARESE, J.K. HOWARD, *et al.* 1998. Leptin modulates the T-cell immune response and reverses starvation-induced immunosuppression. Nature **394:** 897–901.
11. SIERRA-HONIGMANN, M.R., A.K. NATH, C. MURAKAMI, *et al.* 1998. Biological action of leptin as an angiogenic factor. Science **281:** 1683–1686.
12. BUSSO, N., A. SO, V. CHOBAZ-PECLAT, *et al.* 2002. Leptin signaling deficiency impairs humoral and cellular immune responses and attenuates experimental arthritis. J. Immunol. **168:** 875–882.
13. FLIER, J.S. 1998. Lowered leptin slims immune response. Nat. Med. **4:** 1124–1125.

14. Pongratz, G., P. Härle, G. Schnellinger, *et al.* 2005. Norepinephrine in mice inhibits secretion of splenic IL-6 during the dark period but stimulates its secretion in the light period: possible role of the corticosterone tone. J. Neuroimmunol. **158:** 120–127.
15. Sarraf, P., R.C. Frederich, E.M. Turner, *et al.* 1997. Multiple cytokines and acute inflammation raise mouse leptin levels: potential role in inflammatory anorexia. J. Exp. Med. **185:** 171–175.
16. Lloyd, R.V., L. Jin, I. Tsumanuma, *et al.* 2001. Leptin and leptin receptor in anterior pituitary function. Pituitary **4:** 33–47.
17. Kruse, M., S.R. Bornstein, K. Uhlmann, *et al.* 1998. Leptin down-regulates the steroid producing system in the adrenal. Endocr. Res. **24:** 587–590.
18. Silswal, N., A.K. Singh, B. Aruna, *et al.* 2005. Human resistin stimulates the pro-inflammatory cytokines TNF-alpha and IL-12 in macrophages by NF-kappaB-dependent pathway. Biochem. Biophys. Res. Commun. **334:** 1092–1101.
19. Yang, W.S., W.J. Lee, T. Funahashi, *et al.* 2001. Weight reduction increases plasma levels of an adipose-derived anti-inflammatory protein, adiponectin. J. Clin. Endocrinol. Metab. **86:** 3815–3819.
20. Iyengar, P., T.P. Combs, S.J. Shah, *et al.* 2003. Adipocyte-secreted factors synergistically promote mammary tumorigenesis through induction of anti-apoptotic transcriptional programs and proto-oncogene stabilization. Oncogene **22:** 6408–6423.
21. Abderrahim-Ferkoune, A., O. Bezy, C. Chiellini, *et al.* 2003. Characterization of the long pentraxin PTX3 as a TNFalpha-induced secreted protein of adipose cells. J. Lipid Res. **44:** 994–1000.
22. Lin, Y., M.W. Rajala, J.P. Berger, *et al.* 2001. Hyperglycemia-induced production of acute phase reactants in adipose tissue. J. Biol. Chem. **276:** 42077–42083.
23. Juge-Aubry, C.E., E. Somm, V. Giusti, *et al.* 2003. Adipose tissue is a major source of interleukin-1 receptor antagonist: upregulation in obesity and inflammation. Diabetes **52:** 1104–1110.
24. Torpy, D.J., S.R. Bornstein & G.P. Chrousos. 1998. Leptin and interleukin-6 in sepsis. Horm. Metab. Res. **30:** 726–729.
25. Ahima, R.S. & J.S. Flier. 2000. Adipose tissue as an endocrine organ. Trends Endocrinol. Metab. **11:** 327–332.
26. Combs, T.P., A.H. Berg, M.W. Rajala, *et al.* 2003. Sexual differentiation, pregnancy, calorie restriction, and aging affect the adipocyte-specific secretory protein adiponectin. Diabetes **52:** 268–276.
27. Rosenbaum, M. & R.L. Leibel. 1999. Clinical review 107: role of gonadal steroids in the sexual dimorphisms in body composition and circulating concentrations of leptin. J. Clin. Endocrinol. Metab. **84:** 1784–1789.
28. Härle, P., G. Pongratz, C. Weidler, *et al.* 2004. Possible role of leptin in hypoandrogenicity in patients with systemic lupus erythematosus and rheumatoid arthritis. Ann. Rheum. Dis. **63:** 809–816.
29. Ahima, R.S. & J.S. Flier. 2000. Leptin. Annu. Rev. Physiol. **62:** 413–437.
30. Trayhurn, P., J.S. Duncan & D.V. Rayner. 1995. Acute cold-induced suppression of ob (obese) gene expression in white adipose tissue of mice: mediation by the sympathetic system. Biochem. J. **311**(Pt 3): 729–733.
31. Gainsford, T., T.A. Willson, D. Metcalf, *et al.* 1996. Leptin can induce proliferation, differentiation, and functional activation of hemopoietic cells. Proc. Natl. Acad. Sci. U.S.A. **93:** 14564–14568.

32. Howard, J.K., G.M. Lord, G. Matarese, *et al.* 1999. Leptin protects mice from starvation-induced lymphoid atrophy and increases thymic cellularity in ob/ob mice. J. Clin. Invest. **104:** 1051–1059.
33. Matarese, G., S. Moschos & C.S. Mantzoros. 2005. Leptin in immunology. J. Immunol. **174:** 3137–3142.
34. Matarese, G., V. Sanna, R.I. Lechler, *et al.* 2002. Leptin accelerates autoimmune diabetes in female NOD mice. Diabetes **51:** 1356–1361.
35. Heiman, M.L., R.S. Ahima, L.S. Craft, *et al.* 1997. Leptin inhibition of the hypothalamic-pituitary-adrenal axis in response to stress. Endocrinology **138:** 3859–3863.
36. Bruun, J.M., S.B. Pedersen, K. Kristensen, *et al.* 2002. Effects of pro-inflammatory cytokines and chemokines on leptin production in human adipose tissue in vitro. Mol. Cell. Endocrinol. **190:** 91–99.
37. Popa, C., M.G. Netea, T.R. Radstake, *et al.* 2005. Markers of inflammation are negatively correlated with serum leptin in rheumatoid arthritis. Ann. Rheum. Dis. **64:** 1195–1198.
38. Straub, R.H., P. Härle, F. Atzeni, *et al.* 2005. Sex hormone concentrations in patients with rheumatoid arthritis are not normalized during 12 weeks of anti-tumor necrosis factor therapy. J. Rheumatol. **32:** 1253–1258.

Induction of Neutrophil Chemotaxis by Leptin

Crucial Role for p38 and Src Kinases

FABRIZIO MONTECUCCO, GIORDANO BIANCHI, PAOLA GNERRE, MARIA BERTOLOTTO, FRANCO DALLEGRI, AND LUCIANO OTTONELLO

First Clinic of Internal Medicine, Department of Internal Medicine, University of Genova Medical School, Genova, Italy

ABSTRACT: Leptin is involved in energy homeostasis, hematopoiesis, inflammation, and immunity. Although hypoleptinemia characterizing malnutrition has been strictly related to increased susceptibility to infection, other hyperleptinemic conditions, such as end-stage renal disease (ESRD), are highly susceptible to bacterial infections. On the other hand, ESRD is characterized by neutrophil functional defects crucial for infectious morbidity, and several uremic toxins capable of depressing neutrophil functions have been identified. In the present study, we investigated leptin's effects on neutrophil function. Our results show that leptin inhibits neutrophil migration in response to classical chemoattractants. Otherwise, leptin is endowed with chemotactic activity toward neutrophils. The two activities, inhibition of the cell response to chemokines and stimulation of neutrophil migration, could be detected at similar concentrations. On the contrary, neutrophils exposed to leptin did not display detectable $[Ca^{2+}]_i$ mobilization, oxidant production, or β_2-integrin upregulation. The results demonstrate that leptin is a pure chemoattractant devoid of secretagogue properties but capable of inhibiting neutrophil chemotaxis to classical neutrophilic chemoattractants. This effect is dependent on the activation of intracellular kinases involved in F-actin polymerization and neutrophil locomotion. Indeed, p38 mitogen-activated protein kinase (MAPK) and Src kinase, but not extracellular-regulated kinase (ERK), were activated by short-term incubation with leptin. Moreover, p38 MAPK inhibitor SB203580 and Src kinase inhibitor PP1, but not MEK inhibitor PD98059, blocked neutrophil chemotaxis toward leptin. Serum from patients with ESRD inhibits migration of normal neutrophils in response to N-formyl-methionine-leucyl-phenylalanine (FMLP) with a strict correlation between serum leptin levels and serum ability to suppress neutrophil locomotion. The serum

Address for correspondence: Luciano Ottonello, M.D., Dipartimento di Medicina Interna e Specialità Mediche, Viale Benedetto XV n. 6, I-16132 Genova, Italy. Voice: +39 010 3538686; fax: +39 010 3538686.

e-mail: otto@unige.it

**Ann. N.Y. Acad. Sci. 1069: 463–471 (2006). © 2006 New York Academy of Sciences.
doi: 10.1196/annals.1351.045**

inhibitory activity can be effectively prevented by immune-depletion of leptin. Taking into account the crucial role of neutrophils in host defense, we show that leptin-mediated ability of ERSD serum to inhibit neutrophil chemotaxis appears to be a mechanism contributing to neutrophil dysfunction in ESRD.

Keywords: neutrophil; leptin; chemotaxis; MAPK; Src kinases; end-stage renal failure; infection

INTRODUCTION

Leptin is a peptide hormone involved in the control of food intake, breakdown of fat, and energy expenditure.[1] Furthermore, leptin also plays a role in innate and acquired immunity[2] by stimulating cytokine production by monocytes and regulating several T lymphocyte responses. Thus, leptin can be considered a part of the recently categorized family of molecules produced by adipose tissue called adipokines, which are capable of linking metabolism and immune homeostasis.[3]

Although hypoleptinemia is related to increased susceptibility to infection secondary to malnutrition,[3,4] other conditions, such as end-stage renal disease (ESRD) and obesity, are characterized by increased susceptibility to bacterial infection[5,6] despite high levels of leptinemia.[7,8] As far as ESRD is concerned, it is generally assumed that the defects in neutrophils play a crucial role in the infectious morbidity[9] and indeed several uremic toxins (i.e., proteins capable of depressing neutrophil functions) have been identified.[10]

Few and contrasting data about leptin and neutrophils, which are different from other immune cells, are presently available.[11–13] The aim of the present work is to clarify whether leptin is actually endowed with the capacity to modulate neutrophil functional activities and, in case of positive results, to investigate the actual role of this hormone in neutrophil dysfunction in ESRD.

PATIENTS AND METHODS

Neutrophils obtained from healthy volunteers after informed consent were isolated by dextran sedimentation and subsequent centrifugation on a Ficoll-Hypaque density gradient. Contaminating erythrocytes were removed by hypotonic lysis. Serum was obtained from 18 patients with ESRD and from eight healthy controls after informed consent. Leptin serum concentrations were determined by a radioimmunoassay method with a kit from DRG Instruments GmbH (Marburg, Germany). Neutrophil locomotion was studied in duplicate according to the leading front method using blind well chambers (NeuroProbe, Cabin John, MD) with a 3-μm pore-size cellulose ester filter (Millipore, Milan, Italy) separating the cells from the chemoattractant. After incubation in the absence or presence of appropriate reagents, the distance (μm) traveled by the leading front of cells was measured at ×400 magnification. Intracellular $[Ca^{2+}]_i$ was determined in fura-2 AM-loaded neutrophils by monitoring fluorescence changes before and after addition of leptin or FMLP. The release of superoxide anion was studied by the method of ferricytochrome *c* reduction determination. The oxidative metabolism was also studied in DCFH-PD098059DA-loaded neutrophils incubated in the presence or absence of leptin and/or FMLP by flow cytometric analysis. Flow cytometric analysis of CD11b expression was carried out in neutrophils labeled with FITC-conjugated anti-CD11b 44 mAb (Biosource International, Camarillo, CA) and exposed or not to FMLP and/or leptin. The activation of intracellular kinases was studied by Western blot and *in vitro* kinase assays with the appropriate specific antibodies (antiphosphorylated ERK sc-7383 and antiphosphorylated p38 mitogen-activated protein kinase [MAPK] mAbs from R&D System, Minneapolis, MN, and anti-Hck N-30 mAb from Santa Cruz Biotechnology, Santa Cruz, CA).

RESULTS

Effects of Leptin on Neutrophil Locomotion

Using blind well chambers, neutrophils were incubated in absence or presence of different doses of leptin in the upper compartment of the chamber, and challenged with 10 nM FMLP placed in the lower compartment. As shown in FIGURE 1A, the chemotactic response of neutrophils was inhibited by leptin in a dose-dependent manner. Similarly, leptin inhibited the chemotactic response to other chemoattractants, such as interleukin-8 (IL-8) and C5a (not shown). When neutrophils were incubated in the upper compartment of migration chambers, and exposed to leptin added to the lower compartment of migration chambers, they displayed a bell-shaped dose–response curve characteristic of chemoattractants (FIG. 1B). It is noteworthy that the stimulatory activity of leptin was detected at concentrations comparable to those found to inhibit the chemotactic response to FMLP.

Effect of Leptin on Neutrophil Activation

A series of experiments were then performed in order to test the capacity of leptin to trigger neutrophil activation and/or to interfere with FMLP-induced functional responses. Firstly, we tested the effects of leptin on the intracellular levels of calcium $[Ca^{2+}]_i$. Neutrophils mounted a rapid increase of $[Ca^{2+}]_i$ in response to FMLP (FIG. 1C, upper line), also in presence of leptin (FIG. 1C, lower line). On the contrary, as shown in FIGURE 1C (lower line), no $[Ca^{2+}]_i$

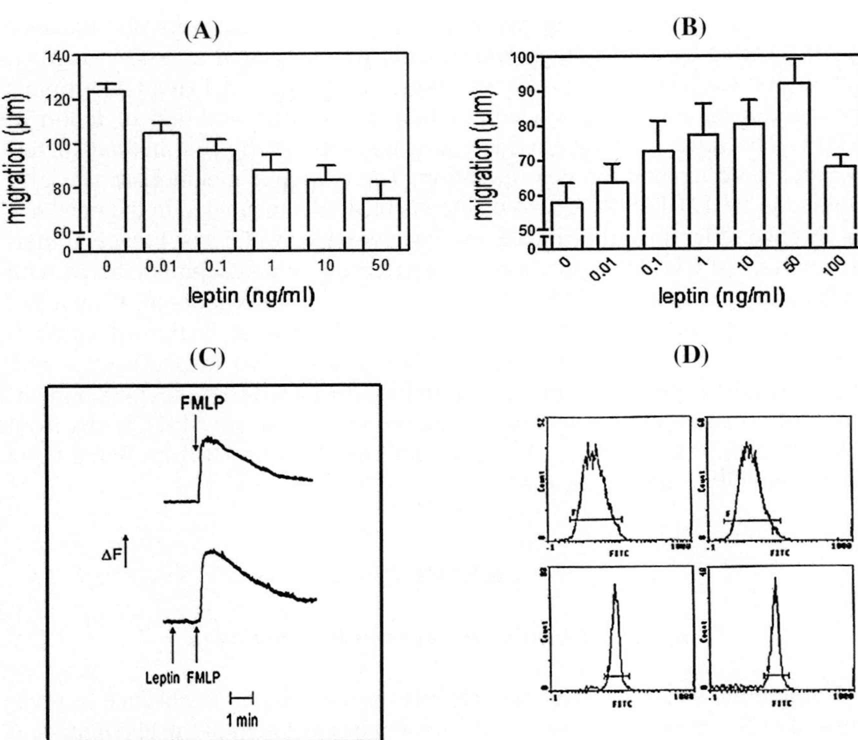

FIGURE 1. (**A**) Dose-dependent inhibition of FMLP-induced neutrophil migration by human recombinant leptin. Neutrophils were incubated in the upper compartment of chemotaxis chamber in absence or presence of various doses of leptin, and their locomotory response to 10 nM FMLP in the lower compartment was tested after 45-min incubation. Results are expressed as mean ± 1 SD of three experiments with neutrophils from different donors. 0 vs. 1: $P < 0.01$; 0 vs. 10: $P < 0.01$; 0 vs. 50: $P < 0.001$. (**B**) Dose-dependent induction of neutrophil migration by various doses of leptin. Neutrophils were incubated in the upper compartment of chemotaxis chamber in medium and their locomotory response in absence or presence of various doses of leptin in the lower compartment was tested after 45-min incubation. Results are expressed as mean ± 1 SD of five experiments with neutrophils from different donors. 0 vs. 1: $P < 0.05$; 0 vs. 10: $P < 0.05$; 0 vs. 50: $P < 0.001$. (**C**) Effects of FMLP and leptin on the intracellular calcium levels in human neutrophils. Neutrophils (2.5×10^6) were loaded with fura-2 AM and fluorescence changes (ΔF) were monitored before and after exposure to 10 nM FMLP (*upper line*) and to 200 ng/mL leptin followed by 10 nM FMLP (*lower line*). *Arrows* indicate the stimulus addition. Results represent one of three experiments that yielded similar results. (**D**) Effect of leptin on neutrophil CD11b expression and FMLP-induced neutrophil CD11b upregulation. *Upper left*: CD11b expression on freshly isolated neutrophils from peripheral blood of healthy donors. *Upper right*: CD11b expression on neutrophils exposed to 200 ng/mL leptin. *Lower left*: CD11b expression on neutrophils exposed to 1 μM FMLP. *Lower right*: CD11b expression on neutrophils pre-incubated with 200 ng/mL leptin and subsequently exposed to 1 μM FMLP. Results represent one of the three experiments that yielded similar results.

mobilization was observed in fura-2 loaded neutrophils exposed to leptin, also after increasing the concentration of leptin or prolonging the exposure of neutrophils to leptin (data not shown). When the oxidative metabolism was studied by the spectrophotometric analysis of superoxide anion production and flow cytometric analysis of intracellular oxidation of 2′-7′-dichloroflourescein in DCFH-DA-loaded neutrophils, leptin did not stimulate the respiratory burst, nor impair the FMLP-triggered oxidative response by neutrophils (data not shown). Finally, leptin did not influence the expression of CD11b on neutrophils and did not affect the CD11b upregulation induced by FMLP (FIG. 1D).

Role of MAPK and Src Kinases in Leptin-Mediated Neutrophil Migration

An attempt was made to investigate the signal transduction pathway(s) involved in leptin-mediated neutrophil migration. We studied MAPK (i.e., ERK-1/2 and p38), which is known to be involved in neutrophil signal transduction in response to classical chemoattractants, such as IL-8,[14] and Src kinases involved in the regulation of F-actin polymerization,[15] an event strictly related to neutrophil locomotion. As shown in FIGURE 1A, neutrophil pretreatment with 1 μM SB203580, a selective inhibitor of p38, and with 20 μM PP1 analog (Src kinase family inhibitor), but not with 25 μM PD098059, a selective inhibitor of MAPK kinase 1 preventing the activation of ERK-1/2, inhibited significantly leptin-triggered neutrophil migration. In accord with these observations, a well-detectable activation of p38 MAPK and Hck Src kinase was observed by Western blot assay and *in vitro* kinase assay, respectively, whereas no ERK 1/2 activation was detected (FIG. 2B). These data suggest that the intracellular signaling by leptin is mediated by p38 MAPK and Src tyrosine kinase pathways.

Inhibition of Neutrophil Chemotaxis by Sera from Patients with Chronic Renal Failure Is Related to Serum Levels of Leptin

Serum from eighteen ESRD patients inhibited the neutrophil chemotactic response to FMLP: neutrophil migration in the presence of 25% ESRD serum in the upper compartment of migration chambers: 82.0 ± 30.0 μm/45 min, $x \pm 1$ SD, $n = 18$; neutrophil migration in the presence of 25% control serum in the upper compartment of migration chambers: 119.3 ± 15.4 μm/45 min, $x \pm 1$ SD, $n = 8$. $P = 0.005$. The concentrations of leptin in sera from ESRD patients were from 1.7 to 137.1 ng/mL, with a mean of 70.10 ± 50.41 ng/mL, $x \pm 1$ SD, $n = 18$. The locomotory values observed for normal neutrophils tested against FMLP in the presence of 25% ESRD sera, and leptin concentrations in the same samples are inversely correlated (Spearman's $r = -0.7110$; $P = 0.0009$).

(A)

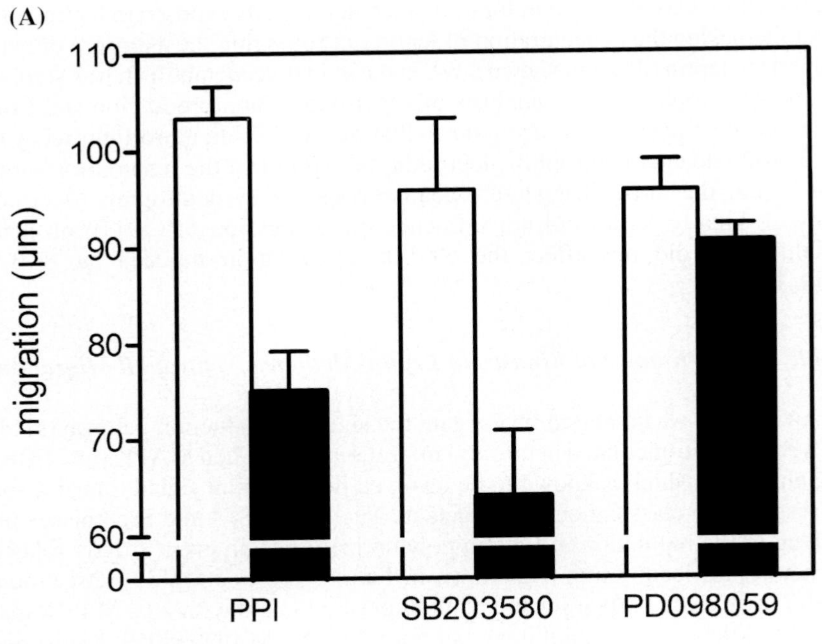
110
100
90
80
70
60
0
migration (µm)
PPI
SB203580
PD098059

(B)

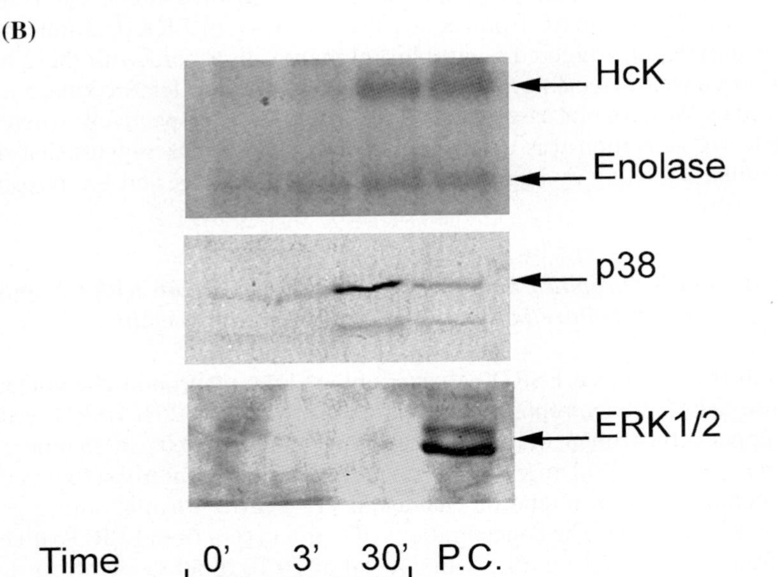
HcK
Enolase
p38
ERK1/2
Time
0'
3'
30'
P.C.

DISCUSSION

In the present work, we confirm and extend previous observations showing that leptin acts as a neutrophil chemoattractant.[11,12] Neutrophil chemotaxins can be classified in two functional groups: (1) classical chemotaxins, including FMLP, C5a, and IL-8, characterized by the ability to induce both chemotaxis and increase of $[Ca^{2+}]_i$;[16] (2) pure chemotaxins, such as TGF-β1, sFasL, and substance P,[17,18] able to induce chemotaxis without causing cell activation (i.e., degranulation and oxidant generation) and without increasing $[Ca^{2+}]_i$. Our results show that neutrophils exposed to leptin, although capable of directed migration, did not display detectable $[Ca^{2+}]_i$ mobilization, nor oxidant production. In other words, leptin can be considered as a pure neutrophil chemotaxin. Consistent with our findings, Zarkesh-Esfahani and coworkers have recently showed that neutrophils do not express the long form Ob-Rb,[13] the receptor isoform mainly involved in the regulation of multiple intracellular signaling cascades, including the classic janus-activating kinase-signal transducer and activator of transcription (JAK-STAT) pathway,[19] which in turn is critical for phospholipase C–dependent $[Ca^{2+}]_i$ rise induced by chemokine stimulation.[20] On the contrary, neutrophils express the short form of the leptin receptor Ob-Ra capable of transducing activating signal to MAPK pathway without JAK-STAT activation.[21] In the present work, we in fact show that leptin is capable of inducing neutrophil locomotion by intracellular pathways involving the activation of p38 MAPK. Accordingly, TGF-β_1, a pure chemoattractant capable of stimulating neutrophil migration in a Ca^{2+}-independent manner, required p38 MAPK

←

FIGURE 2. (**A**) Effect of Src inhibitor PP1, and MAPK inhibitors PD098059 and SB203580 on the locomotory response of neutrophils to leptin. Neutrophils were incubated in the upper compartment of chemotaxis chamber in absence (*open bars*) or presence (*black bars*) of 20 μM PP1 (Src kinase inhibitor), 1 μM SB20358 (p38 MAPK inhibitor), and 25 μM PD098059 (ERK-1/2 inhibitor), and their locomotory response to 50 ng/mL leptin in the lower compartment was tested after 45-min incubation. Data are expressed as mean ± 1 SEM, $n = 3$. Migration in absence vs. migration in presence of PP1: $P < 0.05$. Migration in absence vs. migration in presence of SB20358: $P < 0.05$. Migration in absence vs. migration in presence of PD098059: n.s. (**B**) *In vitro* kinase assay of Hck activity and Western blot analysis of MAPK phosphorylation in human neutrophils. Neutrophils were treated with 50 ng/mL leptin for 0, 3, and 30 min (lane 1–3), or 10 nM IL-8 (for Hck activity) and 300 U/mL GM-CSF (for MAPK activity) as positive controls (PC). For *in vitro* kinase assay, the lysates were immunoprecipitated with specific anti-Hck Ab, incubated with acid-denaturated enolase, and resolved by gel electrophoresis. The *arrows* indicate the bands of Hck autophosphorylation and enolase phosphorylation. For Western blot assay, the lysates were resolved by gel electrophoresis, transferred to nitrocellulose membranes, and incubated with specific antiphosphorylated p38 and antiphosphorylated ERK-1/2 Abs. Results represent one of the three experiments that yielded similar results.

activation.[22] Furthermore, our results show that leptin-mediated signal transduction in neutrophils is strictly dependent on Src kinase activation (i.e., Hck kinase), unveiling a novel role for these kinases in the regulation of neutrophil locomotion toward pure chemoattractant.

A second crucial point from the present work to be highlighted is the capacity of leptin to inhibit the locomotory response of neutrophils to classical chemoattractants, such as FMLP, C5a, and IL-8. This can be considered a potential immunosuppressive activity of leptin, taking into account the crucial role of neutrophils in front-line defense against bacterial infections. In fact, bacterial infections are a major cause of morbidity and mortality among patients with ESRD,[23] a pathologic condition characterized by hyperleptinemia. A critical role in the pathogenesis of increased susceptibility to infections in ESRD is exerted by functional abnormalities of neutrophils.[24] These dysfunctions are considered secondary to diverse causes, such as accumulation of calcium within the cells, iron overload, interactions with biocompatible dialysers and dialysis solutions, and low molecular weight proteins (LMWPs),[24] a recently categorized class of proteins involved in the pathogenesis of uremic syndrome.[25] Among LMWPs, six so-called granulocyte-inhibiting proteins (GIPs) inhibit different functional activities of neutrophils, including oxidative metabolism, chemotaxis, degranulation, and phagocytosis, with consequent impairment of neutrophil-dependent antibacterial defense.[10] Also, leptin has been categorized as a LMWP, and indeed a role has been suggested for this protein in some uremic manifestations, such as anorexia and weight loss.[25] The demonstrated leptin-mediated ability of serum from ESRD patients to inhibit neutrophil chemotaxis appears as a potential mechanism contributing to the establishment of infections in ESRD. In other words, leptin must be considered a *bona fide* GIP detectable in serum of ESRD patients.

In conclusion, the results suggest that: (1) leptin activates intracellular pathways involved in the regulation of the locomotory machinery of neutrophils, such as p38 MAPK and Src kinases; (2) leptin behaves like a chemokine, capable of stimulating neutrophil locomotion and desensitizing the cells to stimulation by another chemoattractant; and (3) leptin is responsible for chemotactic desensitization of neutrophils by sera from patients with chronic renal failure, taken as a disease model of hyperleptinemia.

REFERENCES

1. FRIEDMAN, J.M. & J.L. HALAAS. 1998. Leptin and the regulation of body weight in mammals. Nature **395:** 763–770.
2. FANTUZZI, G. & R. FAGGIONI. 2000. Leptin in the regulation of immunity, inflammation, and hematopoiesis. J. Leukoc. Biol. **68:** 437–446.
3. MATARESE, G. & A. LA CAVA. 2004. The intricate interface between immune system and metabolism. Trends Immunol. **25:** 193–200.
4. LORD, G.M. *et al.* 1998. Leptin modulates the T-cell immune response and reverses starvation-induced immunosuppression. Nature **394:** 897–901.

5. SARNAK, M.J. & B.L. JABER. 2000. Mortality caused by sepsis in patients with end-stage renal disease compared with the general population. Kidney Int. **58:** 1758–1764.
6. LAMAS, O., A. MARTI & J.A. MARTINEZ. 2002. Obesity and immunocompetence. Eur. J. Clin. Nutr. **56:** S42–S45.
7. WIDJAJA, A. *et al.* 2000. Free serum leptin but not bound leptin concentrations are elevated in patients with end-stage renal disease. Nephrol. Dial. Transplant. **15:** 846–850.
8. MANTZOROS, C.S. 1999. The role of leptin in human obesity and disease: a review of current evidence. Ann. Intern. Med. **130:** 671–680.
9. VANHOLDER, R. & S. RINGOIR. 1993. Infectious morbidity and defects of phagocytic function in end-stage renal disease: a review. J. Am. Soc. Nephrol. **3:** 1541–1554.
10. HAAG-WEBER, M., G. COHEN & W.H. HORL. 2000. Clinical significance of granulocyte-inhibiting proteins. Nephrol. Dial. Transplant. **15:** S15–S16.
11. CALDEFIE-CHEZET, F. *et al.* 2001. Leptin: a potential regulator of polymorphonuclear neutrophil bactericidal action? J. Leukoc. Biol. **69:** 414–418.
12. CALDEFIE-CHEZET, F., A. POULIN & M.P. VASSON. 2003. Leptin regulates functional capacities of polymorphonuclear neutrophils. Free Rad. Res. **37:** 809–814.
13. ZARKESH-ESFAHANI, H. *et al.* 2004. Leptin indirectly activates human neutrophils via induction of TNF-α. J. Immunol. **172:** 1809–1814.
14. KNALL, C., G.C. WORTHEN & G.L. JOHNSON. 1997. Interleukin 8-stimulated phosphatidylinositol-3-kinase activity regulates the migration of human neutrophils independent of extracellular signal-regulated kinase and p38 mitogen-activated protein kinases. Proc. Natl. Acad. Sci. USA **194:** 3052–3057.
15. CHODNIEWICZ, D. & D.V. ZHELEV. 2003. Novel pathways of F-actin polymerization in the human neutrophil. Blood **102:** 2251–2258.
16. RICHARDSON, R.M. *et al.* 1995. Cross-desensitization of chemoattractant receptors occurs at multiple levels: evidence for a role for inhibition of phospholipase C activity. J. Biol. Chem. **27:** 27829–27833.
17. HAINES, K.A. *et al.* 1993. Chemoattraction of neutrophils by substance P and transforming growth factor-β1 is inadequately explained by current models of lipid remodeling. J. Immunol. **151:** 1491–1499.
18. OTTONELLO, L. *et al.* 1999. Soluble Fas ligand is chemotactic for human neutrophilic polymorphonuclear leukocytes. J. Immunol. **162:** 3601–3606.
19. ZABEAU, L. *et al.* 2003. The ins and outs of leptin receptor activation. FEBS Lett. **546:** 45–50.
20. SORIANO, S.F. *et al.* 2003. Chemokines integrate JAK/STAT and G-protein pathways during chemotaxis and calcium flux responses. Eur. J. Immunol. **33:** 1328–1333.
21. BJORBAEK, C. *et al.* 1997. Divergent signalling capacities of the long and short isoforms of the leptin receptor. J. Biol. Chem. **272:** 32686–32695.
22. HANNIGAN, M. *et al.* 1998. The role of p38 MAP kinase in TGF-b1-induced signal transduction in human neutrophils. Biochem. Biophys. Res. Comm. **246:** 55–58.
23. UNITED STATES RENAL DATA SYSTEM. 2003. USRDS 2003 Annual Data Report. National Institutes of Health, Diabetes and Digestive and Kidney Diseases. Bethesda, MD.
24. HAAG-WEBER, M. & W.H. HORL. 1996. Dysfunction of polymorphonuclear leukocytes in uremia. Semin. Nephrol. **16:** 192–201
25. VANHOLDER, R. *et al.* 2003. Review on uremic toxins: classification, concentration, and interindividual variability. Kidney Int. **63:** 1934–1943.

Cell Stress Response in Skeletal Muscle Myofibers

ELENA TARRICONE,[a,b] ANNA GHIRARDELLO,[b] SANDRA ZAMPIERI,[b] RAMPUDDA MARIA ELISA,[b] ANDREA DORIA,[b] AND LUISA GORZA[a]

[a]*Department of Biomedical Sciences, University of Padova, 35121 Padova, Italy*

[b]*Department of Clinical and Experimental Medicine, Division of Rheumatology, University of Padova, 35121 Padova, Italy*

ABSTRACT: Cells respond to conditions that impair homeostasis through *ex novo* synthesis of stress proteins, which differ in subcellular localization and biological function and whose differential expression depends on the type of the stressing stimulus and on the involvement of the specific stress-response signaling cascade. The biological significance of such an event is the increased resistance against further perturbations of cell homeostasis, and thus, enhanced survival. We will review briefly the available evidence concerning stress response of skeletal muscle cells, including recent results indicating the involvement of endoplasmic reticulum stress response and proteins in skeletal muscle cell differentiation and in progression of muscle diseases.

KEYWORDS: skeletal muscle; differentiation; heat-shock protein; endoplasmic reticulum; myositis

STRESSING STIMULI AND STRESS RESPONSES IN SKELETAL MUSCLE CELLS

According to the nature of the stressing stimuli, at least three types of responses are differently recruited for stress-protein upregulation. Heat, exercise, ischemia, and reperfusion induce a predominantly cytosolic response, which leads to increased expression of heat-shock proteins (Hsps) in skeletal myofibers.[1–3] Metabolic stresses secondary to glucose deprivation, protein accumulation in rough endoplasmic reticulum (ER) due to either glycosylation inhibition or increased protein synthesis or misfolding of mutated proteins, or impaired Ca^{2+} homeostasis may evoke an ER stress response, which mediates upregulation of ER chaperones, among which are the glucose-regulated

Address for correspondence: Dr. Elena Tarricone, Department of Clinical and Experimental Medicine, Division of Rheumatology, via Giustiniani, 2, 35121 Padova, Italy. Voice: 3333701009; fax: 390498212191.
e-mail: elena.tarricone@unipd.it

Ann. N.Y. Acad. Sci. 1069: 472–476 (2006).
doi: 10.1196/annals.1351.046

proteins (Grps).[4] Interest in the stimuli that lead to the activation of this stress-response cascade in skeletal muscle cells is quickly increasing and, as will be described in detail in the subsequent paragraphs, the occurrence of ER stress has been recently demonstrated during muscle differentiation (Ref. 5 and this work) and disease.[6–8] The third pathway concerns oxidative stress, which induces the expression of enzymes involved in antioxidant defense and is activated in skeletal muscle by atrophy from disuse.[9]

ROLES OF STRESS PROTEINS IN MUSCLE BIOLOGY AND PATHOLOGY

Most Hsps and Grps function in physiologic conditions as molecular chaperones, aiding the proper folding of nascent polypeptides in their secondary and tertiary structures. Although protein folding is dictated by the linear amino acidic sequence, the complexity of cellular environment requi res the auxiliary role of chaperones, which prevent the aggregation of nascent polypeptides and favor the right formation of intramolecular interactions (see Ref. 10 for a review). Thus, an increased number of interactions between chaperones and client proteins avoids aggregate formation and becomes extremely relevant in conditions where correct protein folding is hampered, resulting in enhanced muscle cell survival[2,11] and in recovery of contractile functions.[3] Also, the ER stress response contributes to the inhibition of aggregate formation by reducing the load of nascent polypeptides through negative regulation of classical translation initiation and enhancing protein degradation associated with ER.[4] Furthermore, most ER stress proteins are high-capacity Ca^{2+}-binding proteins; hence, their upregulation may influence the amount of releasable Ca^{2+} and affect Ca^{2+} homeostasis.[11]

ER stress response, however, may not result always in cell protection. When ER stress is persistent or ER functions are severely impaired, apoptotic pathways are activated to protect the organism by eliminating the damaged cells. One of the stress proteins involved in mediating ER-stress-induced apoptosis is the C/EBP homologous protein, CHOP, a proapoptotic transcription factor expressed at very low levels in the cytosol of unstressed cells.[4,12]

ER STRESS RESPONSE AND PROTEINS AND SKELETAL MUSCLE DIFFERENTIATION

We previously showed that the ER stress protein Grp94, which is considered to be ubiquitous, is not expressed in myofibers of mammalian adult skeletal muscle, including that of humans.[6,13] Indeed, we provide evidence that this protein is required for maturation of skeletal myoblasts because it participates in myotube formation[14] by reaching myoblast surface only after tyrosine-phosphorylation.[15]

Such a peculiar involvement of Grp94 becomes less striking when considering the recent findings reported by Nakanishi *et al.*,[5] part of which was also independently obtained in this laboratory (FIG. 1). The body of evidence demonstrates that ER stress is activated during and is required for differentiation of the murine myogenic cell line C2C12. As shown by FIGURE 1, 24-h differentiating C2C12 cells showed intense nuclear labeling for CHOP, a marker of ER stress response, at variance with proliferating ones. Consistent with that reported by Nakanishi *et al.*,[5] immunostaining for CHOP disappeared from the nuclei of 4-day differentiating myotubes, whereas it remained detectable in the cytosol.

STRESS RESPONSE IN SKELETAL MUSCLE PATHOLOGY

The ER stress response occurs in degenerative muscle diseases secondary to accumulation of intracellular protein aggregates, and appears to play an important role in the progression of inflammatory myopathies, included autoimmune myositis.

In sporadic inclusion body myositis, characterized by intracellular inclusions containing amyloid-β, phosphorylated tau, and several other aggregated proteins, the amount of the ER chaperones, calnexin, calreticulin, BiP/Grp78, Grp94, and ERp72, is increased compared with that in control unaffected muscle. These ER chaperones accumulate in the inclusions with the structures formed by amyloid-β and its precursor, suggesting their participation in folding and removal of the protein.[8] Increased amounts of Grp94 and Grp78 were also observed in muscle diseases that are characterized by the presence of tubular aggregates and dysferlin overexpression, such as periodic paralysis, myalgia/cramp syndrome, and malignant hyperthermia. Dysferlin is a Ca^{2+}-binding sarcolemmal protein and the co-localization with ER stress proteins suggests the occurrence of an ER stress response and might explain the Ca^{2+}-loading capacity of tubular aggregates.[6]

Although stress proteins and stress response may play a relevant role in the development of immune response,[16] recent data suggested a nonimmune contribution of the ER stress response in the progression of myositis. Upregulation of the ER stress protein Grp78 was observed in transgenic mice overexpressing class I major histocompatibility complex (MHC) in skeletal muscle fibers and developing myositis.[7] The same study demonstrated increased expression of CHOP and other ER stress regulatory genes by microarray analyses of biopsies obtained from myositis patients, which also display class I MHC upregulation in skeletal muscle fibers. These findings suggest that both ER stress and ER overload, initiated by class I MHC overexpression, activate responses that contribute to muscle fiber damage.[7]

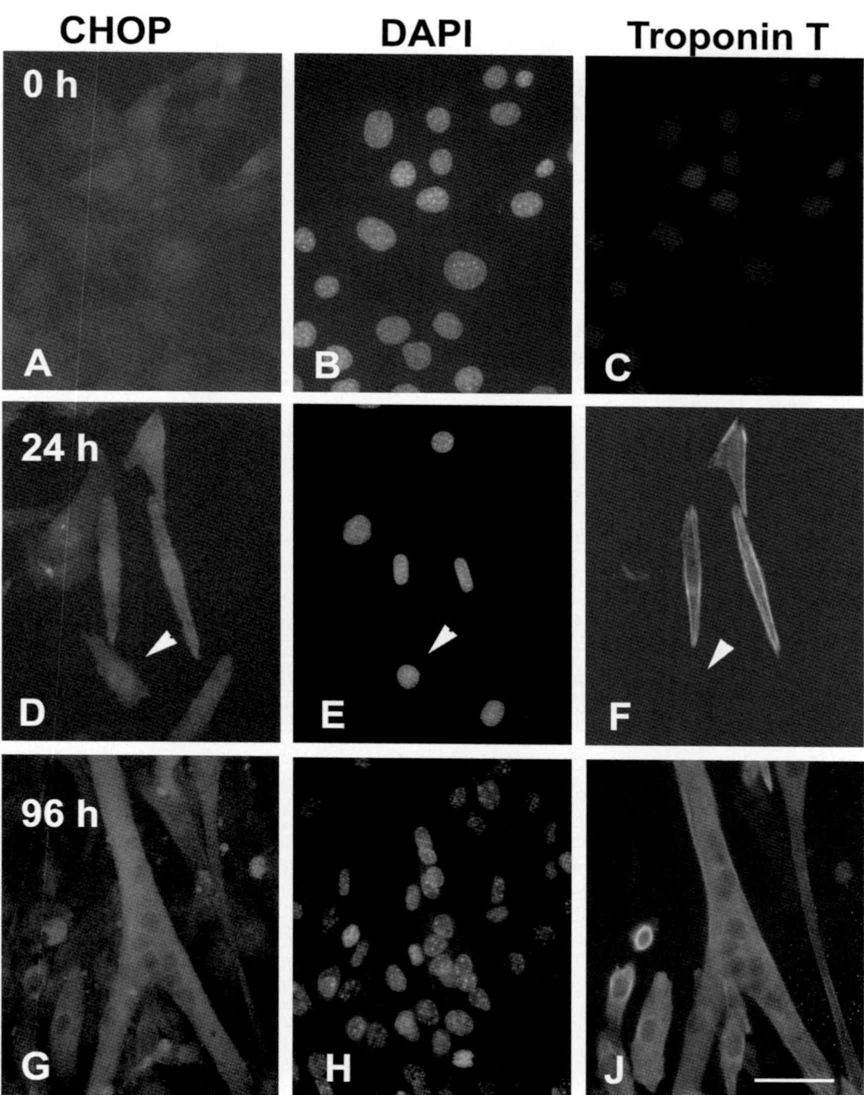

FIGURE 1. Immunofluorescence micrographs illustrating triple immunofluorescence labeling of C2C12 cells grown in proliferation medium (0 h; **A–C**) and after 24 (**D–F**) and 96 h (**G–J**) of growth in differentiation medium. The same cells were stained with polyclonal anti-CHOP antibody (**A, D, G**), nuclear stain DAPI (**B, E, H**), and with monoclonal anti-troponin T antibody (**C, F, J**). CHOP staining increased in intensity and localized in nuclei of 24-h differentiating cells, before the expression of muscle-specific genes (*arrowheads*). Bar: 20 μm.

ACKNOWLEDGMENTS

This work was supported by a grant from MIUR (FIRB 2001, grant number RBAU015R84 to L.G.).

REFERENCES

1. LIU, Y. & J.M. STEINACKER. 2001. Changes in skeletal muscle heat shock proteins: pathological significance. Front. Biosci. **6:** 12–25.
2. MAGLARA, A.A., A. VASILAKI, M.J. JACKSON, *et al.* 2003. Damage to developing mouse skeletal muscle myotubes in culture: protective effect of heat shock proteins. J. Physiol. **548:** 837–846.
3. MCARDLE, W., H. DILLMANN, R. MESTRIL, *et al.* 2004. Overexpression of HSP70 in mouse skeletal muscle protects against muscle damage and age-related muscle dysfunction. FASEB J. **18:** 355–357.
4. KAUFMAN, R.J. 2002. Orchestrating the unfolded protein response in health and disease. J. Clin. Invest. **110:** 1389–1398.
5. NAKANISHI, K., T. SUDO & N. MORISHIMA. 2005. Endoplasmic reticulum stress signalling transmitted by ATF6 mediates apoptosis during muscle development. J. Cell Biol. **169:** 555–560.
6. IKEZOE, K., H. FURUYA, Y. OHYAGI, *et al.* 2003. Dysferlin expression in tubular aggregates: their possible relationship to endoplasmic reticulum stress. Acta. Neurophathol. **105:** 603–609.
7. NAGARAJU, K., L. CASCIOLA-ROSEN, I. LUNDEBERG, *et al.* 2005. Activation of the endoplasmic reticulum response in autoimmune myositis. Arthritis Rheum. **52:** 1824–1835.
8. VATTEMI, G., W.K. ENGEL, J. MCFERRIN, *et al.* 2004. Endoplasmic reticulum stress and unfolded protein response in inclusion body myositis muscle. Am. J. Pathol. **164:** 1–7.
9. HUNTER, R.B., H. MITCHELL-FELTON, D.A. HESSIG, *et al.* 2001. Expression of endoplasmic reticulum stress proteins during skeletal muscle disuse atrophy. Am. J. Physiol. Cell Physiol. **281:** 1285–1290.
10. GORZA, L. & F. DEL MONTE. 2005. Protein unfolding in cardiomyopathies. Heart Fail. Clin. **1:** 237–250.
11. VITADELLO, M., D. PENZO, V. PETRONILLI, *et al.* 2003. Overexpression of the stress-protein Grp94 reduces cardiomyocyte necrosis due to calcium overload and simulated ischemia. FASEB J. **17:** 923–925.
12. OYADOMARI, S. & M. MORI. 2004. Roles of CHOP/GADD153 in endoplasmic reticulum stress. Cell Death Differ. **11:** 381–389.
13. VITADELLO, M., P. COLPO & L. GORZA. 1998. Rabbit cardiac and skeletal myocytes differ in constitutive and inducible expression of the glucose-regulated protein GRP94. Biochem. J. **332:** 351–359.
14. GORZA, L. & M. VITADELLO. 2000. Reduced amount of the glucose-regulated protein GRP94 in skeletal myoblasts results in loss of fusion competence. FASEB J. **14:** 461–475.
15. BRUNATI, A. M., M. VITADELLO, M. FRASSON, *et al.* Submitted for publication.
16. SRIVASTAVA, P. 2002. Interaction of heat shock proteins with peptides and antigen presenting cells: chaperoning of the innate and adaptive immune responses. Ann. Rev. Immunol. **20:** 395–425.

Impact of Thiopurine Methyltransferase Activity and 6-Thioguanine Nucleotide Concentrations in Patients with Chronic Inflammatory Diseases

JÖRG SCHEDEL,[a] ANDREA GÖDDE,[a] EKKEHARD SCHÜTZ,[b] TIM A. BONGARTZ,[a] BERNHARD LANG,[c] JÜRGEN SCHÖLMERICH,[a] AND ULF MÜLLER-LADNER[a,d]

[a]*Department of Internal Medicine I, University Hospital of Regensburg, D-93042 Regensburg, Germany*

[b]*Department of Clinical Chemistry, Georg-August University of Göettingen, 37073 Göettingen, Germany*

[c]*Rheumatology Outpatient Center, Nuremberg, Germany*

[d]*Department of Internal Medicine and Rheumatology, University of Giessen, Kerckhoff Clinic, D-35392 Bad Nauheim, Germany*

ABSTRACT: As azathioprine is one of the standard immunosuppressive drugs used for treatment of patients with different chronic inflammatory diseases, the effect of the azathioprine metabolizing enzyme thiopurine methyltransferase (TPMT) activity on incidence of adverse events (AE) was examined. In addition, potential correlations between the concentration of the azathioprine metabolite 6-thioguanine nucleotide (6-TGN) in erythrocytes (RBC) and inflammatory disease activity as well as hematological AE were investigated. TPMT activities were investigated prospectively in 139 patients (35 male, 104 female) with chronic inflammatory diseases [systemic lupus erythematosus (SLE, 38), progressive systemic sclerosis (PSS, 13), Wegener's granulomatosis (4), rheumatoid arthritis (RA, 5), and other chronic inflammatory diseases (79)]. In addition, 6-TGN concentrations were investigated in a second cohort of 58 patients (17 patients with SLE, 5 with PSS, 5 with vasculitides, 4 with undifferentiated connective tissue diseases, 1 with dermatomyositis, 1 with Sjögren's syndrome, 1 with RA, 20 with Crohn's disease, and 4 with ulcerative colitis) prior to and during therapy with azathioprine. The distribution of activities of TPMT in 139 patients showed a normal Gaussian distribution in the Caucasian population. Within the group of 96 patients taking azathioprine, known azathioprine-related AE could be observed: minor

Address for correspondence: Dr. Jörg Schedel, M.D., Department of Internal Medicine I, Division of Rheumatology and Clinical Immunology, University Hospital of Regensburg, D-93042 Regensburg, Germany. Voice: 49-941-944-7003; fax: 49-941-944-7127.
e-mail: joerg.schedel@klinik.uni-regensburg.de

**Ann. N.Y. Acad. Sci. 1069: 477–491 (2006). © 2006 New York Academy of Sciences.
doi: 10.1196/annals.1351.048**

AE (sickness, rash, and increase in cholestasis parameters) in 11 patients (11.4%), and severe AE (bone marrow toxicity) in 7 patients (7.3%). Below a "cutoff" value of 11.9 nmol/mL RBC × h of TPMT activity, AE were significantly more frequent. In the second cohort of patients, no significant correlations could be observed between 6-TGN concentrations and parameters of disease activity. Reduced activity of TPMT in patients with chronic inflammatory diseases requiring immunosuppressive therapy with azathioprine, especially below a distinct cutoff, appears to inherit a substantial risk for development of AE.

Keywords: thiopurine methyltransferase; 6-thioguanine nucleotide; azathioprine; chronic inflammatory diseases

INTRODUCTION

Azathioprine, as an immunosuppressive agent, has started to be used in rheumatoid arthritis (RA) about 40 years ago. Since then, it has been applied to patients suffering from a variety of rheumatological diseases including systemic lupus erythematosus (SLE), systemic vasculitides, as well as to inflammatory bowel diseases. Azathioprine is a nitroimidazole derivative of 6-mercaptopurin, and is metabolized in the liver to its active agent 6-thioguanine nucleotide (6-TGN) via an enzymatic cascade involving 6-mercaptopurin. Azathioprine and its metabolic derivatives inhibit the proliferation of B and T lymphocytes,[1,2] decrease the production of immunoglobulins dependent on the underlying disease,[3] the production of interleukin-2 (IL-2), the function of natural killer cells, the production of autoantibodies by B lymphocytes,[4] and are able to induce apoptosis in T cells.[5] *In vitro*, azathioprine exhibits also antiphlogistic properties.[6] It is not known if the latter are of clinical significance—the relatively long latency to clinical efficacy, however, does not support a clinically significant antiphlogistic effect. The therapeutic effect of azathioprine can be expected 6–12 weeks after initiation of therapy. Usually, azathioprine is applied orally in doses ranging from 1 to 3 mg/kg body weight per day. Oral bioavailability of azathioprine is 88%,[7] and its biological half-life approximately 24 h.[8] The metabolism of azathioprine can be inhibited significantly by allopurinol,[9] therefore its dose has to be reduced to at least 25% in case both agents need to be administered at the same time.

As the efficacy of azathioprine is established in the majority of rheumatological entities and inflammatory bowel diseases, adverse events (AE) have to be taken into account and monitored closely. It has long been known that genetic polymorphisms of the enzyme thiopurine methyltransferase (TPMT), an enzyme downstream in the azathioprine metabolism, can result in lower enzymatic activity leading to profound toxicity when azathioprine is administered.[10,11] One out of 300 Caucasians exhibits homozygosity for TPMT deficiency, and 11% of this population are heterozygous, which results in intermediate TPMT activity.[12] Differences in ethnic groups have been described.[13] TPMT activity can be measured in erythrocytes (red blood cells [RBC]) and reflects the enzymatic activity in liver, kidney, or leukemic lymphoblasts.[14] The most frequent side effects of azathioprine are gastrointestinal (sickness, vomiting, diarrhea, cholestasis, and pancreatitis), hematological (leukopenia, lymphopenia, megaloblastic anemia, and pancytopenia), and neurological (dizziness). In a cohort study investigating azathioprine in 528 patients with RA, treatment had to be stopped on account of AE in 16% of the patients.[15] In another study with 546 RA patients, gastrointestinal intolerance accounted for about 60% of treatment interruptions.[16]

During the first weeks and months after initiation of therapy with azathioprine, regular laboratory controls are mandatory. In the last years, measurement of the 6-TGN concentration has been developed and has enabled clinicians to control treatment efficacy by monitoring both the patient's compliance and the dosage of medication.[17,18] From clinical experience, a correlation between the concentration of 6-TGN in RBC and clinical efficacy has been postulated. In addition, an association between the concentration of 6-TGN and the toxicity of azathioprine has been assumed. Therefore, in the present study, the effect of TPMT activity on the incidence of AE in patients with chronic inflammatory diseases was examined prospectively. Furthermore, potential correlations between 6-TGN concentrations, inflammatory disease activity, and hematological side effects were investigated.

PATIENTS, MATERIALS, AND METHODS

Measurement of TPMT Activity

To examine the relationship between TPMT activity and AE, TPMT activities were investigated in 139 patients with the following disease entities: SLE ($n = 38$), systemic sclerosis ($n = 13$), Wegener's granulomatosis ($n = 4$), RA ($n = 5$), and other chronic inflammatory diseases, such as mixed connective tissue disease, Crohn's disease, ulcerative colitis, or autoimmune hepatitis ($n = 79$). TPMT enzyme activities were measured using a radiochemical assay at the Department of Clinical Chemistry, Georg-August University of Goettingen. For patients under azathioprine therapy, the cutoff value by which patients are supposed to be heterozygous for TPMT deficiency, is 12.0 nmol/mL RBC $\times$ h.

Ninety-six of these patients were treated with azathioprine. The patients were evaluated both clinically and serologically at the Division of Rheumatology and Clinical Immunology, Department of Internal Medicine I, University Hospital of Regensburg/Germany. AE as well as laboratory parameters were determined using the respective medical records.

Measurement of 6-TGN

In addition, 6-TGN concentrations in RBC were investigated prospectively in a second cohort of 58 patients (17 patients with SLE, 5 with systemic sclerosis, 5 with vasculitides, 4 with undifferentiated connective tissue diseases, 1 with dermatomyositis, 1 with Sjögren's syndrome, 1 with RA, 20 with Crohn's disease, and 4 with ulcerative colitis) at two different time points during therapy with azathioprine to examine clinical efficacy and laboratory side effects. The patients were evaluated both clinically and serologically at the University of Regensburg. Prospectively, the systemic lupus erythematosus activity index (SLEDAI) in patients with SLE, and the Crohn's disease activity index (CDAI) in patients with Crohn's disease were calculated. The concentrations of 6-TGN were measured at the University of Goettingen as described elsewhere.[19,20] Of note, the preliminary therapeutic range in transplant patients has been suggested to be 100–450 pmol/0.8 $\times$ 10^9 RBC.[21]

Statistics

For statistical analysis, the following tests were performed using SPSS 10.0 for windows software: Spearman's Rho rank correlation, chi-square test, and Mann–Whitney U-test for nonparametric variables, Wilcoxon's correlation test for paired, nonparametric samples, and receiver operator curve (ROC) analysis; P values < 0.05 were regarded as significant.

RESULTS

Distribution of TPMT Activity in a Cohort of Patients with Chronic Inflammatory Diseases

The distribution of TPMT activities in 139 patients (35 male, 104 female patients) analyzed showed a normal Gaussian distribution curve in the Caucasian population (mean TPMT activity 13.18 $\pm$ 3.69 nmol/mL RBC $\times$ h; FIG. 1). The mean activity in women was 12.90 $\pm$ 3.60 (mean $\pm$ standard deviation), in men 13.98 $\pm$ 3.88 nmol/mL RBC $\times$ h, which was not significantly different ($P = 0.30$; data not shown). TPMT activity in SLE patients was slightly lower (12.21 $\pm$ 3.25) when compared to all other patient groups (13.40 $\pm$ 3.59; $P =$ 0.095).

Correlation Between TPMT Activity and Incidence of Clinically Severe AE

Within the group of the 96 patients taking azathioprine, known azathioprine-related AE could be observed: minor AE (sickness, rash, hair loss, increase

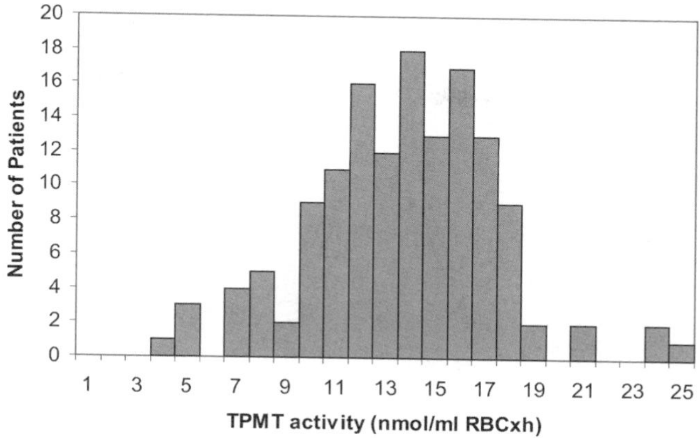

FIGURE 1. Distribution of TPMT activities in 139 patients with different chronic inflammatory diseases (see "Patients, Materials, and Methods").

in mean corpuscular volume [MCV], and increased cholestasis parameters) in 11 patients (11.4%), severe AE (leukopenia and pancytopenia) in 7 patients (7.3%; TABLES 1 and 2). With respect to gender and age, no difference could be noted in patients with and without AE. The mean TPMT activity in patients showing severe AE was 9.76 ± 4.03 nmol/mL RBC × h and, thus, significantly lower compared to the mean TPMT activity in patients exhibiting no AE (13.99 ± 3.19 nmol/mL RBC × h; $P = 0.011$) but did not differ when compared with those exhibiting minor AE (13.57 ± 5.04 nmol/mL RBC × h; $P = 0.085$). When comparing the group with clinically severe AE with both the combined group with no and with minor AE, TPMT activity was also significantly different ($P = 0.012$; FIG. 2).

Below a cutoff value of 11.9 nmol/mL RBC × h, which was determined by a ROC analysis and which approximately corresponds to 12.0 nmol/mL RBC × h representing the upper limit of the reference interval of patients heterozygous for TPMT deficiency during therapy, clinically severe AE were seen significantly more frequently ($P < 0.05$). The sensitivity of this cutoff value

TABLE 1. Demographic data and TPMT activity of 96 patients with different chronic inflammatory diseases on azathioprine therapy who developed AE

	No AE	Minor AE	Severe AE
Number of AEs	78	11	7
Age (mean ± SD) [years]	41.3 ± 14.8	50.0 ± 16.8	47.4 ± 16.4
Sex (male/female)	23/55	3/8	1/6
TPMT [nmol/mL RBC × h]	13.99 ± 3.19	13.57 ± 5.04	9.76 ± 4.03

TPMT = thiopurine methyltransferase; AE = adverse event.

TABLE 2. Demographic data and AE of the 18 out of 96 patients with different chronic inflammatory diseases on azathioprine therapy

Patient no.	Age [years]	Sex f=female, m=male	Dose of azathioprine [mg/day]	TPMT [nmol/mL RBC × h]	Minor AE +=yes, −=no	Severe AE +=yes, −=no	AE
1	25	f	150	25.50	+	−	acne, nausea
2	79	m	nk	15.60	+	−	cholestasis
3	70	f	150	15.50	+	−	elevated alkaline phopshatase
4	41	m	100	15.30	+	−	arthralgia, exanthema, dizziness
5	49	m	100	15.10	−	+	pancytopenia
6	44	f	150	14.10	+	−	elevated transaminases
7	32	f	100	13.90	+	−	erythema
8	44	f	150	13.10	+	−	hair loss
9	58	m	50	10.70	+	−	increase of MCV
10	58	f	150	10.60	−	+	leukopenia
11	61	f	150	11.90	−	+	pancytopenia
12	40	f	150	11.70	+	−	nausea
13	29	f	150	10.10	−	+	dizziness/exanthema/edema of lips and eye lids/elevated transaminases
14	61	f	100	11.90	−	+	leukopenia
15	68	f	100	7.40	+	−	increase in MCV
16	49	f	150	6.50	+	−	myalgia
17	54	f	100	4.70	−	+	leukopenia
18	20	f	150	4.00	−	+	leukopenia

nk = not known; TPMT = thiopurine methyltransferase; AE = adverse event.

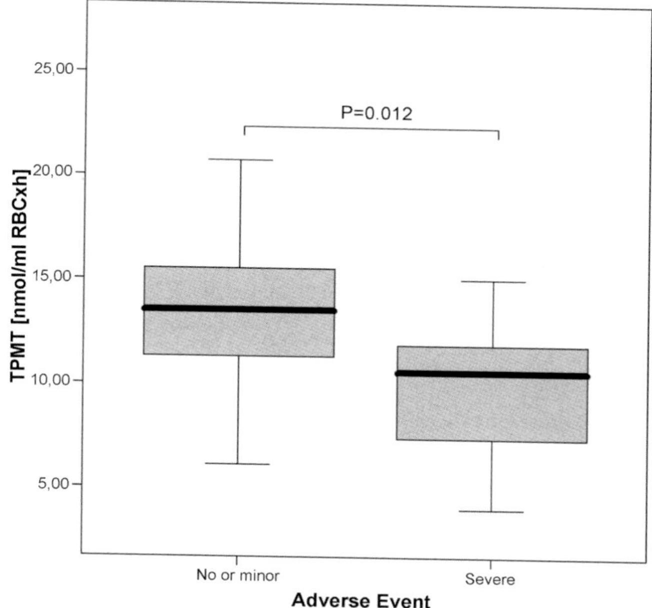

FIGURE 2. Difference of TPMT activity in patients with severe and in patients without/with minor AE. The mean TPMT activity in patients showing severe AE was significantly lower compared to the mean TPMT activity in the combined group of patients without or with minor AE.

was 88%, its specificity 69%, and the accuracy 70% (FIG. 3). Conversely, of the 65 patients under azathioprine treatment with a TPMT activity >11.9 nmol/mL RBC × h, only 1 patient developed a clinically severe AE, whereas below this threshold, 6 of 31 faced severe AE ($P = 0.001$; FIG. 4).

Efficiency of Therapy and Hematological AE under Azathioprine Treatment with Respect to 6-TGN Concentrations

In 58 patients with different chronic inflammatory diseases, who were treated with azathioprine for a mean duration of 38.5 ± 26.2 weeks, 6-TGN concentrations could be determined. The demographic data including laboratory parameters are summarized in TABLE 3. In the subgroup of 17 patients with SLE (demographic data, disease activity score, and laboratory parameters of this subgroup are presented in TABLE 4), the mean SLEDAI was 13.0 ± 6.1 at study entry (time point 0), and 14.1 ± 6.7 after a mean follow-up period of 41.7 ± 23.9 weeks (time point 1), the respective 6-TGN levels were 119.6 ± 72.9 and 157.9 ± 69.8 pmol/0.8 × 10^9 RBC, respectively. Correlations could

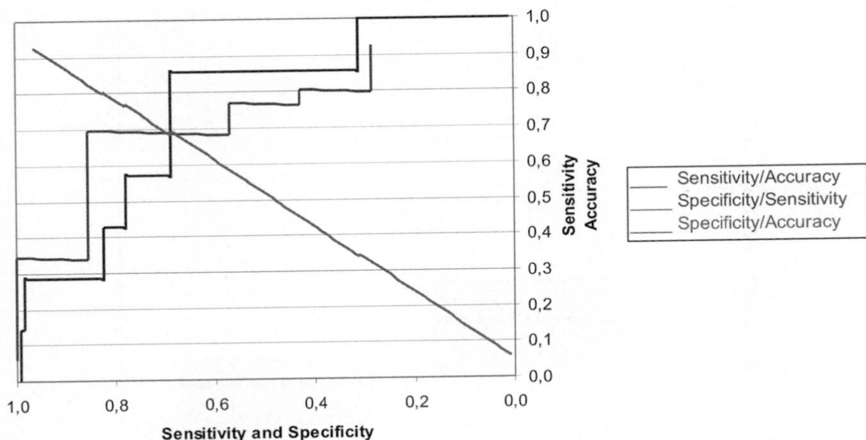

FIGURE 3. Sensitivity and specificity of a cutoff TPMT activity with respect to the occurrence of AE in patients treated with azathioprine. Using a ROC analysis, a cutoff value of 11.9 nmol/mL RBC × h of TPMT activity was identified indicating the optimal relationship between sensitivity and specificity with respect to severe AE in 96 patients treated with azathioprine.

not be demonstrated between the 6-TGN levels measured and any parameters of disease activity or hematological side effects.

In the subgroup of 20 patients with Crohn's disease, the mean CDAI decreased from 234 ± 122.9 at study entry (time point 0) to 166.6 ± 146.2 after a mean treatment duration of 31.4 ± 19.5 weeks (time point 1; $P = 0.14$). The respective 6-TGN values were 212.6 ± 130.9 pmol/0.8 × 10^9 RBC and

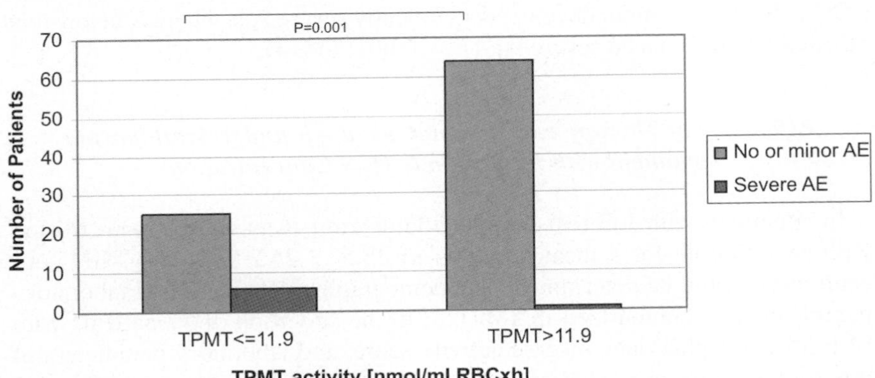

FIGURE 4. AE in dependence of classified TPMT activity. Whereas only 1 patient out of 65 patients with a TPMT activity > 11.9 nmol/mL RBC × h under azathioprine treatment developed a clinically severe AE, under this threshold, 6 of 31 faced a severe AE.

TABLE 3. Demographic and laboratory data of 58 patients with different chronic inflammatory diseases treated with azathioprine in whom 6-TGN concentrations were measured (for diagnoses see "Patients, Materials, and Methods")

	Time point 0	Time point 1
Age [years]	37.6 ± 14,6	
male/female	20/38	
6-TGN [pmol/0.8×10e9 RBC]	130.13 ± 101.04	174.37 ± 89.52
ESR 1st h	33.8 ± 25.91	35.38 ± 24.15
CRP [mg/L]	21.83 ± 36.65	10.84 ± 17.48
Leukocytes [/nL]	8.72 ± 3.47	7.1 ± 2.65
Lymphocytes [%]	13.71 ± 8.56	14.27 ± 9.85
Hemoglobin [g/dL]	1206 ± 2.2	12.7 ± 1.8
MCV [fL]	89.5 ± 12.1	89.1 ± 9.7
Thrombocytes [/nL]	339.3 ± 112.0	329.8 ± 131.7
ALAT [U/L]	10.7 ± 4.6	9.9 ± 4.5
ASAT [U/L]	13.0 ± 8.6	11.0 ± 7.4
Alkaline phosphatase [U/L]	97.8 ± 44.6	110.4 ± 65.4
Gamma-GT [U/L]	28.9 ± 35.7	37.6 ± 84.5
Creatinine [mg/dL]	0.97 ± 1.43	0.98 ± 1.28

6-TGN = 6-thioguanine nucleotide; ESR = erythrocyte sedimentation rate; CRP = C-reactive protein; ASAT = aspartate transferase; ALAT = alanine transferase.

221.4 ± 96.1 pmol/0.8 × 10^9 RBC ($P = 0.59$; TABLE 4). Positive correlations between these parameters, other markers of disease activity, or with hematological side effects could not be established either (data not shown).

DISCUSSION

Azathioprine is widely used as immunosuppressive drug in chronic inflammatory and autoimmune diseases, such as SLE[22,23] or Crohn's disease.[24] Even though lack of efficiency appears to constitute a major factor of azathioprine withdrawal,[25] side effects, such as myelosuppression, notably leukopenia and pancytopenia, often result in discontinuation of treatment. Moreover, fatal outcomes have been reported.[26] Intracellularly, azathioprine and its metabolite 6-mercaptopurin are metabolized to 6-TGN via a cascade of several enzymes. Most frequently, toxic side effects are caused by genetic polymorphisms of the metabolizing enzyme TPMT resulting in decreased enzymatic activity and accumulation of azathioprine metabolites, such as 6-TGN.[10] In recent years, it has become a useful tool to measure TPMT activities prior to therapy, however, these measurements are not yet a standardized clinical procedure and limited to specialized laboratories.[27,28] Nevertheless, evaluation of TMPT status has shown cost-effectiveness,[29,30] and the number needed to avoid one serious AE over a period of 6 months has been estimated to be 20.[29,31] In the first part of the present study, TPMT activities were measured in patients with rheumatic

TABLE 4. Laboratory findings and disease activity indices of the subgroups of patients with SLE ($n = 17$) and with Crohn's disease ($n = 20$) who were treated with azathioprine

	Time point 0 SLE	Time point 1 SLE		Time point 0 Crohn's disease	Time point 1 Crohn's disease
Age [years]	38.4 ± 15.8		Age [years]	31.1 ± 10.2	
male/female	4/13		male/female	9/11	
6-TGN [pmol/ $0.8\times10e^9$ RBC]	120.1 ± 83.3	146.6 ± 79.2	6-TGN [pmol/0.8×10e9 RBC]	164.4 ± 134.2	219.6 ± 97.8
SLEDAI	12.5 ± 5.9	14.1 ± 6.7	CDAI	234.0 ± 122.9	166.6 ± 146.2
ESR [1st h]	30.3 ± 20.2	35.8 ± 24.3	ESR [1st h]	30.1 ± 27.2	54.8 ± 20.7
CRP [mg/L]	8.8 ± 14.5	2.9 ± 5.8	CRP [mg/L]	33.2 ± 43.1	14.9 ± 18.1
Leukocytes [/nL]	10.7 ± 3.5	5.7 ± 2.1	Leukocytes [/nL]	10.7 ± 3.5	8.1 ± 3.0
Lymphocytes [%]	10.2 ± 7.1	11.9 ± 8.9	Lymphocytes [%]	15.3 ± 8.5	15.5 ± 10.0
Hemoglobin [g/dL]	12.5 ± 1.7	12.0 ± 2.0	Hemoglobin [g/dL]	12.1 ± 2.3	12.4 ± 1.6
MCV [fL]	94.8 ± 7.2	92.6 ± 6.6	MCV [fL]	81.0 ± 14.6	85.3 ± 13.3
Thrombocytes [/nL]	271.8 ± 75.0	243.1 ± 54.6	Thrombocytes [/nL]	419.0 ± 109.9	432.0 ± 136.1
ALAT [U/L]	10.2 ± 3.7	10.0 ± 5.6	ALAT [U/L]	9.4 ± 4.6	10.1 ± 4.7
ASAT [U/L]	11.1 ± 6.8	11.1 ± 9.5	ASAT[U/L]	11.7 ± 7.6	9.7 ± 5.6
Alkaline phosphatase	90.1 ± 54.1	91.3 ± 61.5	Alkaline phosphatase	101.7 ± 42.0	141.5 ± 78.5
Gamma-GT [U/L]	37.8 ± 48.9	59.4 ± 112.2	Gamma-GT [U/L]	29.2 ± 37.7	38.4 ± 92.6
Creatinine [mg/dL]	1.52 ± 2.51	1.54 ± 2.24	Creatinine [mg/dL]	0.69 ± 0.13	0.73 ± 0.23

SD = standard deviation; SLEDAI = systemic lupus erythematosus disease activity index; CDAI = Crohn's disease activity index. For other abbreviations see TABLE 3.

and gastrointestinal chronic inflammatory diseases. As expected, a normal distribution of TPMT activities could be found. This distribution corresponds to the usually seen trimodal distribution in the Caucasian population reflecting three different TPMT phenotype subgroups with very low, intermediate, and normal/high activity.[32] As reported in the literature, the mean TPMT activity was slightly (though not significantly) lower in female patients.[33] Similarly, TPMT activity was lower in SLE patients when compared to all other patient groups, which is in accordance with a published report.[34] One explanation for this fact could be the higher prevalence of SLE in female patients and the higher incidence of renal impairment in those patients.[35]

An additional intention of the study was to evaluate the relationship between TPMT activity and potential AE in patients undergoing azathioprine treatment. When applying a cutoff value of 11.9 nmol/mL (RBC) × h of TPMT activity as determined by ROC analysis, severe AE could be detected significantly more frequently in patients below this cutoff. In these patients, genetic polymorphisms were not investigated because at the time of initiation of the study, the examination of genetic TPMT alterations was not an available diagnostic tool. However, since a positive correlation has been established between TPMT mutations and lower TPMT activity,[32,36] one could speculate about underlying TPMT mutations in these patients resulting partly in less than half of the reference TPMT activity defined in our laboratory. This idea is underlined by a study published recently in which a clear concordance rate of 98.4% could be demonstrated between TPMT phenotype and genotype in 1214 healthy blood donors.[37]

Of note, patient 5 developed pancytopenia though not exhibiting a reduced TPMT activity. This situation may be explained by a study in which TPMT activity was investigated in 120 patients with SLE. In this study, 11 drug-associated neutropenias were detected whereas only 1 out of these 11 patients was homozygous for an underlying TPMT polymorphism. It was concluded that wild-type TPMT activity does not preclude the majority of leukopenias seen in patients on azathioprine therapy.[35] Other factors potentially accounting for this phenomenon include the fact that in SLE, disease-related leukopenias are often difficult to distinguish from drug-induced leukopenias. Furthermore, TPMT activity is induced by azathioprine or 6-mercaptopurine, and on the contrary, its activity can be reduced by concomitant medications, such as nonsteroidal anti-inflammatory drugs, diuretics, acetylsalicylic acid, or sulfasalazine.[11,20] Moreover, TPMT constitutes only one of the several enzymes involved in the metabolism of azathioprine, so factors influencing these enzymes could potentially also affect the production of toxic thioguanine nucleotides.

To address this question, in a second cohort of patients, the relationship of disease activity with 6-TGN levels was investigated in azathioprine-treated patients. In the subgroup of patients with SLE, a significant correlation between parameters of disease activity and concentrations of 6-TGN could not be demonstrated. Thus, the concentration of 6-TGN does not appear to facilitate the prediction of a therapeutic response in patients with SLE when treated with azathioprine. Furthermore, a correlation between TPMT activity and 6-TGN levels could not be found, which is in line with a study by Decaux *et al*. In this study, 26 patients with SLE in remission had lower TPMT activities and higher 6-TGN concentrations, but failed to show a correlation between both parameters.[34] This missing correlation might be on account of the fact that 6-TGN can be influenced by several factors, for example, the comedication of the patient. In this respect, the comedication of our patients consisted in steroids, other immunosuppressants, such as cyclosporine or cyclophosphamide, or ACE inhibitors.

Interestingly, in contrast to Decaux *et al*., who described a positive correlation of TGN with an increase in the MCV of RBC,[38] we could not confirm this finding nor other correlations with 6-TGN levels. Whereas the authors claimed MCV to increase after 3 months of therapy, the missing effect on MCV in our study might be explained by the fact that some of our patients had just started azathioprine therapy or had to be dose-adjusted, while in the study mentioned, most patients had been on stable azathioprine doses for more than 2 years, thus, rendering a direct comparison between the two groups difficult.

Reliable data on 6-TGN as indicator of treatment efficacy in rheumatic diseases have not been established yet. A report from transplant medicine, however, suggests that concentrations below 450 pmol/0.8 $\times$ 10^9 RBC are not associated with a higher risk for myelosuppression.[21] Experience from patients with inflammatory bowel diseases indicates that optimal levels of 6-TGN in the treatment of Crohn's disease are above 235 pmol/0.8 $\times$ 10^9 RBC.[39] In our patients with SLE, given the mean 6-TGN levels 119.6 $\pm$ 72.9 pmol/0.8 $\times$ 10^9 RBC and 157.9 $\pm$ 69.8 pmol/0.8 $\times$ 10^9 RBC at two different time points after a mean duration of 41.7 $\pm$ 23.9 weeks, respectively, azathioprine treatment may therefore have been relatively underdosed and may explain the lack of further improvement of disease activity. At present, however, the "therapeutic range" of 6-TGN serum concentrations for rheumatic diseases has still to be fully determined.[31]

In the subgroup of patients with Crohn's disease treated with azathioprine, no correlations between TPMT activity and 6-TGN concentrations could be demonstrated. This might be on account of the relatively low mean initial disease activity (CDAI 234 $\pm$ 122.9 at study entry and 166.6 $\pm$ 146.2 after 31.4 $\pm$ 19.5 weeks), since CDAI values of 150 and below are regarded as quiescent disease.[40] So even though disease activity decreased over time and the standard deviation of 6-TGN was high, 6-TGN levels remained relatively stable. This missing correlation is in line with a study by Lowry *et al*. in which 170 patients with inflammatory bowel disease were treated with azathioprine or 6-mercatopurine, and in which no such correlation between 6-TGN levels and disease activity could be found; moreover, 6-TGN concentrations were similar in patients with active disease and in patients in remission.[41] The decrease in

CDAI as such might be interpreted as treatment success, and 6-TGN levels in the suggested range of about 230 pmol/0.8 $\times$ 10^9 RBC, as referred to in the literature,[42] might account for this development.

In conclusion, our data support the measurement of TPMT activity prior to azathioprine therapy to identify patients with TPMT polymorphisms and avoid severe AE.[43,44] In contrast, measurement of 6-TGN concentration during azathioprine treatment does not appear to constitute a feasible tool to monitor treatment response but studies with higher patient numbers will have to confirm this finding.

REFERENCES

1. YY, D.T. *et al.* 1974. Lymphocyte characteristics in rheumatic patients and the effect of azathioprine therapy. Arthritis Rheum. **17:** 37–45.
2. BACH, M.A. & J.C. BACH. 1972. Activities of immunosuppressive agents vitro. II. Different timing of azathioprine and methotrexate in inhibition and stimulation of mixed lymphocyte reaction. Clin. Exp. Immunol. **11:** 89–98.
3. LEVY, J. *et al.* 1972. The effect of azathioprine on gammaglobulin synthesis in man. J. Clin. Invest. **53:** 2233–2238.
4. FOX, D.A. & W.J. MC CUNE. 1994. Immunosuppressive drug therapy of systemic lupus erythematosus. Rheum. Dis. Clin. North Am. **20:** 265–299.
5. TIEDE, I. *et al.* 2003. CD28-dependent Rac1 activation is the molecular target of azathioprine in primary human CD4+ T lymphocytes. J. Clin. Invest. **111:** 1133–1145.
6. HOMO-DELARCHE, F. *et al.* 1988. In vitro inhibition of prostaglandin production by azathioprine and 6-mercaptopurine. Prostaglandins **35:** 479–491.
7. CHAN, G.L.C. *et al.* 1989. Pharmacokinetics of 6-thiouric acid and 6-mercaptopurine in renal allograft recipients after oral administration of azathioprine. Eur. J. Clin. Pharmacol. **36:** 265–271.
8. CALABRESI, P. *et al.* 1980. Antiproliferative agents and drugs used for immunosuppression. *In* The Pharmacologic Basis of Therapeutics. I.S. Goodman & A. Gilman, Eds.: 265–271. Macmillian. New York.
9. GOADSBY, P.J. *et al.* 1986. 6-mercaptopurine-related leucopenia and in vivo xanthine oxidase activity. Lancet **2:** 869–870.
10. LENNARD, L. *et al.* 1989. Pharmacogenetics of acute azathioprine toxicity: relationship to thiopurine methyltransferse genetic polymorphism. Clin. Pharmacol. Ther. **46:** 149–154.
11. LENNARD, L. 1998. Clinical implications of thiopurine methyltransferase—optimization of drug dosage and potential drug interactions. Ther. Drug Monit. **20:** 527–531.
12. WEINSHILBOUM, R.M. & S. SLADEK. 1980. Mercaptopurin pharmacogenetics: monogenic inheritance of erythrocyte thiopurine methyltransferase activity. Am. J. Human. Genet. **32:** 651–662.
13. COLLIE-DUGUID, E.S. *et al.* 1999. The frequency and distribution of thiopurine methyltransferase alleles in Caucasian and Asian populations. Pharmacogenetics. **9:** 37–42.

14. Szumlanski, C.L. *et al.* 1992. Human liver thiopurine methyltransferase pharmacogenetics: biochemical properties, liver-erythrocyte correlation and presence of isozymes. Pharmacogenetics **2:** 148–159.
15. Keysser, M. 1993. Therapie der Rheumatoid-Arthritis (RA) mit Azathioprin—Ergebnisse einer offenen Langzeitstudie über mindestens 4 Jahre bei 528 Patienten. Z. Rheumatol. **52:** 133–137.
16. Singh, G. *et al.* 1989. Toxic effects of azathioprine in rheumatoid arthritis. A national post-marketing perspective. Arthritis Rheum. **32:** 837–843.
17. Lennard, L. & J.L. Maddocks. 1983. Assay of 6-thioguanine nucleotide, a major metabolite of azathioprine, 6-mercaptopurine and 6-thioguanine, in human red blood cells. J. Pharm. Pharmacol. **35:** 15–18.
18. Schmiegelow, K. & N.J. Kriegbaum. 1993. 6-thioguanine nucleotide accumulation in erythrocytes during azathioprine treatment for systemic connective tissue diseases: a possible index for monitoring treatment. Ann. Rheum. Dis. **52:** 152–154.
19. Schütz, E. *et al.* 1996. Azathioprine pharmacogenetics: the relationship between 6-thioguanine nucleotides and thiopurine methyltransferase in patients after heart and kidney transplantation. Eur. J. Clin. Chem. Clin. Biochem. **34:** 199–205.
20. Dewit, O. *et al.* 2002. Interaction between azathioprine and aminosalicylates: an in vivo study in patients with Crohn's disease. Aliment. Pharmacol. Ther. **167:** 79–85.
21. Schütz, E. *et al.* 1996. Should 6-thioguanine nucleotides be monitored in heart transplant recipients given azathioprine? Ther. Drug Monit. **18:** 228–233.
22. Abu-Shakra, M. & Y. Shoenfeld. 2001. Azathioprine therapy for patients with systemic lupus erythematosus. Lupus **10:** 152–153.
23. Nossent, H.C. & W. Koldingsnes. 2001. Long-term efficacy of azathioprine treatment for proliferative lupus nephritis. Rheumatology **39:** 969–974.
24. Scribano, M. & C. Prantera. 2003. Review article: medical treatment of moderate to severe Crohn's disease. Aliment. Pharmacol. Ther. **17**(Suppl 2): 23–30.
25. Corominas, H. *et al.* 2003. Is thiopurine methyltransferase genetic polymorphism a major factor for withdrawal of azathioprine in rheumatoid arthritis patients? Rheumatology **42:** 40–45.
26. Connell, W.R. *et al.* 1993. Bone marrow toxicity caused by azathioprine in inflammatory bowel disease: 27 years of experience. Gut **34:** 1081–1085.
27. Black, A.J. *et al.* 1998. Thiopurine methyltransferase genotype predicts therapy-limiting severe toxicity from azathioprine. Ann. Intern. Med. **129:** 716–718.
28. Clunie, G.P.R. & L. Lennard. 2004. Relevance of thiopurine methyltransferase status in rheumatology patients receiving azathioprine. Rheumatology **43:** 13–18.
29. Marra, C.A. *et al.* 2002. Practical pharmacogenetics: the cost effectiveness of screening for thiopurine S-methyltransferase polymorphisms in patients with rheumatological conditions treated with azathioprine. J. Rheumatol. **29:** 2507–2512.
30. Oh, K.T. *et al.* 2004. Pharmacoeconomic analysis of thiopurine methyltransferase polymorphism screening by polymerase chain reaction for treatment with azathioprine in Korea. Rheumatology **43:** 156–163.
31. Seidman, E.G. & D.E. Furst. 2002. Pharmacogenetics for the individualization of treatment of rheumatic disorders using azathioprine. J. Rheumatol. **29:** 2484–2487.

32. SCHAEFFELER, E. *et al.* 2004. Comprehensive analysis of thiopurine S-methyltransferase phenotype-genotype correlation in a large population of German-Caucasians and identification of novel TPMT variants. Pharmacogenetics **14:** 407–417.
33. MCLEOD, H.L. *et al.* 1995. Higher activity of polymorphic thiopurine S-methyltransferase in erythrocytes from neonates compared to adults. Pharmacogenetics **5:** 281–286.
34. DECAUX, G. *et al.* 2001. High 6-thioguanine nucleotide levels and low thiopurine methyltransferase activity in patients with lupus erythematosus treated with azathioprine. Am. J. Ther. **8:** 147–150.
35. NAUGHTON, M.A. *et al.* 1999. Identification of thiopurine methyltransferase (TPMT) polymorphisms cannot predict myelosuppression in systemic lupus erythematosus patients taking azathioprine. Rheumatology **38:** 640–644.
36. TAI, H.L. *et al.* 1997. Enhanced proteolysis of thiopurine S-methyltransferase (TPMT) encoded by mutant alleles in humans (TPMT*3A, TPMT*2): mechanisms for the genetic polymorphism of TPMT activity. Proc. Natl. Acad. Sci. USA **94:** 6444–6449.
37. ANSARI, A. *et al.* 2002. Thiopurine methyltransferase activity and the use of azathioprine in inflammatory bowel disease. Aliment. Pharmacol. Ther. **16:** 1743–1750.
38. DECAUX, G. *et al.* 2000. Relationship between red cell mean corpuscular volume and 6-thioguanine nucleotides in patients treated with azathioprine. J. Lab. Clin. Med. **135:** 256–262.
39. DUBINSKY, M.C. *et al.* 2000. Pharmacogenomics and metabolite measurements of 6-mercaptopurine therapy in inflammatory bowel disease. Gastroenterology **118:** 705–713.
40. BEST, W.R. *et al.* 1976. Development of a Crohn's disease activity index. National cooperative Crohn's disease study. Gastroenterology **70:** 439–444.
41. LOWRY, P.W. *et al.* 2001. Measurement of thiopurine methyltransferase activity and azathioprine metabolites in patients with inflammatory bowel disease. Gut **49:** 665–670.
42. MARDINI, H.E. & G.L. ARNOLD. 2003. Utility of measuring 6-methylmercaptopurine and 6-thioguanine nucleotide levels in managing inflammatory bowel disease patients treated with 6-mercaptopurine in a clinical practice setting. J. Clin. Gastroenterol. **36:** 390–395.
43. SANDERSON, J. *et al.* 2004. Thiopurine methyltransferse: should it be measured before commencing thiopurine drug therapy? Ann. Clin. Biochem. **41**(Pt 4): 294–302.
44. ASANUMA, Y. *et al.* 2005. Pharmacogenetics and rheumatology. Molecular mechanisms contributing to variability in drug response. Arthritis Rheum. **52:** 1349–1359.

Index of Contributors